W9-BHS-920

PET and PET/CT: A Clinical Guide

Second Edition

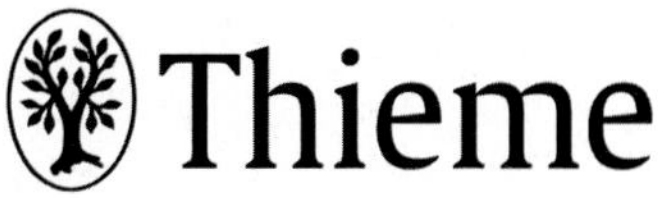

PET and PET/CT: A Clinical Guide

Second Edition

Eugene C. Lin, MD
Clinical Assistant Professor of Radiology
Department of Radiology
University of Washington
Virginia Mason Medical Center
Seattle, Washington

Abass Alavi, MD, MD(Hon), PhD(Hon)
Professor of Radiology and Neurology
Director of Research Education
Department of Radiology
Hospital of the University of Pennsylvania
Philadelphia, Pennsylvania

Thieme
New York • Stuttgart

Thieme Medical Publishers, Inc.
333 Seventh Ave.
New York, NY 10001

Executive Editor: Timothy Hiscock
Vice President, Production and Electronic Publishing: Anne T. Vinnicombe
Production Editor: Heidi Grauel, Maryland Composition
Vice President, International Marketing and Sales: Cornelia Schulze
Chief Financial Officer: Peter van Woerden
President: Brian D. Scanlan
Compositor: Manila Typesetting Company
Printer: Everbest Printing Co.

Library of Congress Cataloging-in-Publication Data

PET and PET/CT : a clinical guide / edited by Eugene C. Lin, Abass Alavi. – 2nd ed.
p. ; cm.
Rev. ed. of: PET and PET/CT / Eugene Lin, Abass Alavi. c2005.
Includes bibliographical references and index.
ISBN 978-1-60406-153-6
1. Tomography, Emission. I. Lin, Eugene. II. Alavi, Abass. III. Lin, Eugene. PET and PET/CT.
[DNLM: 1. Positron-Emission Tomography – methods. 2. Fluorodeoxyglucose F18 – diagnostic use. WN 206 P4765 2008]
RC78.7.T62L56 2008
616.07'575 – dc22

2008048664

Important note: Medical knowledge is ever-changing. As new research and clinical experience broaden our knowledge, changes in treatment and drug therapy may be required. The authors and editors of the material herein have consulted sources believed to be reliable in their efforts to provide information that is complete and in accord with the standards accepted at the time of publication. However, in view of the possibility of human error by the authors, editors, or publisher of the work herein or changes in medical knowledge, neither the authors, editors, nor publisher, nor any other party who has been involved in the preparation of this work, warrants that the information contained herein is in every respect accurate or complete, and they are not responsible for any errors or omissions or for the results obtained from use of such information. Readers are encouraged to confirm the information contained herein with other sources. For example, readers are advised to check the product information sheet included in the package of each drug they plan to administer to be certain that the information contained in this publication is accurate and that changes have not been made in the recommended dose or in the contraindications for administration. This recommendation is of particular importance in connection with new or infrequently used drugs.

Printed in China

5 4 3 2 1

ISBN 978-1-60406-153-6

I would like to thank my colleagues at Virginia Mason Medical Center for providing an environment which allowed me to write this book and Drs. Marie Lee and Paul Sicuro for help in obtaining many of the images in this book. My parents instilled in me a love of learning and working with residents and fellows throughout my career has inspired me to continually seek out new knowledge.

Eugene C. Lin

I wish to dedicate this book to my mother Fatemeh and my wife Jane for sacrifices they have made to make my life most rewarding; I cannot thank them enough for their enormous encouragements all along.

Abass Alavi

Contents

Preface .... **xi**

Contributors .... **xiii**

I Basic Science **1**

Chapter 1: The Physics of PET/CT Scanners
Ruth E. Schmitz, Adam M. Alessio, and Paul E. Kinahan 3

Chapter 2: Basics of Fluorodeoxyglucose Radiochemistry and Biology
Neale S. Mason and Eugene C. Lin 15

Chapter 3: The Role of Glucose and FDG Metabolism in the Interpretation of PET Studies
Ronald L. Korn, Alison Coates, and John Millstine 22

II Clinical Basics **31**

Chapter 4: Patient Preparation
Eugene C. Lin and Abass Alavi 33

Chapter 5: Standardized Uptake Value
Eugene C. Lin, Abass Alavi, and Paul E. Kinahan 38

Chapter 6: Normal Variants and Benign Findings
Eugene C. Lin and Abass Alavi 42

Chapter 7: The Interpretation of FDG PET Studies
Eugene C. Lin and Abass Alavi 78

Chapter 8: The Value of PET/CT
Eugene C. Lin, Paul E. Kinahan, and Abass Alavi 88

Chapter 9: Levels of Evidence for Clinical Indications of FDG PET
Eugene C. Lin. 99

III Oncologic Applications. 101

Chapter 10: Oncologic PET by Anatomical Region
Eugene C. Lin and Abass Alavi 103

Chapter 11: Therapy Response
Eugene C. Lin and Abass Alavi 117

Chapter 12: Brain Neoplasms
Eugene C. Lin and Abass Alavi 121

Chapter 13: Head and Neck Cancer
Eugene C. Lin and Abass Alavi 127

Chapter 14: Thyroid Cancer
Eugene C. Lin and Abass Alavi 136

Chapter 15: Thoracic Neoplasms
Eugene C. Lin and Abass Alavi 142

Chapter 16: Breast Cancer
Eugene C. Lin, Marie E. Lee, and Abass Alavi 155

Chapter 17: Gastric, Esophageal, and Gastrointestinal Stromal Tumors
Eugene C. Lin and Abass Alavi 164

Chapter 18: Lymphoma
Eugene C. Lin and Abass Alavi 173

Chapter 19: Melanoma
Eugene C. Lin and Abass Alavi 181

Chapter 20: Hepatobiliary Tumors
Eugene C. Lin and Abass Alavi 185

Chapter 21: Pancreatic Cancer
Eugene C. Lin and Abass Alavi 190

Chapter 22: Gynecologic Tumors
Eugene C. Lin and Abass Alavi 196

Chapter 23: Urologic Tumors
Eugene C. Lin and Abass Alavi 204

Chapter 24: Colorectal Cancer
Eugene C. Lin and Abass Alavi 212

Chapter 25: Musculoskeletal Tumors
Eugene C. Lin and Abass Alavi 220

IV Nononcologic Applications 229

Chapter 26: Pediatric PET/CT
M. Beth McCarville 231

Chapter 27: PET and PET/CT in Radiation Therapy Planning
Sandip Basu, Guobin Song, Abass Alavi, and Eugene C. Lin 239

Chapter 28: FDG PET in the Evaluation of Infection and Inflammation
Sandip Basu, Abass Alavi, and Eugene C. Lin 245

Chapter 29: Neurologic Applications
Eugene C. Lin and Abass Alavi 257

Chapter 30: Cardiac PET and PET/CT
*Amol Takalkar, Eugene C. Lin, Elias Botvinick,
Adam M. Alessio, and Luis Araujo* 263

Index 275

Preface

Since the publication of the first edition of *PET and PET/CT: A Clinical Guide*, PET and PET/CT have been increasingly used as effective imaging techniques for managing patients with cancer, neurologic diseases, and cardiovascular disorders. Imaging modalities such as CT, which up until recent years were referred to as "conventional" imaging modalities, are being replaced by PET/CT as an alternate and essential imaging modality.

The goal of the first edition was to provide an overview of the clinical applications of FDG PET and PET/CT that was both practical and scientifically rigorous in order to provide busy practitioners and trainees in medical imaging disciplines with the essential information about PET and at the same time reflect the breadth of the scientific literature. The second edition has been updated to reflect advances that have occurred since the publication of first edition. A large number of novel PET/CT images have been added. New chapters related to FDG biology, pediatric PET/CT, and PET/CT in radiation therapy and in inflammatory and infectious disorders have been added. We hope this new edition will continue to serve as a valuable reference source for both the trainees and practitioners who are actively involved in utilizing this powerful modality in their daily practice.

Eugene C. Lin, MD
Abass Alavi, MD

Contributors

Abass Alavi, MD, MD(Hon), PhD(Hon)
Professor of Radiology and Neurology
Director of Research Education
Department of Radiology
Hospital of the University of Pennsylvania
Philadelphia, Pennsylvania

Adam M. Alessio, PhD
Research Assistant
Department of Radiology
University of Washington
Seattle, Washington

Luis Araujo, MD
Department of Radiology
Hospital of the University of Pennsylvania
Philadelphia, Pennsylvania

Sandip Basu, MBBS(Hons), DRM, DNB, MNAMS
Head, Nuclear Medicine Academic Programme
Department of Radiation Medicine Centre
Bombay, India

Elias Botvinick, MD
Professor of Medicine and Radiology
Department of Cardiology
University of California, San Francisco
San Francisco, California

Edgar Cheng, MD
Progressive Physician Associates
Easton, Pennsylvania

Alison Coates
Department of Nuclear Medicine, Research, and PET/CT
Scottsdale Medical Imaging Ltd.
Scottsdale, Arizona

Janet Eary, MD
Department of Radiology
University of Washington
Seattle, Washington

Paul E. Kinahan, PhD
Associate Professor of Radiology, Bioengineering, and Electrical Engineering
Director of PET/CT Physics
Department of Radiology
University of Washington
Seattle, Washington

Ronald L. Korn, MD, PhD
Director of Research and Molecular Imaging
Department of Radiology
Scottsdale Medical Imaging Ltd.
Scottsdale, Arizona

Marie E. Lee, MD
Section Chief, Nuclear Medicine
Department of Radiology
Virginia Mason Medical Center
Seattle, Washington

Eugene C. Lin, MD
Clinical Assistant Professor of Radiology
Department of Radiology
University of Washington
Virginia Mason Medical Center
Seattle, Washington

Neale S. Mason, PhD
Research Assistant Professor of Radiology
Department of Radiology
University of Pittsburgh
Pittsburgh, Pennsylvania

M. Beth McCarville, MD
Associate Member
Division of Diagnostic Imaging
Department of Radiological Sciences
St. Jude Children's Research Hospital
Memphis, Tennessee

Carolyn Meltzer, MD
Professor and Chair
Department of Radiology
Emory University Hospital
Atlanta, Georgia

John Millstine, MD
Director of Clinical Nuclear Medicine
Department of Radiology and Nuclear Medicine
Scottsdale Medical Imaging Ltd.
Scottsdale, Arizona

Ruth E. Schmitz, PhD
Senior Fellow, Department of Radiology
University of Washington
Seattle, Washington

Guobin Song, MD, PhD
Department of Radiation Oncology
Virginia Mason Medical Center
Seattle, Washington

Sinisa Stanic, MD
Resident, Department of Radiation Oncology
University of California Davis
Sacramento, California

Amol Takalkar, MD
Assistant Professor of Clinical Radiology
Department of Radiology
Louisiana State University
Associate Medical Director
PET Imaging Center
Biomedical Research Foundation of Northwest Louisiana
Shreveport, Louisiana

I

Basic Science

1

The Physics of PET/CT Scanners

Ruth E. Schmitz, Adam M. Alessio, and Paul E. Kinahan

◆ What Makes PET Useful?

Positron emission tomography (PET) offers several unique advantages compared with other imaging modalities. PET measures the two annihilation photons that are produced back-to-back after positron emission from a radionuclide tagged tracer molecule, which is chosen to mark a specific function in the body on a biochemical level (**Fig. 1.1**). Hence, PET provides molecular imaging of biological function instead of anatomy. The detection of both annihilation photons in coincidence yields increased sensitivity over single photon imaging and provides inherent collimation and accurate attenuation correction either from a dedicated transmission scan or from computed tomography (CT) information. This allows extraction of accurate quantitative as well as qualitative information from PET images. Only minute amounts of imaging substrate need to be injected (tracer principle) because of the high sensitivity of PET. In addition, positron emitters (^{11}C, ^{13}N, ^{15}O, ^{18}F, etc.) are relatively short-lived, which enables optimal use of imaging photons while keeping patient radiation dose low. Furthermore, many of these isotopes can be incorporated into biological substrates (glucose, H_2O, NH_3, CO_2, O_2, etc.) and pharmaceuticals, without altering their biological activity.

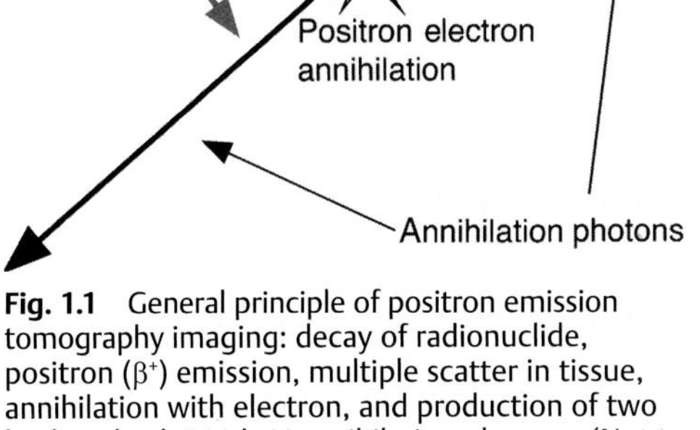

Fig. 1.1 General principle of positron emission tomography imaging: decay of radionuclide, positron (β^+) emission, multiple scatter in tissue, annihilation with electron, and production of two back-to-back 511 keV annihilation photons. (Not to scale.)

Compared with CT scans and magnetic resonance images (MRIs), PET images appear much blurrier or noisier, due to the relatively limited number of photons that can be collected during an imaging study. In addition, detector resolution is poorer due to the detector physics. X-ray CT scanners can easily resolve points < 1 mm in size, whereas PET scanners cannot reliably resolve point sources < 4 to 5 mm at best, and closer to 10 mm in practice. However, this does not impair their high sensitivity to focal tracer concentrations or their usefulness in accurate quantitative functional imaging.

In this chapter, we introduce the physics of PET imaging. Several textbooks provide a more in-depth treatment and are included in the References.[1–3]

◆ Radioactive Decay

General Principles

Radioactive isotopes are atoms whose inner core, their nucleus, is unstable, in a state with too much energy. Nuclei consist of a densely packed arrangement of protons and neutrons. By undergoing decay, the nuclei change their composition and properties to arrive in a less energetic and more stable state.

The decay process follows an exponential law: the number of decays per second is always proportional to the number of undecayed nuclei present. The same is true for the rate of decay, also called activity, which is determined by the half-life of the particular nuclide—the time it takes for half of the original nuclei to decay. Most common in PET is fluorine 18 (^{18}F), which has a half-life of 109 minutes. After some time, t, the activity left, $A(t)$, is proportional to the initial number, $A(0)$, and an exponential term involving the half-life, τ, of the nuclide:

$$A(t) = A(0)e^{-t(\ln 2/\tau)}$$

Radioactive rates (or activity) are measured in units of becquerel (1 Bq = 1 decay/s) in the International System of Units (SI) or the traditional curie (1 Ci = 3.7×10^{10} decay/s). A common scale factor used in the clinic is 1 mCi = 37 MBq.

Positron Emission and Annihilation

In β^+ (positron) decay (**Fig. 1.1**), a nuclide transforms one of its core protons (p) into a neutron (n) and emits a positron (β^+), essentially a positively charged electron, and a neutrino (ν): $p \rightarrow n + \beta^+ + \nu$. The average positron range in matter depends on the positron's energy and material characteristics, such as the density and the atomic number. For [fluorine 18]fluorodeoxyglucose ([^{18}F]FDG), positron ranges are rather short, typically < 1 mm.

At the end of its path, the positron, being antimatter to electrons, will annihilate (recombine) with an atomic electron. In the annihilation, electron and positron convert their mass into energy and produce a pair of 511 keV annihilation photons traveling in opposite directions. The 511 keV photon energy (E) comes from Einstein's famous equation $E = mc^2$, where m is the mass of the electron or positron (a very small number), and c is the speed of light (a very large number squared). This annihilation radiation is what is detected in PET and what is used to form images of tracer concentration in the body.

Interaction of Photons with Matter

The dominant annihilation photon interaction in human tissue is *Compton scatter*. The photon interacts with an electron, ejecting it from its atomic shell. The photon experiences a loss of energy and an associated change of direction, typically out of the detector, and so is unavailable for image formation.

Compton scatter and other interactions lead to an attenuation of the annihilation photons. The number of photons that are observed in a straight line from where they were produced decreases exponentially with increasing length of the material traversed. The thickness of soft tissue required to reduce the intensity of a beam by one half is ~7 cm, as opposed to 3 to 4 cm for x-rays. Thus, for ~14 cm of soft tissue, the 511 keV annihilation photon flux would be reduced to one fourth of its original intensity; through the abdomen the photon flux can be reduced to 1/50 of its original intensity. Thus, attenuation is often the dominant factor in PET image quality, especially for thicker patients.

◆ Data Acquisition

Photon Detection and Scintillation Detectors

The general goal of photon detection is to measure the total energy deposited by the photon when it traverses the detector. For highest sensitivity and accuracy, all of the photon's energy should be deposited, but in practice this is not always possible.

In most PET scanners today, scintillation detectors are used as detection elements. They couple inorganic scintillation crystals that emit visible or near ultraviolet light after interaction with an incident high-energy (511 keV) photon to photo detectors that detect and measure the scintillation photons.

In scintillation crystals, the incident annihilation photon (nominally 511,000 eV energy) interacts and creates tens of thousands of visible wavelength photons (~1 eV energy each) in a very short flash, or "scintillation." The number of scintillation photons produced in the crystal is proportional to the energy deposited by the annihilation photon.

Scintillators for PET photon detection can be rated on four of their characteristic properties:

The *stopping power* is the inverse of the mean distance traveled by photons before they deposit energy in the crystal. This length depends on density and effective atomic number (Z) of the material. A short travel distance is favorable because it will yield more interactions with the 511 keV photons and a better efficiency for detecting them in crystal of fixed size.

The *decay constant* describes how long the scintillation flash lasts in the crystal. Shorter decay constants are desirable because they allow for counting higher photon rates and lower background rates.

Good *energy resolution*—a small ratio of energy variance over energy—means that there are only small fluctuations in the energy measurement. This gives a means to distinguish against PET photons that have Compton scattered (and lost energy) before being measured. The energy resolution depends on the light output and the intrinsic energy resolution of the crystal.

The *light output*, as the name indicates, is the number of scintillation photons produced by each incident photon. Again, this should be as high as possible, allowing the best spatial and energy resolution.

The most commonly used PET scintillators are listed in **Table 1.1**. Other materials are being evaluated (e.g., lanthanum bromide [LaBr]). Manufacturers are divided on the choice of material: currently, BGO (bismuth germinate) is favored by General Electric (GE Healthcare, Chalfont St. Giles, UK), LSO (lutetium oxyorthosilicate) by Siemens (Berlin/Munich, Germany), and GSO (gadolinium orthosilicate) by Philips (Philips Medical Systems, Andover, MA). Time-of-flight PET scanners (TOF-PET) use the scintillator LYSO (lutetium yttrium orthosilicate), which has properties that are very similar to LSO.

The most commonly used photodetectors for PET are photomultiplier tubes (PMTs). PMTs are vacuum tubes with a photocathode, which produce electrons from incoming light photons that are accelerated and amplified. The resulting electrical current is proportional to the number of initial scintillation photons and therefore to the energy deposited in the scintillation crystal by the PET photon.

By segmenting the scintillator blocks, using many small PMTs, or exploiting the properties

Table 1.1 Scintillators Used in PET Scanners

Material	Cost	Light Output*	Effective Density†	Decay Time‡	Comments
NaI(Tl)	Cheap (relatively)	Highest	Lowest	Long	Hygroscopic, no longer used in PET
BGO	Expensive	Lowest	Highest	Long	Workhorse
LSO (or LYSO)	More expensive	High	High	Very short	Patented by CTI/Siemens
GSO	More expensive	Very high	Somewhat lower than LSO	Very short	

* Determines energy and spatial resolution
† Determines scanner sensitivity
‡ Determines dead time and random coincidences rate
Abbreviations: BGO, bismuth germinate; GSO, gadolinium orthosilicate; LSO, lutetium oxyorthosilicate; LYSO, lutetium yttrium orthosilicate; NaI(Tl), thallium-doped sodium iodide; PET, positron emission tomography.

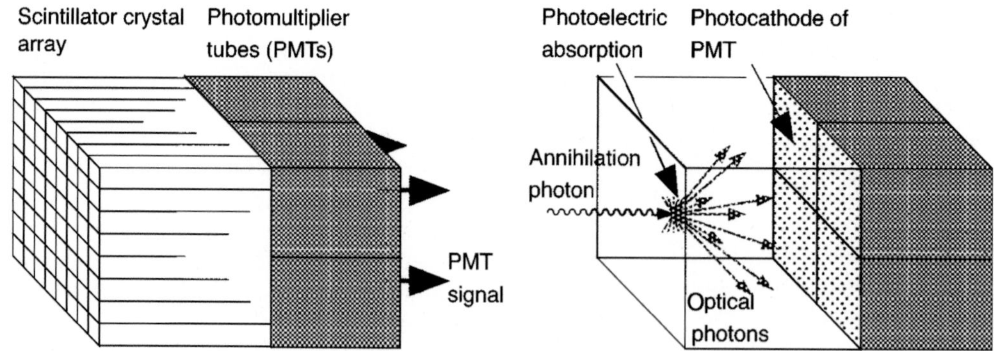

Fig. 1.2 Schematic of a block detector with finely segmented scintillator crystals read out by four photomultiplier tubes.

of position-sensitive PMTs, the location of the photon detection can be determined. The most commonly used setup today is the *block detector* (**Fig. 1.2**). Here, small individual scintillation crystals, a few millimeters in size where they face the patient, are tightly packed into blocks, which are typically coupled to four or more small photomultiplier tubes. To determine the interaction position of the annihilation photon from the spread-out scintillation photon signals, the relative outputs from the PMT signals are compared. The calculated location then determines the crystal element to which the photon is assigned.

Spatial resolution (in the detector) of a few millimeters is possible with this scheme, as it is determined by the size of the crystal cross section.

A full PET scanner is constructed as a cylindrical assembly of block detectors in a ring structure several blocks deep. The sensitive volume inside the detector cylinder that a patient can occupy is called the field of view (FOV), which in human scanners is typically 70 cm in diameter and 16 to 18 cm in axial length (**Fig. 1.3**).

Coincident Photon Events

Because of the positron annihilation, we expect to observe two photons at roughly the same time (in coincidence) in the detector ring. The annihilation event, the radioactive tracer, will then be located somewhere on the line connecting the two photon-detection points, as on the left side of **Fig. 1.3**. This knowledge of the photon direction is a huge advantage over single-photon emission computed tomography (SPECT), where collimators have to be used to restrict possible photon directions at the detectors at the cost of a large reduction in sensitivity.

Several factors lead to the photon detections not occurring at the exact same time: the annihilation may occur closer to one detector surface than the other, which will result in a slight

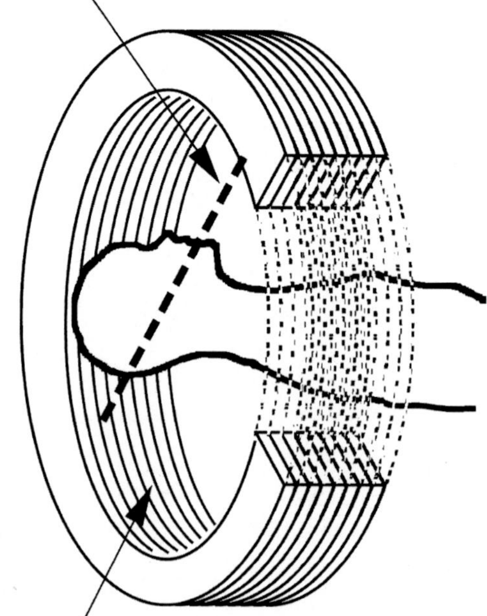

Fig. 1.3 Positron emission tomography scanner schematic with a possible line of response.

but measurable delay of one photon, where the photons travel at the speed of light, or 1 m in 3.3 nanoseconds. Most important for temporal mismatches is the finite timing resolution of the detector, its timing uncertainty, which arises from the decay time of the scintillation in the crystal and the processing time of the PMT signals. These effects lead to the use of a coincidence time window on the order of 6 to 10 nanoseconds.

If two photons are detected within each other's coincidence window, they are assumed to be arising from the same annihilation, and an event is attributed to the line of response (LOR) that connects the two detection points in the sensitive imaging volume (**Fig. 1.4**).

With TOF-PET imaging, the relative time difference (Δt) between the detection of the two annihilation photons is used to determine the most likely location (d) of the annihilation event along the LOR (**Fig. 1.4**), where c is the speed of light. TOF-PET imaging was previously investigated, but it was never adopted. The recent development of scintillators suitable for TOF-PET (i.e., LYSO) combined with advances in timing resolution and timing stability of detector electronics has led to a resurgence of interest in TOF-PET scanners, with commercial models being introduced. The advantage of TOF-PET, however, remains to be evaluated over the next few years.

The detected coincidence events (called *coincidences*) can be classified into true coincidences and background events (**Fig. 1.5**). The latter are distinguished as either accidental (or random) coincidences, where the two photons did not arise from the same annihilation event, or coincidences that did originate from the same annihilation, but where the true annihilation position does not lie on the line connecting the two photon positions because one photon has experienced Compton scatter within the patient and therefore has had a change of direction (scattered coincidences).

Sinograms

In the scanner, coincidence events are observed and identified along their LORs between pairs of detector elements (**Fig. 1.5A**). To organize these raw data as they are acquired, the LORs are stored in such a way that all the LORs passing through a single point in the patient trace a sinusoid curve in the raw data histogram; hence the term *sinogram* for the raw data format. The formation of sinograms is an important middle step in the PET data acquisition

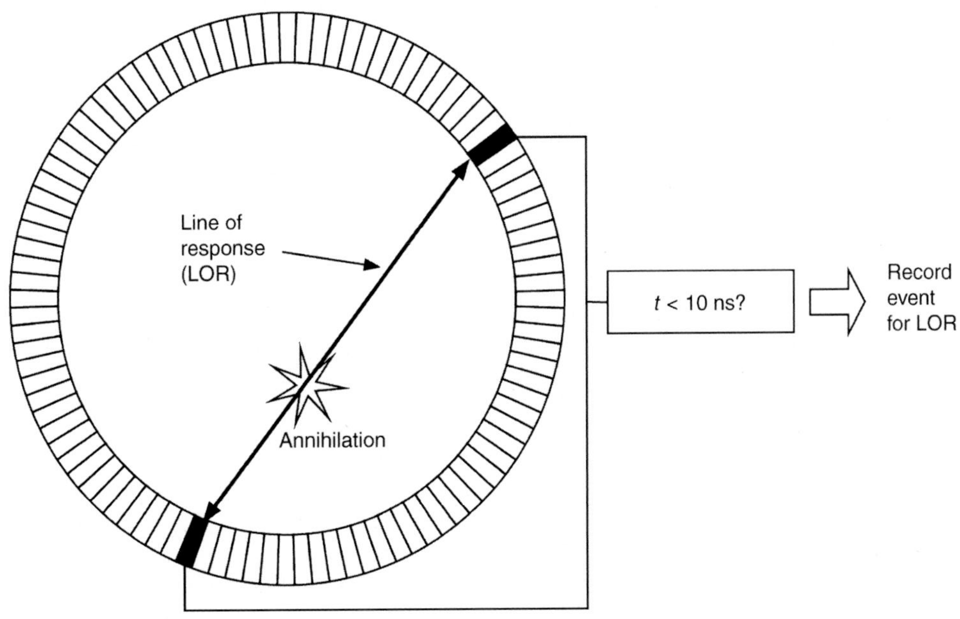

Fig. 1.4 Coincidence processing in positron emission tomography data acquisition.

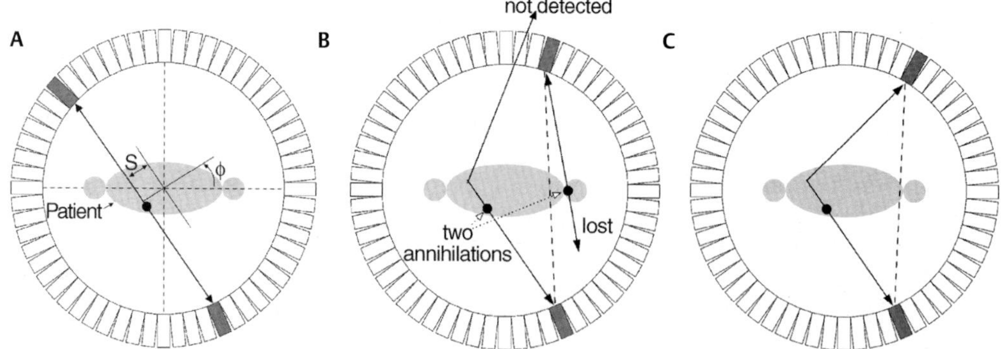

Fig. 1.5 Types of coincident events. From left to right: **(A)** True coincidence, **(B)** random (accidental) coincidence, and **(C)** scattered coincidence. In the last two types, the annihilation event (*black circle*) does not lie on the apparent line of response between the two photon detections.

process because necessary corrections are often applied at this level.

Corrections

The PET data acquisition process is not a perfect one. Interactions in the patient attenuate the emitted photons, detector elements vary in their detection efficiency, and random and scattered coincidences are recorded along with the true coincidence events. These effects need to be corrected to obtain clinically useful images and accurate quantitative information from PET studies.

The most important of the corrections is *attenuation correction* (AC): photons that encounter more or denser material on their path from the annihilation site to the detectors are more likely to be absorbed or scattered (i.e., attenuated) than photons that travel through sparser parts of the body. If images are reconstructed from sinograms without AC, this can lead to less dense areas, like the lungs, appearing darker (emitting more photons) than surrounding denser tissue, like the mediastinum (**Fig. 1.6**). This is clearly an artifact that arises from the fact that lung tissue exhibits lower attenuation, not higher uptake. It not only impairs the visual appearance of the image, but also leads to wildly inaccurate quantitation of tracer uptake. To apply attenuation correction, it is necessary to determine the attenuation through the patient for all LORs. On stand-alone PET scanners, this is done with a *transmission scan*, where an external positron source is rotated around the patient, and the attenuation of the transmitted photons is determined. In PET/CT scanners, the acquired CT image is used for PET attenuation correction.

Two-Dimensional versus Three-Dimensional Acquisitions

Axially, PET scanners consist of several rings of detector elements that may or may not be separated by thin annular rings or septa of photon-absorptive material, typically tungsten, that provide collimation. With collimation, all data are acquired in two-dimensional slices between the septa. This type of acquisition is therefore called 2D, even though the reconstructed stack of images gives three-dimensional (3D) information about the tracer uptake throughout the patient. When a scanner is operated without collimation (i.e., no septa), coincidences from all axial angles in the FOV will be accepted, making this a fully 3D acquisition protocol. Data storage, correction, and image reconstruction are considerably more complex in the fully 3D case. Current PET scanners operate in either 2D-only or 3D-only mode, or in a 2D/3D mode for those with retractable septa.

Figure 1.7 shows the effect that collimation has on the acquisition of coincidence counts: the septa block a large number of true coincidences from ever reaching the detector surface, decreasing sensitivity. However, they also reduce scattered and random coincidences, thus improving contrast. Of special importance here are accidental counts that partly originate from

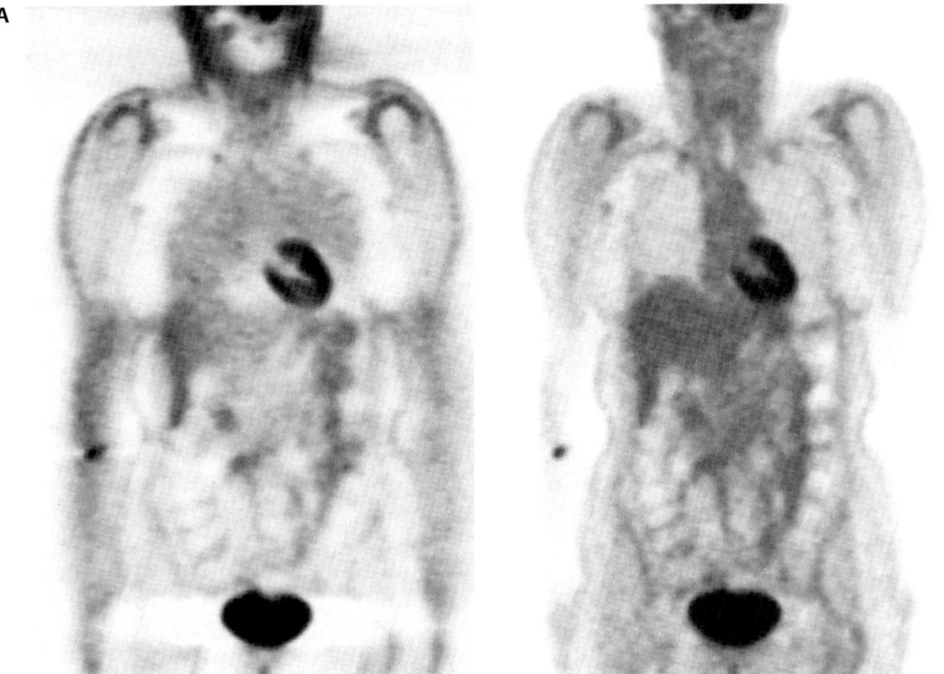

Fig. 1.6 Whole-body positron emission tomography image **(A)** without and **(B)** with attenuation correction. Artifacts from not performing attenuation correction include the lungs and skin showing higher tracer uptake than muscle. In these images, darker regions represent higher tracer uptake using the common inverse-gray color table.

outside the area between the detector surfaces (true FOV) because without collimation, the scanner is sensitive to activity from a very large area outside the true FOV. The decision on whether to use 2D or fully 3D acquisitions is still under debate, weighing the reduction of background counts against the loss of sensitivity. Brain imaging—typically with small activity concentrations outside the true FOV—is a clear indication for 3D imaging with increased sensitivity, whereas whole-body imaging—with usually much more activity directly surrounding the true FOV—does not show a clear preference and is usually done in 2D mode on scanners with 2D/3D capabilities.

◆ Image Reconstruction

After the acquisition of PET data in sinograms and their corrections for attenuation and other effects, as described above, the next stage in the PET processing chain is to reconstruct an estimate of the in vivo tracer distribution. This process of *image reconstruction* is the most mathematically complex step and is well described elsewhere.[1–3] Here we point out the differences between the two most common methods: filtered backprojection (FBP), which is a well-established method, and ordered-subsets expectation maximization (OSEM), which is a more recent iterative approach that allows for a more accurate model of the PET acquisition process. **Figure 1.8** shows a visual comparison of FBP and OSEM images, reconstructed from the same patient sinogram.

FBP is well understood and robust (it is also used in CT), but it does not account for noise.

Modeling the noise in the datasets generates much more complicated sets of equations that can only be solved iteratively, such as with the expectation maximization (EM) algorithm. This process is too slow for clinical needs, but with the advent of the ordered-subsets acceleration of the EM algorithm (OSEM) and faster processors, iterative methods are becoming more common. In many PET centers OSEM is now the reconstruction method of choice.

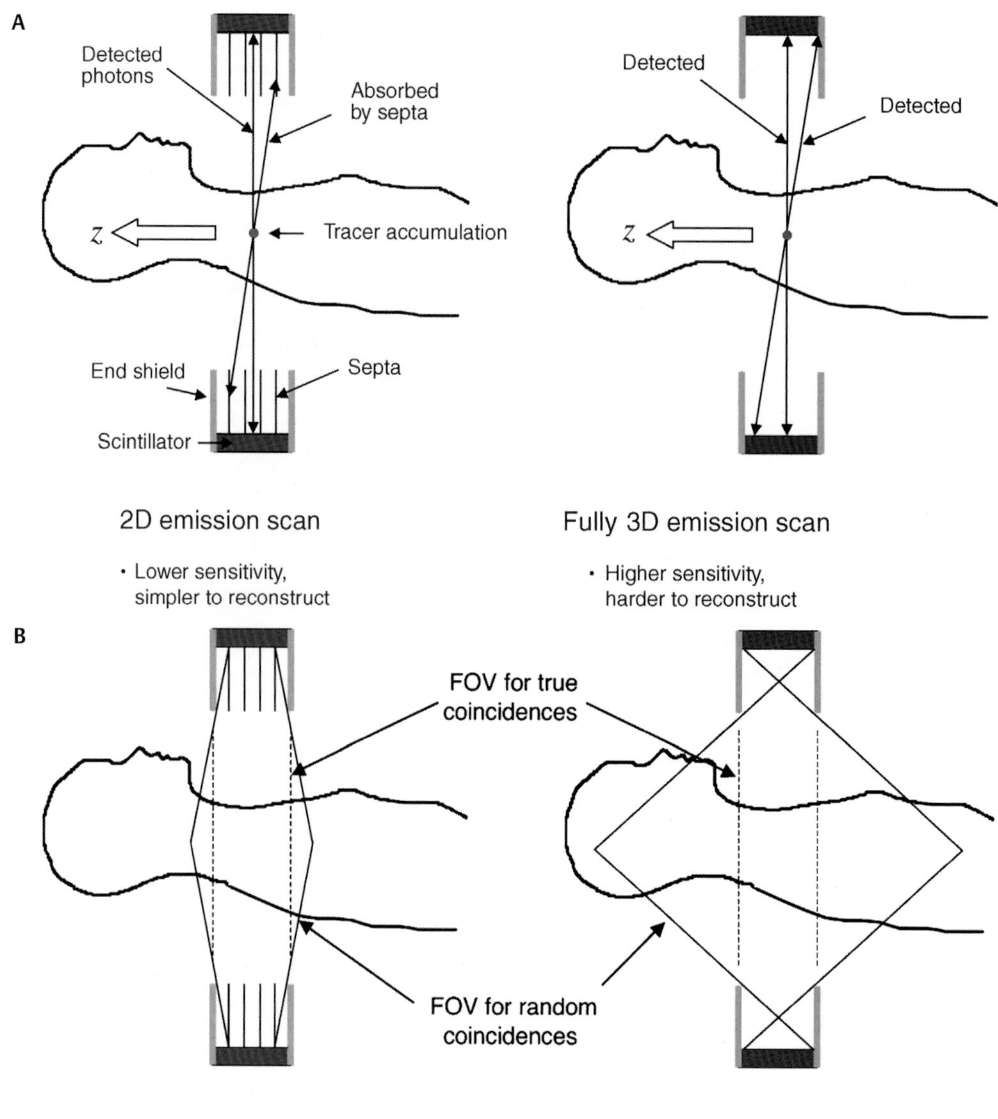

Fig. 1.7 Effect of two-dimensional and three-dimensional acquisition protocols on true and background coincidence counts. FOV, field of view.

Noise/Resolution Trade-offs and Image Quality

If images appear very noisy after reconstruction, they may be *smoothed* in a further step to give the eye an easier task, especially for localizing disease. However, because smoothing averages together neighboring image pixels, it is connected to a loss of resolution, so small structures may not be distinguishable anymore (**Figs. 1.9** and **1.10**). It is task-dependent, observer-dependent, and nontrivial to define an optimal region in the noise/resolution space. Currently there are no standards for adjusting this trade-off.

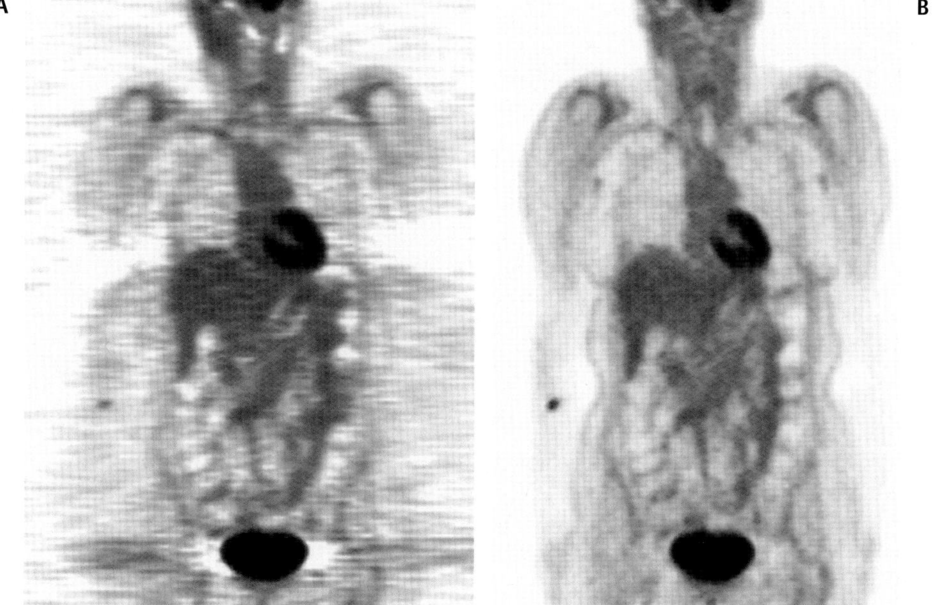

Fig. 1.8 Comparison of coronal sections of positron emission tomography images reconstructed with **(A)** filtered backprojection (FBP) and **(B)** ordered-subsets expectation maximization (OSEM). The FBP image shows characteristic streak artifacts and appears overall noisier than the OSEM image.

PET/CT Scanner Components and Function

The primary purpose of combining CT and PET systems in a single scanner is the precise anatomical localization of regions identified on the PET tracer uptake images. Although it is possible to use nonrigid image registration to align separately acquired whole-body PET and CT images, challenges remain in the practical implementation and validation of software-based methods. In recent years, the advent of combined PET/CT systems has pushed dedicated pure PET scanners almost completely off the market due to the convenience and ease of creating coregistered PET and CT images for

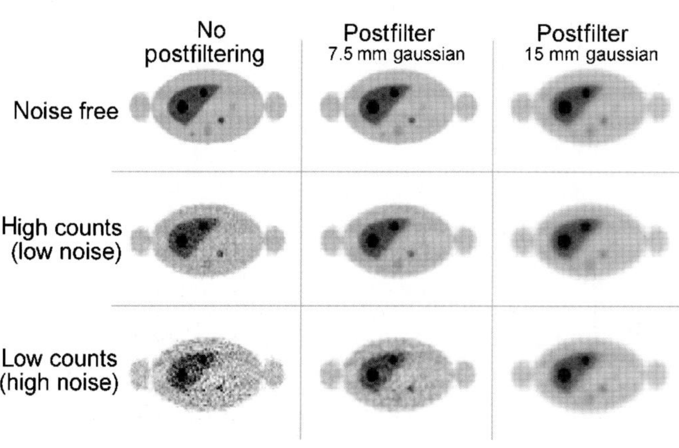

Fig. 1.9 Ordered-subsets expectation maximization images showing the trade-offs between noise (increases downward) and smoothing (increases to the right).

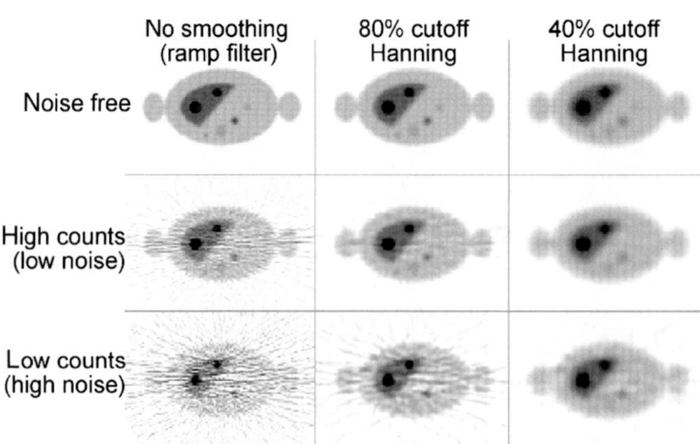

Fig. 1.10 Filtered backprojection images showing the trade-offs between noise (increases downward) and smoothing (increases to the right).

oncology, radiation oncology, and cardiology applications.

In this section we give a brief overview of this new technology; for more details, the reader is referred to Alessio et al.[4]

Basic Components

PET/CT systems are combinations of standalone CT and PET scanners in one gantry with a shared patient bed. They must be able to be very accurately aligned. The patient bed is an important and nontrivial component because there should be no differential bending in the bed between the PET and CT scans. **Fig. 1.11** shows a schematic of a PET/CT scanner.

The typical PET/CT protocol begins with a CT scout scan to define the scan area, followed by a helical CT scan, and finally the PET scan. The entire acquisition sequence is typically controlled from the CT console. However, each subsystem has its separate acquisition system with three or more databases overall (CT, PET, and PET/CT display), making the process somewhat complicated with the current generation of scanners.

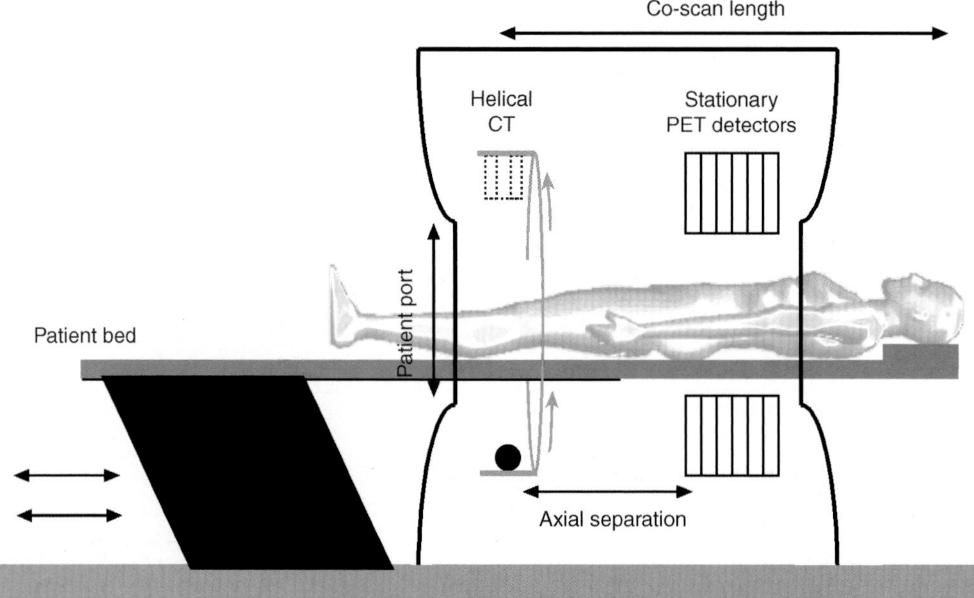

Fig. 1.11 Illustration of the main components of a positron emission tomography/computed tomography (PET/CT) scanner.

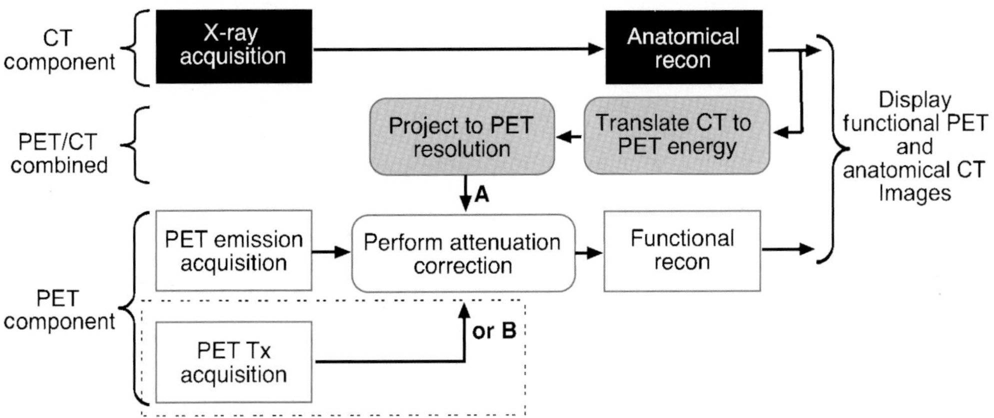

Fig. 1.12 Data flow in a positron emission tomography/computed tomography (PET/CT) scanner.

The data flow in the combined PET/CT acquisition is outlined in the schematic in **Fig. 1.12**. The x-ray CT scan provides anatomical images that after some processing can also be used for attenuation correction in PET, and the PET/CT software can display both images side-by-side or overlaid (fused) (**Fig. 1.13**). It is to be noted that there are no "fused" images in PET/CT—the PET and CT images always remain separate entities. Displaying them together is an overlay process rather than creating a new type of image.

CT-based Attenuation Correction

An important synergy of PET/CT scanners is the use of the CT images for attenuation correction of the PET emission data. All manufacturers of PET/CT scanners incorporate x-ray CT-based attenuation correction (CTAC) algorithms in their systems, and for newer PET/CT scanners it is the only option offered. CT-based attenuation correction offers the significant advantage that the CT data have much lower statistical noise and can be acquired in a shorter time than a

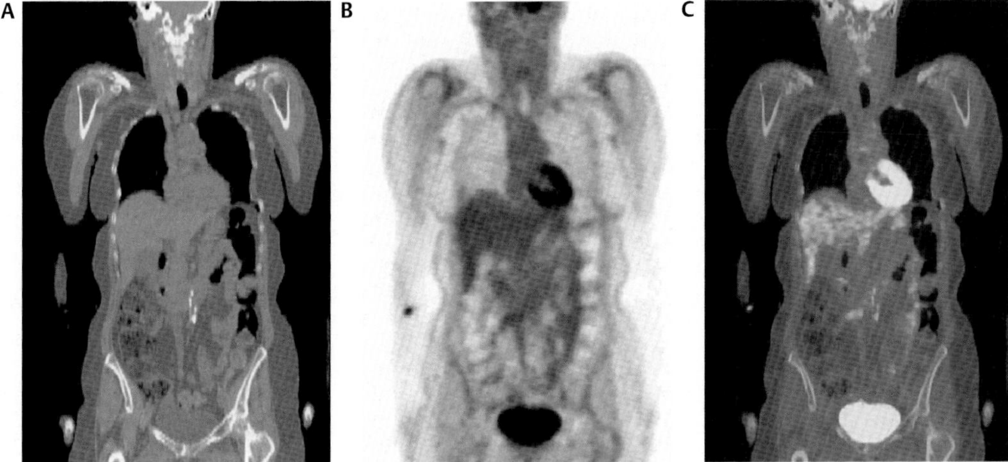

Fig. 1.13 Images from a positron emission tomography/computed tomography (PET/CT) scanner: **(A)** anatomical CT image, **(B)** functional PET image, and **(C)** overlaid image of a whole-body scan.

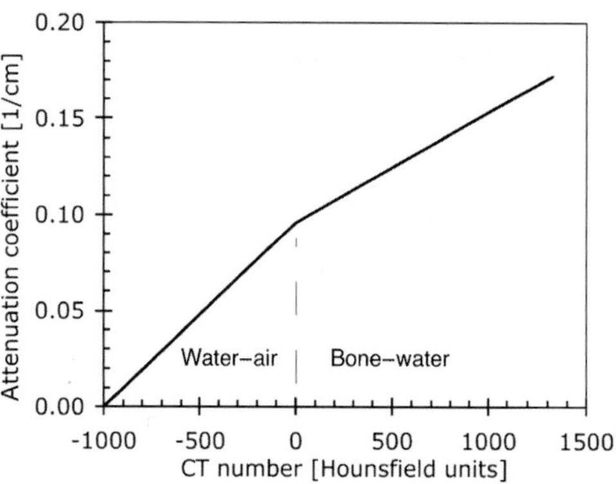

Fig. 1.14 Bilinear scaling transform used to convert computed tomography (CT) image values to positron emission tomography attenuation coefficients.

standard PET transmission scan. CT transmission scans can also be acquired after the PET tracer is injected, giving the ability to collect unbiased postinjection transmission scans. This shortens the time spent by a patient on the scanner bed and provides more efficient use of scanner time.

To be used for attenuation correction, the CT data must be transformed to an estimate of the attenuation coefficients at 511 keV. In the bilinear scaling method,[4] the attenuation map at 511 keV is estimated by using separate scaling factors for bone and nonbone components based on the CT image values (**Fig. 1.14**).

There is, however, no unique transformation from CT energies (~30 to 140 keV) to 511 keV due to the possibility of independent variations in density and atomic number *Z*, which can allow two materials with different atomic numbers to have similar CT values and different attenuation coefficients at 511 keV. Conversely, it is possible for two distinct materials with the same value of attenuation coefficient at 511 keV to yield different CT numbers, and errors in the CTAC image will propagate to errors in the PET image in the same location. This case arises if contrast agent or metallic or high-density implants are present in the CT image. Also, if there are positional mismatches between the PET and CT images due to, for example, respiratory motion, there will also be errors introduced into the PET image. Thus, although CT-based attenuation correction can lead to significant improvements in PET image quality, artifacts can arise from the presence of contrast agent, metallic or high-density implants, and respiratory motion.

References

1. Cherry SR, Sorensen JA, Phelps ME. Physics in Nuclear Medicine. Orlando, FL: Grune & Stratton; 2003
2. Valk PE, Bailey DE, Townsend DW, Maisey MN. Positron Emission Tomography: Basic Science and Clinical Practice. London: Springer-Verlag; 2003
3. Wernick MN, Aarsvold JN. Emission Tomography. San Diego, CA: Elsevier Academic Press; 2004
4. Alessio AM, Kinahan PE, Cheng PM, Vesselle H, Karp JS. PET/CT scanner instrumentation, challenges, and solutions. Radiol Clin North Am 2004;42(6):1017–1032

2

Basics of Fluorodeoxyglucose Radiochemistry and Biology

Neale S. Mason and Eugene C. Lin

Without question, [fluorine 18]fluorodeoxyglucose ([^{18}F]FDG) is the most commonly used positron emission tomography (PET) radiotracer and has demonstrated utility in a variety of applications, including neuroscience, cardiology, and oncology.[1–4] A brief discussion regarding the historical development of [^{18}F]FDG will be presented, but more detailed discussions can be found in several other recent publications.[5,6] In general, there are several chemistry concerns inherent in the production of PET radiotracers. A primary concern is the impact of the relatively short half-lives of the radionuclides on the synthetic process. As a matter of practical necessity, PET radiosyntheses are designed so that the radionuclide is introduced as close to the end of the synthesis as possible. Although it is clearly advantageous to have the incorporation of the radionuclide occur as the final step in the synthetic method, this is sometimes not feasible (as is the case in the production of [^{18}F]FDG). In most circumstances, the radiopharmaceutical for injection must be isolated from the crude reaction mixture using a variety of methods, including solid-phase extraction methods, high-performance liquid chromatography (HPLC) methods, or some combination of the two methods.

The design of 2-fluoro-2-deoxy-D-glucose was predicated upon the utility of [^{14}C]-2-DG, a derivative of glucose where a hydrogen atom replaces the ^{2}C hydroxyl group (**Fig. 2.1**).

In many ways, 2-DG (and by extension FDG) and glucose are very similar. Both compounds

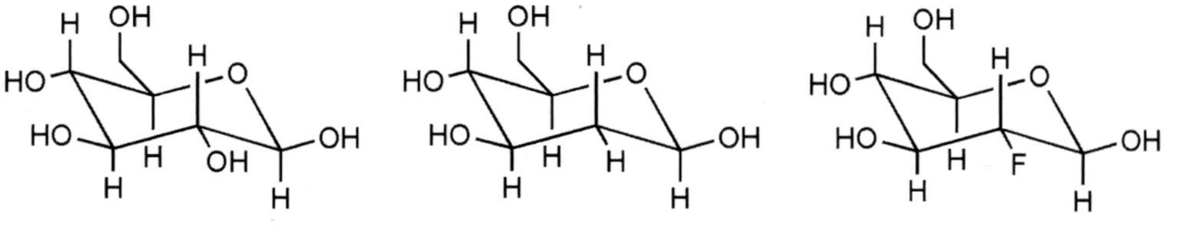

D-glucose   2-deoxy-D-glucose   2-fluoro-2-deoxy-D-glucose

Fig. 2.1 Chemical structures of glucose analogues.

are transported from the plasma via facilitated transport, and both compounds serve as substrates for phosphorylation by the enzyme hexokinase. However, the next enzyme in the metabolic route for these sugars, phosphohexose isomerase, requires the presence of a hydroxyl group on ^{2}C. Consequently, 2-DG and in a similar fashion FDG are trapped in the cell as their respective 6-phosphate derivatives that are not substrates for either phosphohexose isomerase or glucose-6-phosphate dehydrogenase. This metabolic trapping leads to the utility of [^{18}F]FDG in imaging and will be discussed further in the brief section concerning rate constants and pharmacokinetics. The demonstration that 2-FDG, in its unlabeled form, was a reasonable substrate for hexokinase and that the potential alternative substitution positions (i.e., ^{3}F and ^{4}F-deoxy-D-glucose, respectively) possessed significantly lower affinities for hexokinase[7,8] further supported the choice of FDG as a reasonable model compound for the development of an in vivo imaging agent.

◆ Synthesis of [^{18}F]FDG

Initial Method of Synthesis of [^{18}F]FDG

The first radiosynthesis of [^{18}F]FDG took place in 1976 as the result of a long collaboration between investigators at the National Institutes of Health, the University of Pennsylvania, and Brookhaven National Laboratory.[6] The first radiosynthesis of [^{18}F]FDG was based upon the availability of [^{18}F]F_2 via the deuterium bombardment of a nickel target loaded with neon 20 [^{20}Ne(d,α)^{18}F, indicating the collision of an accelerated deuteron (d) with the stable nuclide neon 20 to produce an α particle (α) and the fluorine 18 radionuclide]. The reaction of [^{18}F]F_2 with a protected D-glucal (3,4,6-tri-O-acetyl-D-glucal) yielded a mixture of mannose and glucose isomers that were separable by preparative gas chromatographic methods. Acidic hydrolysis of the glucose derivative yielded [^{18}F]FDG in amounts sufficient for human studies (**Fig. 2.2**).[9]

Later Method of Synthesis of [^{18}F]FDG

Electrophilic Route

A variety of different approaches for the optimization of an electrophilic route to [^{18}F]FDG were investigated.[10–12] The use of [^{18}F]acetyl hypofluorite ([^{18}F]CH_3CO_2F) became one of the methods of choice. However, it was eventually demonstrated that the use of [^{18}F]acetyl hypofluorite yielded varying amounts of the undesired isomer (2-deoxy-2[^{18}F]fluoro-D-mannose), depending on the reaction conditions.[13]

One drawback of the electrophilic method (either [^{18}F]F_2 or [^{18}F]CH_3CO_2F) is that only half of the label is available for incorporation into the target molecule. Another drawback is the use of carrier fluorine gas in the production that leads to reductions in specific activity. A third drawback, especially in light of the increasing utilization of [^{18}F]FDG, was the yield limitation of the production of fluorine 18 from the ^{20}Ne(d,α)^{18}F reaction. The cross-sectional energies for particles in the 10 to 18 MeV range for this reaction are ~60 to 90 mCi/uA. This is significantly lower than the corresponding

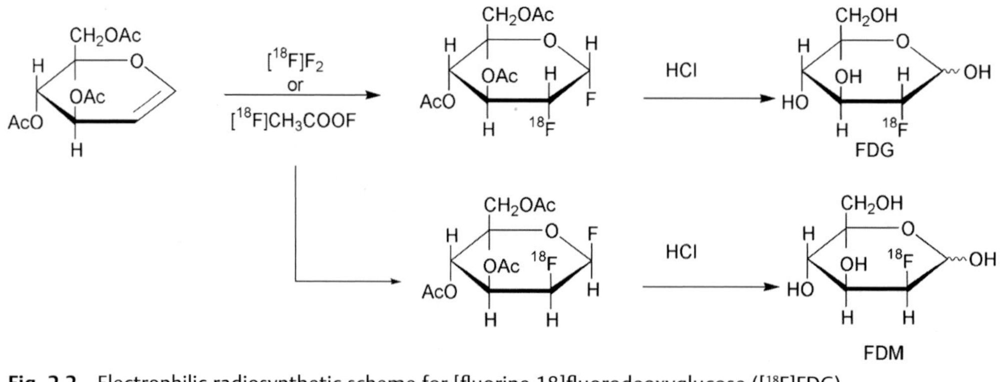

Fig. 2.2 Electrophilic radiosynthetic scheme for [fluorine 18]fluorodeoxyglucose ([^{18}F]FDG).

cross section for the $^{18}O(p,n)^{18}F$ reaction (150 to 260 mCi/uA).[14] Interest in a nucleophilic radiolabeling route to [^{18}F]FDG increased with the development of [^{18}O] water targets capable of producing [^{18}F]fluoride in high yield and with high specific activity. The most common method to produce nucleophilic [^{18}F]fluoride is the $^{18}O(p,n)^{18}F$ reaction (indicating the collision of an accelerated proton (p) with the stable nuclide oxygen 18 to produce a neutron (n) and the fluorine 18 radionuclide). The oxygen 18 target material most commonly consists of enriched [^{18}O]water.[15,16] Irradiation of enriched [^{18}O]water is capable of producing multicurie (> 70 GBq) quantities of [^{18}F]fluoride with high specific activity in relatively short irradiation times depending on target load volumes and beam geometry. In addition, there are now methods for the separation and recovery of the enriched target material from the [^{18}F]fluoride.[17–19]

Higher Yield Nucleophilic Route

The potential for higher [^{18}F]fluoride yields prompted significant efforts aimed at the development of a reliable, high-yielding nucleophilic route to [^{18}F]FDG. In most instances [^{18}F]FDG is synthesized using an adaptation of the Julich method (**Fig. 2.3**).[20] In the original application of this method, aqueous [^{18}F]fluoride is added to a solution consisting of Kryptofix 2.2.2 (Merck-Schuhardt OHG, Hohenbrunn, Germany) and potassium carbonate dissolved in aqueous acetonitrile. The residual water is removed by azeotropic distillation using anhydrous acetonitrile and a stream of inert gas such as nitrogen or argon. A relatively small amount of precursor (~10 to 20 mg of 1,3,4,6-tetra-O-acetyl-2-O-trifluoromethanesulfonyl-β-D-mannopyranose) dissolved in anhydrous acetonitrile is added to the dried [^{18}F]fluoride. The reaction mixture is heated to reflux for several minutes. Ethyl ether is used to transfer the reaction solution after cooling across a Sep-Pak silica cartridge (Waters Corporation, Milford, MA) into a second reaction vessel. This preliminary purification removes the unreacted [^{18}F]fluoride and the Kryptofix 2.2.2. The solvents are removed, and aqueous hydrochloric acid is added to the intermediate product, 2-deoxy-2-[^{18}F]fluoro-1,3,4,6-tetra-O-acetyl-β-D-glucopyranose. The aqueous acid solution is heated to reflux for a short period of time and then purified by passage across an ion-retardation resin followed by an alumina-N Sep-Pak and a C-18 Sep-Pak. Several aliquots of water are subsequently used to transfer all the product material from the hydrolysis vessel across the purification columns. This methodology leads to the presence of D-mannose, D-glucose, and 2-chloro-2-deoxy-D-glucose as chemical impurities in the radiosynthesis of FDG.[21]

This reaction scheme has been used as the basis of a computer-controlled automated synthesizer[22] for the routine production of [^{18}F]FDG (CTI, Knoxville, TN, now part of Siemens). Further modifications of this methodology have led to the development of "one-pot" syntheses for the production of [^{18}F]FDG. These modifications include the substitution of tetramethylammonium carbonate for Kryptofix 2.2.2/potassium carbonate as the phase-transfer reagent and subsequent elimination of the silica Sep-Pak purification step. Because of these modifications, the acidic hydrolysis was performed in the same reaction vessel.[23] A similar one-pot modification was reported that retained Kryptofix 2.2.2 as the phase-transfer reagent. This method also eliminated the intermediate silica Sep-Pak purification step, as well as adding a cation exchange resin to the purification column (to remove the unwanted Kryptofix 2.2.2) and an alumina N Sep-Pak to prevent fluoride ion breakthrough.[24]

The toxicity concerns associated with Kryptofix 2.2.2 (LD_{50} in rats of 35 mg/kg) have prompted the use of other phase-transfer agents such as tetrabutylammonium hydroxide or tetrabutylammonium bicarbonate. This modification has been incorporated into a commercially available synthesizer produced by Nuclear Interface. The Nuclear Interface

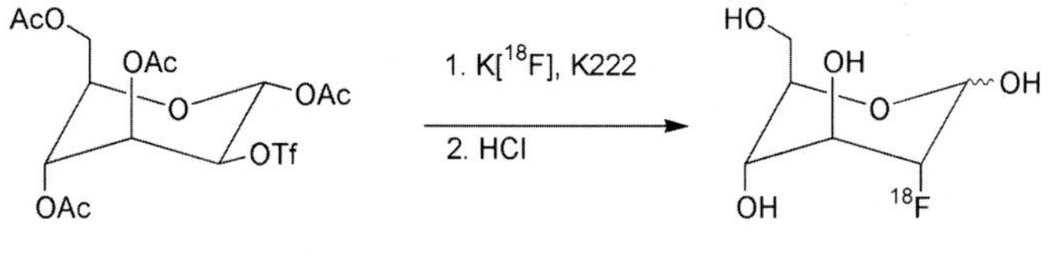

AcO OAc O OAc OTf OAc — 1. K[^{18}F], K222 / 2. HCl → HO OH O OH OH ^{18}F

Fig. 2.3 Nucleophilic radiosynthetic scheme for [fluorine 18]fluorodeoxyglucose ([^{18}F]FDG).

synthesis module is flexible in that it can be set up to use either tetrabutylammonium bicarbonate or Kryptofix 2.2.2 as the phase-transfer reagent. In addition, the module can perform the hydrolysis of the radiolabeled intermediate, 2-deoxy-2-[^{18}F]fluoro-1,3,4,6-tetra-O-acetyl-β-D-glucopyrranose, under either acidic or basic conditions. There are several other variations of this radiolabeling scheme. One variation is the use of an immobilized quaternary 4-aminopyridinium resin material for the isolation of the [^{18}F]fluoride and subsequent incorporation into the [^{18}F]-radiolabeled intermediate. In this process the [^{18}F]fluoride solution is passed across the resin column, where [^{18}F]fluoride is trapped and the bulk of the ^{18}O-enriched water is recovered downstream. The resin-bound [^{18}F]fluoride is dried by passing anhydrous acetonitrile across the resin column while heating the column. A solution of the precursor in anhydrous acetonitrile is then passed over the heated resin column in either a slow single pass or a reciprocating flow across the resin column. The solution containing the radiolabeled intermediate is then transferred to a hydrolysis vessel, where the acetonitrile is removed. Following the acid hydrolysis, the [^{18}F]FDG is purified in an analogous manner to the original method described above.[25] This methodology formed the basis of one commercially available synthesis unit (PET-trace FDG MicroLab, GE Medical Systems, Uppsala, Sweden). This unit uses a disposable cassette system for the reaction column, as well as transfer and addition lines that facilitate the set-up of the unit.

A solid-phase supported basic hydrolysis step[26] has been implemented in the FDG synthesizer marketed by Coincidence Technologies, Inc. (now part of GE Healthcare, Chalfont St. Giles, UK). The basic hydrolysis conditions allow for a faster reaction time as compared with the standard acidic hydrolysis conditions with no evidence of epimerization under the conditions employed (2 minutes at room temperature). Using this system, over 7 Ci of FDG has been produced in a single production run.

Quality Control in Synthesis

The production of [^{18}F]FDG entails not only the generation of the radionuclide ([^{18}F]fluoride) and the radiosynthetic procedure, but also the quality control determination that ensures the final product formulation is suitable for human use. There are several criteria that must be met for a radiopharmaceutical to be deemed suitable for human use. Routine quality control and release criteria for PET radiopharmaceuticals may include tests for radiochemical purity, chemical purity, stereochemical purity, radionuclidic identity, residual organic solvent contamination, pH, sterility, and apyrogenicity of the final formulation. The *United States Pharmacopeia* (USP) Chapter 823, Radiopharmaceuticals for Positron Emission Tomography–Compounding, provides a more detailed presentation of these concerns.[27] In addition, there are currently several USP monographs for individual PET radiotracers [^{18}F]FDG.

Although the majority of the quality control issues already mentioned are relatively straightforward in their application to the routine quality control of [^{18}F]FDG, a few deserve some elaboration. One of these is the determination of residual volatile organic solvents. The two primary organic solvents in question are acetonitrile and ethanol with release limits of 0.04 and 0.5% by volume, respectively. Within the USP framework, there is no allowance made for multiple batch testing for residual volatile organic solvents; that is, the determination of the levels of these solvents is to be made as part of the release criteria for each individual batch of [^{18}F]FDG produced. In addition, there are two chemical purity issues regarding the standard nucleophilic radiosynthetic method that uses an acidic hydrolysis process. The first of these is the determination of residual Kryptofix 2.2.2 in the final product preparation of [^{18}F]FDG. A color spot test method has been reported in the literature for the detection of this impurity at the detection limit specified in the USP.[28] It should be noted that a false-positive is possible with this test and that a confirmatory thin-layer chromatography test (USP method) should be performed to confirm the identity of the suspected impurity. In addition, the amount of 2-chloro-2-deoxy-D-glucose in the final product is to be determined (USP limit of 1 mg of 2-chloro-2-deoxy-D-glucose per total volume of final product formulation). The USP Chapter 823 and the monograph "Fludeoxyglucose F-18 Injection" are the current regulatory framework under which the production of [^{18}F]FDG is to be produced until such time as the Food and Drug Administration releases final current good manufacturing practice guidelines in accordance with the provisions of Section 121 of the Food and Drug Administration Modernization Act of 1997.

◆ Biologic Basis of FDG's Use in Imaging

The utility of [^{18}F]FDG for noninvasive in vivo imaging is based as much upon the pharmacokinetics of the tracer as it is upon the relative ease (at the present time) of production and delivery of [^{18}F]FDG to the end user. The general model for [^{18}F]FDG is the two-tissue compartmental model based upon the work of Sokoloff et al using [^{14}C]-DG[29] and later adopted for use with [^{18}F]FDG. More detailed discussions of the modeling of [^{18}F]FDG can be found in several other publications, but a brief description follows.[30,31] The model consists of three compartments: $C_p(t)$, arterial plasma concentration; $C_f(t)$, unmetabolized or free FDG; and $C_m(t)$, metabolized FDG trapped as FDG-6-phosphate (**Fig. 2.4**).

K_1 represents the rate constant for transport from arterial plasma to the tissue compartment. The rate constant k_2 is defined as the rate constant for transport from the free tissue compartment to arterial plasma. The rate constant k_3 represents the rate of phosphorylation, which is a measure of hexokinase activity. The rate constant k_4 represents the rate of dephosphorylation, and k_5 is the rate constant for further metabolism. In general, both k_4 and k_5 are ignored for [^{18}F]FDG, as the rate of dephosphorylation is very low compared with phosphorylation, and further metabolism by glucose-6-phosphate dehydrogenase is not possible due to the lack of a hydroxyl group at ^{2}C.

By definition, the metabolic rate of glucose is the net rate of the conversion of glucose to glucose-6-phosphate. However, in a PET study one measures the rate constants not for glucose, but rather for [^{18}F]FDG, and through the use of a "lumped constant" that represents the ratio of metabolic rates of FDG and glucose, one then calculates the metabolic rate of glucose in absolute terms (μmol/min/100 g).

The kinetics of FDG allows for an even simpler approach that was ultimately based on the autoradiography work of Sokoloff et al using [^{14}C]DG.[29] This approach is based on the presumption that [^{18}F]FDG is trapped in the tissue following phosphorylation. The fraction of trapped radioactivity continually increases throughout a study, whereas clearance from tissue of the free component is relatively rapid. Consequently, a single static image at 40 to 60 minutes postinjection reflects, to a very close degree, the relative metabolic rate of glucose.

Phosphorylation by hexokinase corresponding to the rate constant k_3 is the rate-limiting step for FDG metabolism, and overexpression of hexokinase may account to a large extent for the increased signal seen in some lesions. However, the etiology of the signal seen on FDG PET images is multifactorial. FDG activity in a lesion may be largely dependent upon blood flow in cases where perfusion is decreased. Cell density in the lesion also plays a factor in the amount of signal seen. Once the FDG reaches a lesion, it must be transported through the cell membrane. There are multiple facilitative mammalian glucose transporters (GLUT). The most important glucose transporter for FDG is GLUT1, which is expressed in almost all cell types. Overexpression of GLUT1 transporters is primarily responsible for the increased FDG signal seen in many lesions, and this may be independent of hexokinase activity. Another glucose transporter significant in FDG PET imaging is the GLUT4 transporter, which is insulin sensitive and present in the myocardium and skeletal muscle. Therefore, insulin will increase FDG uptake in the myocardium and

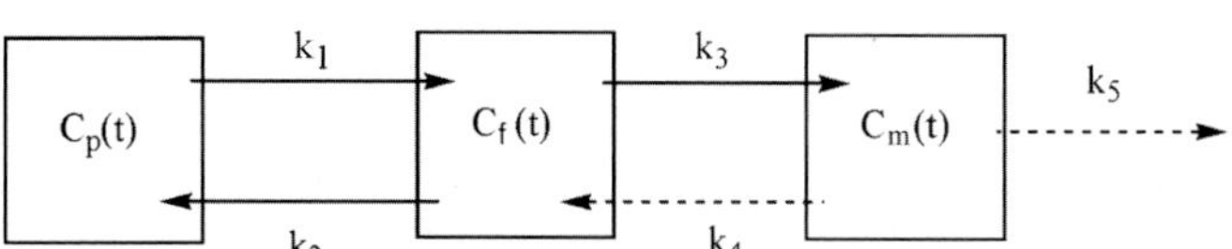

Fig. 2.4 Schematic representation of the two-tissue compartmental model for [fluorine 18]fluorodeoxyglucose ([^{18}F]FDG). For a more detailed description of C_P, C_F, C_M, and K_{1-5}, see the text.

skeletal muscle, with important implications for patient preparation for FDG PET studies and cardiac imaging with FDG (see Chapter 4). In general, the etiology of a hot spot seen on clinical FDG PET studies is a complex interaction of multiple factors, and interpreters should be cautious in ascribing the uptake to one specific physiological or molecular mechanism.

◆ Summary

The development of high yield [^{18}O]-enriched water targets for the production of [^{18}F]fluoride, the capabilities of current generation of cyclotrons to perform dual-target irradiations at relatively high target currents, and the availability of automated synthesis modules for the production of [^{18}F]FDG now makes possible the production of multicurie amounts of [^{18}F]FDG in a single production run. This capability has significantly increased the utilization of [^{18}F]FDG and has led to the introduction of production facilities dedicated to the synthesis and distribution of FDG to end users with only imaging capabilities.

References

1. Antonini A, Kazumata K, Feigin A, et al. Differential diagnosis of parkinsonism with [^{18}F]fluorodeoxyglucose and PET. Mov Disord 1998;13(2):268–274
2. Bar-Shalom R, Valdivia AY, Blaufox MD. PET imaging in oncology. Semin Nucl Med 2000;30(3):150–185
3. Fazekas F, Payer F. F-18 fluorodeoxyglucose positron emission tomography in neurology. Wien Med Wochenschr 2002;152(11–12):293–297
4. Saab G, Dekemp RA, Ukkonen H, Ruddy TD, Germano G, Beanlands RS. Gated fluorine 18 fluorodeoxyglucose positron emission tomography: determination of global and regional left ventricular function and myocardial tissue characterization. J Nucl Cardiol 2003;10(3):297–303
5. Beuthien-Baumann B, Hamacher K, Oberdorfer F, Steinbach J. Preparation of fluorine-18 labelled sugars and derivatives and their application as tracer for positron-emission-tomography. Carbohydr Res 2000; 327(1–2):107–118
6. Fowler JS, Ido T. Initial and subsequent approach for the synthesis of 18FDG. Semin Nucl Med 2002;32(1):6–12
7. Bessell EM, Courtenay VD, Foster AB, Jones M, Westwood JH. Some in vivo and in vitro antitumour effects of the deoxyfluoro-D-glucopyranoses. Eur J Cancer 1973;9(7):463–470
8. Machado de Domenech EE, Sols A. Specificity of hexokinases towards some uncommon substrates and inhibitors. FEBS Lett 1980;119(1):174–176
9. Ido T, Wan CN, Fowler JS, Wolf AP. Fluorination with F_2: a convenient synthesis of 2-deoxy-2-fluoro-D-glucose. J Org Chem 1977;42:2341–2342
10. Adams MJ. A rapid, stereoselective, high yielding synthesis of 2-deoxy-2-fluoro-D-hexopyranoses: reaction of glycals with acetyl hypofluorite. J Chem Soc Chem Commun 1982;13:730–732
11. Ehrenkaufer RE, Potocki JF, Jewett DM. Simple synthesis of F-18-labeled 2-fluoro-2-deoxy-D-glucose: concise communication. J Nucl Med 1984;25(3): 333–337
12. Sood S, Firnau G, Garnett ES. Radiofluorination with xenon difluoride: a new high yield synthesis of [^{18}F]2-fluro-2-deoxy-D-glucose. Int J Appl Radiat Isot 1983;34(4):743–745
13. Bida GT, Satyamurthy N, Barrio JR. The synthesis of 2-[F-18]fluoro-2-deoxy-D-glucose using glycals: a reexamination. J Nucl Med 1984;25(12):1327–1334
14. Ruth TJ, Wolf AP. Absolute cross sections for the production of ^{18}F via the ^{18}O(p,n)^{18}F reaction. Radiochim. Acta 1979;26:21–24
15. Kilbourn MR, Hood JT, Welch MJ. A simple ^{18}O water target for ^{18}F production. Int J Appl Radiat Isot 1984;35(7):599–602
16. Wieland B, Hendry G, Schmidt D, Bida G, Ruth T. Efficient small-volume ^{18}O-water targets for producing ^{18}F-fluoride with low energy protons. J Labelled Comp Radiopharm 1986;23:1205–1207
17. Jewett DM, Toorongian SA, Mulholland GK, Watkins GL, Kilbourn MR. Multiphase extraction: rapid phase-transfer of [^{18}F]fluoride ion for nucleophilic radiolabeling reactions. Int J Rad Appl Instrum [A] 1988;39(11):1109–1111
18. Schlyer DJ, Bastos M, Wolf AP. A quantitative separation of fluorine-18 fluoride from oxygen-18 water. J Nucl Med 1987;28:764
19. Schlyer DJ, Bastos M, Alexoff D, Wolf A. Separation of [^{18}F]fluoride from [^{18}O]water using anion exchange resin. Int J Rad Appl Instrum [A] 1990;41: 531–533
20. Hamacher K, Coenen HH, Stocklin G. Efficient stereospecific synthesis of no-carrier-added 2-[^{18}F]-fluoro-2-deoxy-D-glucose using aminopolyether supported nucleophilic substitution. J Nucl Med 1986;27(2): 235–238
21. Alexoff DL, Casati R, Fowler JS, et al. Ion chromatographic analysis of high specific activity 18FDG preparations and detection of the chemical impurity 2-deoxy-2-chloro-D-glucose. Int J Rad Appl Instrum [A] 1992;43(11):1313–1322
22. Padgett HC, Schmidt DG, Luxen A, Bida GT, Satyamurthy N, Barrio JR. Computer-controlled radiochemical synthesis: a chemistry process control unit for the automated production of radiochemicals. Int J Rad Appl Instrum [A] 1989;40(5):433–445
23. Mock BH, Vavrek MT, Mulholland GK. Back-to-back "one-pot" [^{18}F]FDG syntheses in a single Siemens-CTI chemistry process control unit. Nucl Med Biol 1996;23(4):497–501
24. Padgett HC, Wilson D, Clanton J, Wolf AP. Paper presented at: *RDS Users Meeting* (Abstr.); 1998
25. Toorongian SA, Mulholland GK, Jewett DM, Bachelor MA, Kilbourn MR. Routine production of 2-deoxy-2-[^{18}F]fluoro-D-glucose by direct nucleophilic exchange on a quaternary 4-aminopyridinium resin. Int J Rad Appl Instrum B 1990;17(3):273–279
26. Lemaire C, Damhaut PH, Lauricella B, et al. Fast [^{18}F]FDG synthesis by alkaline hydrolysis on a low

polarity solid phase support. J Labelled Comp Radiopharm 2002;45:435–447

27. The United States Pharmacopeial Convention. Radiopharmaceuticals for positron emission tomography—compounding. In: United States Pharmacopeia 20/National Formulary 25. Rockville, MD: The United States Pharmacopeial Convention, Inc.;2002:2068–2071
28. Mock BH, Winkle W, Vavrek MT. A color spot test for the detection of Kryptofix 2.2.2 in [^{18}F]FDG preparations. Nucl Med Biol 1997;24(2):193–195
29. Sokoloff L, Reivich M, Kennedy C, et al. The [^{14}C]deoxyglucose method for the measurement of local cerebral glucose utilization: theory, procedure, and normal values in the conscious and anesthetized albino rat. J Neurochem 1977;28(5):897–916
30. Phelps ME, Huang SC, Hoffman EJ, Selin C, Sokoloff L, Kuhl DE. Tomographic measurement of local cerebral glucose metabolic rate in humans with (F-18)2-fluoro-2-deoxy-D-glucose: validation of method. Ann Neurol 1979;6(5):371–388
31. Reivich M, Kuhl D, Wolf A, et al. The [^{18}F]fluorodeoxyglucose method for the measurement of local cerebral glucose utilization in man. Circ Res 1979; 44(1):127–137

3

The Role of Glucose and FDG Metabolism in the Interpretation of PET Studies

Ronald L. Korn, Alison Coates, and John Millstine

Ask most physicians to recall the enzymatic pathways of glucose metabolism, and you will likely provoke memories of premedical or medical school biochemistry classes where the common dictum was, "Glucose metabolism? Why do I need to know this stuff? I will never use this information again!"

Fortunately, a few students of science and medicine have had the astuteness to realize that even the most mundane and obscure fact could someday come in handy. Such is the story of glucose metabolism and its relationship to [fluorine 18]fluorodeoxyglucose ([^{18}F]FDG) positron emission tomography (PET) imaging. In 1924, Otto Warburg, a famous German biochemist, made a fundamental observation that would forever change the course of our understanding of the role of glucose metabolism in cancer biology. In an article published in the journal *Biochemische Zeitschrift*,[1] he and his colleagues noted that cancer cells consume more glucose and produce more lactic acid than normal (resting) cells. This straightforward observation, later termed the Warburg effect in his honor, was apparent even under aerobic conditions. Because of his pioneering work, Warburg was awarded the Nobel Prize for Medicine and is considered one of the central figures in positron emission tomography (PET) imaging.

One glucose molecule metabolized in the presence of adequate oxygen can lead to the production of 36 adenosine triphosphate (ATP) molecules with CO_2 and H_20 as its by-products (so-called tricarboxylic acid, or TCA, cycle). However, in hypoxic conditions and in many cancer cell types, only two ATPs are formed from glucose metabolism, with lactic acid (glycolysis) produced as its by-product. These observations have given rise to several theories about the survival and tenacity of cancer even under the most formidable conditions.[2–8] Yet it is the rather simplified pathway of glucose metabolism through the glycolytic pathway that has been responsible for the explosion of FDG PET imaging over the last few decades.

Although a detailed understanding of the role of glucose metabolism in the context of the critical changes that occur to transform a normal cell into a malignant one is beyond the scope of this chapter, we will briefly focus on the biology of FDG imaging in the framework of what the clinician needs to know for everyday interpretation of FDG PET studies. We will attempt to provide a basic understanding of the changes that occur at the molecular level that account for the increased glucose metabolism in cancer cells and other benign inflammatory conditions. It is hoped that this chapter will serve as a starting point for our readers to delve further into the complex biology of glucose and FDG metabolism and to begin to appreciate the central role of glucose metabolism as a molecular probe in oncology imaging. Furthermore, this chapter will focus almost exclusively on the biology of FDG oncology imaging, but it will not address the biological changes that occur in cardiac or neurologic diseases. Finally, we hope that this chapter will help answer question the age-old question of "why you need to know this stuff."

◆ The Breakdown of Glucose/FDG from Injection to Cell Entry

The importance of glucose metabolism in malignancy has provided a foundation for understanding cancer biology. A decisive advantage of FDG in oncology imaging is that it behaves in so many ways like glucose. For example, glucose metabolism in most organs like the brain, heart, and visceral structures is closely coupled to blood flow. In some malignancies, such as breast cancer,[9] there is an uncoupling of the flow–metabolism cycle with subsequent elevated glucose metabolism compared with surrounding normal tissue. This elevated glucose metabolic rate seems to be a vital mechanism needed to feed the various biological alterations that have transformed the host cell into a malignant one.

Sanjiv Gambhir, in his chapter on the quantitative assay development for PET,[10] directs his readers to pretend to be a molecule of FDG and then asks the readers to think about all of the different directions that they can go once they are injected into the body. If we play along with his thought experiment, we would begin our journey from the syringe into the bloodstream (plasma). Once in the blood, we would either leave the plasma space to enter the interstitium or travel in the blood to the kidneys, where we would be excreted because of our ^{18}F atom on the 2-carbon position of the deoxyglucose molecule. If not excreted by the kidneys, we would be transported into the cell, and then we would proceed down the chemical reaction pathway of our journey. Once in the cell, most of us would be phosphorylated and chemically trapped by the glycolytic pathway and end up with our ^{18}F moiety decaying; some of us would be kicked back out of the cell into the interstitium, eventually migrating back into the bloodstream and kidneys. If we brought a PET scanner to take pictures of our journey, we would inevitably find that many of us are congregating in a tumor against a low background of FDG in host tissues due to the rapid clearance of FDG from the bloodstream and body.

When thought about in this way, we can begin to divide our journey into at least four different phases or spaces: (1) the vascular space, (2) the interstitial space, (3) the intracellular space, and (4) the FDG-6-phosphate (FDG-6-P) or glucose-6-phosphate (Gluc-6-P) space. The concentration (or, more precisely, the mass) of FDG in each of these compartments can be accurately measured by the PET scanner through kinetic analysis for detailed quantitative PET imaging, a feature that is unique to this modality. As kinetic analysis is cumbersome in routine clinical practice, a semiquantitative estimate of FDG concentration also exists in the form of the standardized uptake value (SUV). The interested reader is referred to many excellent review articles on this subject.[11–14]

Similarities between Glucose and FDG

It is very fortunate, if not fortuitous, that FDG behaves very similarly if not identically to glucose in the first three phases or compartments of the journey. FDG is circulated in the blood like glucose (vascular space). It migrates from the plasma space into the interstitium similarly to glucose (interstitial space). It is transported into the cells (intracellular space) via facilitated transport (whether malignant or not) just like glucose, utilizing a family of glucose transport proteins (GLUT). Although there are approximately 13 GLUTs,[15] it is GLUT1 that is found in most noncardiac tissue, including tumors. This is important to remember because the translocation of GLUT1 from the cytosol to the cell membrane in tumors is an insulin independent process, whereas GLUT4 (whose presence predominates on the cell membrane in myocytes) requires insulin for it to translocate on the cell membrane. This phenomenon helps to explain why one needs to either inject a patient with insulin to perform myocardial viability PET studies with FDG or give an exogenous glucose load (initiates a spike in endogenous insulin production) to drive the tracer into the myocytes; however, this is not required for oncology or neurology PET imaging.

Once glucose or FDG is internalized into the cell, it is acted upon by hexokinase II (HK II) in a similar way to glucose. HK II phosphorylates both glucose and FDG to glucose-6-phosphate (G-6-P) or FDG-6-phosphate (FDG-6-P), respectively. Once in the G-6-P form, this moiety can be further degraded through the glycolysis or TCA cycle to produce ATP for cellular energy and metabolism. However, FDG-6-P cannot undergo further metabolism. Furthermore, the negative charge from the phosphate group on FDG-6-P serves to trap it in the cell. Because cancer cells me-

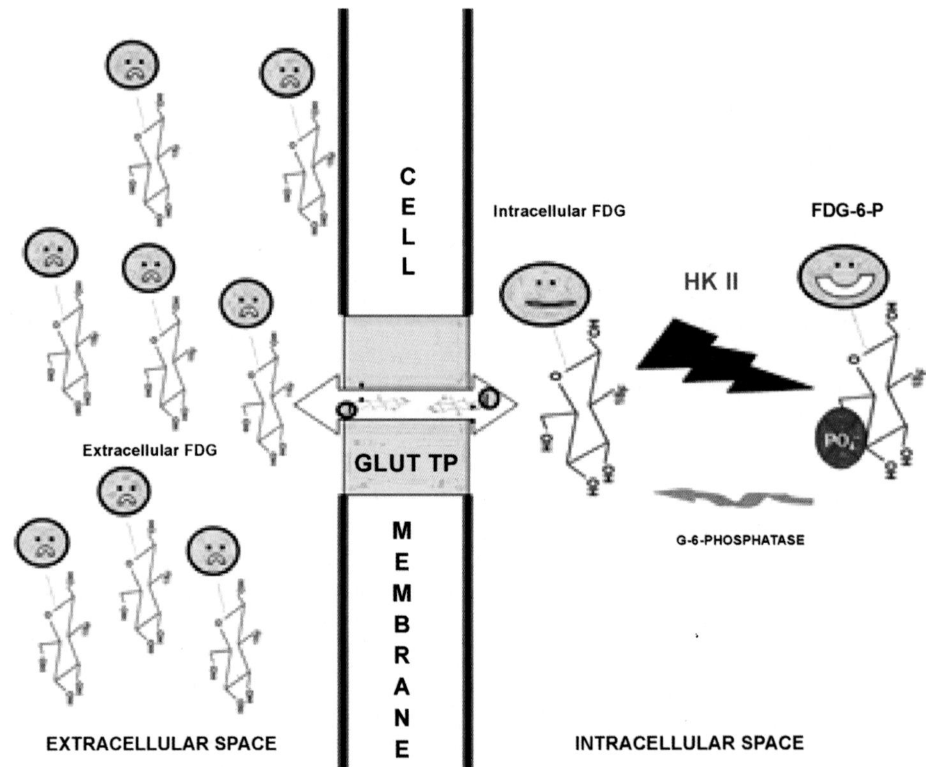

Fig. 3.1 Metabolism of [fluorine 18]fluorodeoxyglucose ([^{18}F]FDG). Cartoon depicts the metabolism of FDG at a very basic level. FDG (stick figure in cartoon with blue head and FDG backbone body) in the extracellular space is taken up by the cell via facilitated transport through the glucose transport protein [GLUT;]. There are at least 13 different types of GLUTs. GLUT1 is the prominent protein that is responsible for most of the FDG uptake in malignant and many inflammatory cells. Once in the cytosol, FDG is phosphorylated by hexokinase II [HK II;] to form FDG-6-P. The FDG-6-P is essentially trapped in the cytosol of the cell and cannot either participate further in metabolism or diffuse out of the cell due to the negative charge on the phosphate group. A small fraction of the intracellular FDG-6-P can be dephosphorylated back to FDG by the action of glucose-6-phosphatase (). This "free" fraction of FDG can diffuse back out of the cell via GLUT. It is the relative balance of these processes that determines the overall FDG activity in a cell.

tabolize more glucose than host cells, they will accumulate more FDG, thus paving the way for detection on PET (**Fig. 3.1**).

This difference in glucose metabolism between host cells and cancer cells is not the only explanation for elevated FDG-6-P activity in the malignant cell. Some cells, such as hepatocytes, have increased glucose-6-phosphatase activity (G-6-Pase). This enzyme is responsible for dephosphorylating both G-6-P and FDG-6-P back into their respective native forms, which then allows them to diffuse back out of the cell. Indeed, some tumors, like low-grade hepatocellular carcinomas, have increased G-6-Pase, which might account for their low metabolic potential (relative lack of FDG accumulation; see next section).[16]

FDG Activity in Different Cells, Tissues, Organs, and Bodies

The presence of FDG in a particular cell, tissue, or organ—and even in the whole body—is dependent on multiple factors and cannot be simplified to a single mechanism. Much of the FDG uptake, however, is dependent upon the balance of local factors and the metabolic behavior occurring at the organ and whole body level.

Cellular Level

At the cellular level, the following components have been implicated in promoting elevated FDG uptake in malignant cells compared with host cells.

1. Increased vascular tumor flow → more tracer is available for uptake
2. Increased GLUT1 on the cellular membrane → more FDG movement into the cell
3. More HK II → more FDG-6-P production, leading to metabolic trapping of FDG in cancer cells
4. Reduced G-6-Pase → less intracellular dephosphorylation of FDG-6-P and less egress of FDG activity out of the malignant cell

All these different mechanisms contribute to FDG uptake in tumors, making PET very sensitive for many tumor types; however, these processes also occur in nonmalignant tissues. For example, inflammatory cells also demonstrate increased GLUT1, which can simulate malignancy when associated FDG uptake is intense.[17] The inflammatory-type uptake has been especially noted in macrophages, neutrophils, histiocytes, and lymphocytes. As noted before, some tumors have higher than average G-6-Pase compared with other tumors, which favors egress of FDG activity out of the cell and, subsequently, diminished lesion conspicuity on the PET scan. In short, the mechanism for increased glucose metabolism can be different for different cells. Thus, FDG uptake can be dependent upon blood flow (cardiac tissue), HK II activity (most tumors), and dephosphorylating activity (brain tissue and hepatocytes).[18,19]

Tissue Level

At the tissue level, FDG uptake is closely linked to the number of viable cells, proliferation activity, tissue perfusion (or neovascularity), hypoxia, and presence of inflammatory cells.[20–22] It is the balance of these factors that can control the overall activity and even heterogeneity of FDG activity in the tissue. For example, some early studies demonstrated a significant FDG accumulation in macrophages and granulation tissue over the tumor cells in patients with non–small cell lung cancers.[23] Finally, there is some preliminary evidence that endothelial cells in tumor vessels can have enhanced FDG metabolism and account for some of the FDG activity observed on PET scans.[24]

Organ Level

At the organ level, the amount of FDG uptake is closely linked to organ perfusion, tumor volume, intrinsic glucose metabolism, and presence of inflammatory responses such as concurrent chemotherapy and radiation therapy or stimulated glucose metabolic activity from the use of medications (e.g., colony-stimulating factors) (**Fig. 3.2**). In addition, some tumors, like well-differentiated thyroid and prostate cancers, have FDG uptake based on their endocrine responsiveness. As these tumors dedifferentiate, their hormone responsiveness decreases while

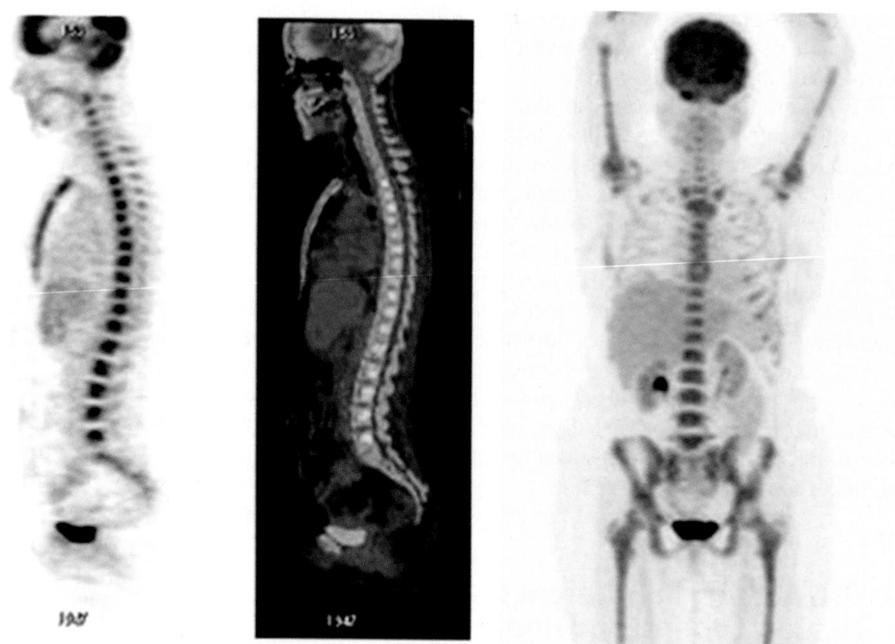

Fig. 3.2 Robust [fluorine 18]fluorodeoxyglucose ([^{18}F]FDG) uptake in the marrow space due to stimulation from colony-stimulating factor therapy. This figure illustrates how FDG metabolism can be influenced at the organ level by multiple factors, including iatrogenically induced conditions. **(A)** A sagittal image showing the intense uptake of FDG activity in the bone marrow. **(B)** A positron emission tomography/computed tomography (PET/CT) fusion image. **(C)** A maximum intensity projection (MIP) of a whole-body scan. A MIP is a computer rendering technique that allows the interpreter to view the PET images in a three-dimensional fashion.

their FDG uptake increases and is an indicator of poor prognosis.[25,26]

Whole-Body Level

On a systemic or whole-body level, the amount of endogenous blood glucose can affect FDG uptake. For example, circulating glucose in the setting of hyperglycemia (blood glucose levels > 200 mg/dL) can effectively compete at the cellular level for FDG uptake, thus reducing the overall uptake of FDG.[27] Patients who have exercised within 24 hours of their scan, recently consumed food or liquid calories, or who arrive in the PET centers intoxicated will have FDG uptake driven preferentially into the skeletal muscles rather than tumors, thus reducing the sensitivity of FDG PET. Also, diabetic patients who have administered short-acting insulin within 3 to 4 hours prior to FDG injection will have preferential uptake of activity in their muscles because of the stimulation of GLUT4 (**Fig. 3.3**). In general, FDG administration should be delayed for about 3 to 4 hours postinsulin administration to reduce this skeletal dominant pattern of uptake for oncology PET scans. Cardiac activity can also be altered based on both dietary and fasting states and insulin levels. In particular, high protein and fat diets consumed the night before an exam can reduce cardiac activity by favoring fatty acid metabolism in the myocytes over glucose metabolism. Finally, the mental state of a patient or cold weather can drive FDG into brown fat deposits in the neck and chest and neuronally activated tissue along the spine.[28] Even in warm states like Arizona, brown fat uptake can be highly stimulated when a patient enters an air-conditioned, 72°F imaging center environment after walking through 120°F heat from the parking lot

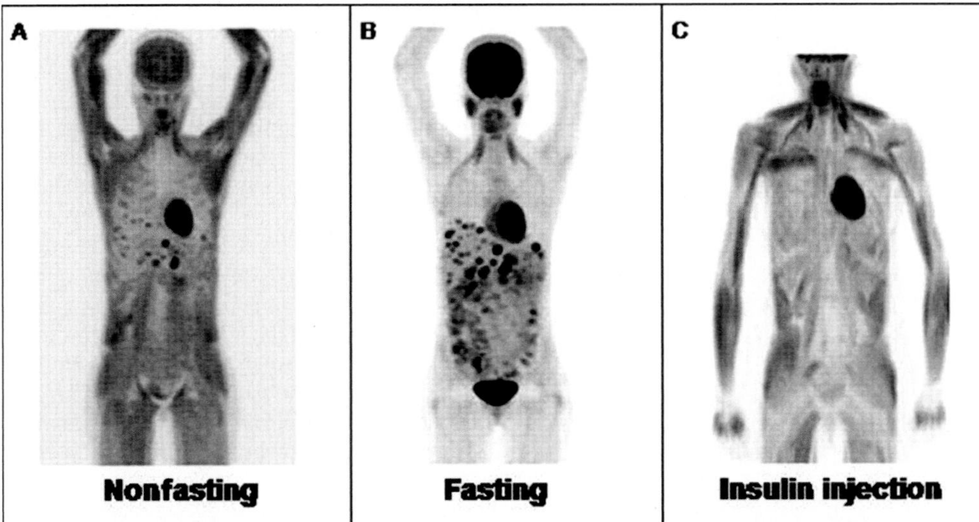

Fig. 3.3 The influence of glucose, insulin, and proper patient preparation on positron emission tomography (PET) scan quality. Maximum intensity projection (MIP) images from different patients are shown. PET scans **(A)** and **(B)** demonstrate two studies in the same patient obtained at different times 1 week apart. They show a 37-year-old with a stage IV gastrointestinal stroma tumor (GIST) who claimed adherence to a 4-hour fast prior to [fluorine 18]fluorodeoxyglucose ([^{18}F]FDG) **(A)**. On further questioning, the patient recalled eating 1 hour before arriving at the PET/CT center. **(B)** PET scan shows the MIP from the repeat study, with the patient having undergone a true 4-hour fast. On both occasions the patient's blood glucose level was normal before FDG injection. Note that the MIP in **(A)** has extensive FDG uptake in the skeletal muscles and heart (presumably due to increased GLUT4 transport protein), with a relative paucity of activity in the brain, hepatic metastases, and urinary tract system compared with **(B)**. This case underlies the need for proper patient preparation for accurate interpretation and illustrates how endogenous insulin release from eating can quickly alter FDG uptake and metabolism. **(C)** MIP image from a separate patient who failed to tell the technologist that he self-administered 5 units of Humulin (Eli Lilly & Co., Indianapolis, IN), 1 hour prior to FDG injection. Notice how similar the MIP image in **(A)** is to **(C)**. Tumor metabolic uptake is reduced in this setting, rendering the study nondiagnostic. Current recommendations suggest at least a 3- to 4-hour hiatus between short-acting insulin dosing and FDG injection for oncologic imaging.

to the facility (**Fig. 3.4**). An awareness of all of these variables can assist the clinician in optimizing PET scan acquisition parameters and interpretation.

Molecular Interactions in the Cellular and Tumor Microenvironment that Promote Glucose Metabolism and FDG Uptake

Cancer has a "molecular sweet tooth"[6] that can be traced to various biological changes that occur at the cellular level during host cell malignant transformation. In addition to activating the Warburg effect, these cellular alterations can result in a series of modifications in the biology of the tumor cell, which can assist tumor survival in a relatively hostile host environment, lead to multidrug resistance and metastasis, and promote the suppression of programmed cellular death (apoptosis). In this section, we will provide an elementary understanding of the altered biological pathways, which will help to explain why FDG is such an ideal tracer for tumor imaging. The reader is encouraged to consult an excellent review on this subject for more details.[29]

Hypoxic Environment

Many tumors exist in a relatively hostile environment of dysfunctional tumor perfusion, low pH, and hypoxia.[2] Their adaptation to this environment is therefore critical for survival and metastasis. Central to tumor survival might be a

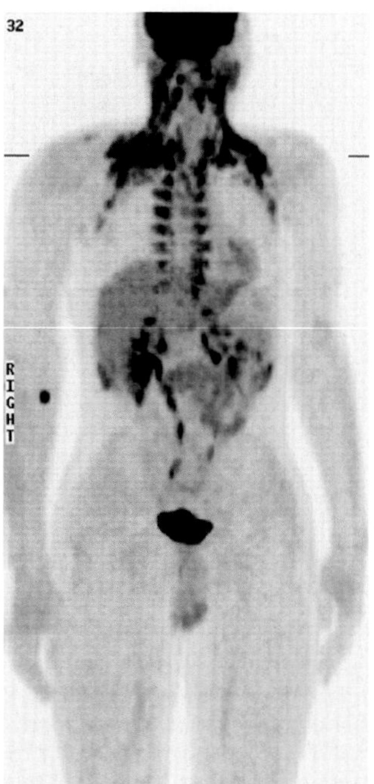

Fig. 3.4 Maximum intensity projection image showing fluorodeoxyglucose (FDG) uptake in brown fat. Note the extensive metabolism in the neck and paraspinal area from neuronal activation of brown fat deposits in these locations. The study was obtained in July when the outside temperature in Scottsdale, Arizona, was 116°F, but ambient temperature was a pleasant 71°F in the injection bay. Such climate changes can alter FDG uptake and metabolism. Keeping the patient warm and comfortable prior to injection can reduce such activity.

protein called hypoxia induction factor (HIF-) 1. HIF-1 is a heterodimer composed of two protein subunits—α and β. In hypoxic conditions, HIF-1α is stabilized, and the HIF-1 heterodimer is reinforced. This stabilization of the HIF-1 protein can lead to the direct production of GLUT1 and HK II. In addition, HIF-1 stimulates the manufacture of vascular endothelial growth factor (VEGF), which promotes tumor neovascularity. As a result, glucose metabolism is increased by enhanced substrate delivery to the tumor via developing neovascularity, elevated glucose (or FDG) flux into the tumor cells due to transactivation of GLUT1, and ultimately higher metabolic activity because of greater HK II dependent conversion of glucose to G-6-P (or FDG-6-P).[30] As elegant as this processsounds, it is clearly not the entire story and does not fully account for the Warburg effect.

Aerobic Glycolysis

For aerobic glycolysis to occur, oxidative phosphorylation in the mitochondria has to be reduced, and the metabolism of glucose into pyruvate and lactic acid needs to be enhanced, even when oxygen is plentiful. Many alterations in the transformed cell biology promote aerobic glycolysis by accentuating the effects of HIF-1. For example, several oncogene and/or tumor suppressor gene products help to stabilize HIF-1, prevent its degradation, or increase its production. These include *Src* oncogene, *H-Ras,* phosphatidylinositol 3-kinase, *VHL, SDH,* and *FH* mutations. However, not all the changes that occur in a cancer cell favor the bolstering of HIF-1 protein. For example, activation of the serine-threonine kinase *AKT* can lead to increased aerobic glycolysis by affecting glucose transport and HK II activity directly, independent of HIF-1.

So, how does one explain the Warburg effect of aerobic glycolysis? Ultimately for this to occur, glucose metabolism will require a switchover from the TCA cycle to glycolysis. Although not fully understood, it appears that the *MYC* oncogene found in many tumors is key to this change: it enhances mitochondrial production, which eventually creates more reactive oxygen species or radicals. As a result, these oxygen radicals can induce local mitochondrial DNA damage, resulting in mitochondrial dysfunction. This process, compounded by the action of the p53 protein found in most tumor cells and several other enzymes involved in the TCA cycle, will favor a switch from oxidative phosphorylation to lactic acid production, leading to dwindling mitochondrial function. Thus, oncogene activation (*AKT, MYC, H-Ras*, etc.) along with HIF-1 stabilization can lead to the immortalization of the cancer cell and activate those changes that Warburg observed over 80 years ago.[6,7]

◆ New Therapies Based on Glycolytic Metabolism

Beginning with Warburg's original speculations that tumorigenesis is the result of mitochondrial dysfunction, to the current concepts of oncogenic and tumor suppression-guided activation of the glycolytic pathway, many investigators are refocusing their attention on glucose metabolism to design cancer therapy. Among the intriguing approaches either currently in trials or under consideration is the use of biological agents that target HIF-1, GLUT1, and ATP citrate lyase. This latter enzyme is involved in lipid synthesis that predominates when aerobic glycolysis is switched on; thus, inhibiting lipid synthesis by targeting ATP citrate lyase can suppress tumor growth. Finally, some investigators have rediscovered the use of deoxyglucose itself for inhibition of glucose uptake in malignant cells.

◆ Summary

Aerobic glycolysis as observed by Otto Warburg in the 1930s has come full circle. The central role of FDG in probing this pathway has made it an almost ideal tracer for cancer detection in PET. Although several benign and inflammatory conditions share elevated glucose metabolism with tumor cells, FDG remains one of the best agents available for cancer imaging. The mechanism of FDG metabolism in tumor cells has been explored in this chapter in a most elementary fashion to give the clinician the flavor of the molecular sweet tooth of a cancer cell and a basic understanding of the meaning of "hot spots" on FDG PET scans. Although aerobic glycolysis might not cause cellular malignant transformation, it is clear that it is necessary to facilitate the cancerous state. Such adaptive responses by the tumor to the host cell can trigger tumor survival, multidrug resistance, and suppression of programmed cell death. Strategies that disrupt the Warburg effect are therefore of top priority in the development of therapeutic agents that can target these survival mechanisms of a cancer cell.

References

1. Warburg O, Posener K, Negelein E. VIII. The metabolism of cancer cells. Biochem Zeitschr 1924;152:129–169
2. Gatenby RA, Gillies RJ. Why do malignant cancers have high levels of glycolysis? Nat Rev Cancer 2004;4:891–899
3. Izuishi K, Kato K, Ogura T, Kinoshita T, Esumi H. Remarkable tolerance of tumor cells to nutrient deprivation: possible new biochemical targets for cancer therapy. Cancer Res 2000;60:6201–6206
4. Graeber TG, Osmanian C, Jacks T, et al. Hypoxia-mediated selection of cells with diminished apoptotic potential in solid tumors. Nature 1996;379:88–91
5. Gatenby RA, Gawlinski ET, Gmitro AF, Kaylor B, Gillies RJ. Acid-mediated tumor invasion: a multidisciplinary study. Cancer Res 2006;66:5216–5223
6. Kim JW, Dang CV. Cancer's sweet tooth and the Warburg effect. Cancer Res 2006;66:8927–8930
7. Dang CV. Role of MYC and HIF in the Warburg effect and tumorigenesis. Paper presented at: American Association for Cancer Research Annual Meeting, April 14, 2007
8. Bomanji JB, Costa DC, Ell PJ. Clinical role of positron emission tomography in oncology. Lancet Oncol 2001;2:157–164
9. Tseng J, Dunnwald LK, Shubert EK, et al. 18 F-FDG kinetics in locally advanced breast cancer: correlation with tumor blood flow and changes in response to neoadjuvant chemotherapy. J Nucl Med 2004;45: 1829–1837
10. Gambhir SS. Quantitative assay development for PET. In: Phelps ME, ed. PET: Molecular Imaging and Its Biological Applications. New York/Heidelberg/Berlin: Springer-Verlag; 2004:125–216
11. Weber WA, Schwaiger M, Avril N. Quantitative assessment of tumor metabolism using FDG-PET imaging. Nucl Med Biol 2000;27:683–687
12. Keyes JW Jr . SUV: standard uptake or silly useless value? J Nucl Med 1995;36:1836–1839
13. Huang SC. Anatomy of SUV. Nucl Med Biol 2000;27: 643–646
14. Mankoff DA, Muzi M, Krohn KA. Quantitative PET imaging to measure tumor response to therapy: what is the best method? Mol Imaging Biol 2003;5:281–285
15. Wood IS, Trayhurn P. Glucose transporters (GLUT and SGLT): expanded families of sugar transport proteins. Br J Nutr 2003;89:3–9
16. Torizuka T, Tamaki N, Inokuma T, et al. In vivo assessment of glucose metabolism in hepatocellular carcinoma with FDG PET. J Nucl Med 1995;36:1811–1817
17. Chung JH, Cho KJ, Lee SS, et al. Overexpression of Glut1 in lymphoid follicles correlates with false-positive ^{18}F-FDG PET results in lung cancer staging. J Nucl Med 2004;45:999–1003
18. Phelps ME, Huang S, Hoffman E. Tomographic measurement of local cerebral glucose metabolic rate in humans with (^{18}F)2-fluoro-2-deoxy-D-glucose: validation of method. Ann Neurol 1979;6:371–388
19. Reivich M, Kuhl D, Wolf A, et al. The [^{18}F] fluorodeoxyglucose method for the measurement of local cerebral glucose utilization in man. Circ Res 1979;44:127–137
20. Brown RS, Leung JY, Fisher S, Frey KA, Ethier SP, Wahl RL. Intratumoral distribution of tritiated-FDG in breast carcinoma: correlation between GLUT-1 expression and FDG uptake. J Nucl Med 1996;37:1042–1047
21. Higashi K, Clavo AC, Wahl RL. Does FDG uptake measure proliferative activity of human cancer cells? In vitro comparison with DNA flow cytometry and tritiated thymidine uptake. J Nucl Med 1993;34:414–419
22. Brown RS, Leung JY, Fisher SJ, Grey KA, Ethier SP, Wahl RL. Intratumoral distribution of tritiated fluorodeoxyglucose in breast carcinoma: I. Are inflammatory cells important? J Nucl Med 1995;36:1854–1861

23. Kubota R, Yamada S, Kubota K, et al. Intratumoral distribution of fluorine-18 fluorodeoxyglucose in vivo. J Nucl Med 1992;33:1972–1980

24. Maschauer S, Prante O, Hoffmann M, Deichen JT, Kuwert T. Characterization of ^{18}F-FDG uptake in human endothelial cells in vitro. J Nucl Med 2004;45: 455460

25. Morris MJ, Akhurst T, Osman I, et al. Fluorinated deoxyglucose positron emission tomography imaging in progressive metastatic prostate cancer. Urology 2002;59:913–918

26. Wang W, Larson SM, Tuttle RM, et al. Resistance of [^{18}F]-fluorodeoxyglucose-avid metastatic thyroid cancer lesions to treatment with high-dose radioactive iodine. Thyroid 2001;11:1169–1175

27. Lindholm P, Minn H, Leskinen-Kallio S, et al. Influence of the blood glucose concentration on FDG uptake in cancer—a PET study. J Nucl Med 1993;34:1–6

28. Hany TF, Gharehpapagh E, Kamel EM, et al. Brown adipose tissue: a factor to consider in symmetrical tracer uptake in the neck and upper chest region. Eur J Nucl Med Mol Imaging 2002;29:1393–1398

29. Mankoff DA, Eary JF, Link JM, et al. Tumor-specific positron emission tomography imaging in patients: ^{18}F fluorodeoxyglucose and beyond. Clin Cancer Res 2007;13:3460–3469

30. Bos R, van der Hoeven JJ, van der Wall E, et al. Biologic correlates of 18fluorodeoxyglucose uptake in human breast cancer measured by positron emission tomography. J Clin Oncol 2002;20:379–387

II

Clinical Basics

4

Patient Preparation

Eugene C. Lin and Abass Alavi

Proper patient preparation prior to and during the positron emission tomography (PET) study is important to ensure maximum diagnostic yield. The most important factors are glucose level, minimizing the effects of physiologic activity, and timing the performance of a scan relative to the type of treatment.

◆ Oncological PET

Glucose Level

Acceptable glucose levels for oncologic PET can be achieved by keeping the patient NPO (nothing by mouth) for a time before the study (see Diet subsection). Diabetic patients may require insulin or other drugs to control their blood glucose levels.

1. ***Acceptable glucose levels.*** High glucose levels can compete with fluorodeoxyglucose (FDG) uptake and can substantially degrade image quality and the accuracy of the results.
   a. Glucose level should be ≤ 150 mg/dL if possible for optimal image quality.
   b. PET usually should not be performed if glucose is above 200 mg/dL.
2. ***Diabetic patients.*** If needed, the physician managing the patient should be consulted for lowering blood glucose levels.
   a. *Type I diabetes:* Scan in morning after overnight fast.
   b. *Type II diabetes:* May require insulin in the morning.
3. ***Insulin administration.*** Insulin (2 to 5 units) can be given if glucose is elevated. Glucose should be rechecked prior to FDG injection.
   a. Insulin administration will increase FDG uptake in the heart, skeletal muscles, and liver (the same pattern is seen if the patient has eaten before FDG administration). This will degrade image quality and therefore the ability to detect lesions (**Fig. 4.1**).
   b. A minimum time interval of 1 hour is necessary between insulin administration and FDG injection to minimize undesirable effects.[1]
4. ***Other diabetic medications.*** Because the mode of action of metformin is a reduction of hepatic gluconeogenesis, this medication should not interfere with FDG uptake. Other oral antidiabetic drugs, such as sulfonylureas (tolbutamide, glyburide, glipizide), lower plasma glucose primarily by stimulating insulin secretion, and it makes sense to stop them before an FDG PET study. Insulin sensitizers, such as rosiglitazone, may not affect FDG uptake because their mode of action is primarily activation of peroxisome proliferator-activated receptors.

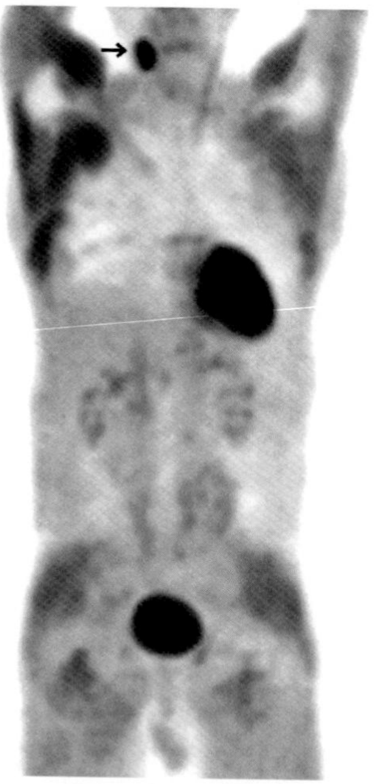

Fig. 4.1 Effects of insulin release on fluorodeoxyglucose uptake. A patient with lymphoma did not follow instructions and ate 1 hour before the exam. Increased uptake is present in the skeletal muscle and heart with minimal activity elsewhere. An abnormal cervical node is seen (*arrow*), but this exam should be repeated, as disease elsewhere could be missed.

Diet

1. The patient should be fasting for at least 4 hours prior to the exam.
2. If there is known or suspected thoracic pathology, fasting for at least 12 hours is desirable to minimize cardiac activity.
3. A low carbohydrate/high protein/high fat diet prior to the exam can optimize uptake and decrease myocardial uptake. This diet should be followed for at least 24 hours before the exam.
4. Caffeine, nicotine, and alcohol should be avoided for 24 hours before the exam.
   - Caffeine can have a variable effect on cardiac uptake; it can increase uptake or stimulate myocardial fatty acid metabolism and decrease FDG uptake.[2]

Hydration

1. ***Oral hydration.*** Oral hydration starting the day before the scan and continued hydration after the scan is recommended.[3] Along with frequent voiding, this reduces bladder radiation dose and possibly improves image quality by reducing urinary artifact.
2. ***Intravenous hydration.*** Intravenous hydration is useful but less frequently employed. If intravenous hydration is used, the fluid should not contain dextrose or lactose.

Minimization of Physiologic Uptake

Physiologic uptake in muscle, brown fat, the urinary tract, and bowel can obscure or mimic disease.

1. ***Muscle uptake***
   a. The patient should avoid strenuous exercise the day of the study.
   b. Muscle relaxants such as diazepam are helpful in reducing muscle uptake from stress. Note that diazepam may be helpful in reducing brown fat uptake as well.
      - Pretreatment with diazepam should be considered for all patients with suspicion of cervical and supraclavicular nodal disease because muscular uptake is most common in these regions.

   c. Laryngeal muscle uptake can be minimized by instructing the patient not to talk 5 minutes before and 20 minutes after the injection.
2. ***Brown fat uptake*** (see Chapter 6). Brown fat uptake can be limited by decreasing adrenergic stimulation. This can be achieved by pharmacologic intervention and/or limiting patient exposure to cold temperatures.
   a. *Pharmacologic interventions*
      - Diazepam. Diazepam may decrease brown fat uptake (brown fat has benzodiazepine receptors; in addition diazepam may decrease general sympathetic activity).
        - However, in one report[4] diazepam did not affect brown fat uptake in rats.
      - Other drugs. Administration of resperine and propanolol has been shown to decrease brown fat uptake in rats.[4]
        - Resperine and propanolol also decrease cardiac activity.

- The indication and appropriate dosage in humans are not currently well established.
- Drugs to avoid. Drugs that stimulate the sympathetic nervous system (e.g., nicotine and ephedrine) can potentially increase brown fat uptake and should be avoided prior to the study if possible.

b. *Minimized exposure to cold temperature.* Patients should dress warmly and avoid cold temperature for 48 hours before the scan. Also, patients should be kept warm between injection and imaging.[5] Temperature control may be helpful even when pharmacologic intervention is unsuccessful.

3. *Urinary activity.* FDG activity is seen in renal collecting systems, ureters, and bladder. The role of intervention to reduce urinary artifacts depends on the pathology being evaluated. Collecting system activity can mimic or obscure renal neoplasms. Reducing ureteral activity is helpful for evaluating retroperitoneal nodes. Reduction of bladder activity is important for evaluating pelvic pathology and nodes (see Chapters 22 and 23). However, in many circumstances, additional intervention is usually not necessary, particularly if the cancer being evaluated does not have a propensity for pelvic or retroperitoneal metastases. A protocol can be designed to reduce bladder activity, collecting system/ureteral activity, or both. Nevertheless, in our experience, these interventions are rarely required. Combined PET/computed tomographic (CT) imaging will also reduce the need for such interventions.

a. *Reducing bladder activity*

- Hydration/diuretics
  - Hydration and/or diuretics dilute urine activity and also result in more frequent voiding.
  - Diuretic administration has a potential additional advantage over hydration alone: both hydration and diuretics increase urine volume, but hydration can also increase FDG delivery to the bladder (potentially offsetting the value of increased voiding).[6]
- Foley catheter
  - Placement of a Foley catheter for drainage will greatly reduce bladder activity and decrease radiation dose to the bladder.
  - However, the bladder may be helpful in certain cases as an anatomic landmark on non-PET/CT studies. If the bladder is filled with saline through the catheter before imaging the pelvis, this will result in a full bladder that can be used as a landmark, but without intense activity that may obscure important findings.
  - Catheter placement has the disadvantage of adding an invasive component to a noninvasive study.
- Bladder irrigation
  - In conjunction with a Foley catheter, warm saline is used to irrigate the bladder during the time of the scan.
  - If bladder irrigation is used, diuretics may not be necessary.[7]

b. *Reducing collecting system/ureteral activity.* Collecting system and ureteral activity can be reduced by diluting the urine with hydration and/or diuretics.

- Sample protocol to reduce urinary activity:[8]
  - Hydrate after FDG injection.
  - Administer furosemide 30 minutes after FDG injection.
  - Place Foley catheter before scanning.
  - Scan the pelvis as the last bed position.
  - Fill the bladder retrograde with normal saline and clamp catheter before scanning the pelvis.

4. *Bowel activity.* Bowel activity is primarily seen in the cecum, right colon, and rectosigmoid and to a lesser extent in the remaining colon and small bowel. Several methods can be used to reduce bowel activity (uptake is mostly in the wall and to a lesser extent the lumen; no one method is completely successful to reduce bowel activity). As with urinary activity, combined PET/CT imaging may reduce the need to minimize bowel activity with interventions.

a. Administer isosmotic solution (e.g., GoLYTELY, Braintree Laboratories, Inc., Braintree, MA) the evening prior to the exam. NPO until the exam.

b. Administration of glucagon or oral spasmolytic medications (e.g., mebeverine) to decrease peristalsis is typically less helpful.[9]

PET Scan Timing

1. ***Postbiopsy.*** 1 week
2. ***Postsurgery.*** 6 weeks
   • Should be adjusted based upon the invasiveness of the procedure.
3. ***Postradiofrequency ablation.*** 4 weeks[10]
4. ***Postchemotherapy.*** 2 to 4 weeks
5. ***Postradiation.*** 2 to 6 months
   a. Both chemotherapy and radiation can cause false-positive results (from inflammation) and false-negative results (from presumed "stunning" of viable tumor). Corticosteroids decrease the inflammatory response after chemotherapy.[11]
   b. False-positive/negative results have been reported up to 3 months postchemotherapy[12] and 5 months postradiation.[13] One study[14] suggests that PET can be accurately performed 1 month after radiotherapy of head and neck cancer. The preceding time intervals represent a general range based upon the published literature.
   c. Baseline studies should be performed before initiation of chemotherapy because FDG uptake can be decreased even 1 day after start of chemotherapy.[15]
6. ***Postgranulocyte colony-stimulating factor (G-CSF).*** 1 week to 1 month
   • The reported time interval after cessation of G-CSF necessary to avoid increased uptake due to the stimulation is variable, ranging from 5 days to 1 month (see Chapter 6).[16,17]

Breastfeeding

1. ***Radiation dose.*** Most of the radiation dose to the baby is from proximity to the mother rather than FDG excretion into breast milk.[18]
2. ***Discontinuation.*** Breastfeeding can be discontinued for 24 hours after FDG injection.

Route of FDG Administration

FDG can be administered orally if intravenous access is not available (**Fig. 4.2**). The same delay before imaging used with intravenous injection can be employed with oral administration.

◆ Cardiac PET

The myocardium metabolizes free fatty acids in the fasting state. To image the myocardium specifically, the nutrient substrate must be switched to glucose. This can be achieved either by oral glucose loading or by hyperinsulinemic-euglycemic clamp. Another approach is to decrease myocardial fatty acid metabolism.[19,20]

Oral Glucose Loading

Twenty-five to 100 g of oral glucose can be administered prior to FDG injection.

1. ***Advantages.*** Glucose loading is very practical to perform compared with hyperinsulinemic–euglycemic clamp.

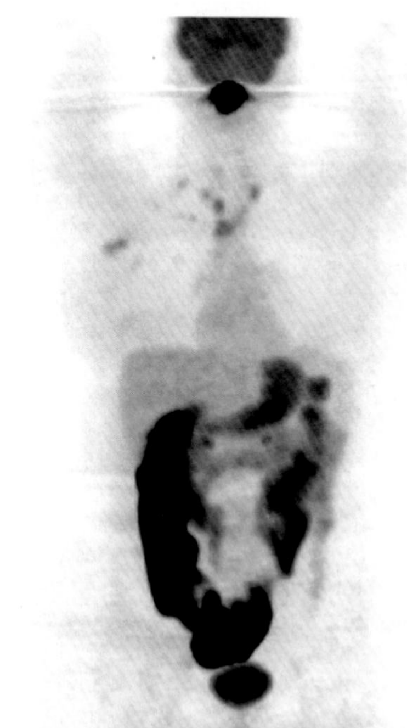

Fig. 4.2 Oral fluorodeoxyglucose (FDG) administration. Coronal positron emission tomography scan performed with oral FDG administration has substantial oral and bowel activity but adequate FDG uptake. (Courtesy of Bruce Higginbotham, Little Rock, AR.)

2. ***Disadvantages.*** Image quality may be suboptimal, particularly in diabetic patients.
3. ***Diabetics.*** Supplemental doses of short-acting insulin after oral glucose loading may be helpful in diabetic patients and patients with blood glucose > 110 mg/dL.
4. ***Glucose level.*** Blood glucose level should be in the 100 to 140 mg/dL level at the time of FDG injection.

Hyperinsulinemic–Euglycemic Clamp

Insulin is infused for the duration of the study. Glucose is infused at the same time to maintain blood glucose at baseline levels (based upon multiple blood glucose determinations).

1. **Advantages.** Using the clamp technique results in greater and more homogeneous myocardial uptake, particularly in diabetic patients.
2. **Disadvantages**
   a. Time and labor intensive procedure
   b. Often requires supplemental potassium due to hypokalemia

Decreasing Free Fatty Acid Metabolism

Niacin and acipimox (nicotinic acid derivatives) lower free fatty acid levels in plasma and therefore increase myocardial glucose uptake.

References

1. Turcotte E, Benard F, Boucher L, Verreault J. Use of IV insulin to reduce blood glucose levels before FDG-PET scanning in diabetic patients. J Nucl Med 2000;41:294
2. Cook GJ, Wegner EA, Fogelman I. Pitfalls and artifacts in 18FDG PET and PET/CT oncologic imaging. Semin Nucl Med 2004;34(2):122–133
3. Hamblen SM, Lowe VJ. Clinical ^{18}F-FDG oncology patient preparation techniques. J Nucl Med Technol 2003;31(1):3–7
4. Tatsumi M, Engles JM, Ishimori T, et al. Intense (18)F-FDG uptake in brown fat can be reduced pharmacologically. J Nucl Med 2004;45(7):1189–1193
5. Cohade C, Mourtzikos KA, Wahl RL. "USA-Fat": prevalence is related to ambient outdoor temperature—evaluation with ^{18}F-FDG PET/CT. J Nucl Med 2003;44(8):1267–1270
6. Moran JK, Lee HB, Blaufox MD. Optimization of urinary FDG excretion during PET imaging. J Nucl Med 1999;40(8):1352–1357
7. Koyama K, Okamura T, Kawabe J, et al. Evaluation of ^{18}F-FDG PET with bladder irrigation in patients with uterine and ovarian tumors. J Nucl Med 2003;44(3):353–358
8. Miraldi F, Vesselle H, Faulhaber PF, et al. Elimination of artifactual accumulation of FDG in PET imaging of colorectal cancer. Clin Nucl Med 1998;23(1):3–7
9. De Barsy C, Daenen F, Benard F, Ishimori T. Is FDG bowel uptake modified by oral spasmolytic premedication? J Nucl Med 2002;43(5):203
10. Okuma T, Matsuoka T, Okamura T, et al. ^{18}F-FDG small-animal PET for monitoring the therapeutic effect of CT-guided radiofrequency ablation on implanted VX2 lung tumors in rabbits. J Nucl Med 2006;47(8):1351–1358
11. Brepoels L, Stroobants S, Vandenberghe P, et al. Effect of corticosteroids on ^{18}F-FDG uptake in tumor lesions after chemotherapy. J Nucl Med 2007;48(3):390–397
12. Akhurst T, Kates TJ, Mazumdar M, et al. Recent chemotherapy reduces the sensitivity of [^{18}F]fluorodeoxyglucose positron emission tomography in the detection of colorectal metastases. J Clin Oncol 2005; 23(34):8713–8716
13. Peng N, Yen S, Liu W, et al. Evaluation of the effect of radiation therapy to nasopharyngeal carcinoma by positron emission tomography with 2-. Clin Positron Imaging 2000;3(2):51–56
14. Kim SY, Lee SW, Nam SY, et al. The feasibility of ^{18}F-FDG PET scans 1 month after completing radiotherapy of squamous cell carcinoma of the head and neck. J Nucl Med 2007;48(3):373–378
15. Yamane T, Daimaru O, Ito S, et al. Decreased ^{18}F-FDG uptake 1 day after initiation of chemotherapy for malignant lymphomas. J Nucl Med 2004;45(11):1838–1842
16. Hollinger EF, Alibazoglu H, Ali A, et al. Hematopoietic cytokine-mediated FDG uptake simulates the appearance of diffuse metastatic disease on whole-body PET imaging. Clin Nucl Med 1998;23(2):93–98
17. Kazama T, Swanston N, Podoloff DA, Macapinlac HA. Effect of colony-stimulating factor and conventional- or high-dose chemotherapy on FDG uptake in bone marrow. Eur J Nucl Med Mol Imaging 2005;32(12):1406–1411
18. Hicks RJ, Binns D, Stabin MG. Pattern of uptake and excretion of (18)F-FDG in the lactating breast. J Nucl Med 2001;42(8):1238–1242
19. Beanlands RSB, Ruddy TD, Mahhadi J. Myocardial viability. In: Wahl RL, ed. Principles and Practice of Positron Emission Tomography. Philadelphia, PA: Lippincott Williams & Wilkins; 2002:334–350
20. Takalkar A, Mavi A, Alavi A, Araujo L. PET in cardiology. Radiol Clin North Am 2005;43(1):107–119

5

Standardized Uptake Value

Eugene C. Lin, Abass Alavi, and Paul E. Kinahan

The standard uptake value (SUV) is also known as

- SUR (standardized uptake ratio)
- DUR (differential uptake value, dose uptake ratio)
- DAR (differential absorption ratio, dose absorption ratio)

◆ SUV Calculation

1. ***Definition.*** The standardized uptake value is the measured activity normalized for body weight/surface area and injected dose. As a reference, if the dose were uniformly distributed over the entire body, the value everywhere would be SUV ~ 1.0. Thus, SUV is a relative uptake measure.[1]
2. ***Formula***

$$\frac{\text{Region of interest (ROI) activity (mCi/mL)} \times \text{body weight (g)}}{\text{injected dose (mCi)}}$$

- Lean body mass or body surface area can be substituted for body weight. This will be more accurate for obese patients (see Pitfalls section).

Pitfalls

The SUV is a semiquantitative measurement. Numerous factors can result in erroneous results.[2]

1. ***Patient size.*** The SUV has a strong positive correlation with weight if calculated using body weight.
   - ***a.*** The SUVs in normal tissues of heavy patients can be twice those in lighter patients. This is secondary to the relatively low fluorodeoxyglucose (FDG) uptake in fat. An obese patient who weighs 300 pounds will not have twice the glucose metabolizing mass of a patient weighing 150 pounds, as much of the additional weight is from fat. Thus, using 300 pounds in the SUV equation for an obese patient is inaccurate because the glucose metabolizing mass in this patient is substantially lower than 300 pounds.
   - ***b.*** If the measured activity in an obese patient is multiplied by body weight, the SUV will be substantially overestimated.
   - ***c.*** The overestimation of SUVs in obese patients can be avoided by using lean body mass or body surface area rather than weight in the calculation.
2. ***Time of measurement.*** FDG uptake in most lesions increases rapidly in the first 2 hours following the administration of FDG, then increases slowly after that.[3]
   - ***a.*** Imaging earlier provides low SUV results.
   - ***b.*** Conversely, delayed scans provide high SUVs.
   - ***c.*** Earlier scans are usually subject to greater measurement error because the SUV in lesions has not yet plateaued.

d. The SUV plateaus earlier following therapeutic interventions.

3. ***Plasma glucose levels.*** Because nonlabeled glucose is competitive with FDG uptake, the higher the plasma glucose, the lower the SUV. Thus, SUVs are underestimated at high glucose levels and should ideally be corrected upward in these situations.
   a. Correction of SUV with the plasma glucose level can be used (e.g., SUV × glucose concentration/100 mg/dL).
   b. This is primarily useful for serial monitoring in the same patient, but interstudy SUV variability in normal tissues will be increased.
4. ***Partial volume effects.*** Small lesions may have artifactually low SUVs from partial volume effects.
   a. Partial volume effects occur when lesions are less than 2 to 3 full-width half-maximum resolution of the scanner (5 to 10 mm in practice for most positron emission scanners [PET] scanners).
   b. On standard PET scanners, partial volume effects will definitely occur below 2 cm. However, any lesion < 3 cm can potentially demonstrate partial volume effects.
   c. Partial volume effects are more prominent for less compact tumors. "Compact" refers to the surface area for a given volume (spheric tumors are most compact). Thus, spheric tumors are least affected by partial volume effects.[4]
5. ***Background activity.*** Another partial volume effect is "spilling in" of background activity. A lung tumor with equal metabolic activity to a liver tumor may have a lower SUV due to less "spilling in" of background activity.[4]
6. ***Dose extravasation.*** Dose extravasation results in an underestimated SUV. If dose extravasation is known to have occurred, it is usually better to use a tumor-to-background ratio, as this is not affected by dose extravasation.
7. ***Reconstruction parameter.*** Both reconstruction parameters and attenuation correction methods can affect SUV values.[5]
   a. Filtered back versus interactive reconstruction. SUVs from images reconstructed with filtered backprojection may be different from images reconstructed with iterative reconstruction.
      - Number of iterations. The SUV of hot spots will increase with more iterations. Most of the increase in average SUV will occur in the first five iterations, with lesser degrees of increase with more iterations. The maximum SUV will increase steadily with more iterations. Thus, the number of iterations will affect the maximum SUV more than the average SUV.[6]

   b. Attenuation correction. The attenuation correction (AC) method can have more of an effect on SUV than the reconstruction method, particularly if there are artifacts introduced by the AC (e.g., due to patient motion).
8. ***Computed tomography- (CT-) based attenuation correction.*** SUVs from CT-attenuation corrected studies may vary from those generated with a radionuclide source. In addition, SUV values on PET/CT may be erroneous due to misregistration or truncation artifact.
   a. CT attenuation-corrected SUVs on early PET/CT scanners were reported to be 4 to 15% higher than those calculated by a germanium 68-corrected source.[7] However, there was no difference in SUVs between PET and PET/CT in a later study.[8]
      - The largest difference is seen in the osseous structures.
      - This may be related to errors associated with converting CT attenuation values to 511 keV positron annihilation values.
      - Caution should be used when comparing SUVs between PET/CT and PET studies.

   b. Measured SUVs can be erroneous due to acquiring CT and PET studies at different respiratory phases (see Chapter 7).
      - CT attenuation-corrected SUVs can vary up to 30% in areas of significant respiratory motion (e.g., the lung bases).[9]

   c. Truncation artifact occurs due to differences in the field of view (FOV) between PET and CT. Obese patients may have part of their anatomy outside the FOV of the CT scan. This truncated portion does not provide data for attenuation correction, resulting in artifactually low SUVs.

Pearls

1. ***SUV ROI.***[10] ROIs placed to measure SUV may vary among centers. However, it is necessary to standardize ROI placement within the same institution and to duplicate the ROI placement method if SUVs from studies at another institution are used for comparison.
   - ***a.*** *Manual definition*
     - Automated methods will decrease variability.
   - ***b.*** *Three-dimensional isocontour at a percentage of maximum pixel value*
     - This is most accurate for noisy data.
     - Yields information on the metabolically active volume of tumor
   - ***c.*** *Maximum pixel value*
     - Used instead of average value for small objects to avoid partial-volume errors.
     - This is most accurate for smoothed (low noise) data and less accurate for noisy data.
     - However, smoothing the data increases partial-volume effect.
     - Uptake is often overestimated at low levels.
   - ***d.*** *Fixed-size ROI centered on maximum pixel value*
     - A fixed-size ROI is useful for following tumors that have changed in size, to avoid partial volume effects related to the size change.
     - This is probably the most robust ROI determination method.
     - However, this technique is inaccurate for small tumors.
   - ***e.*** *Volumetric versus two-dimensional (2D) ROI.* Volumetric ROIs should be performed if possible. 2D ROIs can result in significant (> 25%) interobserver variability.[11] To improve reproducibility with 2D ROIs, the interpreter should remeasure the SUVs on the prior exams rather than relying on prior reports.
2. ***Maximum versus mean SUV.*** Either maximum or mean SUV in a region of interest can be used.
   - ***a.*** *Maximum SUV.* This is preferred when using a large region of interest, as areas of necrosis and structures outside the lesion can result in an artifactually low SUV if a mean value is employed. However, maximum SUV is more prone to be artifactually elevated due to noise, and thus is substantially affected by the reconstruction algorithm. Typically, SUV will be overestimated, but occasionally it can be underestimated. The maximum SUV is least affected by partial volume effects.[4]
   - ***b.*** *Mean SUV.* If mean SUV is used, a small region of interest should be placed around the most intense area of the region.
3. ***SUV cutoff values.*** Caution must be taken when using SUV cutoffs from published literature in clinical practice.
   - ***a.*** The specifics of the data acquisition and analysis used to determine these SUV cutoffs are often not available in the published literature. As already noted, variations in data acquisition and analysis can have substantial effects upon measured SUVs. Also, the patient population varies from center to center.
   - ***b.*** In general, the reproducibility of SUV measurements between institutions is poor.
   - ***c.*** Given these factors, it is often advisable to use published SUV cutoffs with caution if at all. Values substantially higher and lower than the cutoff are significant, but values close to the cutoff value may be of questionable value for diagnostic purposes.
4. ***Interpretation.*** SUVs should be just one of many criteria used for interpretation, including visual uptake, lesion size relative to uptake, pattern of uptake, and clinical history. There is no evidence that SUVs in isolation are superior to visual interpretation for optimal diagnosis.
5. ***Therapy response.*** Some form of relative quantitation is necessary for accurately assessing therapy response, and SUV is a practical method for this purpose. Therefore, it is important that the acquisition and analysis schemes for generating PET images are kept the same between exams. Because protocols can be standardized within an institution, SUVs may be more helpful for monitoring response to treatment rather than primary diagnosis.[10] If SUVs are used for monitoring therapy response, then it is

essential to control the factors that influence SUV. In addition, calibration between the scanner and the dose calibrator, as well as the longitudinal stability of the scanner global scale factors, should have rigorous quality assurance/quality control (QA/QC) monitoring procedures. SUVs are most useful in primary diagnosis if the cutoff values are derived from data at the interpreting institution.

6. ***Reporting.*** For patients with cancer, it is important to report SUVs of chosen index lesions, even if these measurements are not used for interpretation of the current study. If the patient is restudied at a later date, the SUVs will be necessary for follow-up interpretation.
7. ***Dual time-point imaging.***[12–14] SUV in malignant lesions will usually increase over time, and uptake in benign lesions will usually decrease or will remain stable. Imaging at two time points and evaluating SUV change between early and delayed imaging can improve accuracy. The disadvantage is decreased patient throughput, although this can be minimized if a limited scan is performed after completion of the whole-body scan.
   - ***a.*** Accuracy improvements have been shown for thoracic and head and neck neoplasms.
     - The primary value of dual time-point imaging in the thorax is in central lesions.
   - ***b.*** Dual time-point imaging may be less valuable in the abdomen.
   - ***c.*** A change in lesion configuration between early and delayed images may indicate a benign etiology.
   - ***d.*** The delay between early and delayed images should be 30 minutes or more.

References

1. Thie JA. Understanding the standardized uptake value, its methods, and implications for usage. J Nucl Med 2004;45(9):1431–1434
2. Keyes JW Jr. SUV: standard uptake or silly useless value? J Nucl Med 1995;36(10):1836–1839
3. Hamberg LM, Hunter GJ, Alpert NM, et al. The dose uptake ratio as an index of glucose metabolism: useful parameter or oversimplification? J Nucl Med 1994;35(8):1308–1312
4. Soret M, Bacharach SL, Buvat I. Partial-volume effect in PET tumor imaging. J Nucl Med 2007;48(6):932–945
5. Schoder H, Erdi YE, Chao K, et al. Clinical implications of different image reconstruction parameters for interpretation of whole-body PET studies in cancer patients. J Nucl Med 2004;45(4):559–566
6. Jaskowiak CJ, Bianco JA, Perlman SB, Fine JP. Influence of reconstruction iterations on ^{18}F-FDG PET/CT standardized uptake values. J Nucl Med 2005;46(3):424–428
7. Nakamoto Y, Osman M, Cohade C, et al. PET/CT: comparison of quantitative tracer uptake between germanium and CT transmission attenuation-corrected images. J Nucl Med 2002;43(9):1137–1143
8. Souvatzoglou M, Ziegler SI, Martinez MJ, et al. Standardised uptake values from PET/CT images: comparison with conventional attenuation-corrected PET. Eur J Nucl Med Mol Imaging 2007;34(3):405–412
9. Erdi YE, Nehmeh SA, Pan T, et al. The CT motion quantitation of lung lesions and its impact on PET-measured SUVs. J Nucl Med 2004;45(8):1287–1292
10. Boellaard R, Krak NC, Hoekstra OS, Lammertsma AA. Effects of noise, image resolution, and ROI definition on the accuracy of standard uptake values: a simulation study. J Nucl Med 2004;45(9):1519–1527
11. Marom EM, Munden RF, Truong MT, et al. Interobserver and intraobserver variability of standardized uptake value measurements in non-small-cell lung cancer. J Thorac Imaging 2006;21(3):205–212
12. Dobert N, Hamscho N, Menzel C, et al. Limitations of dual time point FDG-PET imaging in the evaluation of focal abdominal lesions. Nuklearmedizin 2004;43(5):143–149
13. Conrad GR, Sinha P. Narrow time-window dual-point 18F-FDG PET for the diagnosis of thoracic malignancy. Nucl Med Commun 2003;24(11):1129–1137
14. Hustinx R, Smith RJ, Benard F, et al. Dual time point fluorine-18 fluorodeoxyglucose positron emission tomography: a potential method to differentiate malignancy from inflammation and normal tissue in the head and neck. Eur J Nucl Med 1999;26(10):1345–1348

6

Normal Variants and Benign Findings

Eugene C. Lin and Abass Alavi

◆ General Principles

As a rule, most inflammatory or infectious processes are visualized by positron emission tomography (PET) because activated white cells have increased glycolysis. Thus, it is not possible to exhaustively list all potential nonneoplastic causes of fluorodeoxyglucose (FDG) uptake. Correlation with clinical data and other imaging studies should alert the interpreter in many cases to potential false-positive findings in such settings. The discussion in this chapter will focus on the range of normal sites of FDG uptake and the common noninfectious/inflammatory causes of increased uptake. Artifacts specific to PET/computed tomography (CT) will be discussed in Chapter 8.

◆ Brain

It is important that physicians who interpret PET brain scans review a large number of normal images before interpreting studies in patients with neuropsychiatric disorders.[1]

1. ***Normal pattern of uptake***
   a. The normal brain has high FDG uptake in the gray matter, with a gray to white matter activity ratio from 2.5 to 4:1.
   b. The basal ganglia usually has slightly more uptake than the cortex.
   c. Mild focal areas of increased activity[2] can be seen normally in the
   - Frontal eye fields
   - Posterior cingulate cortex
   - Wernicke region (posterosuperior temporal lobe)
   - Visual cortex (see Chapter 29)
2. ***Age-related changes.*** Cortical metabolism decreases with age, particularly in the frontal lobes. In contrast, metabolic activity of the basal ganglia, visual cortices, and cerebellum remain unchanged.
3. ***Renal function.*** Patients with renal failure have decreased FDG uptake in the cortex and white matter compared with those with normal renal function.[3]
4. ***Symmetry of uptake.*** There are often minimal asymmetries in uptake between areas in the left and right hemispheres. Asymmetric uptake should be interpreted with caution unless
   a. There is a significant difference between the two sides that correlates with clinical findings. For example, any level of asymmetry in the temporal lobes in a patient with epilepsy should be considered a potential focus for seizure activity. Quantitatively, a difference of 10 to 15% is often considered significant, but clinical correlation is paramount.
   b. The asymmetry is fairly extensive and seen on multiple slices.

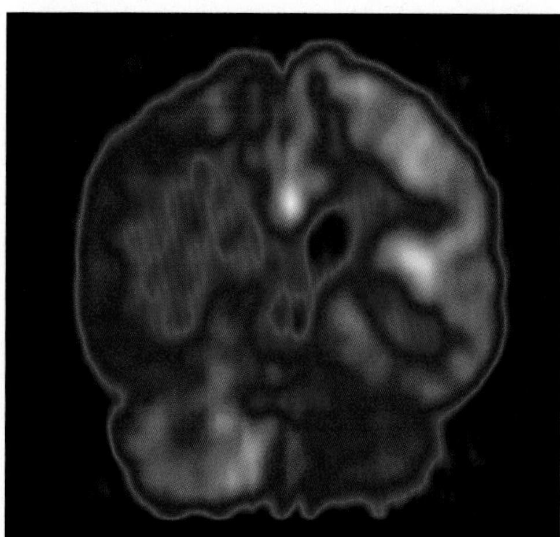

Fig. 6.1 Crossed cerebellar diaschisis. Coronal positron emission tomography scan demonstrates decreased activity in the right cerebral hemisphere secondary to infarct. There is decreased left cerebellar metabolism secondary to crossed cerebellar diaschisis.

5. ***Comparison with single-photon emission computed tomography (SPECT)***
   a. FDG uptake usually correlates with uptake of SPECT perfusion tracers, except in cases where metabolism and perfusion are uncoupled (e.g., luxury perfusion postinfarct).
   b. The magnitude of hypometabolism seen on PET is usually greater than that of hypoperfusion seen on SPECT.
   c. Cerebellar uptake of FDG is variable but in general is less than that seen on SPECT. This differs from brain SPECT images, where consistently the cerebellum appears more active than other brain structures.
6. ***Crossed cerebellar diaschisis.*** The glucose metabolism in the cerebellar hemisphere contralateral to a supratentorial abnormality (tumor, infarct, or trauma) is frequently decreased (**Fig. 6.1**) in the acute phase of the disease and may change over time. This does not indicate cerebellar pathology.
   a. Diaschisis is thought to be related to interruption of the corticopontocerebellar pathway.
   b. Ipsilateral pontine hypometabolism and preservation of metabolism in the contralateral dentate nucleus have been reported.[4]

◆ Spinal Cord

Spinal cord uptake is variable. Mild spinal cord uptake is normal.

◆ Heart

1. ***Ventricular uptake***
   a. Fasting state. For noncardiac PET studies done during fasting, myocardial metabolism shifts from utilizing glucose to utilizing fatty acids. Therefore, in theory myocardial uptake on fasting PET studies should be minimal. However, in many cases there will be substantial myocardial FDG uptake on fasting PET studies.
   - Outpatients, men, younger patients, patients with heart failure, and patients receiving benzodiazepines tend to have more myocardial uptake.[5,6] Diabetic patients and patients receiving bezafibrate or levothyroxine tend to have less myocardial uptake.[5,7]
   - An irregular pattern of ventricular uptake is not uncommon. Focal areas of increased and decreased uptake should not be considered sites of disease in the absence of a supporting cardiac history.
   - The myocardial uptake pattern demonstrates a large spatial and temporal variability, and a patient without cardiac disease can demonstrate substantially different patterns of myocardial FDG uptake on serial studies (**Fig. 6.2**).[8]
   - Decreased septal activity has been noted as a common normal variant in fasting patients (**Fig. 6.3**). However, left bundle branch block can also cause decreased septal uptake.[9]

   b. Insulin effect. Increased myocardial activity is seen after insulin administration or insulin release secondary to a recent meal (myocardial glucose receptors are insulin sensitive). This is seen in conjunction with intense skeletal muscle uptake (as seen in **Fig. 4.1**, p. 34).

c. *Right ventricular uptake.* There is greater uptake in the left ventricle than the right ventricle. Typically, right ventricular uptake is minimal unless there is hypertrophy.

d. *Papillary muscle uptake.* Papillary muscle uptake is often seen in conjunction with uptake in the left ventricular wall. Occasionally, papillary muscle uptake can be seen in isolation (**Fig. 6.4**).[10] In these cases, the uptake could mimic an intraventricular neoplasm or thrombus. Note that there are no septal left ventricular papillary muscles, and left ventricular uptake arising from the septum cannot represent papillary muscle (**Fig. 6.4**).

2. ***Atrial uptake***
   a. Atrial uptake can be irregular and focal. Focal atrial FDG uptake can mimic a mediastinal node (**Fig. 6.5**). This is particularly true on axial images in the subcarinal region. Therefore, correlation with sagittal and coronal PET images and CT is necessary before diagnosing subcarinal nodal uptake on axial images.
   b. Ringlike atrial uptake can mimic a large necrotic subcarinal node (**Fig. 6.6**). This is easily differentiated by correlation with all imaging planes and CT.
   c. Increased right and left atrial uptake is associated with atrial fibrillation.[11–13] Right atrial uptake (**Fig. 6.7**) is usually more prominent.[12]
3. ***Perfusion imaging.*** If perfusion imaging is performed with nitrogen 13 ammonia, lateral wall activity is normally decreased compared with the septum.[14] This is of unknown etiology.

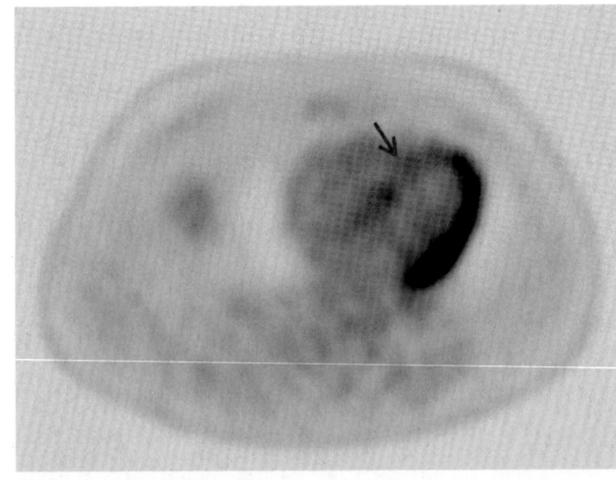

Fig. 6.3 Normal variant decreased septal uptake. Axial positron emission tomography scan demonstrates decreased septal uptake (*arrow*), which is a normal variant in this patient. In the majority of cases, this finding is a normal variant, but an infarct or left bundle branch block could also cause this appearance and cannot be differentiated from normal variant decreased uptake without clinical history.

◆ Head and Neck

1. ***Normal uptake (sagittal).*** On sagittal images, there is normally an inverted C shape composed of the mylohyoid muscles and sublingual glands, soft palate, and tonsils (**Fig. 6.8**). These are the most common areas of normal uptake.

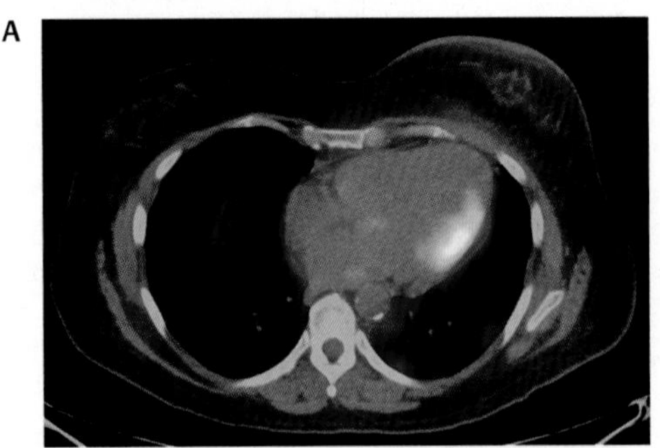

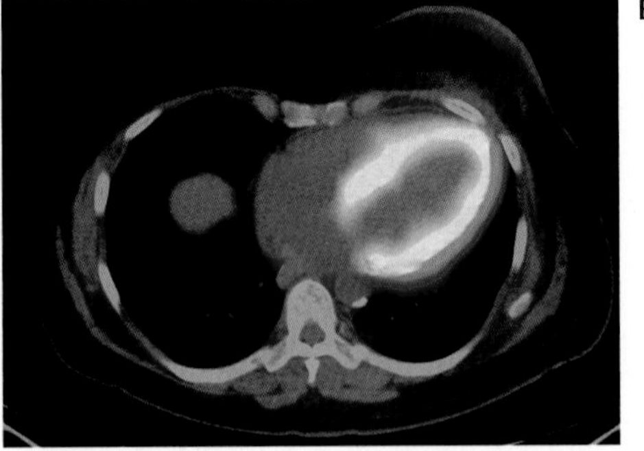

Fig. 6.2 Changing pattern of cardiac uptake. **(A)** Axial positron emission tomography/computed tomography (PET/CT) scan demonstrates absent fluorodeoxyglucose (FDG) uptake in the septum, anterior wall, and apex. This should not be interpreted as an infarct in the absence of a supporting clinical history, and this patient did not have a history of cardiac disease. **(B)** Axial PET/CT scan in the same patient done at a later date demonstrates homogeneous myocardial uptake.

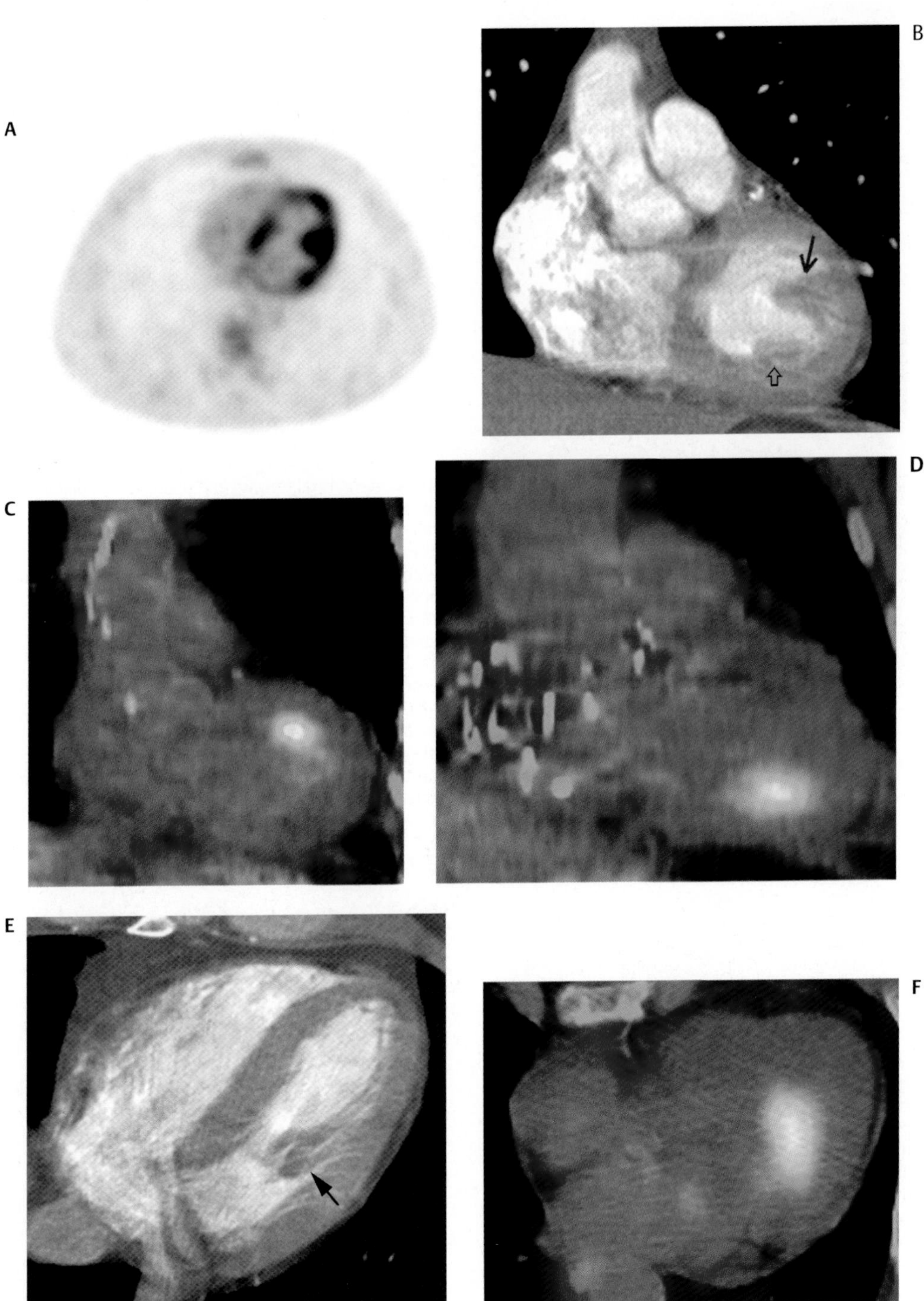

Fig. 6.4

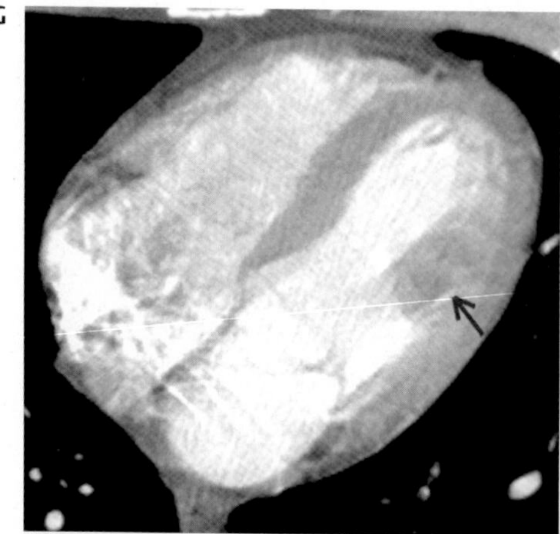

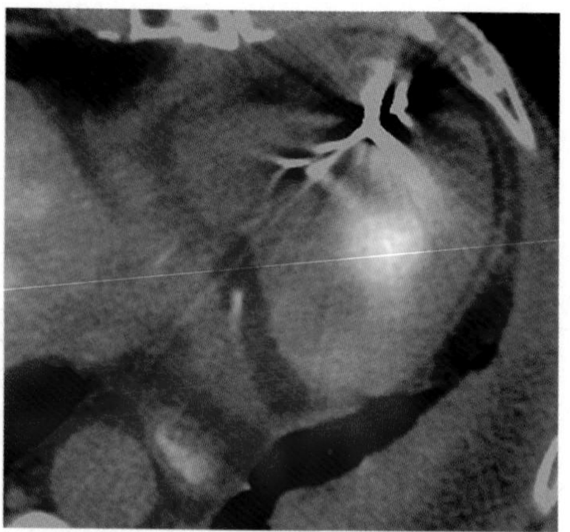

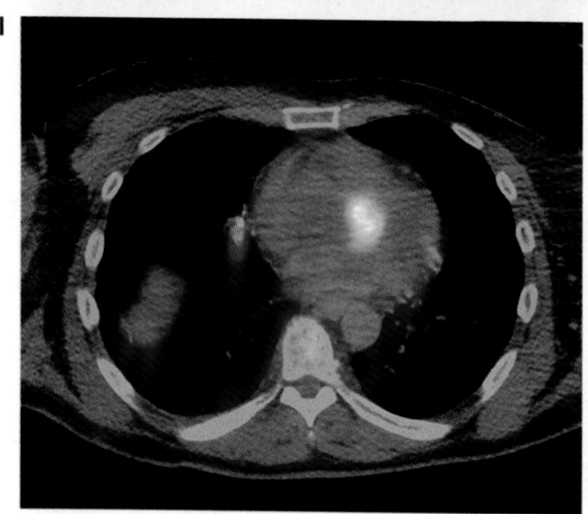

Fig. 6.4 (*Continued*) Isolated papillary muscle uptake versus cardiac metastasis. **(A)** Axial positron emission tomography (PET) scan demonstrates uptake in the left ventricular myocardium and a papillary muscle. However, papillary muscle uptake is sometimes seen without myocardial uptake. **(B)** Coronal computed tomography (CT) scan demonstrates the anterior lateral (*arrow*) and posterior medial (*open arrow*) papillary muscles. **(C)** Coronal PET/CT scan demonstrates isolated uptake in the anterior lateral papillary muscle. **(D)** Coronal PET/CT scan demonstrates isolated uptake in the posterior medial papillary muscle. **(E)** Axial CT scan demonstrates the anterior lateral papillary muscle (*arrow*). **(F)** Axial PET/CT scan demonstrates isolated anterior lateral papillary muscle uptake. **(G)** Axial CT scan demonstrates the posterior medial papillary muscle (*arrow*). **(H)** Axial PET/CT scan demonstrates isolated posterior medial papillary muscle uptake. **(I)** Focal uptake is noted in a left ventricular metastasis. Note that this cannot represent papillary muscle, as it arises from the septum, and there are no left ventricular septal papillary muscles. (From Lin EC. Isolated papillary muscle uptake on FDG PET/CT. Clin Nucl Med 2007;32(1):76–78. Reprinted with permission.)

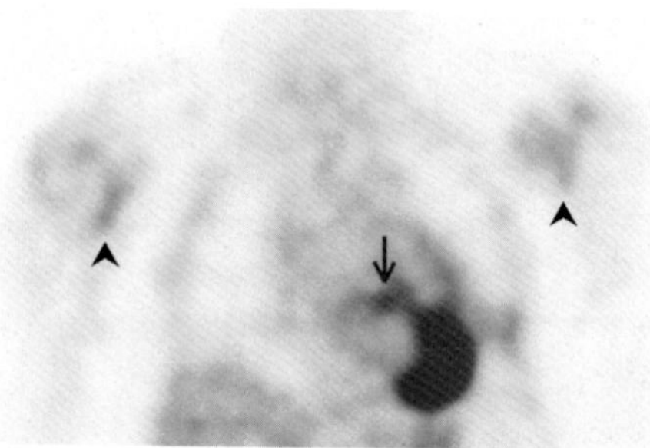

Fig. 6.5 Focal left atrial uptake mimicking nodal uptake and glenohumeral joint uptake. Coronal positron emission tomography scan demonstrates focal increased uptake in the left atrium (*arrow*). This could mimic abnormal subcarinal node uptake on an axial slice through this focus. On the coronal image, the uptake can be seen to be contiguous with the left atrium. Increased glenohumeral joint uptake (*arrowheads*) is noted. Although this can mimic adenopathy, it can be distinguished by its linear appearance and location immediately medial to the humeral heads.

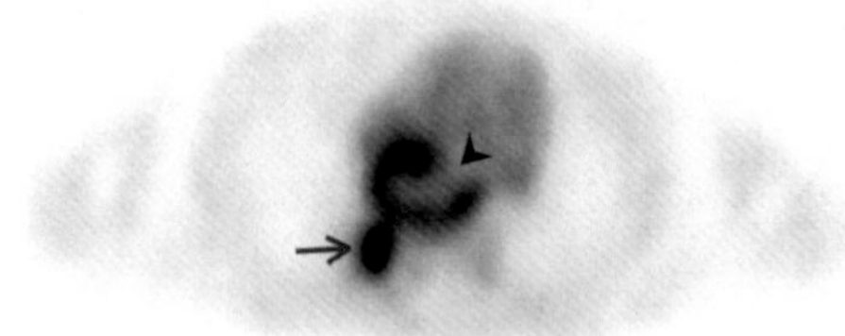

Fig. 6.6 Diffuse left atrial uptake mimicking a necrotic node. Axial positron emission tomography scan in a patient with lung cancer (*arrow*) demonstrates a circular area of uptake medially suggestive of a necrotic mediastinal node. This is uptake in the left atrium, which can be suspected, given the lack of uptake in the region of the valve plane (*arrowhead*).

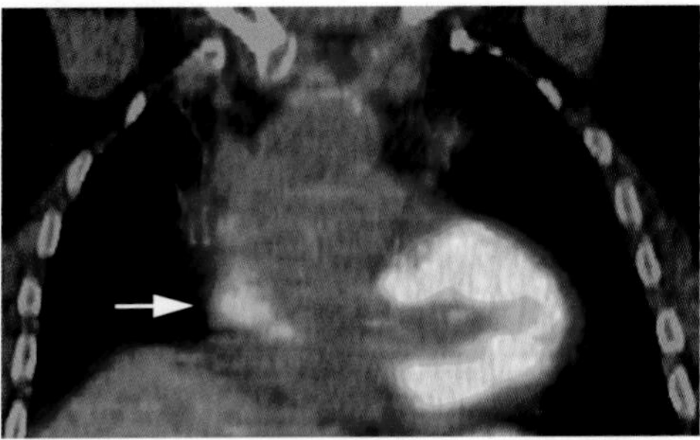
Fig. 6.7 Right atrial uptake. Coronal positron emission tomography/computed tomography scan demonstrates uptake in the right atrium (*arrow*).

2. ***Mylohyoid muscles and sublingual glands (axial).*** On axial images, uptake in the mylohyoid muscles and/or sublingual glands can form an inverted V medial to the mandible. Due to their proximity, it is difficult to distinguish whether uptake is in the sublingual glands, mylohyoid muscles, or both. Sublingual uptake is more superior and focal (**Fig. 6.9**), whereas mylohyoid uptake is more inferior and linear (see **Fig. 8.6**, p. 92).
3. ***Soft palate (axial).*** The soft palate can appear as a prominent focus of activity on axial images (**Fig. 6.10**).
   - Soft palate uptake is more prominent in males.[15]
4. ***Tonsils (coronal).*** Normal uptake in the palatine and lingual tonsils (**Figs. 6.8** and **6.11**) forms two vertical linear bands of uptake on coronal images. This may be prominent in

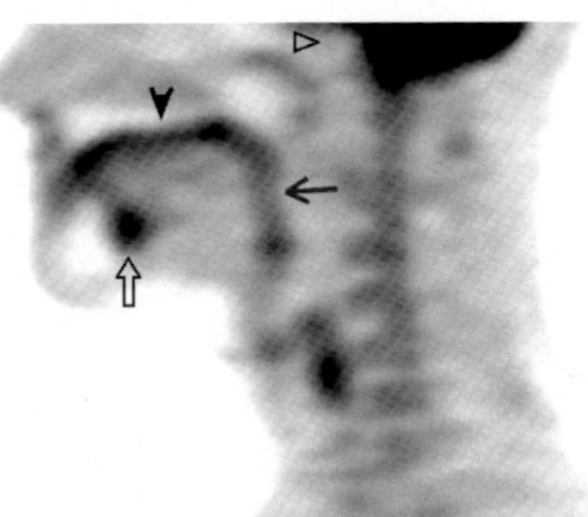
Fig. 6.8 Normal sagittal head and neck. Sagittal positron emission tomography scan demonstrates a typical inverted U-shaped pattern of uptake in the tonsils (*solid arrow*), soft palate (*arrowhead*), mylohyoid muscle, and sublingual glands (*open arrow*). Nasopharyngeal uptake (*open arrowhead*) is also seen.

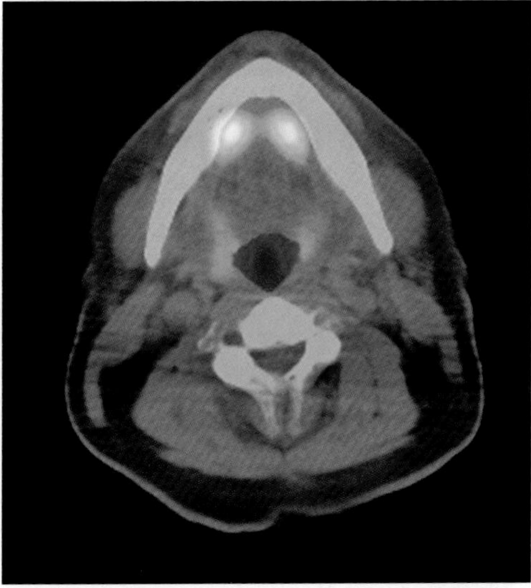
Fig. 6.9 Sublingual gland uptake. Axial positron emission tomography/computed tomography scan demonstrates normal inverted V-shaped uptake in the sublingual glands. Mylohyoid muscle uptake can have a similar appearance, but it is slightly inferior and more linear.

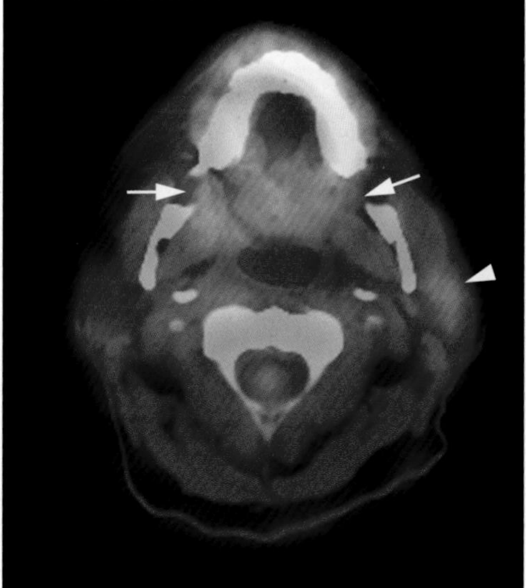
Fig. 6.10 Soft palate, parotid gland, and spinal cord uptake. Axial positron emission tomography/computed tomography scan demonstrates normal soft palate uptake (*arrows*), which can appear very prominent on axial images. There is normal uptake in the left parotid gland (*arrowhead*). This is more prominent than right parotid uptake, as this patient has more left parotid tissue at this level. Normal spinal cord uptake is also seen.

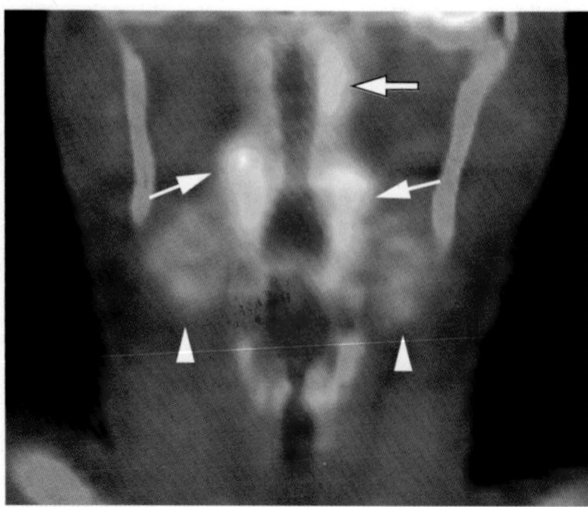

Fig. 6.11 Tonsil and submandibular gland uptake and nasopharyngeal carcinoma. Coronal positron emission tomography scan demonstrates typical vertical bands of tonsillar uptake (*arrows*). Mild submandibular gland uptake is seen (*arrowheads*). Tonsil uptake is usually greater than salivary gland uptake. There is asymmetric uptake in the left nasopharynx (*open arrow*) secondary to nasopharyngeal carcinoma. However, in populations where nasopharyngeal carcinoma is not endemic, asymmetric uptake is often inflammatory. If this uptake were symmetric, it could be a normal variant or secondary to inflammation.

cold/temperate climates and is also prominent in children.

- There is less uptake with increasing age in the palatine tonsils.[15]

5. ***Salivary glands.*** Salivary gland uptake is more variable than tonsillar uptake.[15] Salivary gland uptake if seen is usually less than tonsillar uptake (**Fig. 6.11**).
   a. There is less uptake with increasing age in the sublingual glands.[15]
   b. The submandibular glands are in close proximity to submandibular nodes, and submandibular nodal uptake can be difficult to distinguish from normal glandular uptake even with PET/CT (**Fig. 6.12**).
6. ***Nasopharyngeal uptake.*** Nasopharyngeal uptake is sometimes seen as a normal variant (**Fig. 6.8**), although larger degrees of uptake could be secondary to inflammation or tumor. Uptake in the lateral pharyngeal recess can be symmetric or asymmetric.
   a. Asymmetric uptake. Asymmetric uptake in the lateral pharyngeal recess (**Fig. 6.11**), cervical nodal uptake, and asymmetric wall thickening in the lateral

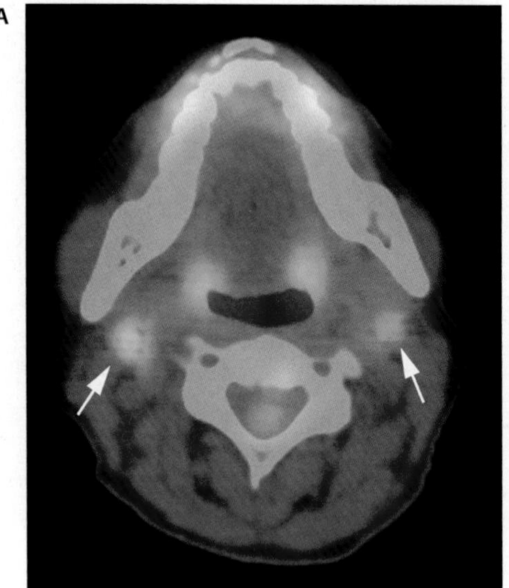

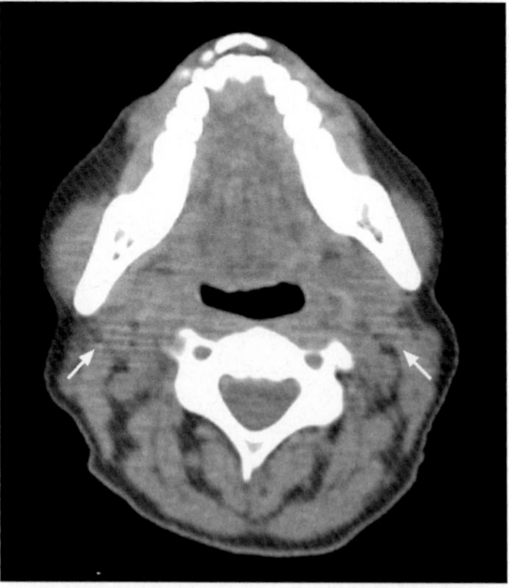

Fig. 6.12 Node or submandibular gland? **(A)** Axial positron emission tomography/computed tomography (PET/CT) scan demonstrates bilateral uptake near the submandibular glands (*arrows*). It is difficult to determine whether this uptake is in nodes or the submandibular glands, particularly as the uptake is bilateral. However, the uptake is relatively posterior, suggesting that it is not in the submandibular glands. **(B)** Axial CT scan demonstrates bilateral nodes (*arrows*) corresponding to the fluorodeoxyglucose (FDG) uptake. Lower density submandibular glands are noted anterior to the nodes.

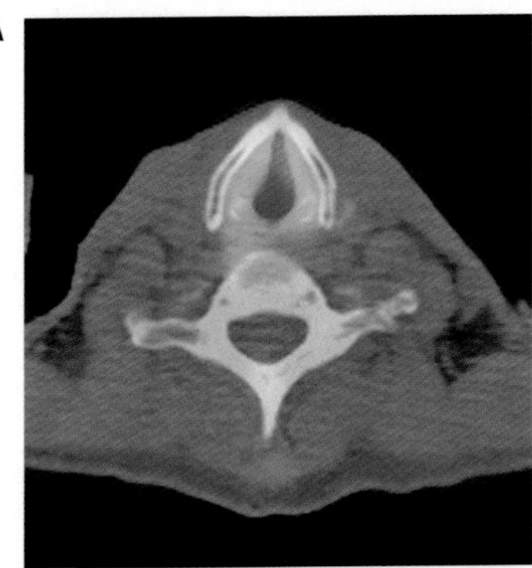

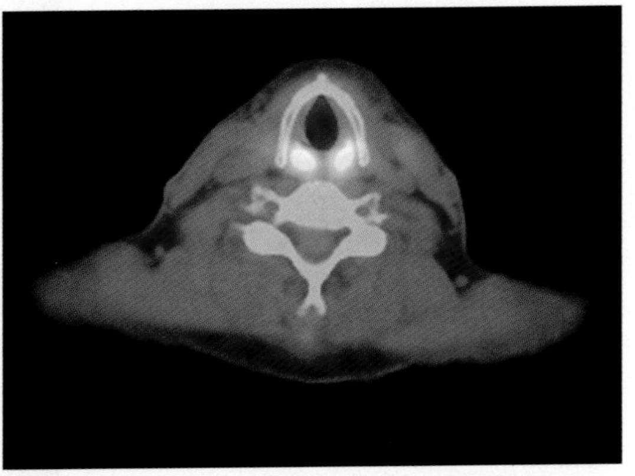

Fig. 6.13 Patterns of laryngeal uptake. **(A)** Axial positron emission tomography/computed tomography (PET/CT) scan demonstrates an inverted V-shaped appearance of the laryngeal uptake secondary to uptake in both the vocal cords and cricoarytenoid muscles. **(B)** Axial PET/CT scan demonstrates two foci of posterior cricoarytenoid uptake. Note the absence of anterior cord uptake in this patient, which is a normal variant. If anterior cord uptake was greater than posterior uptake, this would be more worrisome for pathology.

pharyngeal recess on CT are associated with nasopharyngeal carcinoma.[16]

- However, in patient populations where nasopharyngeal carcinoma is less frequent, asymmetric uptake in the lateral pharyngeal recesses is often inflammatory.

b. An SUV cutoff of < 3.9 and a lateral pharyngeal recess to palatine tonsil uptake ratio of < 1.5 are helpful in differentiating benign from malignant lateral pharyngeal recess uptake.[16]

7. ***Tongue.*** Tongue uptake can occasionally be seen, particularly if the patient speaks after FDG injection. In children, adenoid tissues are commonly visualized at the base of the tongue.
8. ***Laryngeal uptake.*** Laryngeal muscle uptake is a normal variant and is pronounced if the patient speaks soon after FDG administration. It can have a horseshoe-like appearance with uptake in both the vocal cords and cricoarytenoid muscles or appear as two foci of posterior uptake in the cricoarytenoid muscles (**Fig. 6.13**). Normal activity is most pronounced posteriorly.
   a. It is better to use asymmetry of uptake rather than absolute uptake in the larynx as a criterion of abnormality.
   b. However, laryngeal uptake may be asymmetric secondary to postoperative changes or vocal cord paralysis (**Fig. 6.14**).
   c. Anterior uptake is more concerning than posterior uptake.
9. ***Muscle uptake.*** Muscular uptake is common, particularly in the sternocleidomastoids. Less commonly, uptake is seen in the longus colli muscles. This can be asymmetric and potentially mimic neoplasm (**Fig. 6.15**).[17] However, before attributing uptake to asymmetric longus colli activity, retropharyngeal adenopathy (**Fig. 6.16**) should

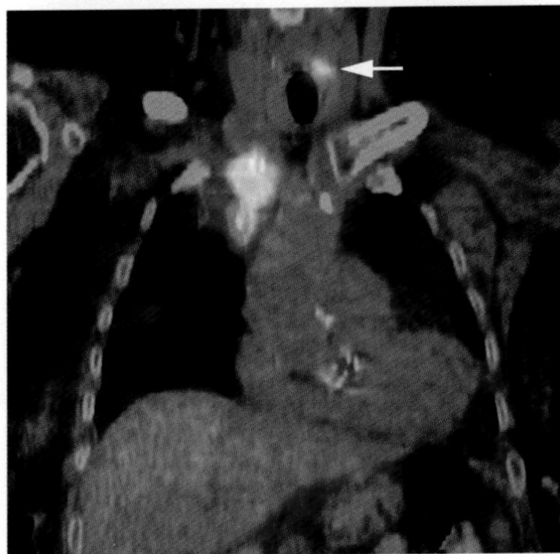

Fig. 6.14 Coronal positron emission tomography/computed tomography scan demonstrates unilateral uptake in the left vocal cord (*arrow*) secondary to right vocal cord paralysis caused by a right apical lung cancer.

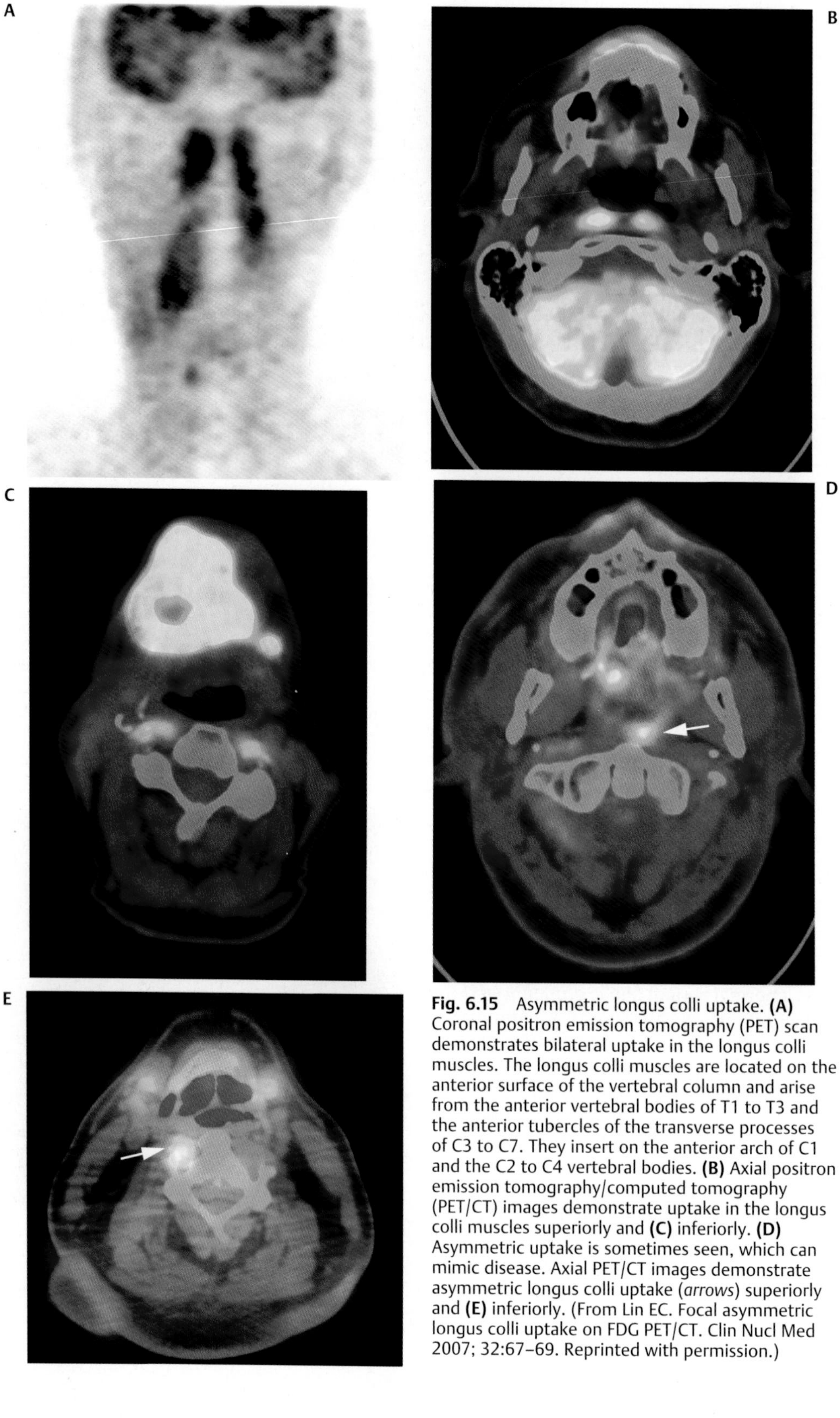

A

B

C

D

E

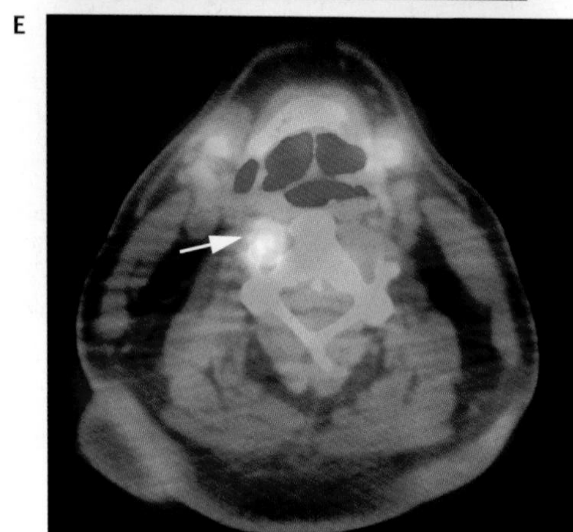

Fig. 6.15 Asymmetric longus colli uptake. **(A)** Coronal positron emission tomography (PET) scan demonstrates bilateral uptake in the longus colli muscles. The longus colli muscles are located on the anterior surface of the vertebral column and arise from the anterior vertebral bodies of T1 to T3 and the anterior tubercles of the transverse processes of C3 to C7. They insert on the anterior arch of C1 and the C2 to C4 vertebral bodies. **(B)** Axial positron emission tomography/computed tomography (PET/CT) images demonstrate uptake in the longus colli muscles superiorly and **(C)** inferiorly. **(D)** Asymmetric uptake is sometimes seen, which can mimic disease. Axial PET/CT images demonstrate asymmetric longus colli uptake (*arrows*) superiorly and **(E)** inferiorly. (From Lin EC. Focal asymmetric longus colli uptake on FDG PET/CT. Clin Nucl Med 2007; 32:67–69. Reprinted with permission.)

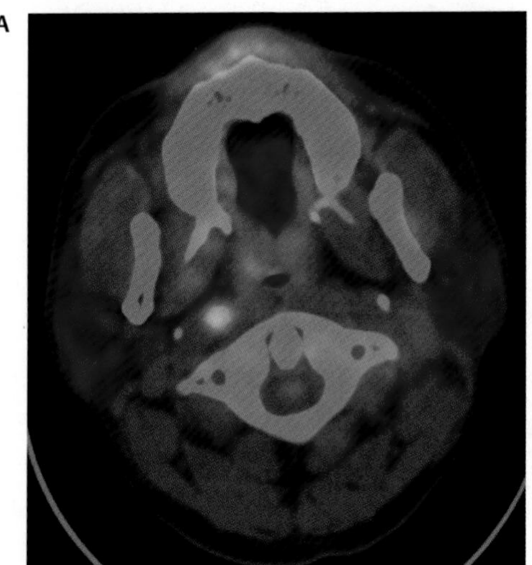

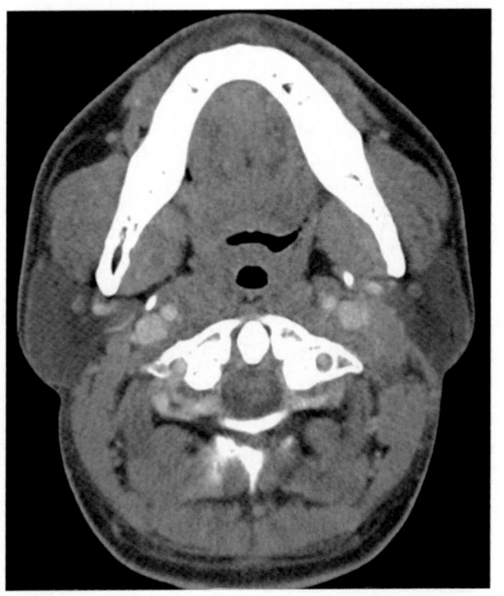

Fig. 6.16 Retropharyngeal node versus longus colli uptake. **(A)** Axial positron emission tomography/computed tomography (PET/CT) scan demonstrates focal uptake in the region of the right longus colli. This could mimic normal variant asymmetric longus colli uptake, but correlation with a **(B)** contrast-enhanced CT scan demonstrates asymmetric soft tissue in this region. The uptake was in a retropharyngeal node.

be excluded, as it can have a similar appearance on axial images.

◆ Thyroid

1. ***Diffuse uptake.*** Mild diffuse thyroid uptake can be a normal variant. Greater degrees of diffuse uptake are seen in Graves disease and chronic thyroiditis (**Fig. 6.17**).[18,19] In particular, diffuse thyroid uptake is often associated with chronic lymphocytic (Hashimoto) thyroiditis. This is not affected by thyroid hormone therapy. The SUV does not correlate with the degree of hypothyroidism.[20]
   a. *SUV.* The normal thyroid has a mean SUV of 1.5 ± 0.2.[21]
   b. *Graves disease.* Increased thyroid uptake in Graves disease is relatively uncommon; increased skeletal muscle and thymus activity is actually more commonly seen in this disorder.[22]
2. ***Focal uptake.*** Focal uptake is nonspecific and can be seen in both benign and malignant nodules (see Chapter 14).
3. ***Thyroid nodule mimics.*** Correlation with anatomic imaging is necessary before diagnosing peripheral thyroid nodules on PET.
   a. *Lymph node.* A medial lymph node adjacent to the thyroid can mimic a thyroid nodule (see Chapter 14).
   b. *Parathyroid abnormality.* Both parathyroid adenomas and hyperplasia can cause focal increased uptake mimicking a thyroid nodule. The normal parathyroids are not visualized on FDG PET.

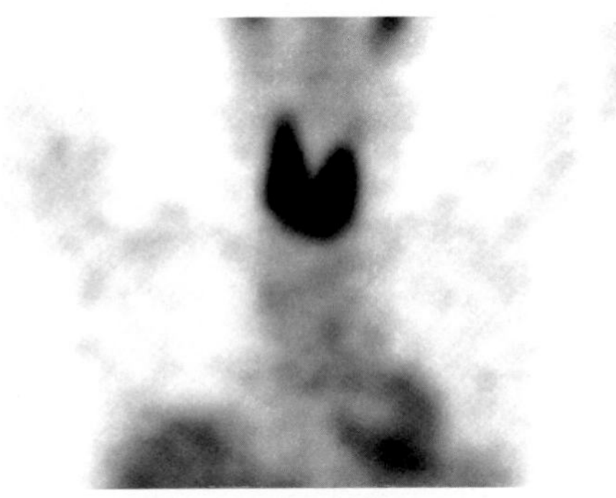

Fig. 6.17 Thyroiditis. Diffuse increased thyroid uptake is secondary to thyroiditis. Lesser degrees of diffuse uptake could be a normal variant.

◆ Axilla

1. ***Glenohumeral joint.*** Glenohumeral joint activity can mimic axillary adenopathy on axial and coronal images (**Fig. 6.18**). It can be distinguished by its linear appearance and location immediately medial to the humeral head. This finding may not always be a normal variant, as it is often associated with joint pain.
2. ***Dose extravasation.*** Extravasation at the injection site can cause ipsilateral axillary node uptake due to particle formation and phagocytosis at the draining lymph nodes.

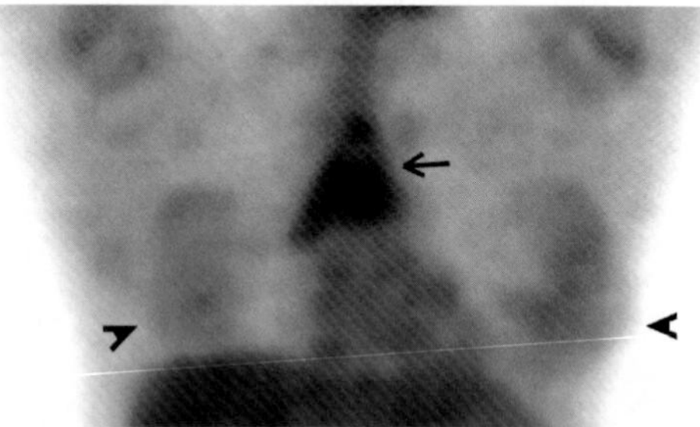

Fig. 6.19 Thymic hyperplasia and normal breast uptake. Coronal fluorodeoxyglucose (FDG) scan demonstrates uptake in a hyperplastic thymus in a 35-year-old woman. This should not be confused with mediastinal adenopathy, as it has an inverted V shape and a horizontal photopenic cleft (*arrow*) characteristic of thymus. A photopenic cleft can sometimes be seen in the vertical direction. Normal uptake in premenopausal glandular breast tissue is seen (*arrowheads*).

◆ Breast

1. ***Premenopausal.*** Diffuse low-grade uptake is seen in glandular breast tissue in premenopausal women (**Fig. 6.19**). The SUV in dense breasts is higher than in nondense breasts; however, the uptake in dense breasts is still very low (SUV around 1).[23]
2. ***Postmenopausal.*** Postmenopausal women on hormone replacement therapy may also have glandular uptake. The breast uptake should be less than the liver in postmenopausal women who are not on hormonal therapy.[24]
3. ***Lactation.*** Prominent diffuse uptake is seen during lactation.
4. ***Nipple.*** Nipple uptake is commonly seen.
5. ***Breast implants.*** Mildly increased uptake can be seen around breast implants, which appear as negative defects.
6. ***Focal uptake.*** Focal uptake is seen due to a wide range of benign conditions but commonly represents malignancy (see Chapter 16).

◆ Thymus

1. ***Children.*** Thymus uptake is a normal variant in children.

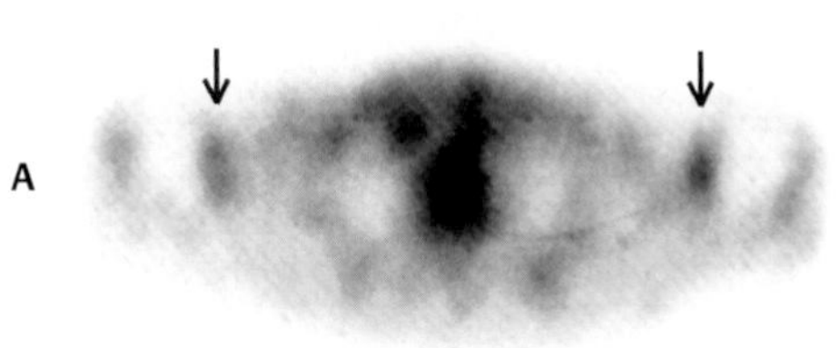

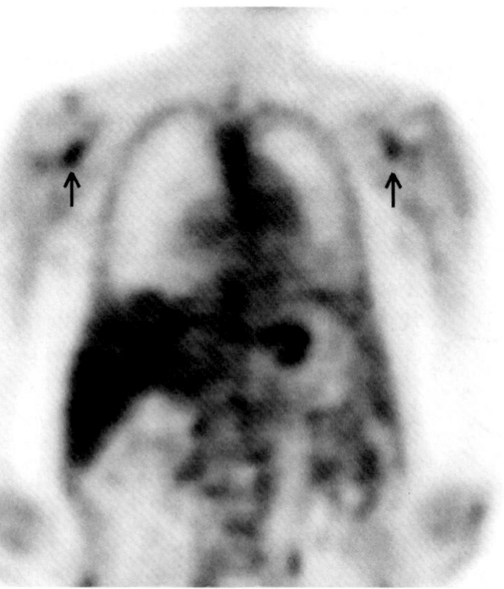

Fig. 6.18 Glenohumeral joint activity mimicking axillary nodal uptake. **(A)** Axial positron emission tomography (PET) scan through the upper thorax demonstrates bilateral glenohumeral joint uptake (*arrows*). **(B)** Coronal PET scan in the same patient demonstrates bilateral glenohumeral joint uptake (*arrows*). Although this uptake could be confused with axillary nodal uptake, it can be distinguished by its linear appearance and location immediately medial to the humeral head.

2. ***Adults.*** In adults, thymic uptake (**Figs. 6.19** and **6.20**) can be seen with thymic hyperplasia or if a substantial amount of normal thymic tissue remains after adolescence. The thymus can be distinguished from anterior mediastinal adenopathy by its characteristic inverted V shape. In addition, photopenic clefts are often seen extending through the thymic tissue.
   a. *Age.* Although thymic uptake is usually seen in young adults, it has been reported in patients up to 54 years old.[25]
   b. *Clinical scenarios.* Thymic uptake is occasionally seen soon after chemotherapy and is common following radioiodine treatment for thyroid cancer.
   c. *Malignancy.* If the uptake is focal, intense (greater than cerebellum or bladder or high SUV), or if the thymic shape is distorted, the possibility of malignancy should be considered.
   d. *SUV*[26]
      - The average SUV in thymic hyperplasia is 1.9.[27] However, SUV measurements as high as 3.8 have been reported in thymic hyperplasia.
      - Thymomas typically have higher SUVs than thymic hyperplasia.[27] However, the SUVs seen in thymic hyperplasia may overlap with those in thymoma.
      - Invasive thymomas do not have higher SUVs than noninvasive thymomas.
      - Thymic carcinoma usually has higher SUVs than thymoma.
      - SUV cutoffs to differentiate thymic carcinoma from thymoma are variable ranging from 5 to 10.[28]
      - Uptake in thymic carcinomas tends to be homogeneous, whereas uptake in thymomas is often heterogeneous.[28]
   e. *Graves disease.* Increased thymus uptake is common in Graves disease. A clue to the diagnosis is seeing increased skeletal muscle uptake and thyroid uptake (less likely) in conjunction with the thymic uptake.[22]
3. ***Superior mediastinal activity.*** A normal variant can be seen secondary to superior extension of the thymus.[29] In these cases there is a soft tissue nodule anteromedial to the left brachiocephalic vein, which can have increased FDG uptake, particularly in children and young adults who have thymic hyperplasia after chemotherapy. Although this nodule may not be connected to the thymus, it should have a similar SUV.

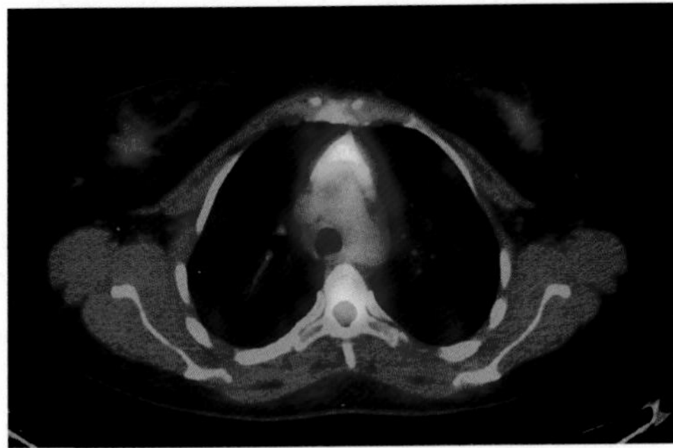

Fig. 6.20 Thymus uptake. Axial positron emission tomography/computed tomography scan demonstrates intense thymic uptake.

Lung

1. ***Normal gradient of uptake.*** The lungs typically have minimal or no activity on attenuation-corrected images. Lung activity increases from the anterior to the posterior and from the superior to the inferior segments, particularly if the lungs are not fully inflated. This is more prominently seen on nonattenuation-corrected images.
2. ***Increased uptake.*** A wide range of infectious/inflammatory processes can cause diffuse or focal increased uptake. Some rare causes of uptake are
   a. *Diffuse uptake.* Drug toxicity in cancer patients, radiation pneumonitis, acute respiratory distress syndrome[30]
      - A neoplastic etiology of diffuse uptake is lymphangitic carcinomatosis (**Fig. 6.21**).[31]
   b. *Nodular uptake.*[32–34] Bronchiolitis obliterans organizing pneumonia, lung infarction, amyloidosis
3. ***Focal uptake without a CT correlate.*** There should almost always be a correlative finding on CT for focal FDG uptake in the lung. If substantial motion artifact is present, small lung nodules may not be identified. If no correlative finding is identified on a CT without motion, a small focus of focal FDG uptake could represent a clot injected during FDG administration (**Fig. 6.22**).

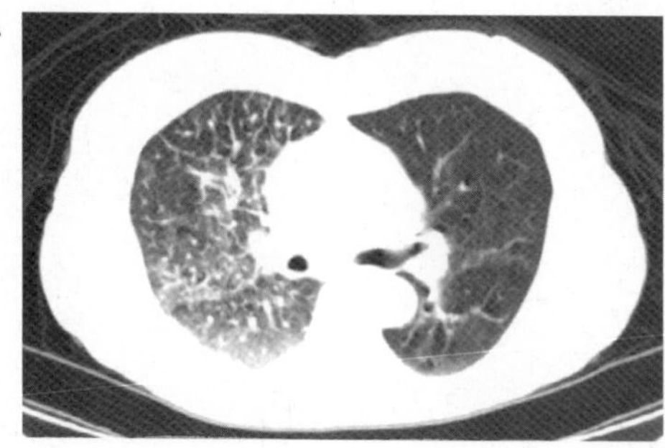

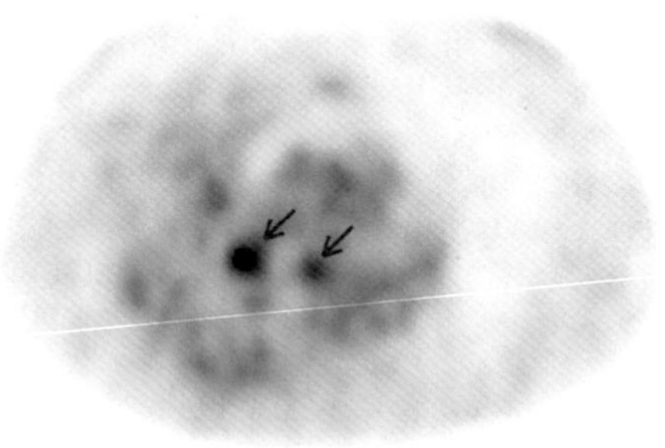

Fig. 6.21 Lymphangitic spread. **(A)** Axial computed tomography scan demonstrates interstitial thickening in the right lung suspicious for lymphangitic spread. **(B)** Corresponding axial positron emission tomography scan demonstrates diffuse right lung uptake secondary to lymphangitic spread. In addition, focal uptake (*arrows*) is present in right hilar and subcarinal nodal metastases.

4. ***Radiation pneumonitis.*** Radiation pneumonitis can cause very intense uptake before radiographic changes are seen. This should be suspected in the proper clinical setting if the uptake has a linear margin (**Fig. 6.23**). However, the lung is a relatively slow-reacting tissue to radiation, and radiation-induced elevation in FDG uptake typically does not occur until months after completion of radiotherapy.[35] Uptake (usually pleural) in the contralateral shielded nonirradiated lung is common after radiation.[36]
5. ***Atelectasis.*** Severely atelectatic lung can have increased activity (**Fig. 6.24**). However, PET is helpful in cases of postobstructive atelectasis, as the central obstructing tumor will have more uptake than the distal atelectasis (**Fig. 6.25**).
6. ***False-positive results.*** Very rare causes of false-positive results are hamartoma, round atelectasis, and pleural fibrosis. In the majority of cases, these entities do not have significant uptake.[37]

◆ Hila

1. Mild bilateral hilar nodal uptake is very common (**Fig. 6.26**). This appearance is almost never associated with malignancy.
2. Uptake in a central pulmonary embolus could mimic hilar adenopathy.

◆ Esophagus

1. ***Patterns of esophageal uptake*** (**Fig. 6.27**)
   a. Mild diffuse esophageal uptake is often a normal variant.

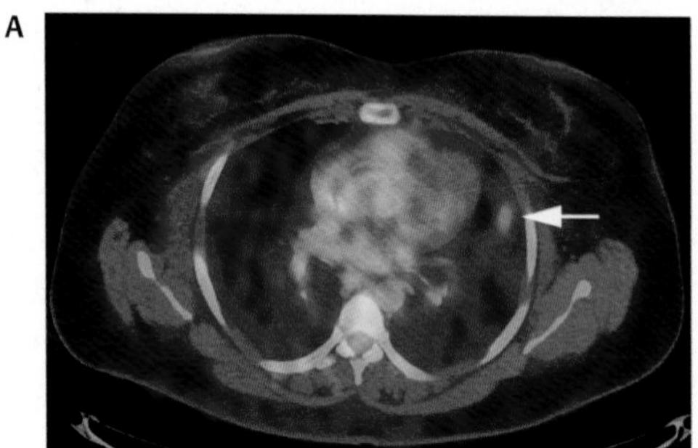

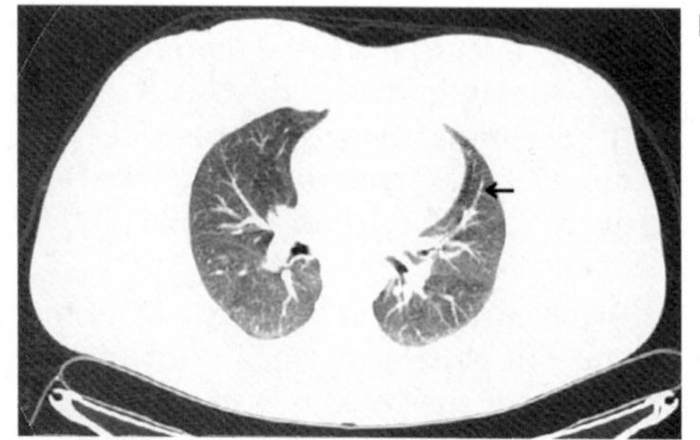

Fig. 6.22 Injected clot. **(A)** Axial positron emission tomography/computed tomography scan demonstrates focal uptake in the lingula (*arrow*). **(B)** Corresponding axial computed tomography scan does not demonstrate a nodule in this region; however, this uptake appears to lie in a vessel (*arrow*). This uptake is likely secondary to injected clumped FDG.

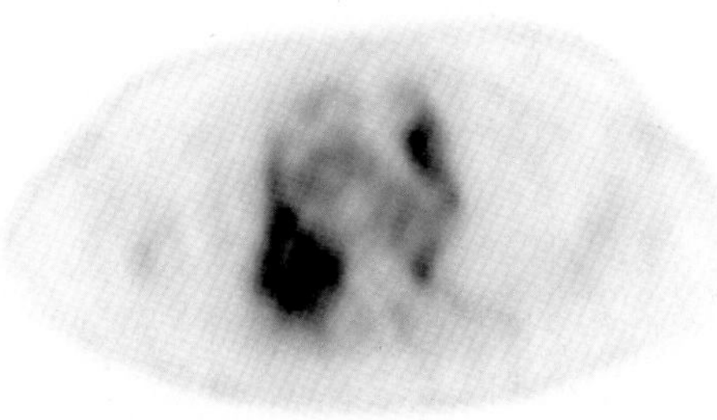

Fig. 6.23 Radiation pneumonitis. Axial positron emission tomography scan demonstrates intense increased uptake around the mediastinum with linear margins corresponding to a radiation field. The appearance is typical for radiation pneumonitis.

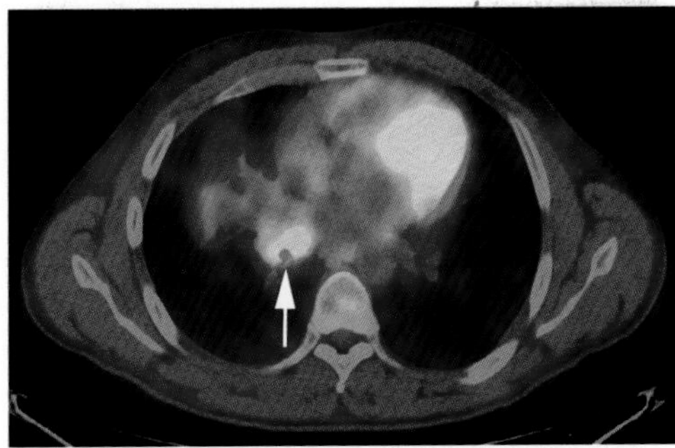

Fig. 6.25 Atelectasis secondary to obstructing tumor. Axial positron emission tomography/computed tomography (PET/CT) scan demonstrates atelectasis secondary to a right hilar mass (*arrow*). The identification of an obstructing mass within an area of atelectasis is a particular strength of PET/CT, as the mass often cannot be separated from the atelectasis by CT.

b. Intense diffuse uptake is usually secondary to esophagitis. Radiation therapy to the thorax can cause a limited area of diffuse intense esophageal uptake in the radiation port.

c. Minimal focal uptake is often seen at the gastroesophageal junction as a normal variant. However, greater degrees of activity at the gastroesophageal junction are worrisome for neoplasm. SUVs greater than 4 at the gastroesophageal junction are worrisome for pathology (see Stomach section).

d. Focal esophageal activity not at the gastroesophageal junction is worrisome for neoplasm.

2. ***Other causes of esophageal uptake.*** Esophageal uptake can be seen with esophageal spasm, reflux, and Barrett esophagus.

3. ***Brown fat mimic.*** Brown fat uptake in the azygoesophageal recess can mimic focal esophageal uptake.[38]

◆ Stomach

1. ***Normal pattern of uptake***
   a. Moderate diffuse stomach uptake is a normal variant.
   b. Physiological gastric uptake is higher proximally (**Fig. 6.28**).
2. ***Abnormal uptake.*** These patterns of uptake are abnormal and should raise suspicion for

A

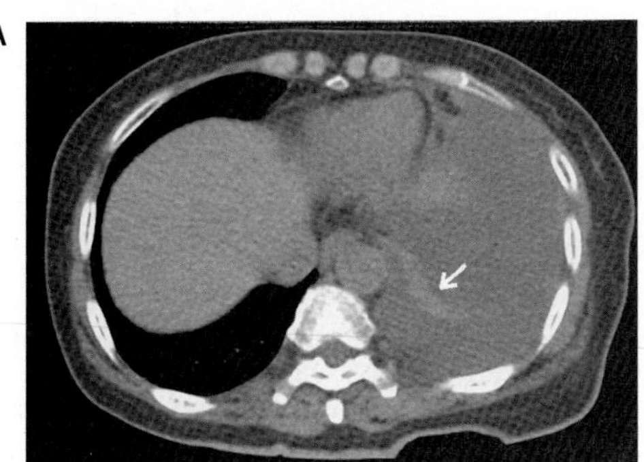

B

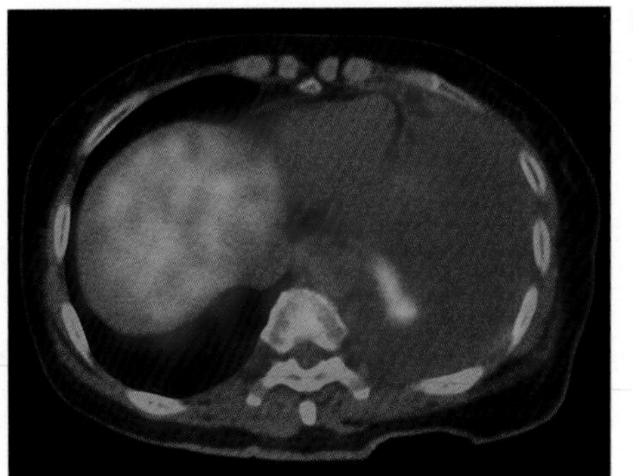

Fig. 6.24 Atelectasis. **(A)** Axial computed tomography (CT) scan demonstrates a sliver of atelectatic lung (*arrow*) in a large left effusion. **(B)** Corresponding positron emission tomography/computed tomography (PET/CT) scan demonstrates focal uptake in the atelectatic lung. This is commonly seen when the atelectasis is severe.

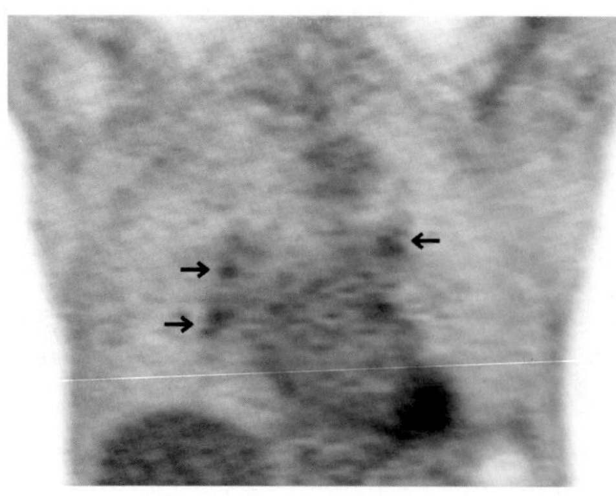

Fig. 6.26 Bilateral hilar uptake. Coronal positron emission tomography (PET) scan demonstrates mild bilateral hilar uptake (*arrows*). This is a common finding on PET and may be related to granulomatous disease or smoking. This degree and pattern of uptake are almost never secondary to malignancy.

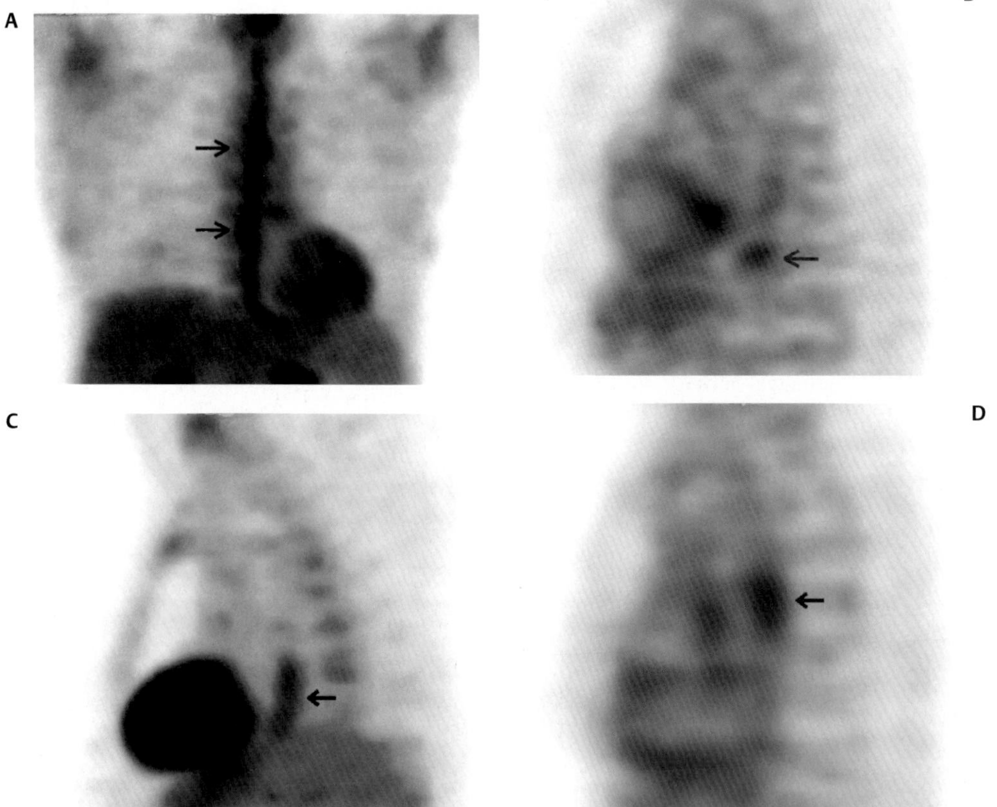

Fig. 6.27 Patterns of normal and abnormal esophageal uptake. **(A)** Normal esophagus. Uptake throughout the esophagus (*arrows*) on coronal positron emission tomography (PET) scan is a normal variant in this patient, although esophagitis could also cause this appearance. **(B)** Normal gastroesophageal junction uptake. Sagittal PET scan demonstrates a small focus of normal variant uptake at the gastroesophageal junction (*arrow*). **(C)** Esophageal cancer. Increased uptake in the distal esophagus (*arrow*) on sagittal PET scan is secondary to esophageal carcinoma. This extends over a longer distance and is more intense than the normal uptake in **(B)**. **(D)** Esophageal cancer. Focal uptake in the midesophagus on sagittal PET scan is secondary to esophageal carcinoma. Focal esophageal uptake not at the gastroesophageal junction is almost never normal.

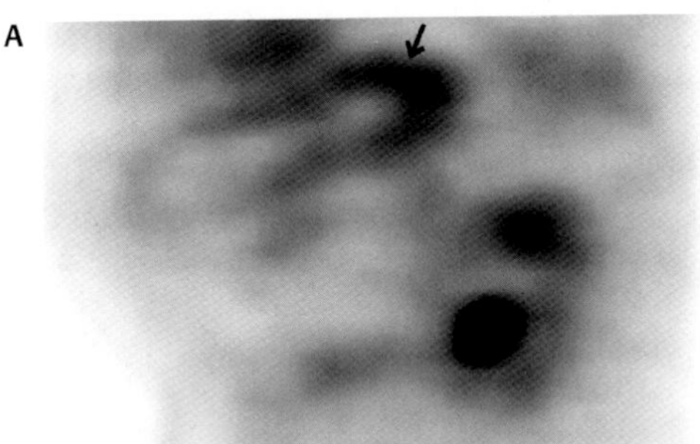

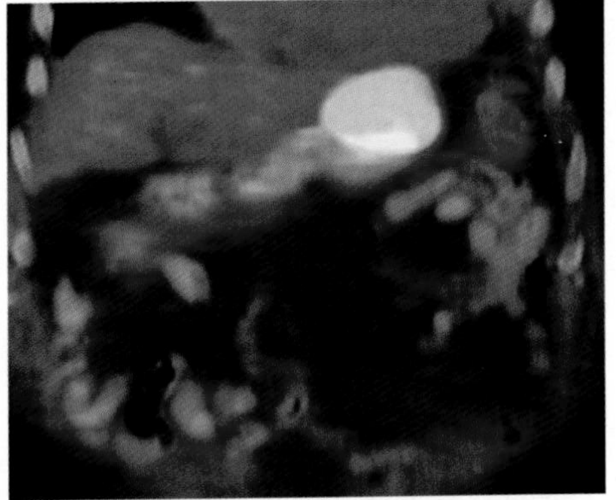

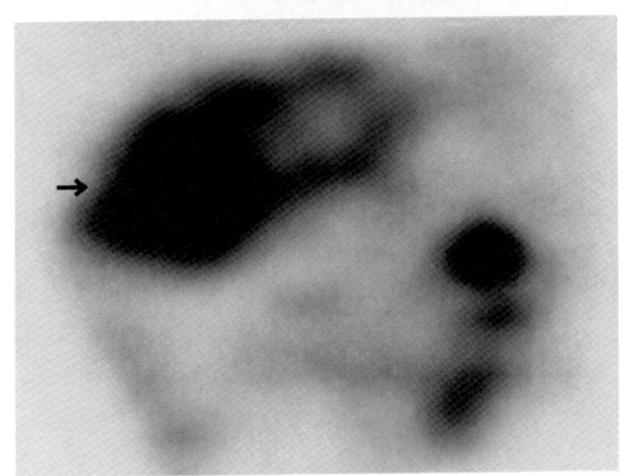

Fig. 6.28 Normal and abnormal gastric uptake. **(A)** Sagittal positron emission tomography (PET) scan demonstrates normal stomach uptake, proximal (*arrow*) greater than distal with no focal uptake. **(B)** Coronal positron emission tomography/computed tomography (PET/CT) scan demonstrates focal uptake in the fundus of the stomach secondary to gastric cancer. Even though this is proximal, it is abnormal because it is focal, and the degree of intensity is much greater than the distal stomach. **(C)** Sagittal PET scan in a patient with gastric cancer demonstrates focal increased uptake in the distal stomach (*arrow*) greater than the normal uptake in proximal stomach. The distal uptake is abnormal because it is both focal and greater than the proximal uptake.

inflammatory or neoplastic processes (**Figs. 6.28** and **6.29**).

a. Focal uptake (benign ulceration (**Fig. 6.29**) as well as malignancy can cause focal uptake)[39]

b. Diffuse intense uptake

c. If distal uptake is more prominent than proximal uptake, a malignancy should be suspected.[40]

3. ***Hiatal hernia.*** Hiatal hernias can cause large foci of uptake at the expected region

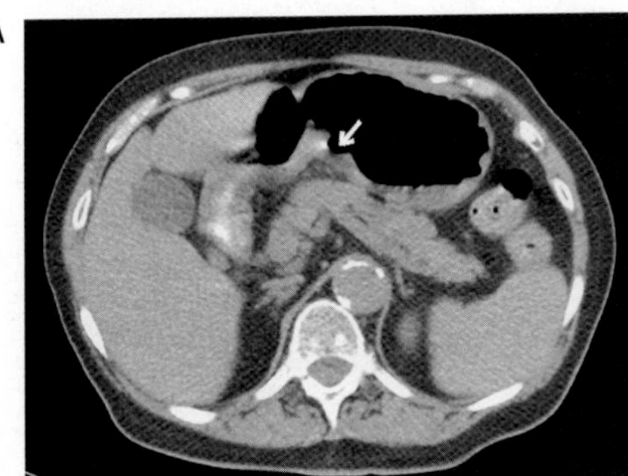

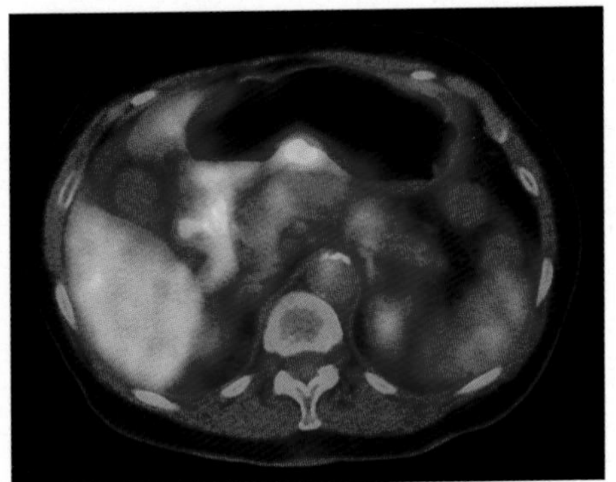

Fig. 6.29 Gastric ulcer. **(A)** Axial computed tomography (CT) scan demonstrates a gastric ulcer (*arrow*). **(B)** Corresponding axial positron emission tomography/computed tomography (PET/CT) scan demonstrates intense uptake in the ulcer. PET cannot differentiate between benign and malignant ulcers. This ulcer was benign. (From Lin E. F-18 fluorodeoxyglucose uptake in a benign gastric ulcer. Clin Nucl Med 2007;32:462–463. Reprinted with permission.)

of the gastroesophageal junction, mimicking a distal esophageal neoplasm or node.

4. ***SUV***[41]
   a. *Without reflux.* An SUV of less than 4 at the gastroesophageal junction or antrum is usually considered a normal variant. An SUV higher than 4 should prompt further work-up.
   b. *Reflux disease.* Patients with reflux may have SUV values slightly higher than 4 at the gastroesophageal junction. However, reflux does not result in SUV values much greater than 4, and further work-up should still be pursued in patients with reflux and very high levels of uptake.

◆ Small and Large Bowel

1. ***Bowel activity.*** Bowel activity is a normal variant; it may be primarily due to bowel wall smooth muscle motility, but lymphoid tissue, mucosal activity, and luminal contents can contribute to visualized activity.
2. ***Small bowel activity.*** Small bowel activity is usually less than large bowel activity.
3. ***Large bowel activity.*** Large bowel activity is most prominent in the right colon (**Fig. 6.30**), particularly the cecum (**Fig. 6.31**), and the rectosigmoid. However, the pattern is unpredictable, and at times the entire colon is visualized. Children often have minimal uptake in the large bowel.
   a. A nodular pattern of uptake is often a normal variant in the ascending colon.[42]
   b. A segmental pattern of uptake is most commonly seen in the rectosigmoid colon (**Fig. 6.32**).[42]
4. ***Oral contrast.*** Oral contrast can cause focal or diffuse increased colonic FDG uptake. This is secondary not only to the high CT density of the contrast (see Chapter 8), but also from accelerated physiologic reaction.[42]

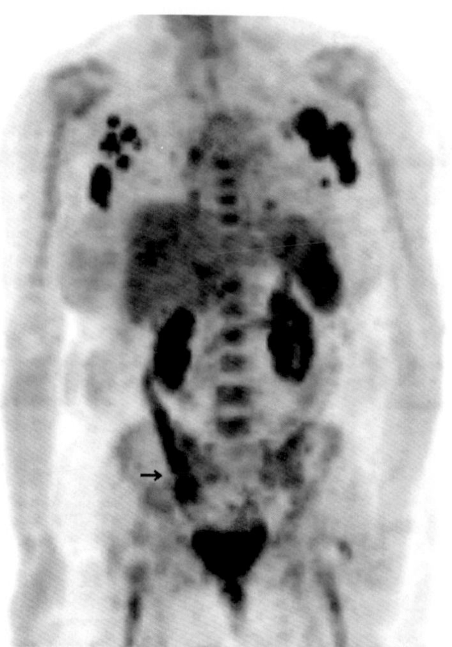

Fig. 6.30 Bone and splenic uptake postgranulocyte colony-stimulating factor (G-CSF) treatment and normal colonic uptake. Coronal positron emission tomography scan in a patient with lymphoma demonstrates bone marrow and splenic uptake post-G-CSF treatment. Bilateral axillary nodal uptake is also noted. Increased uptake in the right colon (*arrow*) is a normal variant.

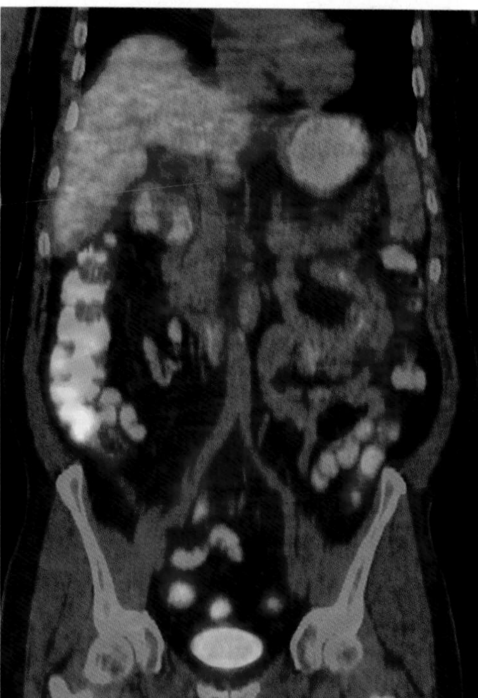

Fig. 6.31 Cecal uptake. Focal cecal uptake on a coronal positron emission tomography/computed tomography scan is a normal variant in this patient. Outside the cecum and ascending colon, focal uptake is more worrisome.

5. ***Focal and segmental uptake.*** Focal or segmental areas of increased uptake are often pathologic. Segmental colonic activity suggests inflammation; focal colonic activity can be secondary to polyps or colon cancer (see Chapter 24).
   a. However, focal uptake in the ascending colon is often a normal variant. In particular, focal cecal uptake (**Fig. 6.31**) is often normal. Focal uptake in the descending colon can be seen in constipated patients. Segmental uptake in the rectosigmoid is often a normal variant (**Fig. 6.32**).[42]
   b. If there is a question whether a focal or segmental area of colonic uptake is abnormal, corresponding CT scans if available should be reviewed for an associated abnormality at the same site. Increased FDG uptake in conjunction with a CT abnormality is associated with a high incidence of cancerous or precancerous lesions.[43]
   c. Focal bowel uptake as noted on PET/CT is associated with gastrointestinal tract pathology in ~70% of cases.[44,45] The incidence of false-positive results is substantially higher with PET alone.
   d. Although SUVs tend to be higher in true-positive findings than false-positive findings, SUVs cannot be used to differentiate physiologic from pathologic gastrointestinal tract uptake.[44,45]

◆ Liver

1. ***SUV.*** The normal liver has a mean SUV of 3.2 ± 0.8.[21]
2. ***Noise artifact.*** On attenuation-corrected images, the liver may appear to have substantial nonuniform uptake (more so than any other visceral organ) secondary to image noise. Therefore, it is possible that the noise associated with attenuation-corrected images could mimic or obscure liver lesions (see Chapter 10).
3. ***Insulin.*** Insulin administration increases liver FDG uptake.[46]
4. ***Lesions.*** Cholestasis and inflammatory biliary tract uptake (**Fig. 6.33**) can cause false-positive liver lesions.

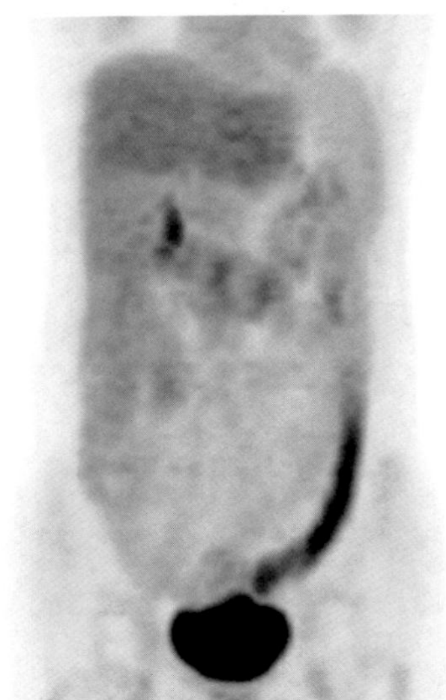

Fig. 6.32 Segmental uptake. Coronal positron emission tomography scan demonstrates segmental distal descending and sigmoid colon uptake. This pattern is often a normal variant in this region but would suggest inflammation if seen in other areas, such as the transverse colon.

◆ Gallbladder/Biliary Tree

1. ***Normal pattern.*** No uptake is seen in the normal gallbladder wall or lumen.
2. ***Gallbladder wall uptake.*** Gallbladder wall uptake is seen in inflammatory conditions such as acute or chronic cholecystitis.
3. ***Focal uptake.*** Focal uptake in the gallbladder is seen with benign polyps, adenomyomatosis,[47] and gallbladder carcinoma.
4. ***Biliary tract uptake.*** Biliary tract uptake can be seen after recent stent placement (**Fig. 6.33**).

◆ Spleen

1. ***SUV.*** The mean SUV is 2.4 ± 0.6.[21] The uptake is usually equal to or less than that of the liver.
2. ***Diffuse increased uptake.*** Diffuse increased uptake can be seen associated with malignancy and also in benign conditions such as congestive splenomegaly and giant cell arteritis. Granulocyte colony-stimulating factor (G-CSF) treatment is another cause of diffuse increased uptake.

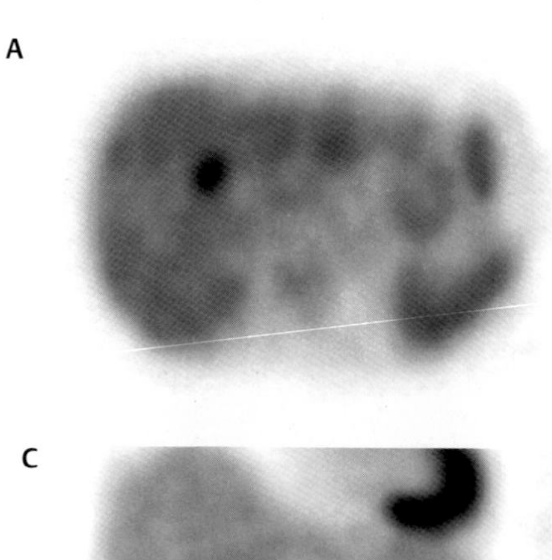

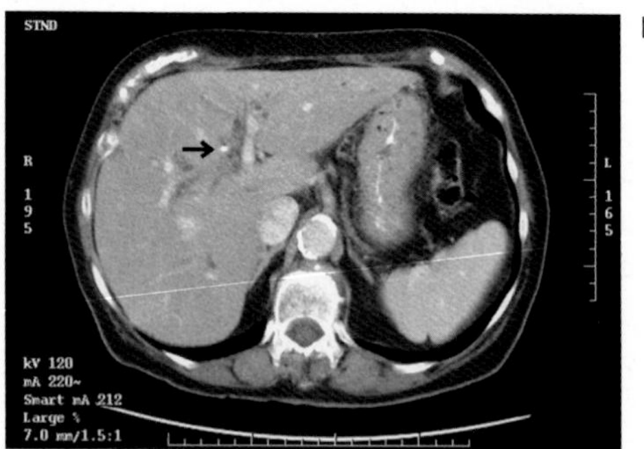

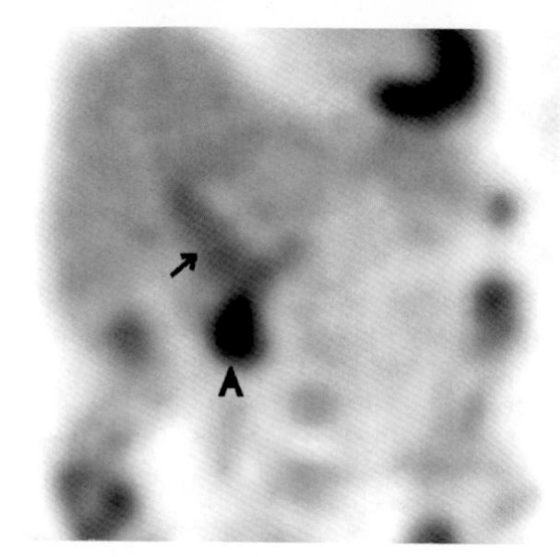

Fig. 6.33 Biliary tract uptake from stent placement. **(A)** Axial positron emission tomography (PET) scan in a patient with pancreatic cancer demonstrates focal liver uptake suspicious for metastasis. **(B)** Computed tomography (CT) scan demonstrates this uptake to correspond to a biliary stent (*arrow*). **(C)** Coronal PET scan demonstrates the full extent of the biliary tract uptake (*arrow*). Uptake is also seen in the pancreatic head cancer (*arrowhead*). (From Lin EC, Studley M. Biliary tract FDG uptake secondary to stent placement. Clin Nucl Med 2003;28:318–319. Reprinted with permission.)

3. ***Granulocyte colony-stimulating factor.*** Splenic uptake is seen in 53% of patients during or immediately after G-CSF treatment (**Fig. 6.30**).[48] The degree of increased uptake is less intense than that seen in bone marrow. Like bone marrow activity, the splenic activity declines after the G-CSF treatment stops, but it is typically seen for at least 10 days.

◆ Pancreas

1. ***SUV.*** The pancreas demonstrates minimal uptake, less than the liver or spleen. The uptake is difficult to visualize if normal. The mean SUV is 2.0 ± 0.5.[21]
2. ***Diffuse uptake.*** Diffuse uptake is seen in acute or chronic pancreatitis.
3. ***Focal uptake.*** Focal uptake is seen in both benign and malignant lesions (see Chapter 21).

◆ Adrenal

1. ***Normal pattern.*** The adrenals are not discretely identified on a normal PET scan. However, they are often visible on PET/CT studies with minimal uptake.
2. ***Focal uptake.*** Focal adrenal uptake is abnormal. Besides metastatic disease, other causes of focal adrenal uptake are
   - ***a.*** Benign and malignant pheochromocytoma (malignant more likely)[49]
   - ***b.*** Giant adrenal myelolipoma[50] (the majority of myelolipomas do not have uptake)
   - ***c.*** Adrenal carcinoma
   - ***d.*** Adrenal hemorrhage
   - ***e.*** Adrenal histoplasmosis
3. ***Bilateral uptake.*** Although bilateral adrenal uptake is worrisome for metastases, this can also be secondary to adrenal hyperplasia (**Fig. 6.34**).

◆ Genitourinary Tract

1. ***FDG excretion.*** Unlike glucose, the kidneys excrete any filtered FDG. There is normally a large amount of activity in the renal collecting systems and bladder, and variable activity in seen in the ureters.
2. ***Renal false-positives***

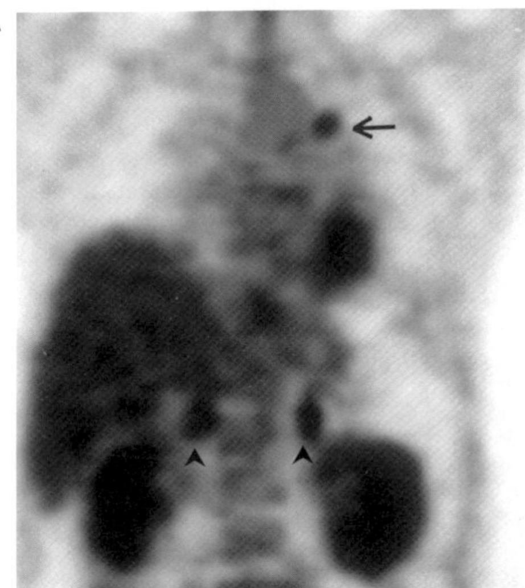

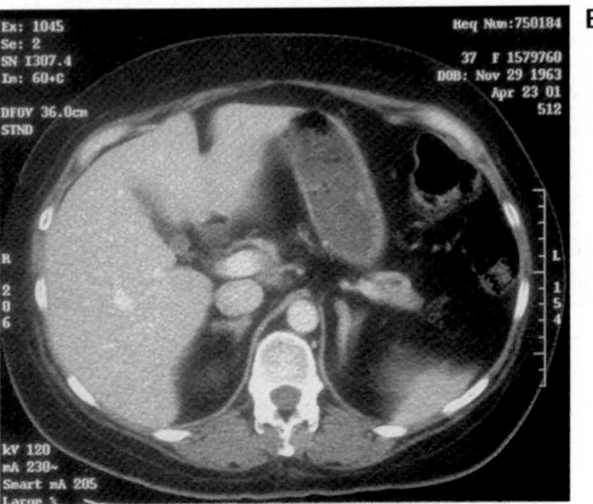

Fig. 6.34 Adrenal hyperplasia. **(A)** Coronal positron emission tomography scan demonstrates uptake in the mediastinum (*arrow*) and both adrenals (*arrowheads*). Although a primary lung cancer with bilateral adrenal metastases would be the first consideration, the adrenal uptake is symmetric, which would be unlikely for metastases. **(B)** Computed tomography scan demonstrates bilateral adrenal hyperplasia. The patient had Cushing syndrome and adrenal hyperplasia secondary to a mediastinal paraganglioma. (From Lin EC, Helgans R. Adrenal hyperplasia in Cushing syndrome demonstrated by FDG positron emission tomographic imaging. Clin Nucl Med 2002;27(7):516–517. Reprinted with permission.)

   a. Pooled activity in the renal collecting system can mimic a renal lesion (see **Fig. 23.2**, p. 205).
   b. Oncocytomas and angiomyolipomas have been reported to have increased uptake despite their benign nature (see Chapter 23).

3. ***Ureteral false-positives***
   a. Focal activity in the ureters can mimic retroperitoneal nodal uptake (**Figs. 6.35** and **6.36**). This is easily differentiated on PET/CT, but it may be difficult to differentiate on PET. Correlation between three imaging planes can often localize this to the ureter.
   b. Even if focal, ureteral activity is usually linear. In addition, the most common location for focal ureteral activity is in the superior pelvis where the ureter crosses the iliac vessels. These findings can aid in determining whether a focus of increased activity is ureteral in origin (**Figs. 6.35** and **6.36**).

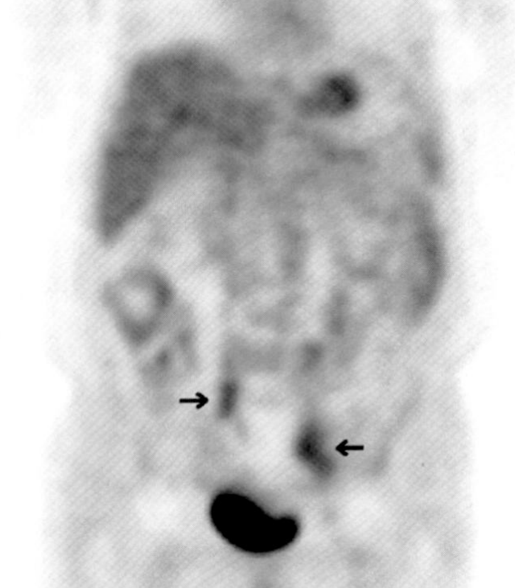

Fig. 6.35 Ureteral activity or node? Coronal positron emission tomography (PET) scan in a lymphoma patient demonstrates two foci of uptake (*arrows*) in the course of the ureters. Unless these foci of uptake can be definitely linked to the ureters, they cannot be differentiated from nodal uptake without computed tomography correlation. However, the linear nature of the uptake on the right suggests that it is ureteral, and the more nodular uptake on the left suggests nodal uptake. In addition, the location of the right-sided activity in the superior pelvis (where the ureter crosses the iliacs) also suggests ureteral activity. In this case the right-sided activity was ureteral, and the left-sided activity was in a node.

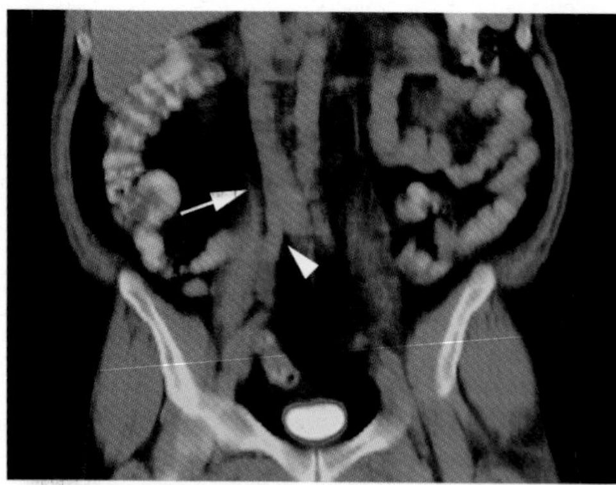

Fig. 6.36 Focal ureteral activity. Coronal positron emission tomography/computed tomography scan demonstrates focal linear activity in the right ureter. Note the characteristic location in the superior pelvis where the ureter crosses the right iliac vein (*arrowhead*). Unopacified ureter (*arrow*) is seen contiguous with the ureteral activity.

◆ Uterus

1. ***Normal pattern.*** The uterus is usually not discretely identified on PET.
2. ***Leiomyomas.*** Leiomyomas are a common cause of focal uterine uptake. As there is no uptake in the remaining uterus, they are often difficult to identify as leiomyomas on PET and can mimic other pelvic masses. Leiomyomas cannot be differentiated from leiomyosarcomas by PET.
   a. In a woman with a large focus of uptake above the bladder, a leiomyoma is a highly likely etiology (**Figs. 6.37** and **6.38**).
   b. An artifactual cause of focal activity above the bladder is bladder filling during imaging if the patient is scanned inferior to superior.
3. ***Endometrial uptake.*** Endometrial uptake is usually a normal variant, most commonly seen during menstruation.[51]
   a. Most prominent at midcycle and menstrual flow phase
   b. Postmenopausal women can have mild endometrial uptake.
   c. Intrauterine devices also cause endometrial uptake.
   d. Scheduling PET a week before or a few days after the menstrual flow phase minimizes physiologic endometrial and ovarian uptake.[52]
4. ***Postpartum.*** The postpartum uterus demonstrates intense diffuse uptake (**Fig. 6.39**).[53]

◆ Ovary

1. ***Normal pattern.*** Normally the ovaries are not visualized on PET.
2. ***Ovarian uptake.*** Ovarian uptake can be seen in malignancy as well as in a wide range of benign conditions (see Chapter 21)

A

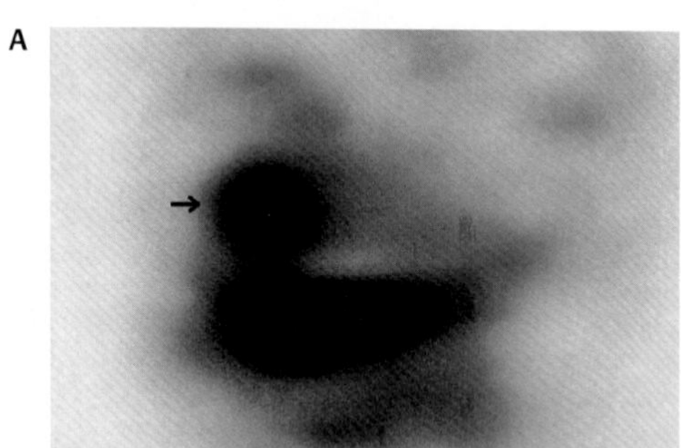

B

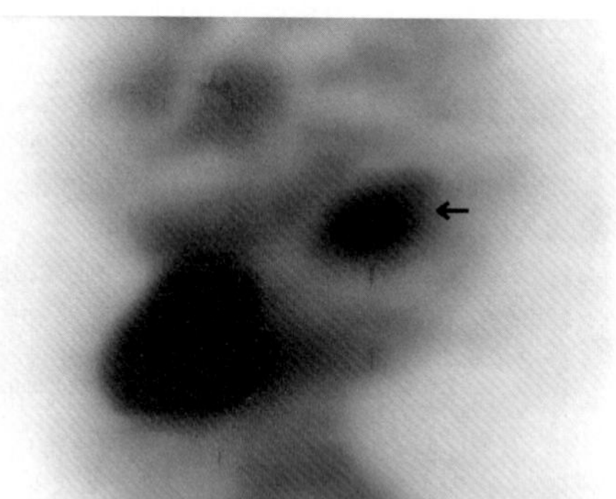

Fig. 6.37 Uterine leiomyomas. Sagittal positron emission tomography scans demonstrate large foci of uptake (*arrows*) in uterine fundal leiomyomas in an **(A)** anteverted and a **(B)** retroverted uterus. When large foci of uptake are seen superior to the bladder, leiomyomas should be suspected, but correlation with anatomic imaging is necessary.

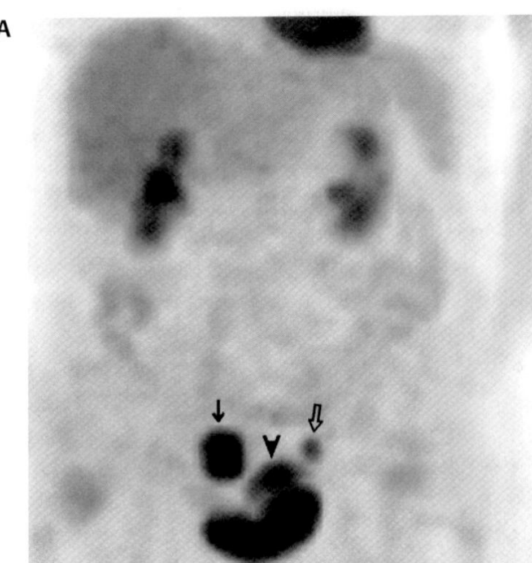
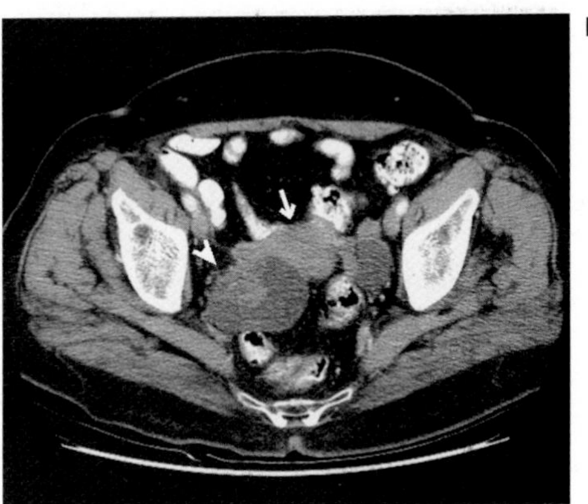

Fig. 6.38 Spectrum of pelvic uptake. **(A)** Coronal positron emission tomography scan in a premenopausal woman demonstrates uptake in a right ovarian carcinoma (*arrow*), fibroid (*arrowhead*), and left ovarian follicular cyst (*open arrow*). The size and degree of the right ovarian uptake is worrisome of malignancy. The left ovarian uptake would be equivocal without imaging correlation in a premenopausal woman. In a postmenopausal woman, the left ovarian uptake would be worrisome for malignancy. **(B)** Axial computed tomography scan in the same patient demonstrates the right ovarian carcinoma and left ovarian follicular cyst. Most of the fibroid is inferior to this level, but the top of the fibroid is seen as an area of minimal hypodensity (*arrow*). A solid component is seen in the right ovarian carcinoma (*arrowhead*).

(**Fig. 6.38**). The most common cause is a follicular cyst. Occasionally, the ovary can be confused with a pelvic lymph node (see Chapter 10).

3. ***Premenopausal uptake.*** In premenopausal women, physiologic ovarian uptake is most common around ovulation and during the early luteal phase of the menstrual cycle.[54] Physiologic uptake can be minimized by scheduling PET a week before or a few days after the menstrual flow phase.[52] However, physiologic ovarian uptake can be seen in women of reproductive age even after hysterectomy.[55]
4. ***Postmenopausal uptake.*** Ovarian uptake in the postmenopausal woman is much more worrisome than in a premenopausal woman, and malignancy should be considered.[51]

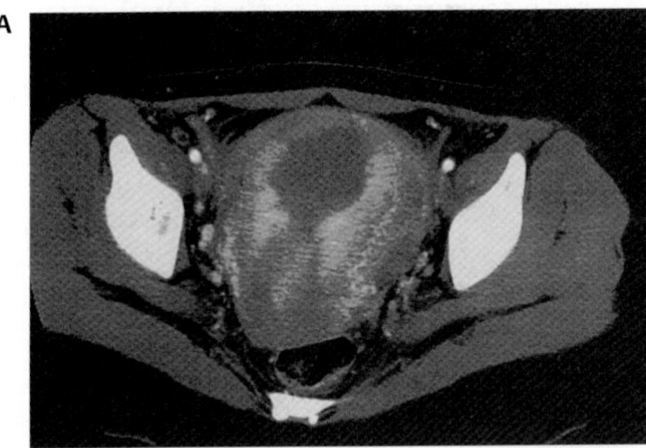
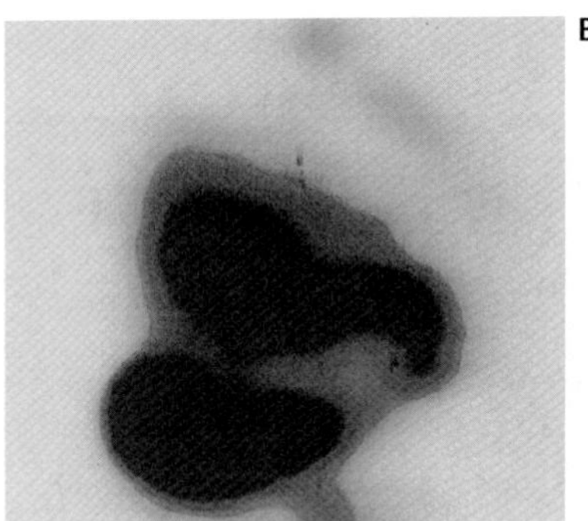

Fig. 6.39 Postpartum uterus. **(A)** Computed tomography scan of the pelvis demonstrates a heterogeneous postpartum uterus with a prominent endometrial cavity. **(B)** Sagittal positron emission tomography scan demonstrates intense diffuse fluorodeoxyglucose uptake in the uterus. (From Lin E. FDG PET appearance of a postpartum uterus. Clin Nucl Med 2006;31:159–160. Reprinted with permission.)

◆ Testes

1. Symmetric testicular uptake is a normal variant that declines with age.
2. The normal testis can have an SUV as high as 5.7 (mean 2.2).[56]

◆ Bone and Bone Marrow

1. ***Normal uptake.*** Normal bone (without red marrow) has very minimal FDG uptake due to low metabolic activity. Red marrow activity is responsible for relatively increased FDG uptake in the axial skeleton.
2. ***Benign fractures.*** Benign fractures can have uptake (**Figs. 6.40** and **6.41**).
   a. *Amount of uptake.* Uptake in fractures is variable and likely depends on the site and severity of the fracture. Some acute fractures may not have significant uptake.
   b. *Duration.* The duration of uptake in fractures is variable, but uptake has been reported up to 6 months after a fracture.[57] Most fractures do not have substantial uptake after 2 to 3 months.[11,37]
   c. *Insufficiency fractures.* Sacral insufficiency fractures can mimic pelvic bone metastases.[58] Usually, they do not have the classic H-shaped pattern of uptake seen on bone scans. The uptake is often linear, rather than nodular, which suggests the diagnosis. Vertebral insufficiency fractures can also have uptake in the more acute phase, which can mimic vertebral metastases. Like sacral insufficiency fractures, a linear appearance suggests the diagnosis (**Fig. 6.42**).
3. ***Granulocyte colony-stimulating factor.*** Diffuse bone marrow uptake is seen in 87% of patients during and immediately after G-CSF treatment (**Fig. 6.30**).[59] The uptake declines after the end of treatment. The reported time interval after treatment necessary to avoid increased uptake is variable, ranging from 5 days to 1 month.[60] However, patients treated with high-dose chemotherapy followed by transplantation and G-CSF often do not have increased marrow uptake, possibly secondary to severely decreased marrow reserve. If marrow uptake is diffusely increased secondary to G-CSF, bone metastases (**Fig. 6.43**) and benign bone lesions such as vertebral hemangiomas (**Fig. 6.44**) can appear as photopenic defects relative to the hyperplastic marrow.[61,62]
4. ***Other causes of diffuse marrow uptake***
   a. *Chemotherapy.* Multiple cycles of chemotherapy may cause decreased bone marrow uptake.[60] Recovery of marrow following chemotherapy may cause a mild increase in bone marrow uptake, although this is not observed in some cases, possibly due to poor marrow reserve.
   b. *Erythropoietin.* Erythropoietin can cause extensive diffuse increased uptake.
   c. Pathological processes such as myelodysplastic syndromes, β-thalassemia, and chronic myeloid leukemia can result in diffuse marrow uptake.[63–65]
5. ***Arthritis.*** There is often minimal or no uptake in arthritic joints (because of this, FDG

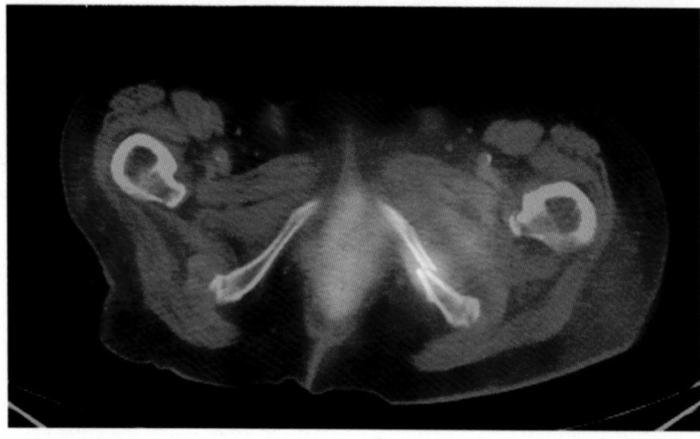

Fig. 6.40 Acute fracture fluorodeoxyglucose (FDG) uptake. Axial positron emission tomography/computed tomography scan demonstrates uptake in an acute pelvic fracture.

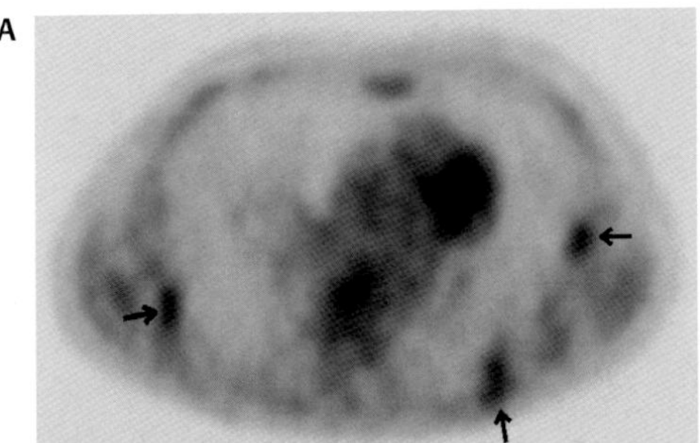

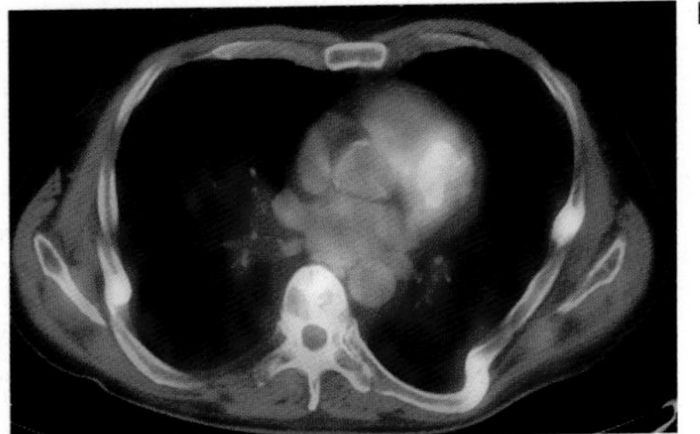

Fig. 6.41 Chronic fracture fluorodeoxyglucose (FDG) uptake. **(A)** Axial positron emission tomography (PET) scan demonstrates multiple foci of uptake in the peripheral thorax (*arrows*). PET has difficulty in localizing peripheral lesions such as these: it cannot be determined whether these foci are in the lungs, pleura, or ribs. Note that these foci are similar in appearance to a peripheral lung neoplasm (see **Fig. 15.1**, p. 116). **(B)** Axial positron emission tomography/computed tomography (PET/CT) scan demonstrates that these foci of uptake correspond to old rib fractures. This degree of uptake in old fractures is unusual.

PET is more specific than bone scan), unless there is an inflammatory component. In the spine, uptake can be seen corresponding to both degenerative disk and facet disease. The degree of uptake weakly correlates with the severity on CT.[66] Inflammatory arthritis can have substantial uptake depending upon the degree of inflammation.

a. Degenerative spurring in the spine can sometimes demonstrate substantial FDG uptake (**Fig. 6.45**).

b. Subchondral cysts can have FDG uptake (**Fig. 6.46**).

c. Uptake in joints affected by rheumatoid arthritis is much more likely than in those affected by osteoarthritis. In rheumatoid arthritis, there is usually uptake if the joint is clinically inflamed.[67]

6. ***Specific joints.*** Uptake is more common in these joints:[18,19]
   a. Glenohumeral joints (**Figs. 6.3** and **6.12**)
   b. Sternoclavicular joints
   c. Costovertebral joints
7. ***Radiation effects.*** Radiation therapy will cause reduced uptake corresponding exactly to the radiation field (**Fig. 6.47**).
8. ***Focal uptake.*** Focal uptake in skeletal structures can be secondary to bone marrow me-

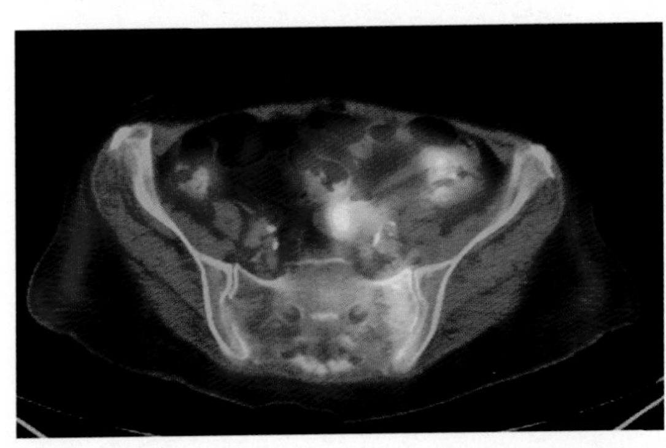

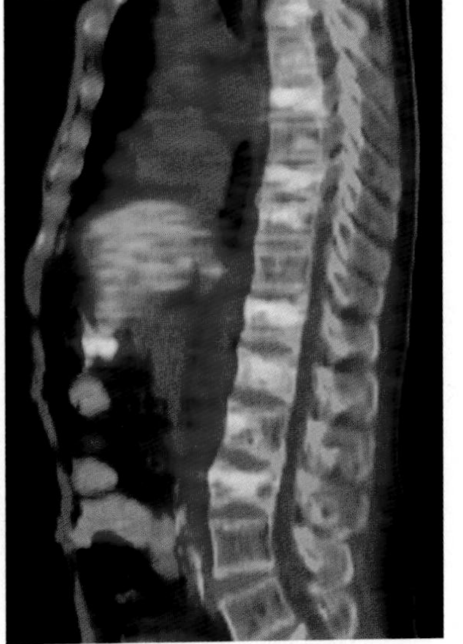

Fig. 6.42 Sacral and vertebral insufficiency fractures. **(A)** Axial positron emission tomography/computed tomography (PET/CT) scan demonstrates linear uptake in a left sacral insufficiency fracture. **(B)** Sagittal PET/CT scan demonstrates multiple horizontal linear areas of uptake in the spine secondary to compression fractures. The location of the uptake is comparable to the location of the fracture lines sometimes seen by magnetic resonance imaging in vertebral insufficiency fractures.

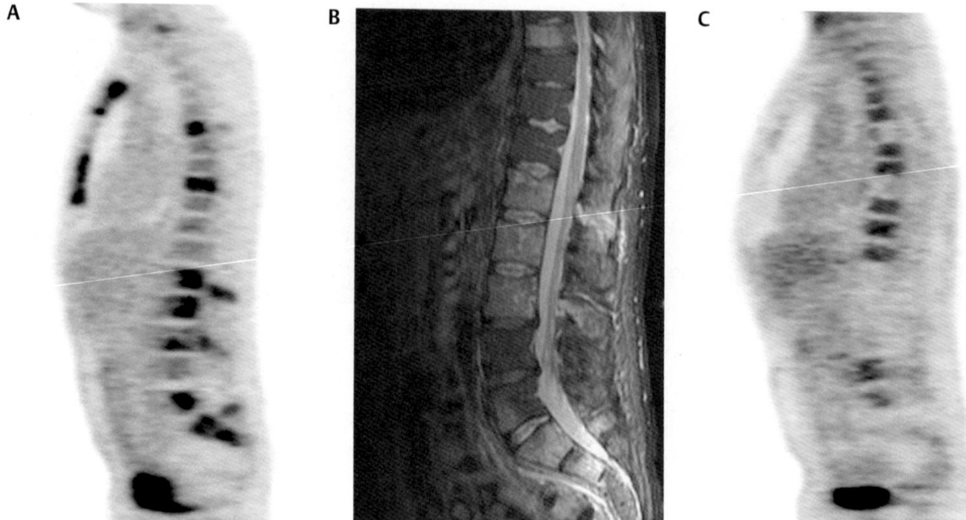

Fig. 6.43 Flip-flop phenomenon of treated bone marrow disease. **(A)** Sagittal positron emission tomography (PET) scan demonstrates bone marrow infiltration from lymphoma involving the sternum, spine, and sacrum. **(B)** The areas of fluorodeoxyglucose (FDG) uptake are seen as abnormal hyperintense signal on sagittal short T1 inversion recovery magnetic resonance imaging (STIR MRI). **(C)** Posttherapy scan demonstrates the previously noted areas of uptake to be photopenic. However, the normal marrow now appears to have increased uptake relative to the treated regions (this appearance could be accentuated by granulocyte colony-stimulating factor or recovery from chemotherapy). If pretherapy studies are not available for comparison, these areas of normal marrow uptake could mimic disease. (From Lin EC. FDG PET/CT flip-flop phenomenon in treated lymphoma of bone. Clin Nucl Med 2006;31:803–805. Reprinted with permission.)

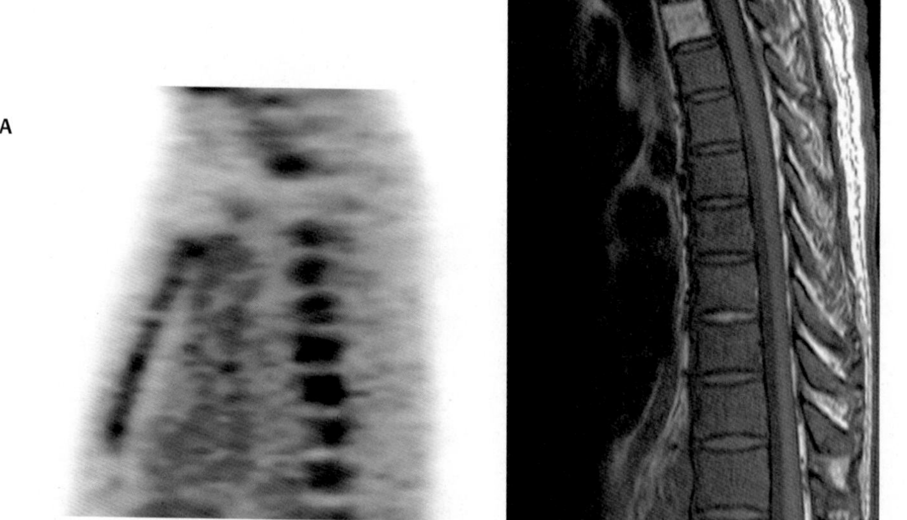

Fig. 6.44 Vertebral body hemangioma. **(A)** Sagittal positron emission tomography (PET) scan in a patient with marrow hyperplasia demonstrates a single vertebral body in the upper thoracic spine, which is relatively photopenic. **(B)** Sagittal T1-weighted magnetic resonance image demonstrates a hyperintense hemangioma in this photopenic vertebral body. The remaining marrow is hypointense, consistent with marrow hyperplasia. Bone lesions that contain little or no red marrow may appear as areas of decreased fluorodeoxyglucose (FDG) uptake in the setting of marrow hyperplasia.

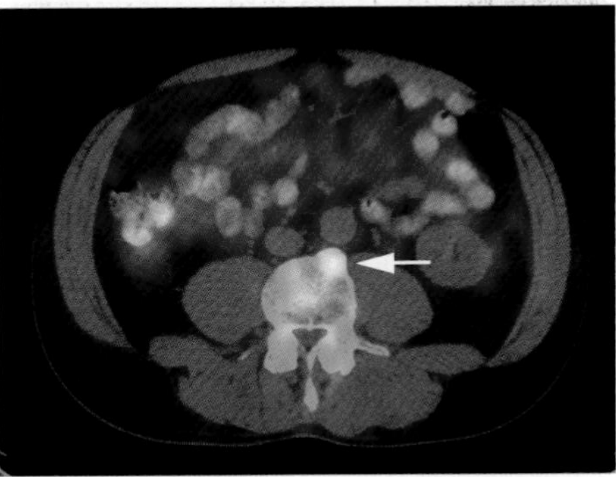

Fig. 6.45 Degenerative spur. Axial positron emission tomography/computed tomography scan demonstrates intense uptake in an anterior vertebral column spur (*arrow*).

tastases or primary bone lesions. Uptake in a bone lesion does not necessarily indicate malignancy, as many benign primary bone lesions have FDG uptake (see Chapter 25).

9. ***Intraspinous bursa uptake.*** Uptake is often seen in the lower lumbar spine in the region of the posterior spinous processes. On axial images, this uptake often appears to be in the spinous process and mimics an osseous lesion, but on sagittal images, it can be seen to lie between the spinous processes.

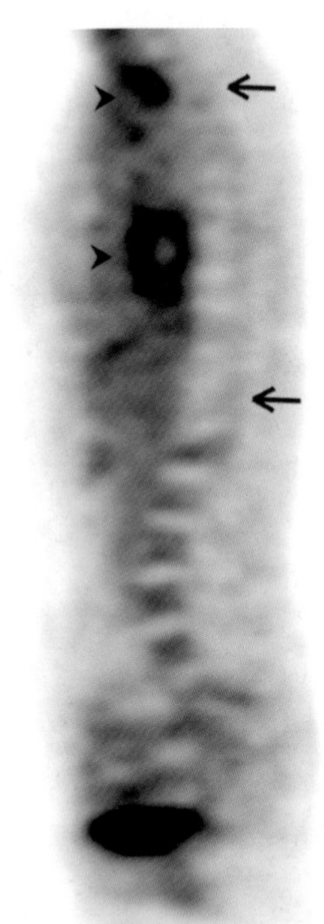

Fig. 6.47 Radiation effects on bone. Sagittal positron emission tomography scan demonstrates a large area of decreased uptake in the thoracic spine (*arrows*) secondary to radiation for thoracic tumors (*arrowheads*).

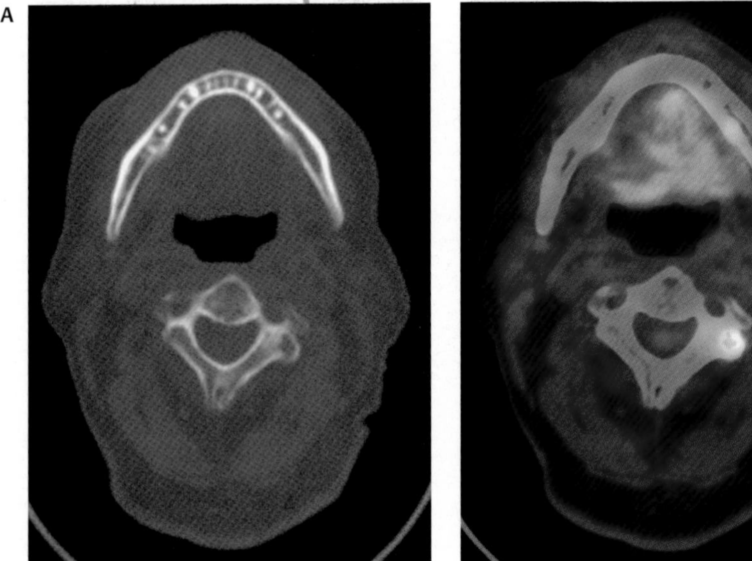

Fig. 6.46 Subchondral cyst. **(A)** Computed tomography (CT) scan demonstrates a subchondral cyst related to a cervical facet joint. **(B)** Axial positron emission tomography/computed tomography (PET/CT) scan demonstrates fluorodeoxyglucose (FDG) uptake in this subchondral cyst.

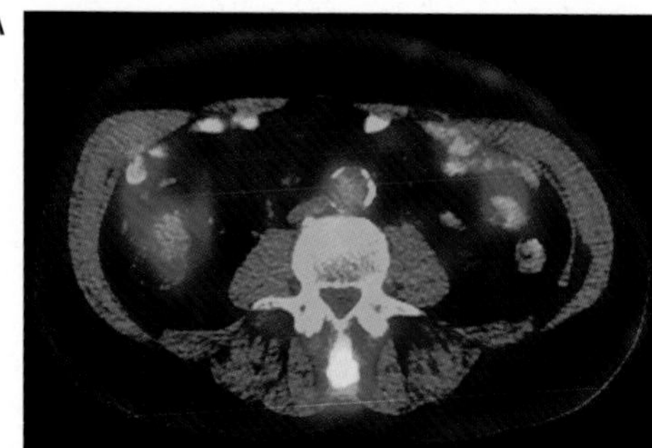

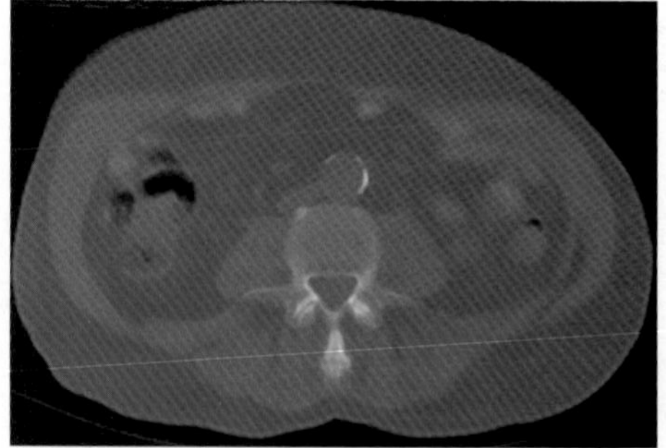

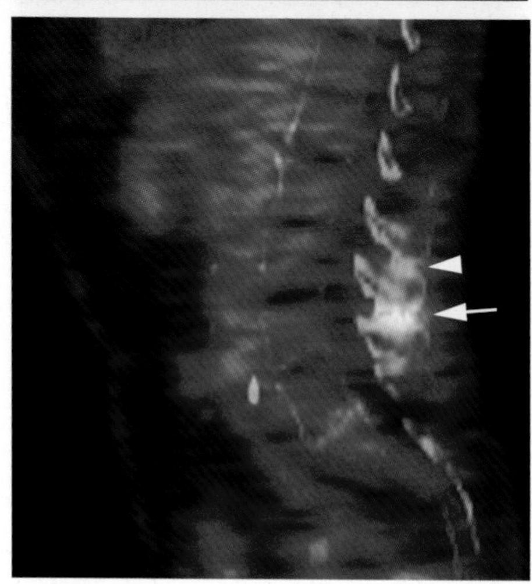

Fig. 6.48 Baastrup disease. **(A)** Axial positron emission tomography/computed tomography (PET/CT) scan demonstrates apparent uptake in a lumbar spinous process. **(B)** Corresponding axial CT scan demonstrates sclerosis, hypertrophy, and flattening involving this spinous process. **(C)** Sagittal PET/CT scan demonstrates that the uptake (*arrow*) lies between spinous processes. Minimal uptake is also noted between the spinous processes just above this level (*arrowhead*). Intraspinous bursal uptake can often appear to lie in the spinous process on axial images. As spinous process metastases are rare, close correlation with sagittal images is necessary. Although the CT findings suggest Baastrup disease in this case, intraspinous bursal uptake on PET is often seen with a normal CT appearance of the spinous processes. (From Lin E. Baastrup's disease (kissing spine) demonstrated by FDG PET/CT. Skeletal Radiology 2008; 37:173–175. Reprinted with permission.)

This uptake is usually secondary to Baastrup disease (kissing spine), where there is inflammation in the intraspinous bursa secondary to close approximation and contact between adjacent spinous processes (**Fig. 6.48**).[68,69]

◆ Skeletal Muscle

1. ***Causes of increased skeletal muscle uptake***
   a. *Insulin.* Skeletal muscle uptake is diffusely increased after insulin administration or insulin release from recent ingestion of food (skeletal muscle glucose receptors are insulin sensitive) (as seen in **Fig. 4.1,** p. 34). This is seen in conjunction with increased myocardial uptake.
   b. *Exercise.* Skeletal muscle uptake is increased after recent exercise.
   c. *Anxiety.* Anxiety will increase skeletal muscle uptake. This is most prominent in the neck, supraclavicular region, and thoracic paravertebral muscles.
   d. *Graves disease.* Skeletal muscle uptake is often increased in Graves disease.
      - Most common in the psoas and rectus abdominis muscles
      - Usually seen in conjunction with increased thymic and less commonly thyroid uptake
2. ***Mimics.*** Skeletal muscle can be difficult to differentiate from nodal and brown fat uptake.
   a. *Nodal uptake.* Skeletal muscle uptake can usually be differentiated from nodal uptake by its linear appearance and symmetry.
      - Skeletal muscle uptake can occasionally be nodular and mimic the appearance of nodes. However, in these cases a symmetric appearance will suggest muscle as the site of uptake.
      - As nodal disease can exist in conjunction with skeletal muscle uptake in the same region, it is important to fur-

ther evaluate all areas of asymmetry for possible disease. Correlation with anatomical imaging is very helpful in these cases (**Figs. 6.49** and **6.50**).

b. Brown fat uptake. Both brown fat (see Brown Fat section) and muscle uptake are usually symmetric. A linear appearance suggests muscle. Fat and muscle uptake often cannot be differentiated without PET/CT (**Fig. 6.49**), but this is usually of no clinical significance.

3. ***Specific muscles***

a. Teres minor uptake can be seen, often unilaterally.[18]

b. Extraocular muscle uptake is often seen due to eye movement.

c. Diaphragmatic crus uptake can be seen with increased respiratory effort. The crus uptake can be diagnosed by its linear appearance. On coronal images, it appears as a continuous vertical line. The right crus is larger and extends more inferiorly than the left crus (**Fig. 6.50**). Occasionally, a retrocrural node can be difficult to distinguish from normal crural uptake (**Fig. 6.51**).

d. Diaphragmatic slips can also have increased uptake.

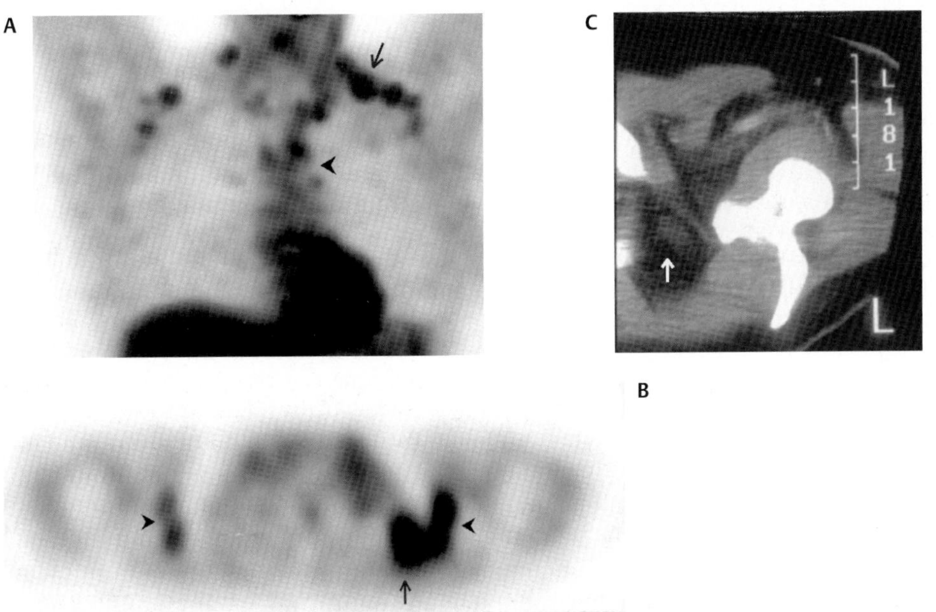

Fig. 6.49 Muscle/brown fat activity obscuring a lymph node. **(A)** Coronal positron emission tomography (PET) scan in a patient with lymphoma demonstrates multiple foci of uptake in the superior mediastinum and supraclavicular region bilaterally. This was not a positron emission tomography/computed tomography (PET/CT) study which makes evaluation more difficult, although a CT scan was available for correlation. The superior mediastinal activity is most consistent with brown fat, as no nodes were seen in this region on CT, and there should not be muscle uptake in the superior mediastinum. In addition, the mediastinal uptake does not extend below the aortic arch (*arrowhead*), which suggests brown fat uptake rather than nodal disease. The supraclavicular activity could either be brown fat or muscle; this could not be differentiated without CT fusion. However, there is an asymmetric focus of increased activity in the left supraclavicular region (*arrow*). Even if brown fat/muscle activity is known to be present, the images should be closely scrutinized for asymmetric activity. **(B)** Axial PET scan shows that the asymmetric focus (*arrow*) corresponds to a left supraclavicular node (*arrow*) seen on CT **(C)**. The bilateral uptake (*arrowheads*) could either be in the subscapularis muscles or the fat just medial to the muscles (fusion would be necessary to exactly localize the activity, as side-by-side correlation is inadequate for this purpose). This case demonstrates the synergy of PET and CT. The supraclavicular node was not detected prospectively on CT. PET detected a potential but equivocal abnormality, and retrospective correlation with the CT was necessary to determine that a node was definitely present.

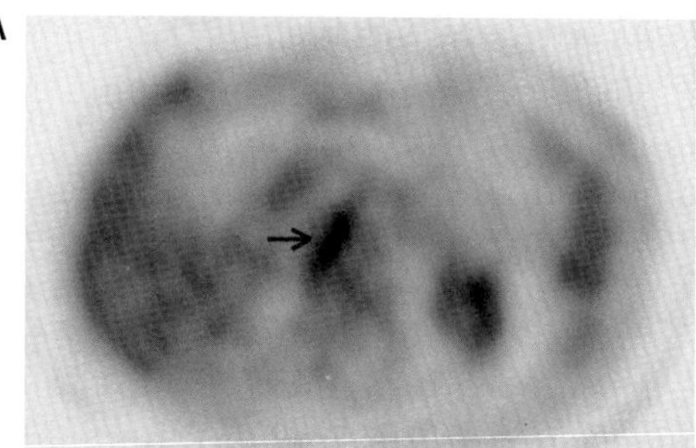

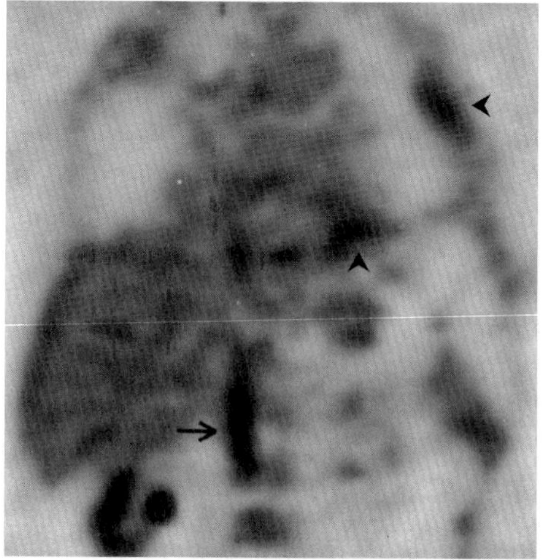

Fig. 6.50 Diaphragmatic crus uptake. **(A)** Axial positron emission tomography (PET) scan demonstrates linear uptake in the right retroperitoneum (*arrow*). **(B)** Coronal PET scan demonstrates linear uptake corresponding to the right diaphragmatic crus (*arrow*). Typically, crus uptake is bilateral and secondary to hyperventilation. In this case, the unilateral uptake is likely secondary to decreased movement of the left hemidiaphragm related to left pleural metastases (*arrowheads*). (From Lin EC, Bhola R. Unilateral diaphragmatic crus uptake on FDG positron emission tomographic imaging. Clin Nucl Med 2001;26(5):479. Reprinted with permission.)

e. Intercostal muscle uptake is more common in smokers and patients with chronic obstructive pulmonary disease.[30]

f. The longus colli muscles in the neck often have asymmetric uptake (**Fig. 6.15**).[10]

◆ Vascular

1. ***Vascular wall***

   a. Atherosclerosis. Uptake in the vascular wall can be seen in atherosclerosis. This is common in the thoracic aorta and iliac and femoral arteries. It usually does not correspond to areas of calcification and may reflect metabolically active macrophages in the atherosclerotic plaques.[70]

   - Focal uptake in atherosclerotic aortic plaque can rarely mimic mediastinal adenopathy (**Fig. 6.52**).

   b. Vasculitis. Vasculitis (**Fig. 6.53**) is another cause of vascular wall uptake.

2. ***Thrombosis.*** Both acute and chronic benign thrombosis can demonstrate signifi-

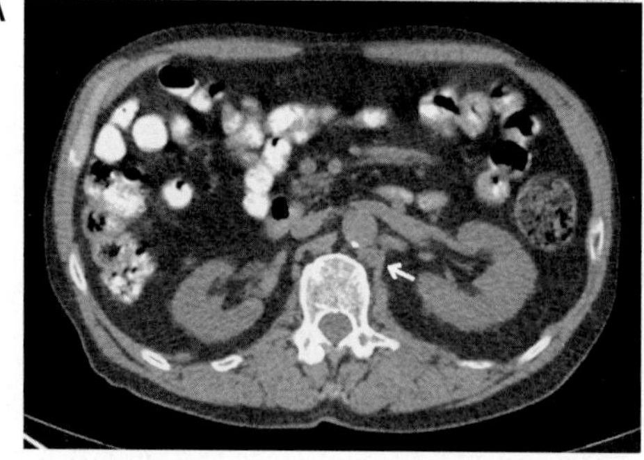

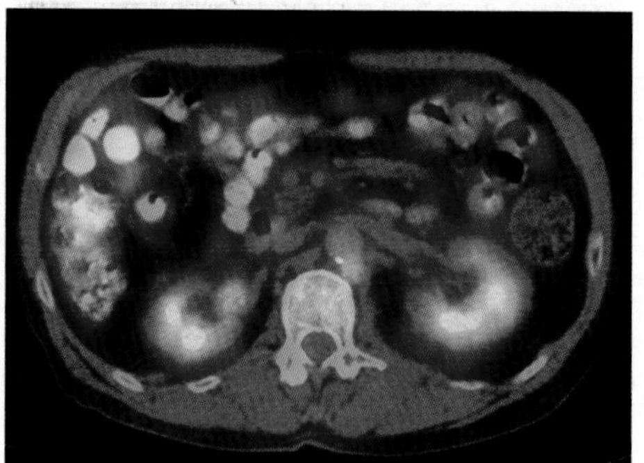

Fig. 6.51 Retrocrural node. **(A)** Axial computed tomography (CT) scan demonstrates slight nodularity in the region of the left crus (*arrow*). Without intravenous contrast, it is difficult to differentiate this from the normal crus. **(B)** Corresponding axial positron emission tomography/computed tomography (PET/CT) scan demonstrates focal uptake in a left retrocrural node.

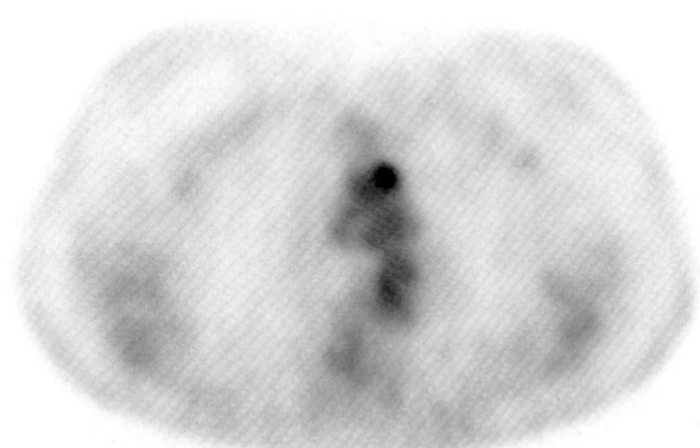

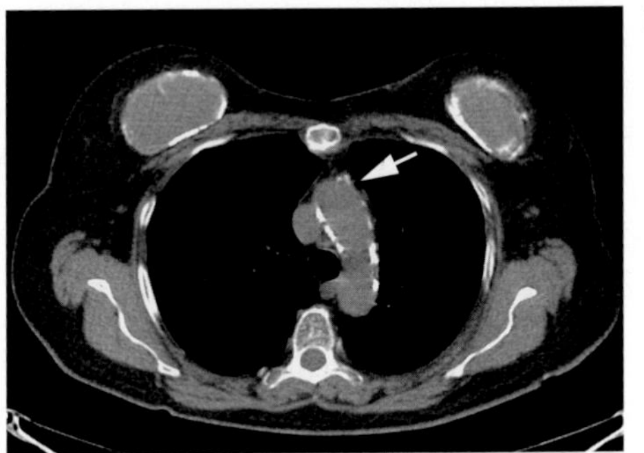

Fig. 6.52 Focal plaque uptake. **(A)** Intense focal uptake is noted on an axial positron emission tomography scan, **(B)** corresponding to an atherosclerotic aortic plaque (*arrow*) seen on a computed tomography scan. Uptake in aortic plaque can occasionally mimic adenopathy.

cant uptake. Uptake in a thrombus does not necessarily indicate tumor thrombosis (**Fig. 6.54**).

- Uptake in a central pulmonary embolus could mimic hilar adenopathy (**Fig. 6.55**).

3. ***Vascular grafts.*** Mild linear uptake along a vascular graft usually does not indicate infection (**Fig. 6.56**); focal uptake is suspicious for infection.[71]

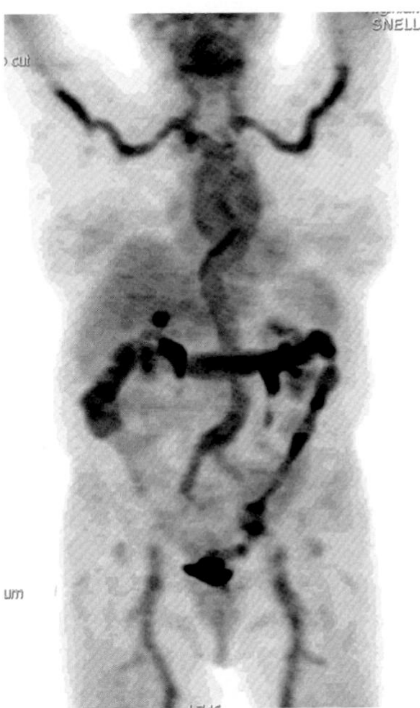

Fig. 6.53 Vasculitis. Coronal positron emission tomography scan demonstrates extensive arterial fluorodeoxyglucose uptake secondary to vasculitis.

4. ***Perivascular tumor infiltration.*** Tumor infiltration along the course of a vessel can have a linear appearance (**Fig. 6.57**). Although a linear appearance usually suggests a benign abnormality or normal variant, perivascular tumor infiltration is one exception.

◆ Soft Tissues

Uptake is common at sites of intervention, such as catheter insertion, ostomies, and surgical scars.

◆ Brown Fat

There are two types of fat in the human body: white and brown fat. White fat stores energy; brown fat generates heat in response to cold exposure. Brown fat can cause focal increased FDG uptake mimicking muscle activity or malignancy.[72–74]

1. ***Locations***
   - ***a.*** Neck
   - ***b.*** Supraclavicular region
   - ***c.*** Axilla
   - ***d.*** Around the large vessels in the mediastinum
   - ***e.*** Interatrial septum (**Fig. 6.58**)
   - ***f.*** Azygoesophageal recess
   - ***g.*** Paraspinal (**Fig. 6.59**)
   - ***h.*** Intercostal spaces
   - ***i.*** Perinephric space

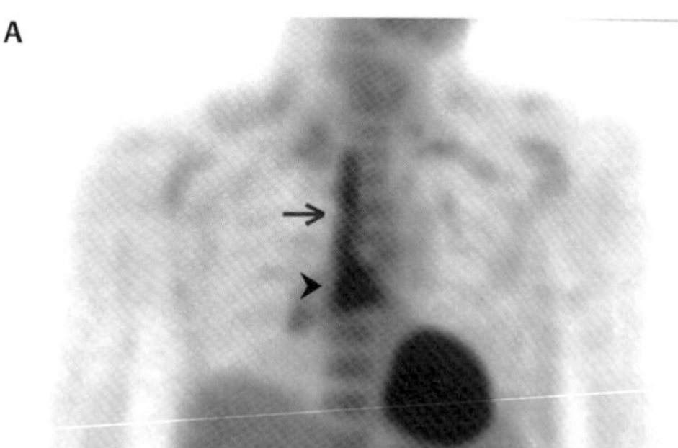

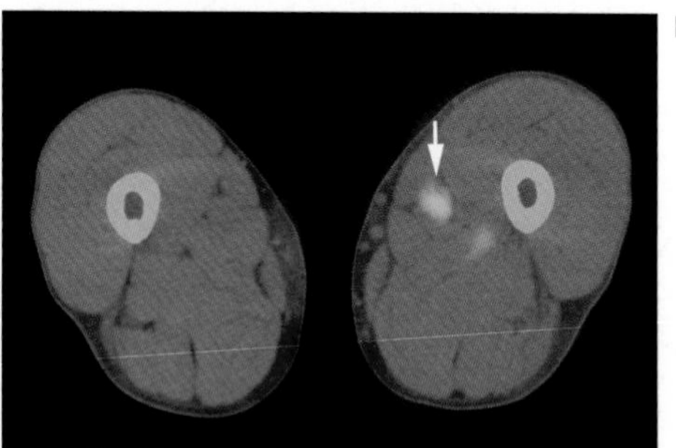

Fig. 6.54 Thrombus uptake. **(A)** Coronal positron emission tomography (PET) scan demonstrates intense uptake in benign superior vena cava thrombus (*arrow*) extending into the right atrium (*arrowhead*). Uptake can be seen in both benign and tumor thrombus. **(B)** Axial positron emission tomography/computed tomography (PET/CT) scan demonstrates uptake in a deep vein thrombus (*arrow*) in the left superficial femoral vein.

j. Paracolic and parahepatic spaces

2. ***Pearls***

a. SUVs cannot differentiate brown fat uptake from malignancy, as SUVs in brown fat can be very high.

b. Neck/supraclavicular uptake is most common. There is usually uptake in the neck/supraclavicular region also when uptake in other brown fat areas is seen.

c. Brown fat uptake in the neck/supraclavicular regions is usually symmetric.

d. Uptake is more common in women and younger patients.

- Low body mass index has been reported to increase uptake in some studies, but not others.[38]

e. Uptake is more common with colder temperatures.

3. ***Differential diagnosis***

a. The diagnosis of brown fat uptake usually requires PET/CT. If PET/CT is not available, the diagnosis can still be suggested

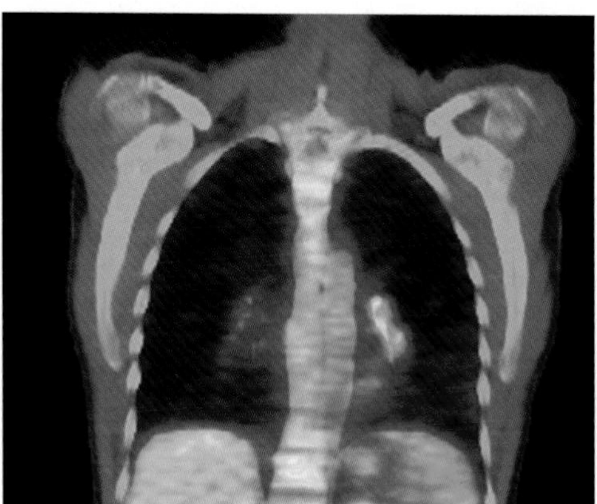

Fig. 6.55 Pulmonary embolus uptake. Coronal positron emission tomography/computed tomography (PET/CT) scan demonstrates left hilar uptake secondary to uptake in a pulmonary embolus. This could mimic nodal disease on PET, but PET/CT can localize the activity to the pulmonary artery.

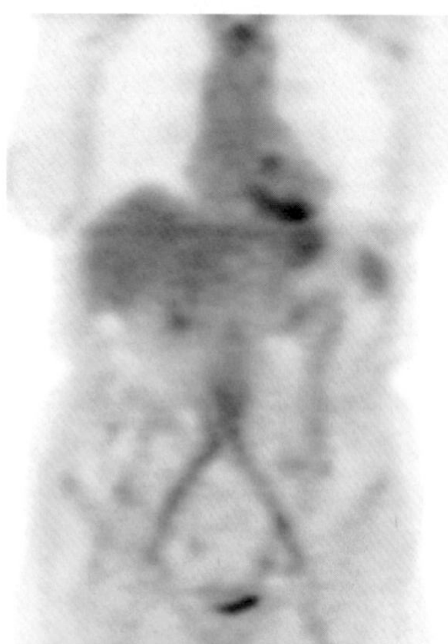

Fig. 6.56 Graft uptake. Coronal positron emission tomography scan demonstrates normal variant uptake in an aortobifemoral graft.

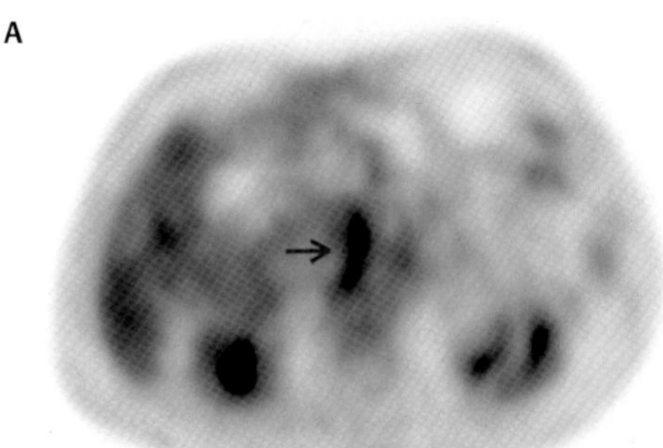

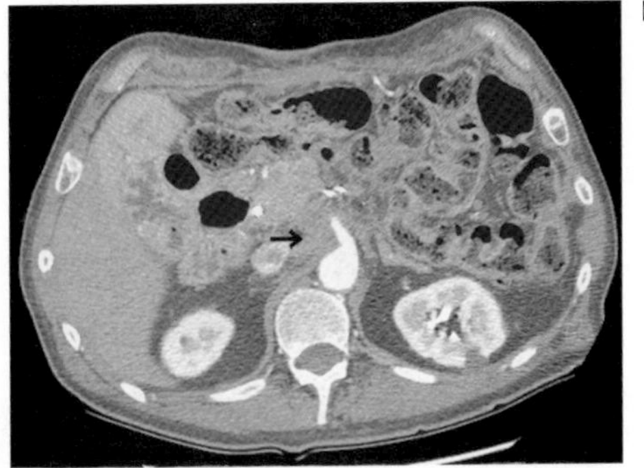

Fig. 6.57 Perivascular tumor uptake. **(A)** Axial positron emission tomography scan demonstrates a linear area of uptake in the posterior abdomen (*arrow*). Although a linear focus of uptake often suggests a benign or physiologic etiology, in this case the uptake was secondary to perivascular tumor infiltration from pancreatic cancer. Note the similarity in appearance of this uptake to the diaphragmatic crus uptake (**Fig. 6.50**). **(B)** Axial computed tomography scan at the same level demonstrates tumor infiltration (*arrow*) around the celiac axis.

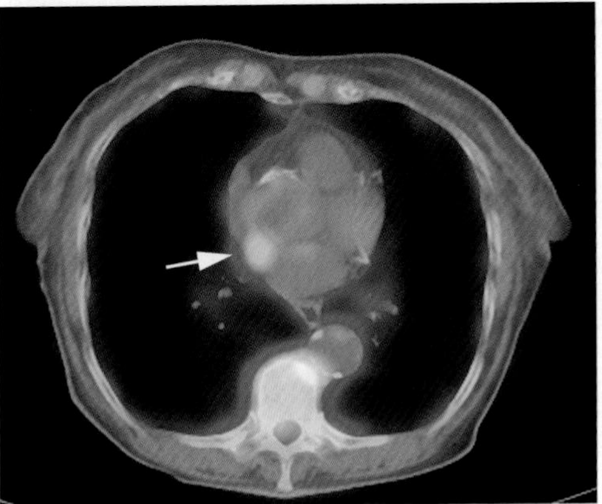

Fig. 6.58 Brown fat uptake in the interatrial septum. Axial positron emission tomography/computed tomography scan demonstrates uptake in the fat of the interatrial septum (*arrow*).

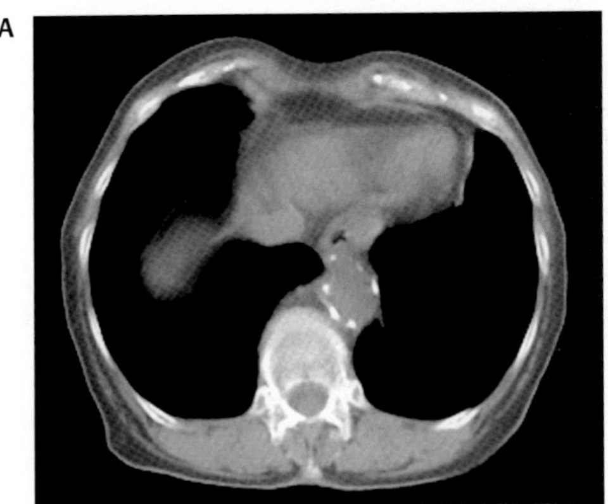

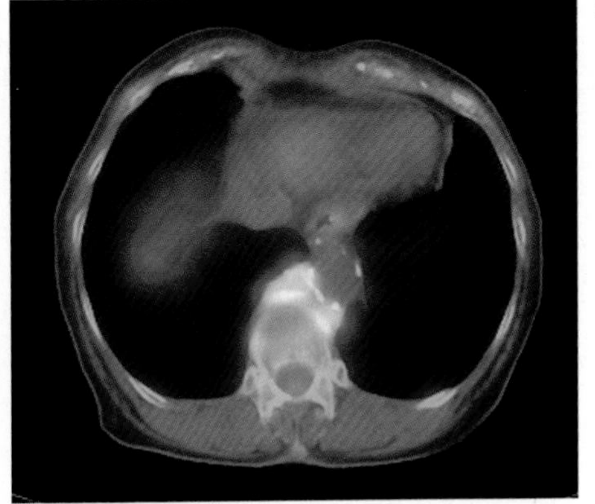

Fig. 6.59 Paraspinal brown fat uptake. **(A)** Axial computed tomography (CT) and **(B)** positron emission tomography/computed tomography (PET/CT) scans demonstrate uptake in paraspinal fat.

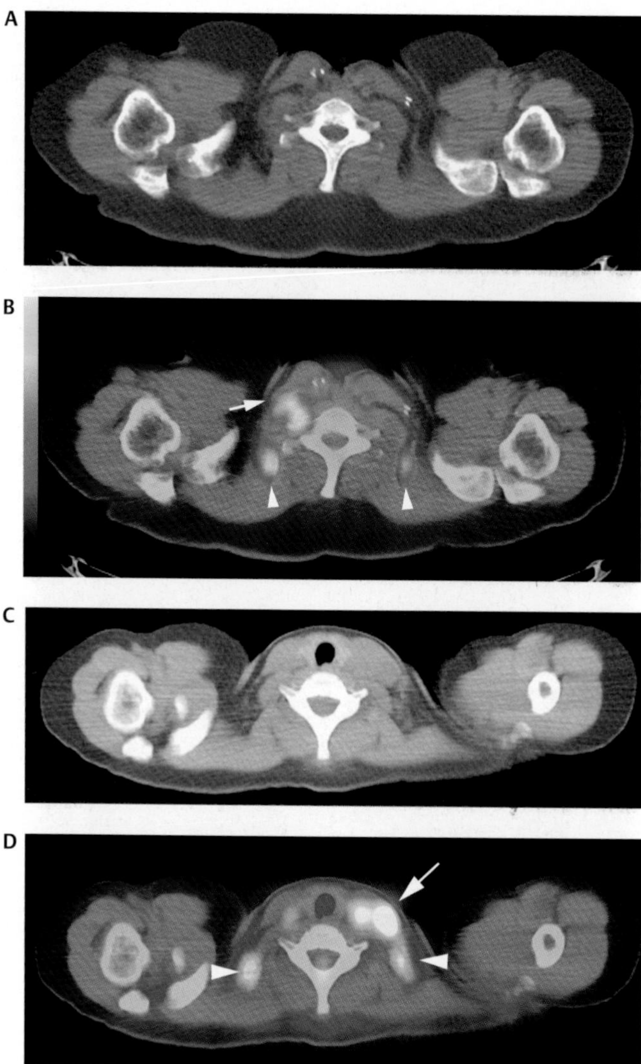

Fig. 6.60 Brown fat, muscle, and node uptake. Brown fat, muscle, and node uptake can have similar locations and appearances and occur in conjunction. **(A)** Computed tomography (CT) and **(B)** positron emission tomography (PET) exams demonstrate uptake in both brown fat (*arrowheads*) and muscle (*arrow*). The muscle uptake is atypical, as it is unilateral and could have been a worrisome finding on PET alone; however, PET/CT localizes it to muscle. In another patient, **(C)** CT and **(D)** PET/CT scans demonstrate uptake in both brown fat (*arrowheads*) and nodes (*arrow*).

in many cases. The other entities that are in the differential diagnosis are muscle uptake and node uptake. Often two or three of these entities (brown fat, muscle, and nodes) exist in conjunction, which can further complicate interpretation (**Figs. 6.49** and **6.60**).

b. *Neck/supraclavicular uptake.* Without PET/CT, brown fat uptake in the neck/supraclavicular region often cannot be differentiated from muscle uptake, but this is not clinically relevant. The usual symmetric appearance will suggest that the uptake is in either fat or muscle rather than nodes. Any area of asymmetry should raise concern for nodal disease (**Figs. 6.49** and **6.60**). If no correlative finding is seen on CT images and there is asymmetric FDG uptake, a follow-up CT is helpful, as adenopathy may be noted on subsequent CT exams (see Chapter 7).

c. Other areas. Uptake outside the neck/supraclavicular region is rarely seen in isolation. Thoracic uptake is usually accompanied by neck/supraclavicular uptake. Infradiaphragmatic uptake is usually seen in conjunction with supradiaphragmatic uptake (in particular, suprarenal uptake is usually seen in conjunction with paravertebral uptake).[75,76]

d. Practical pointers. In practice the hardest area to differentiate from nodal disease without PET/CT is mediastinal fat uptake. Usually, there is also neck/supraclavicular uptake in addition, which suggests the diagnosis, but very rarely isolated mediastinal brown fat uptake is seen.
   - A correlative CT is helpful even if fusion is not available. If no nodes are seen on CT, the uptake is likely in the mediastinal fat.
   - A useful pattern for making the diagnosis of mediastinal brown fat is involvement of only the superior mediastinum. With brown fat, the uptake will usually not extend below the aortic arch (**Figs. 6.49** and **6.61**), which would be an uncommon pattern for nodal disease.

e. If differentiation from disease is not possible, the study can be repeated with premedication (e.g., diazepam) and/or keeping the patient in a warm environment for 48 hours before the study is repeated.

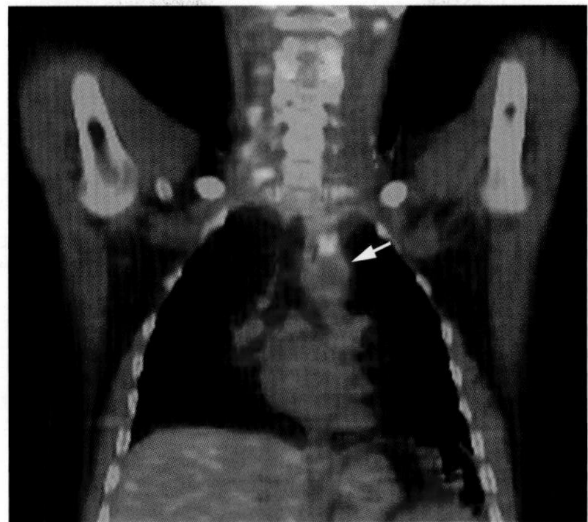

Fig 6.61 Neck and mediastinal brown fat uptake. Coronal positron emission tomography/computed tomography scan demonstrates neck and mediastinal brown fat uptake. The mediastinal brown fat uptake does not extend below the top of the aortic arch (*arrow*).

◆ Metallic Prostheses

Artifactually increased uptake can be seen around a metallic prosthesis on attenuation-corrected images. This could potentially mimic prosthesis infection. In the head and neck, areas of increased activity adjacent to the metallic dental implants (see Chapter 8) could cause false-positive tumor localization.

1. This artifact is seen with both CT and radionuclide-based attenuation-corrected images.[77] However, it is more prominent when CT-based attenuation correction is used, particularly in metallic dental implants.
2. The artifacts are enhanced by patient motion.

References

1. Bohnen N. Neurological applications. In: Wahl RL, ed. Principles and Practice of Positron Emission Tomography. Philadelphia, PA: Lippincott Williams & Wilkins; 2002:276–297
2. Loessner A, Alavi A, Lewandrowski KU, Mozley D, Souder E, Gur RE. Regional cerebral function determined by FDG-PET in healthy volunteers: normal patterns and changes with age. J Nucl Med 1995; 36(7):1141–1149
3. Minamimoto R, Takahashi N, Inoue T. FDG-PET of patients with suspected renal failure: standardized uptake values in normal tissues. Ann Nucl Med 2007;21(4):217–222
4. Fulham MJ, Brooks RA, Hallett M, Di CG. Cerebellar diaschisis revisited: pontine hypometabolism and dentate sparing. Neurology 1992;42(12):2267–2273
5. Israel O, Weiler-Sagie M, Rispler S, et al. PET/CT quantitation of the effect of patient-related factors on cardiac ^{18}F-FDG uptake. J Nucl Med 2007;48(2):234–239
6. Kaneta T, Hakamatsuka T, Takanami K, et al. Evaluation of the relationship between physiological FDG uptake in the heart and age, blood glucose level, fasting period, and hospitalization. Ann Nucl Med 2006;20(3):203–208
7. Khandani AH, Isasi CR, Donald BM. Intra-individual variability of cardiac uptake on serial whole-body ^{18}F-FDG PET. Nucl Med Commun 2005;26(9):787–791
8. Inglese E, Leva L, Matheoud R, et al. Spatial and temporal heterogeneity of regional myocardial uptake in patients without heart disease under fasting condi-

tions on repeated whole-body ^{18}F-FDG PET/CT. J Nucl Med 2007;48(10):1662–1669

9. Zanco P, Desideri A, Mobilia G, et al. Effects of left bundle branch block on myocardial FDG PET in patients without significant coronary artery stenoses. J Nucl Med 2000;41(6):973–977
10. Lin EC. Isolated papillary muscle uptake on FDG PET/CT. Clin Nucl Med 2007;32(1):76–78
11. Cook GJ, Wegner EA, Fogelman I. Pitfalls and artifacts in 18FDG PET and PET/CT oncologic imaging. Semin Nucl Med 2004;34(2):122–133
12. Fujii H, Ide M, Yasuda S, Takahashi W, Shohtsu A, Kubo A. Increased FDG uptake in the wall of the right atrium in people who participated in a cancer screening program with whole-body PET. Ann Nucl Med 1999;13(1):55–59
13. Nguyen BD. PET demonstration of left atrial appendage in chronic atrial fibrillation. Clin Nucl Med 2005;30(3):177–179
14. Beanlands RS, Muzik O, Hutchins GD, Wolfe ER Jr, Schwaiger M. Heterogeneity of regional nitrogen 13-labeled ammonia tracer distribution in the normal human heart: comparison with rubidium 82 and copper 62-labeled PTSM. J Nucl Cardiol 1994;1(3):225–235
15. Nakamoto Y, Tatsumi M, Hammoud D, Cohade C, Osman MM, Wahl RL. Normal FDG distribution patterns in the head and neck: PET/CT evaluation. Radiology 2005;234(3):879–885
16. Chen YK, Su CT, Chi KH, Cheng RH, Wang SC, Hsu CH. Utility of ^{18}F-FDG PET/CT uptake patterns in Waldeyer's ring for differentiating benign from malignant lesions in lateral pharyngeal recess of nasopharynx. J Nucl Med 2007;48(1):8–14
17. Lin EC. Focal asymmetric longus colli uptake on FDG PET/CT. Clin Nucl Med 2007;32(1):67–69
18. Shreve PD, Anzai Y, Wahl RL. Pitfalls in oncologic diagnosis with FDG PET imaging: physiologic and benign variants. Radiographics 1999;19(1):61–77
19. Shreve PD, Wahl RL. Normal variants in FDG PET Imaging. In: Wahl RL, ed. Principles and Practice of Positron Emission Tomography. Philadelphia, PA: Lippincott Williams & Wilkins; 2002;111–136
20. Karantanis D, Bogsrud TV, Wiseman GA, et al. Clinical significance of diffusely increased ^{18}F-FDG uptake in the thyroid gland. J Nucl Med 2007;48(6):896–901
21. Zincirkeser S, Sahin E, Halac M, Sager S. Standardized uptake values of normal organs on 18F-fluorodeoxyglucose positron emission tomography and computed tomography imaging. J Int Med Res 2007;35(2):231–236
22. Chen YK, Chen YL, Liao AC, Shen YY, Kao CH. Elevated ^{18}F-FDG uptake in skeletal muscles and thymus: a clue for the diagnosis of Graves' disease. Nucl Med Commun 2004;25(2):115–121
23. Kumar R, Chauhan A, Zhuang H, Chandra P, Schnall M, Alavi A. Standardized uptake values of normal breast tissue with 2-deoxy-2-[F-18]fluoro-D-glucose positron emission tomography: variations with age, breast density, and menopausal status. Mol Imaging Biol 2006;8(6):355–362
24. Lin CY, Ding HJ, Liu CS, Chen YK, Lin CC, Kao CH. Correlation between the intensity of breast FDG uptake and menstrual cycle. Acad Radiol 2007;14(8):940–944
25. Alibazoglu H, Alibazoglu B, Hollinger EF, et al. Normal thymic uptake of 2-deoxy-2[F-18]fluoro-D-glucose. Clin Nucl Med 1999;24(8):597–600
26. Ferdinand B, Gupta P, Kramer EL. Spectrum of thymic uptake at ^{18}F-FDG PET. Radiographics 2004;24(6):1611–1616
27. El-Bawab H, Al-Sugair AA, Rafay M, Hajjar W, Mahdy M, Al-Kattan K. Role of flourine-18 fluorodeoxyglucose positron emission tomography in thymic pathology. Eur J Cardiothorac Surg 2007;31(4):731–736
28. Sung YM, Lee KS, Kim BT, Choi JY, Shim YM, Yi CA. ^{18}F-FDG PET/CT of thymic epithelial tumors: usefulness for distinguishing and staging tumor subgroups. J Nucl Med 2006;47(10):1628–1634
29. Smith CS, Schoder H, Yeung HW. Thymic extension in the superior mediastinum in patients with thymic hyperplasia: potential cause of false-positive findings on ^{18}F-FDG PET/CT. AJR Am J Roentgenol 2007;188(6):1716–1721
30. Jacene HA, Cohade C, Wahl RL. F-18 FDG PET/CT in acute respiratory distress syndrome: a case report. Clin Nucl Med 2004;29(12):786–788
31. Digumarthy SR, Fischman AJ, Kwek BH, Aquino SL. Fluorodeoxyglucose positron emission tomography pattern of pulmonary lymphangitic carcinomatosis. J Comput Assist Tomogr 2005;29(3):346–349
32. Kamel EM, McKee TA, Calcagni ML, et al. Occult lung infarction may induce false interpretation of ^{18}F-FDG PET in primary staging of pulmonary malignancies. Eur J Nucl Med Mol Imaging 2005;32(6):641–646
33. Lyburn ID, Lowe JE, Wong WL. Idiopathic pulmonary fibrosis on F-18 FDG positron emission tomography. Clin Nucl Med 2005;30(1):27
34. Ollenberger GP, Knight S, Tauro AJ. False-positive FDG positron emission tomography in pulmonary amyloidosis. Clin Nucl Med 2004;29(10):657–658
35. Kong FM, Frey KA, Quint LE, et al. A pilot study of [^{18}F]fluorodeoxyglucose positron emission tomography scans during and after radiation-based therapy in patients with non small-cell lung cancer. J Clin Oncol 2007;25(21):3116–3123
36. Hassaballa HA, Cohen ES, Khan AJ, Ali A, Bonomi P, Rubin DB. Positron emission tomography demonstrates radiation-induced changes to nonirradiated lungs in lung cancer patients treated with radiation and chemotherapy. Chest 2005;128(3):1448–1452
37. Asad S, Aquino SL, Piyavisetpat N, Fischman AJ. False-positive FDG positron emission tomography uptake in nonmalignant chest abnormalities. AJR Am J Roentgenol 2004;182(4):983–989
38. Truong MT, Erasmus JJ, Munden RF, et al. Focal FDG uptake in mediastinal brown fat mimicking malignancy: a potential pitfall resolved on PET/CT. AJR Am J Roentgenol 2004;183(4):1127–1132
39. Lin E. F-18 fluorodeoxyglucose uptake in a benign gastric ulcer. Clin Nucl Med 2007;32(6):462–463
40. Koga H, Sasaki M, Kuwabara Y, et al. An analysis of the physiological FDG uptake pattern in the stomach. Ann Nucl Med 2003;17(8):733–738
41. Salaun PY, Grewal RK, Dodamane I, Yeung HW, Larson SM, Strauss HW. An analysis of the ^{18}F-FDG uptake pattern in the stomach. J Nucl Med 2005;46(1):48–51
42. Otsuka H, Graham MM, Kubo A, Nishitani H. The effect of oral contrast on large bowel activity in FDG-PET/CT. Ann Nucl Med 2005;19(2):101–108
43. Kamel EM, Thumshirn M, Truninger K, et al. Significance of incidental ^{18}F-FDG accumulations in the gastrointestinal tract in PET/CT: correlation with endoscopic and histopathologic results. J Nucl Med 2004;45(11):1804–1810

44. Gutman F, Alberini JL, Wartski M, et al. Incidental colonic focal lesions detected by FDG PET/CT. AJR Am J Roentgenol 2005;185(2):495–500
45. Israel O, Yefremov N, Bar-Shalom R, et al. PET/CT detection of unexpected gastrointestinal foci of ^{18}F-FDG uptake: incidence, localization patterns, and clinical significance. J Nucl Med 2005;46(5):758–762
46. Iozzo P, Geisler F, Oikonen V, et al. Insulin stimulates liver glucose uptake in humans: an ^{18}F-FDG PET Study. J Nucl Med 2003;44(5):682–689
47. Maldjian PD, Ghesani N, Ahmed S, Liu Y. Adenomyomatosis of the gallbladder: another cause for a "hot" gallbladder on ^{18}F-FDG PET. AJR Am J Roentgenol 2007;189(1):W36–W38
48. Sugawara Y, Zasadny KR, Kison PV, Baker LH, Wahl RL. Splenic fluorodeoxyglucose uptake increased by granulocyte colony-stimulating factor therapy: PET imaging results. J Nucl Med 1999;40(9):1456–1462
49. Shulkin BL, Thompson NW, Shapiro B, Francis IR, Sisson JC. Pheochromocytomas: imaging with 2-[fluorine-18]fluoro-2-deoxy-D-glucose PET. Radiology 1999;212(1):35–41
50. Ludwig V, Rice MH, Martin WH, Kelley MC, Delbeke D. 2-Deoxy-2-[^{18}F]fluoro-D-glucose positron emission tomography uptake in a giant adrenal myelolipoma. Mol Imaging Biol 2002;4(5):355–358
51. Lerman H, Metser U, Grisaru D, Fishman A, Lievshitz G, Even-Sapir E. Normal and abnormal ^{18}F-FDG endometrial and ovarian uptake in pre- and postmenopausal patients: assessment by PET/CT. J Nucl Med 2004;45(2):266–271
52. Nishizawa S, Inubushi M, Okada H. Physiological ^{18}F-FDG uptake in the ovaries and uterus of healthy female volunteers. Eur J Nucl Med Mol Imaging 2005;32(5):549–556
53. Lin E. FDG PET appearance of a postpartum uterus. Clin Nucl Med 2006;31(3):159–160
54. Kim SK, Kang KW, Roh JW, Sim JS, Lee ES, Park SY. Incidental ovarian ^{18}F-FDG accumulation on PET: correlation with the menstrual cycle. Eur J Nucl Med Mol Imaging 2005;32(7):757–763
55. Nishizawa S, Inubushi M, Ozawa F, Kido A, Okada H. Physiological FDG uptake in the ovaries after hysterectomy. Ann Nucl Med 2007;21(6):345–348
56. Pandit-Taskar N, Sinha A, Gonen M, et al. Testicular uptake in [18]FDG PET scan. J Nucl Med 2001;5:287
57. Gorospe L, Raman S, Echeveste J, Avril N, Herrero Y, Herna Ndez S. Whole-body PET/CT: spectrum of physiological variants, artifacts and interpretative pitfalls in cancer patients. Nucl Med Commun 2005;26(8):671–687
58. Fayad LM, Cohade C, Wahl RL, Fishman EK. Sacral fractures: a potential pitfall of FDG positron emission tomography. AJR Am J Roentgenol 2003;181(5):1239–1243
59. Hollinger EF, Alibazoglu H, Ali A, Green A, Lamonica G. Hematopoietic cytokine-mediated FDG uptake simulates the appearance of diffuse metastatic disease on whole-body PET imaging. Clin Nucl Med 1998;23(2):93–98
60. Kazama T, Swanston N, Podoloff DA, Macapinlac HA. Effect of colony-stimulating factor and conventional- or high-dose chemotherapy on FDG uptake in bone marrow. Eur J Nucl Med Mol Imaging 2005;32(12):1406–1411
61. Basu S, Nair N. "Cold" vertebrae on F-18 FDG PET: causes and characteristics. Clin Nucl Med 2006;31(8):445–450
62. Lin EC. FDG PET/CT flip flop phenomenon in treated lymphoma of bone. Clin Nucl Med 2006;31(12):803–805
63. Aflalo-Hazan V, Gutman F, Kerrou K, Montravers F, Grahek D, Talbot JN. Increased FDG uptake by bone marrow in major beta-thalassemia. Clin Nucl Med 2005;30(11):754–755
64. Inoue K, Okada K, Harigae H, et al. Diffuse bone marrow uptake on F-18 FDG PET in patients with myelodysplastic syndromes. Clin Nucl Med 2006;31(11):721–723
65. Takalkar A, Yu JQ, Kumar R, Xiu Y, Alavi A, Zhuang H. Diffuse bone marrow accumulation of FDG in a patient with chronic myeloid leukemia mimics hematopoietic cytokine-mediated FDG uptake on positron emission tomography. Clin Nucl Med 2004;29(10):637–639
66. Rosen RS, Fayad L, Wahl RL. Increased ^{18}F-FDG uptake in degenerative disease of the spine: characterization with ^{18}F-FDG PET/CT. J Nucl Med 2006;47(8):1274–1280
67. Elzinga EH, van der Laken CJ, Comans EF, Lammertsma AA, Dijkmans BA, Voskuyl AE. 2-Deoxy-2-[F-18]fluoro-D-glucose joint uptake on positron emission tomography images: rheumatoid arthritis ver HIF-1sus osteoarthritis. Mol Imaging Biol 2007;9(6):357–360
68. Lin E. Baastrup's disease (kissing spine) demonstrated by FDG PET/CT. Skeletal Radiol 2008;37(2):173–175
69. Resnick D. Degenerative diseases of the vertebral column. Radiology 1985;156(1):3–14
70. Tatsumi M, Cohade C, Nakamoto Y, Wahl RL. Fluorodeoxyglucose uptake in the aortic wall at PET/CT: possible finding for active atherosclerosis. Radiology 2003;229(3):831–837
71. Keidar Z, Engel A, Hoffman A, Israel O, Nitecki S. Prosthetic vascular graft infection: the role of ^{18}F-FDG PET/CT. J Nucl Med 2007;48(8):1230–1236
72. Cohade C, Mourtzikos KA, Wahl RL. "USA-fat": prevalence is related to ambient outdoor temperature-evaluation with ^{18}F-FDG PET/CT. J Nucl Med 2003;44(8):1267–1270
73. Cohade C, Osman M, Pannu HK, Wahl RL. Uptake in supraclavicular area fat ("USA-fat"): description on ^{18}F-FDG PET/CT. J Nucl Med 2003;44(2):170–176
74. Yeung HW, Grewal RK, Gonen M, Schoder H, Larson SM. Patterns of (18)F-FDG uptake in adipose tissue and muscle: a potential source of false-positives for PET. J Nucl Med 2003;44(11):1789–1796
75. Bar-Shalom R, Gaitini D, Keidar Z, Israel O. Non-malignant FDG uptake in infradiaphragmatic adipose tissue: a new site of physiological tracer biodistribution characterised by PET/CT. Eur J Nucl Med Mol Imaging 2004;31(8):1105–1113
76. Kim S, Krynyckyi BR, Machac J, Kim CK. Concomitant paravertebral FDG uptake helps differentiate supraclavicular and suprarenal brown fat uptake from malignant uptake when CT coregistration is not available. Clin Nucl Med 2006;31(3):127–130
77. Goerres GW, Ziegler SI, Burger C, Berthold T, Von Schulthess GK, Buck A. Artifacts at PET and PET/CT caused by metallic hip prosthetic material. Radiology 2003;226(2):577–584

7

The Interpretation of FDG PET Studies

Eugene C. Lin and Abass Alavi

Optimal fluorodeoxyglucose positron emission tomography (FDG PET) interpretation requires attention to many details both before and after the examination is performed.

◆ Limitations of PET

PET has a wide range of potential applications, with varying degrees of scientific evidence for the efficacy of each application. It is helpful to have a process for screening less common requests for PET (e.g., the "C" level indications in this text). Knowledge of PET is somewhat variable among referring physicians, and it is not uncommon to receive requests for indications for which PET would be unlikely to provide the expected answers. In cases where PET is of marginal value, the referring physician should be made aware of the potential limitations before the examination is performed. This is important to avoid generalization of the information provided in these settings to the overall role of the test in other indications. Screening unusual requests will avoid situations where the referring physician believes that PET will provide specific information that it is unlikely to provide based upon available knowledge. Possible limitations of PET include the following.

1. ***Limited/inadequate evidence***
   a. *Limited accuracy*. There are disease processes where PET has either or both poor sensitivity and specificity (e.g., FDG PET for detection of metastatic prostate cancer).
   b. *Limited management effect/cost-effectiveness*. PET may not change management for some potential applications regardless of the results, or it may not be cost-effective relative to other options (e.g., PET is not cost-effective in differentiating benign from malignant thyroid nodules, and it does not change management, as it is not accurate enough to preclude biopsy).
   c. *Limited evidence*. There are many potential applications for which the literature is limited at this time. In these cases, PET may be potentially useful, but it may be unclear what additive benefit PET would have over conventional imaging techniques.
2. ***Technical limitations.*** PET is limited in the evaluation of small lesions. In some cases, PET may be limited for lesions < 1 cm. This can be used as a threshold, but it is not a definite cutoff. Lesions < 1 cm are detectable, but with lower sensitivity. Detectability of lesions in the 5 to 7 mm range has been

reported in clinical studies; in our experience, lesions < 5 mm in size can be detected if metabolically active and in locations where motion and background activity are limited.

a. Lesion detectability is dependent largely upon location. Lesion detectability is increased in areas with minimal motion (e.g., the retroperitoneum, neck, and extremities) and minimal background physiologic activity (e.g., the lungs and retroperitoneum). It is often possible to easily detect uptake in lesions < 1 cm in certain locations (see Chapter 23). Areas with large amounts of physiologic activity (e.g., the liver) will have decreased detection rates for small lesions. In the lungs, background activity is low, but respiratory motion decreases detection, particularly in the lung bases. Respiratory misregistration artifact specific to PET/computed tomography (CT) scans would further limit lesion detection in the lung bases.

b. PET is sometimes requested for evaluation of equivocal lesions that may be too small to detect by PET. It is optimal to evaluate larger lesions, but lesions < 1 cm in size could be considered for evaluation depending upon the location. In these cases the referring physician should be made aware that false-negative results are possible, and only positive results are reliable. The PET study may be very helpful if positive, as this is very specific for malignancy in small lesions. Standardized uptake values (SUVs) will likely be of limited value due to partial volume effects.

3. ***Patient limitations.*** Patient factors such as recent chemotherapy or radiation or inability to lie still may limit optimal examination. In most cases, these situations can be resolved with further communication with the referring physician and instituting measures such as delaying the exam or sedation.

◆ Interpretation of PET

In general, FDG PET is a very sensitive but less-specific modality (although PET can be very specific in certain settings). Therefore, an approach to optimal interpretation is to maximize specificity. Specificity can be maximized by

- Correlation with clinical data
- Correlation between all available PET data
- Correlation with anatomical imaging

Correlation with Clinical Data

It is essential that pertinent information about the history of the illness and relevant ancillary studies are collected before interpreting PET. This is especially true for PET compared with other imaging modalities, given the numerous potential pitfalls. Although the interpreting physician may choose to review the images initially without benefit of patient history, the final interpretation should take into consideration all available and pertinent data related to the disease process. Clinical pretest probability is often useful in the interpretation of PET findings.

1. If the pretest probability of disease is low (e.g., the incidence of mediastinal metastases in peripheral lung cancer or residual disease after treatment of early-stage Hodgkin disease), then a negative PET is highly predictive of lack of disease, and a positive PET is more likely to be false-positive.
2. If the pretest probability of disease is high (e.g., a spiculated lung nodule), a negative PET is more likely to be false-negative, and a positive PET is highly predictive of disease.

Correlation among All PET Data

For typical PET scans, three sets of data are provided: maximum intensity projection (MIP), nonattenuation corrected (NAC), and attenuation corrected (AC). The NAC and AC images are typically reconstructed in axial, sagittal, and coronal planes. Findings on all datasets should be closely correlated.

1. ***MIP images.*** The MIP image is reviewed in a rotating format and allows review of the entire volume imaged in different projections. In general, MIP images are less sensitive than the tomographic sets, but they allow a

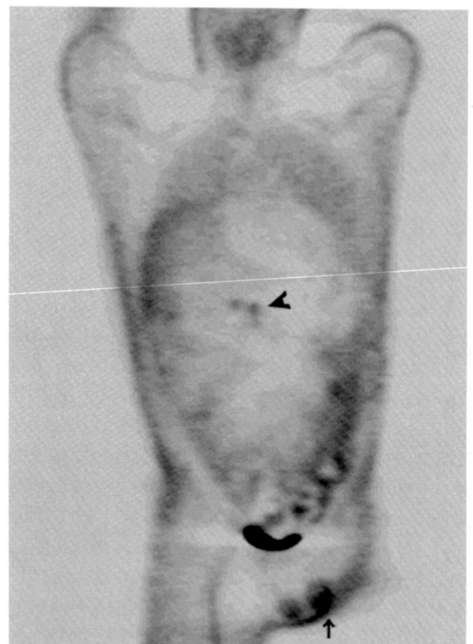

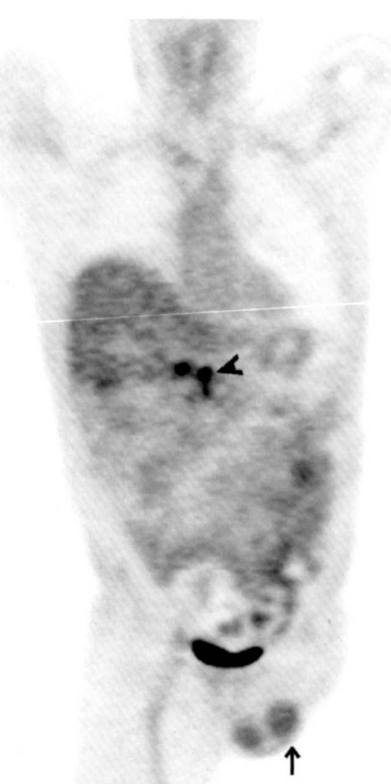

Fig. 7.1 Differences between nonattenuation-corrected and attenuation-corrected positron emission tomography images. **(A)** Coronal nonattenuation-corrected image demonstrates increased skin activity, increased lung activity, and central decreased activity, including a photopenic mediastinum. Note that the superficial testes (*arrow*) appear more intense than central abdominal nodes (*arrowhead*). **(B)** Coronal attenuation-corrected image at the same level demonstrates that the central nodes (*arrowhead*) are actually more intense than the testes (*arrow*).

complete overview of the extent of disease and help define relationships of the abnormalities to each other and to anatomical sites.

2. ***NAC images.*** NAC images can be distinguished from AC images (**Fig. 7.1**) by
   - High skin activity
   - High lung activity
   - Decreased central activity (e.g., low activity in the deep structures of the mediastinum and abdomen)
3. ***NAC advantages***
   - *Low noise.* AC adds noise to the study, which can cause false-positive results. In addition, dense areas can cause artifacts on AC images if CT is used for AC (see Chapter 8). Review of NAC images may be vital to identify these false-positive findings.
   - If a potential lesion is seen on AC images but not on NAC images, the possibility of a false-positive secondary to artifact (noise or dense material) should be considered. This is more of a consideration if the lesion is peripheral (because a central lesion may not be visualized on NAC images secondary to attenuation).
   - *Detectability*. Some lesions are better detected on NAC images. In our experience, detection of lung (**Fig. 7.2**), bone (**Fig. 7.3**), or superficial lesions may be superior on NAC images.
     - o A clinical study suggests that NAC may be superior for lung lesion detection,[1] but a phantom study suggests that NAC may be superior for abdominal lesions and inferior for lung lesions.[2] A clinical PET/CT study[3] did not demonstrate a difference between AC and NAC images in the detection of pulmonary metastases.
     - o Lesions in areas of uniform attenuation (e.g., the abdomen) will demonstrate greater contrast on NAC images, but lesions in areas of nonuniform attenuation (e.g., the thorax) will demonstrate greater contrast on AC images.[2]

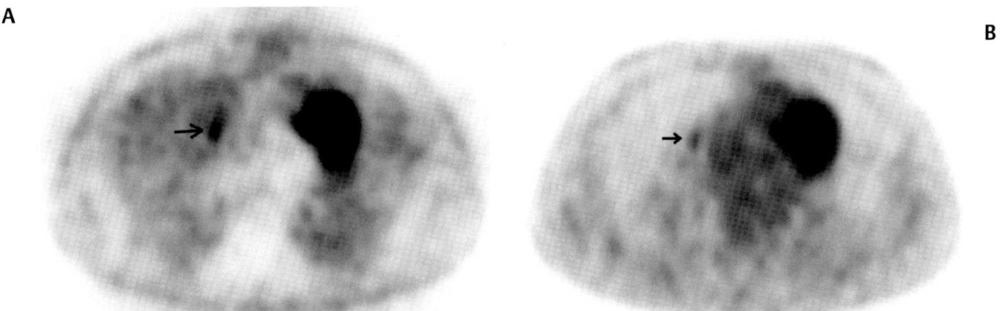

Fig. 7.2 Lung nodule detection—attenuation corrected versus nonattenuation corrected. **(A)** A right lung nodule (*arrow*) is much better visualized on a nonattenuation-corrected axial positron emission tomography scan than on **(B)** an attenuation-corrected scan.

- o Superficial lesions may be better visualized on NAC images due to the increased activity of peripheral structures. However, if these lesions are close to the intense skin activity on NAC images, they may be obscured.

4. ***AC images.*** AC images are the standard format for review of PET studies, but AC images should not be reviewed alone without also reviewing the NAC data.

a. *AC advantages*[4]

- *Anatomical localization.* Without AC, it is often difficult to localize lesions accurately. In particular, AC is very helpful for side-by-side CT correlation.
- *SUV measurement.* AC must be performed if SUV is measured (otherwise the measured SUV would depend upon the amount of attenuation).
- *Lesion detection.* Although there is no published evidence that AC images detect more lesions in most clinical settings, NAC images can potentially miss deeply seated lesions secondary to attenuation.
- *Accurate lesion size/shape.* NAC images will distort lesion size and shape (the lesion is elongated in the direction with the least attenuation) (**Fig. 7.4**).

b. *AC disadvantages*

- *Image noise.* AC images are noisier than NAC images.
- *Additional time.* Generating an attenuation map for AC takes additional time. This is less of an issue with CT-based AC.
- *Artifacts.* Typically, these artifacts are created at areas of high density (barium, iodine, metal) and appear with falsely high intensity; they are most pronounced with CT-based AC (see Chapters 6 and 8). Misregistration artifacts are specific to the use of CT for AC (see Chapter 8).

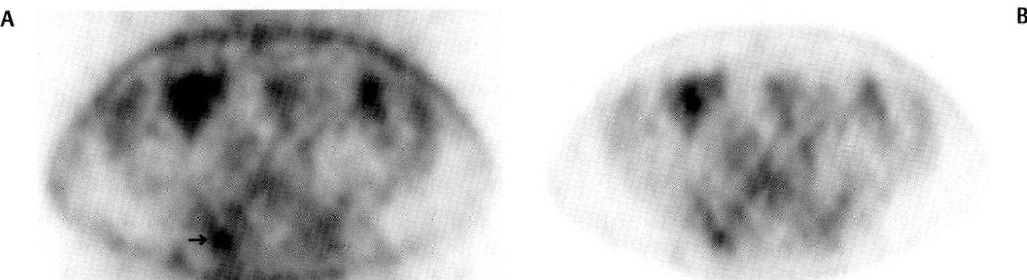

Fig. 7.3 Bone lesion detection—attenuation corrected versus nonattenuation corrected. **(A)** A bone metastasis to the sacrum (*arrow*) is seen on a nonattenuation-corrected axial positron emission tomography scan but **(B)** was not identified prospectively on an attenuation-corrected scan.

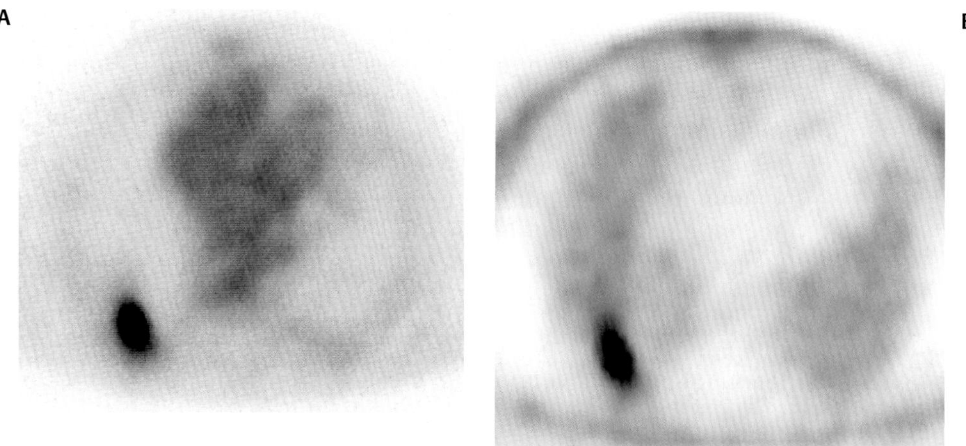

Fig. 7.4 Distortion of lesion shape on nonattenuation-corrected positron emission tomography images. **(A)** Axial attenuation-corrected image demonstrates a right lung nodule. **(B)** Axial nonattenuation-corrected image of the same nodule demonstrates that nodule appears smaller in the horizontal dimension due to more attenuating tissue in this direction. The overall shape of the nodule is more elongated.

Correlation with Anatomical Imaging

Correlation with cross-sectional modalities such as CT and magnetic resonance imaging (MRI) can be very helpful in improving the specificity of PET. This can be done visually, with image fusion, or with a dedicated PET/CT scanner.

1. It is important not to rely on reports, but to actually view the anatomical images in all cases even if the anatomical study was interpreted as negative. The contrast between the lesion and background is usually much greater with PET than with other imaging modalities. As a result, many abnormalities on anatomical images will be seen only retrospectively, after attention is directed to the specific region by a positive PET scan (**Fig. 7.5**).

2. Anatomical correlation is primarily helpful in

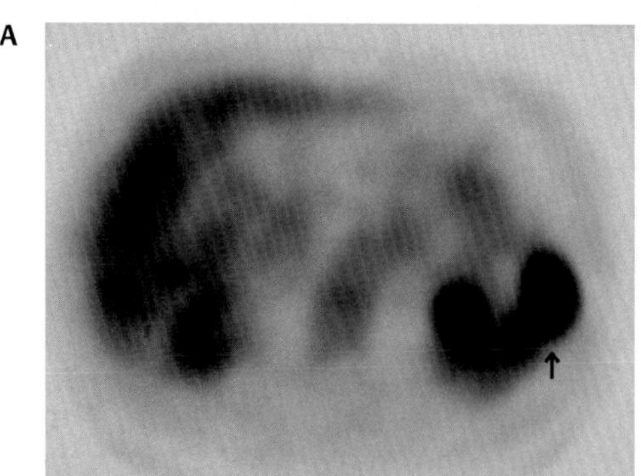

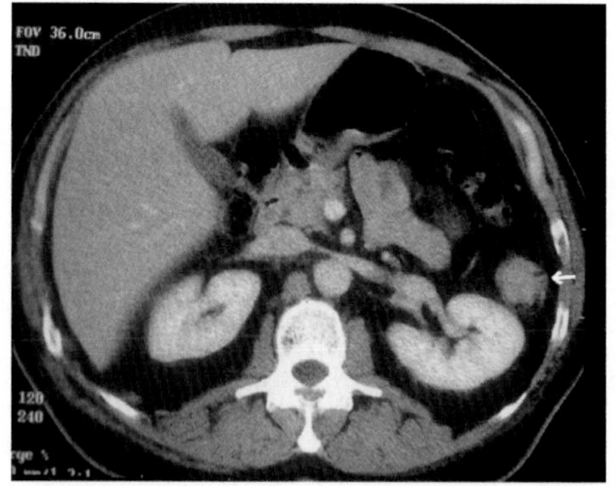

Fig. 7.5 Colon cancer found incidentally. **(A)** Axial positron emission tomography (PET) scan shows an intense focus of uptake (*arrow*) lateral to the left kidney. This was thought initially to be exophytic from the kidney. **(B)** Computed tomography (CT) scan at the same level demonstrates soft tissue filling the colonic lumen (*arrow*). This was not seen prospectively on the CT, as there was no associated colonic wall thickening or pericolonic abnormality. Both PET and CT scans were necessary to make this diagnosis: the lesion was obvious on PET but not seen on CT; however, the initial anatomical localization on PET was incorrect, and retrospective correlation with CT was necessary to localize the uptake correctly.

a. *Localizing lesions.* In many cases, anatomical correlation is necessary to localize a lesion seen on PET correctly to a specific site (**Fig. 7.5**). This is particularly true with lesions that are peripheral in location (see **Fig. 6.41**, p. 65).

b. *Identifying false-positives.* Many false-positive sources of uptake can be identified as such after anatomical correlation.

c. *Confirming equivocal PET findings/increasing interpretation confidence.* Interpreter confidence in a PET finding improves considerably by identifying a corresponding abnormality on anatomical imaging (which is often seen only retrospectively). Although both the PET and CT findings may be equivocal in isolation when combined, they can be confidently interpreted as a positive finding (**Fig. 7.6**).

Pearls

1. ***Lesion size.*** Lesion size on anatomical imaging should influence how the PET findings are interpreted.
   a. *Small lesions.* PET has decreased sensitivity but increased specificity in small lesions.
      - A small lesion (e.g., < 1 cm) with increased uptake is more likely to be malignant. Any definite uptake should be considered worrisome for malignancy because visible increased uptake in a small focus suggests a highly hypermetabolic lesion (see Chapter 24).
      - SUVs in small lesions should be interpreted with caution because SUVs are often low even in malignancy secondary to partial volume effects. Similarly, the degree of uptake as judged by visual criteria may be relatively minimal and of limited value in a small malignant lesion.
      - A small lesion with no uptake may be falsely negative. A small malignant focus with a mild to moderate degree of uptake may go undetected due to confounding factors, such as motion and partial volume effects.
   b. *Large lesions.* PET has increased sensitivity but possibly decreased specificity in large lesions.
      - A large lesion with a negative PET study is more likely to be benign. A malignant focus large enough to result in a substantial structural abnormality should be detectable on PET if it is metabolically active. Note that this may not apply to mildly enlarged lesions (e.g., a 1.5 cm lymph node); in these cases, the amount of tumor burden causing the mild enlargement may not be

A

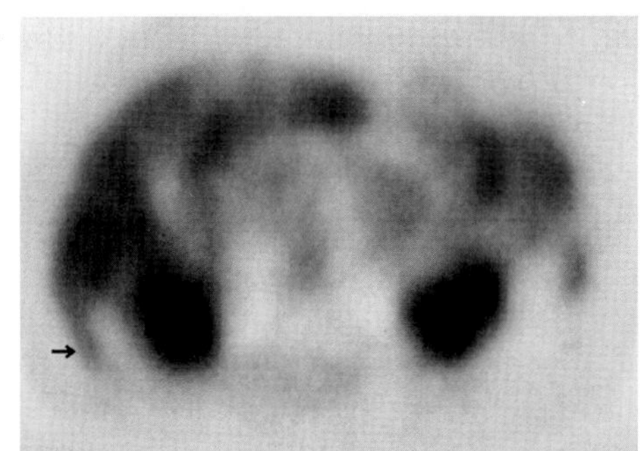

B

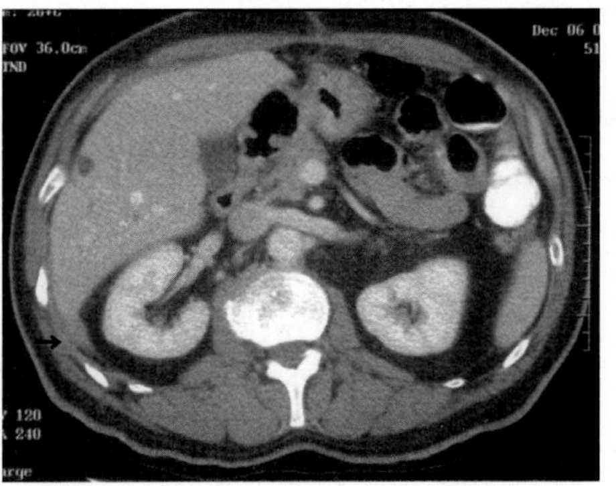

Fig. 7.6 Peritoneal metastasis from colon cancer. **(A)** Axial fluorodeoxyglucose positron emission tomography (FDG PET) scan shows a vertical linear area of uptake posterior to the right liver (*arrow*). This was detected on initial review of the PET, but it would be difficult to call it definitively abnormal as it is not different in intensity from the liver (potentially it could represent an unusual configuration of the liver). **(B)** Computed tomography (CT) scan at the same level shows abnormal soft tissue with the same linear configuration (*arrow*) as seen on PET. This was not detected prospectively on CT, but in conjunction with the PET findings, it is definitely abnormal, as there should be no normal soft tissue in this location. The CT correlation in this case greatly increases interpreter confidence in the PET finding.

substantial, and a negative PET in these situations should still raise concern for false-negative results.
  - A large lesion with a positive PET study may be falsely positive. Infectious or inflammatory processes severe enough to cause substantial anatomical enlargement may have substantial FDG uptake.

2. ***Lesion location.*** The value of CT correlation often depends upon the location of the lesion. A true-positive PET finding may have no anatomical correlate in some areas and almost always has a correlate in other areas. Two questions to consider are
   a. What are the potential etiologies for the positive PET finding?
   b. Would these potential etiologies be detected by CT?
   - In certain anatomical sites, it is very unlikely that a true-positive PET finding would have no CT correlate. A focal area of mediastinal uptake should have a CT correlate (e.g., a normal-sized node on CT). If correlation is accurate, a node large enough to cause PET uptake should be detected by CT, unless it is in an area where small nodes may be difficult to visualize (e.g., the hilum). For example, an area of increased uptake in the mediastinum without a corresponding node, localizing to mediastinal fat, can be interpreted as mediastinal brown fat uptake.
   - In other anatomical sites, there may be no CT correlate for true-positive PET findings. For example, unexplained focal PET uptake in the abdomen is often due to colonic adenomas or less likely peritoneal metastases. Colonic adenomas are not usually detected on CT, and detection of peritoneal metastases by CT is limited. In these cases, further work-up is usually necessary.[5]

Pitfalls

There are several potential pitfalls when correlating PET and anatomical imaging studies:

1. ***Motion.*** Because PET scan is performed during free breathing, whereas a CT scan may be acquired during a breath hold, inaccurate localization of lesions may result. Other structures such as the head and breast may also change in position between the CT and PET examinations. This is predominantly a factor during PET/CT scans, but it may affect side-by-side PET and CT interpretation as well.
2. ***Importance of correlation with recent studies.*** Correlation with old examinations can result in interpretive error, particularly in posttherapy states (**Fig. 7.7**).
3. ***Delayed resolution of PET findings.*** It is common for inflammatory processes to have increased FDG uptake weeks or months after resolution of the process on anatomical images. This may result in an apparent discrepancy between PET and recent anatomical imaging. Thus, if a current anatomical study does not demonstrate a corresponding finding, it is important to review preceding anatomical studies as well (**Fig. 7.8**).
4. ***Difficulty in correlation.*** In the head, neck, and pelvis, visual correlation of PET and CT can be difficult due to lack of anatomical landmarks or physiologic activity (e.g., bladder). In these cases, PET/CT or fusion imaging is usually necessary. Accurate correlation in the abdomen and pelvis is often possible with side-by-side reading of PET and CT images.

◆ Reporting

1. ***SUV.*** For oncological patients with lesions, it is important to report SUVs of index lesions, even if these measurements are not used for interpretation of the current study. If the patient is restudied at a later date, the SUVs will be necessary to assess the course of the disease and response to treatment. In addition, it may be helpful to report the method of SUV calculation and the time of imaging after injection, as these factors may be helpful for comparison of SUVs if the patient is evaluated at another institution in the future.
2. The impression should state clearly any potential limitations of PET for the specific

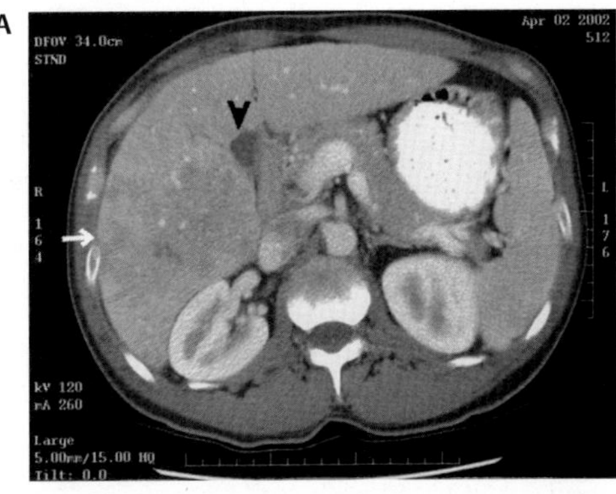

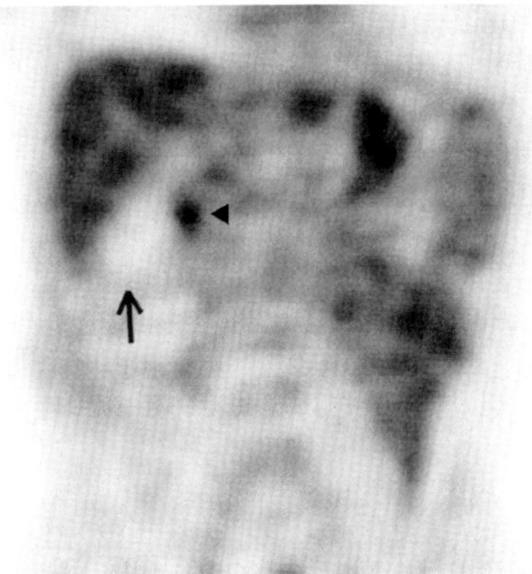

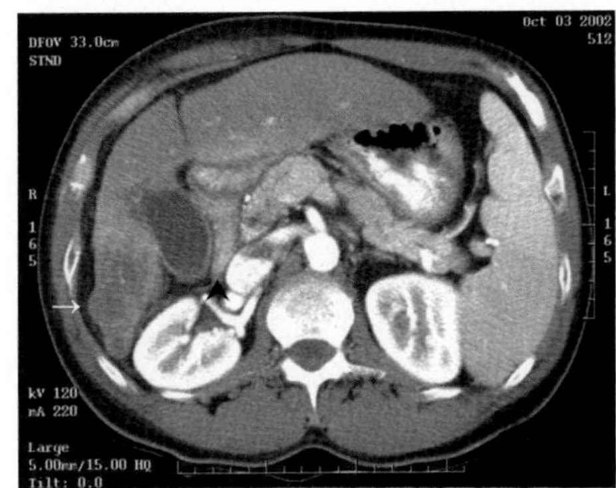

Fig. 7.7 False-positive from correlation with old examination—hepatocellular carcinoma status postradiofrequency (RF) ablation. **(A)** Computed tomography (CT) scan demonstrates a large mass in the right lobe of the liver (*arrow*). The gallbladder (*arrowhead*) is small. The patient underwent RF ablation of the mass after this CT. **(B)** Coronal positron emission tomography (PET) scan performed 3 months after the ablation demonstrates a large photopenic area (*arrow*) with a focus of uptake at the medial margin (*arrowhead*). As a recent CT scan was not available, correlation was made by the CT scan in **(A)**. The photopenic area was initially thought to represent the ablated mass, with the medial activity representing residual tumor. **(C)** However, CT performed a day after the PET scan demonstrates that the right lobe of the liver has greatly decreased in size postablation (*arrow*). The gallbladder is much larger than on the previous CT scan. The photopenic area on the PET scan is actually the gallbladder, and the medial activity thought to represent residual tumor is in the duodenum (*arrowhead*).

disease process in question. For example, if there is a small lesion seen on CT that could potentially be missed on PET due to size, the report should state that a negative PET study does not exclude active disease due to the limited resolution of this modality.

3. The relevance of PET findings should be stated explicitly. For example, if the patient has had a recent CT with a nonspecific 1.5 cm hypodense liver lesion, rather than reporting that no abnormal liver uptake is identified, it is more helpful to report "the 1.5 cm hypodense liver lesion seen on CT does not demonstrate increased uptake on PET, suggesting that it is most likely a benign lesion. However, a low-grade hepatocellular carcinoma may appear hypometabolic on PET imaging."
4. Lesion size is not well evaluated by PET, as the apparent size is largely dependent upon the intensity of uptake (see Chapter 24). Unless obvious changes are present, comments about changes in lesion size evaluated by PET alone should be avoided.

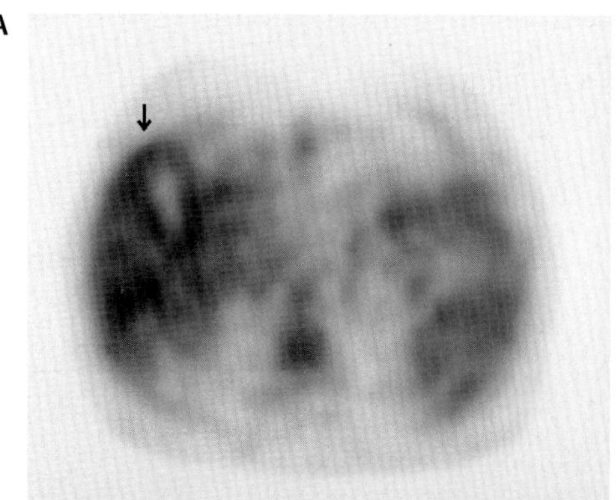

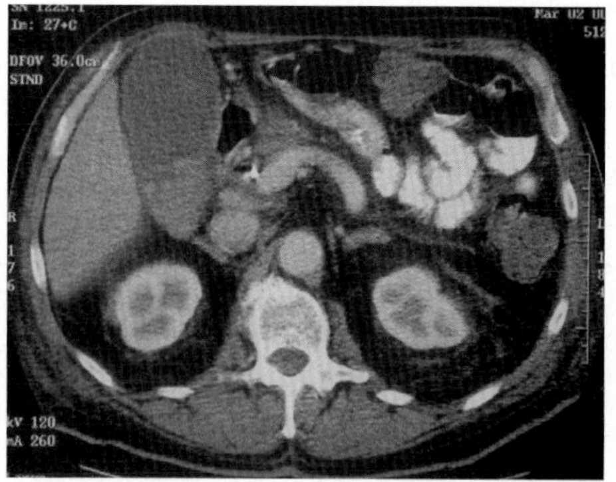

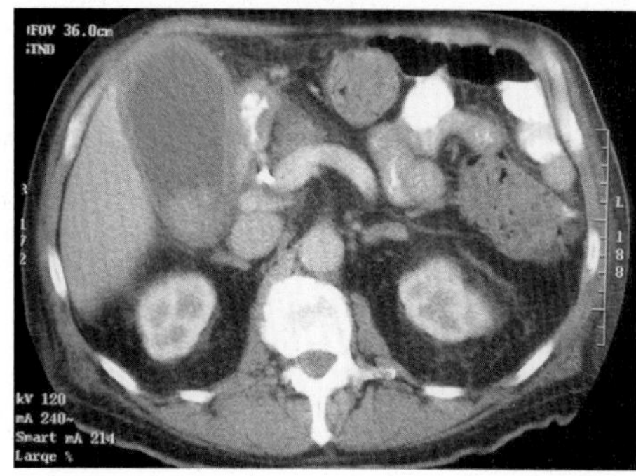

Fig. 7.8 Gallbladder wall inflammation. **(A)** Axial fluorodeoxyglucose positron emission tomography (FDG PET) scan shows increased uptake in the gallbladder wall (*arrow*). **(B)** Computed tomography (CT) scan at the same level done 1 day before the PET shows sludge in the gallbladder but a normal-appearing gallbladder wall. **(C)** CT scan done 1 month before shows a thickened gallbladder wall. Inflammatory processes will often resolve on anatomical imaging before PET imaging.

◆ Follow-up

The first step toward follow-up of abnormalities noted on PET should include correlation with recent or concurrent (PET/CT) anatomical imaging studies. Often, findings seen with the superior contrast resolution of PET can be seen retrospectively on other imaging studies. If no recent anatomical imaging studies are available, they should be requested.

1. ***Unexpected findings.*** Findings that are not clearly related to the known disease process for which PET is requested are not uncommon. These findings often represent clinically undiagnosed malignant or premalignant disorders, and in most cases they should be pursued further.[6]
2. ***PET finding without imaging correlate.*** In the experience of the primary author, the majority of true-positive PET findings has a corresponding structural abnormality, which is often seen in retrospect. If no corresponding abnormalities are seen, further work-up might depend upon the location of the abnormality and clinical history (see Pearls section). A PET finding without imaging correlate could be false-positive or represent a pathology that is usually not visible anatomically at an early stage. In some cases, a follow-up CT at a short interval can be help-ful because some processes seen on PET that are not visualized on initial CT may be visualized on follow-up CT (**Fig. 7.9**).

   Example. Focal lung uptake without a corresponding finding on chest CT is very unlikely to represent a lung neoplasm. One possibility might be false-positive activity from a radiolabeled clot. On the other hand, a diffuse pattern of uptake can represent radiation pneumonitis or even early pneumonia with a negative CT. In the former situation, no further imaging or follow-up is necessary. In the latter situation, a follow-up CT exam at a short interval may be helpful.

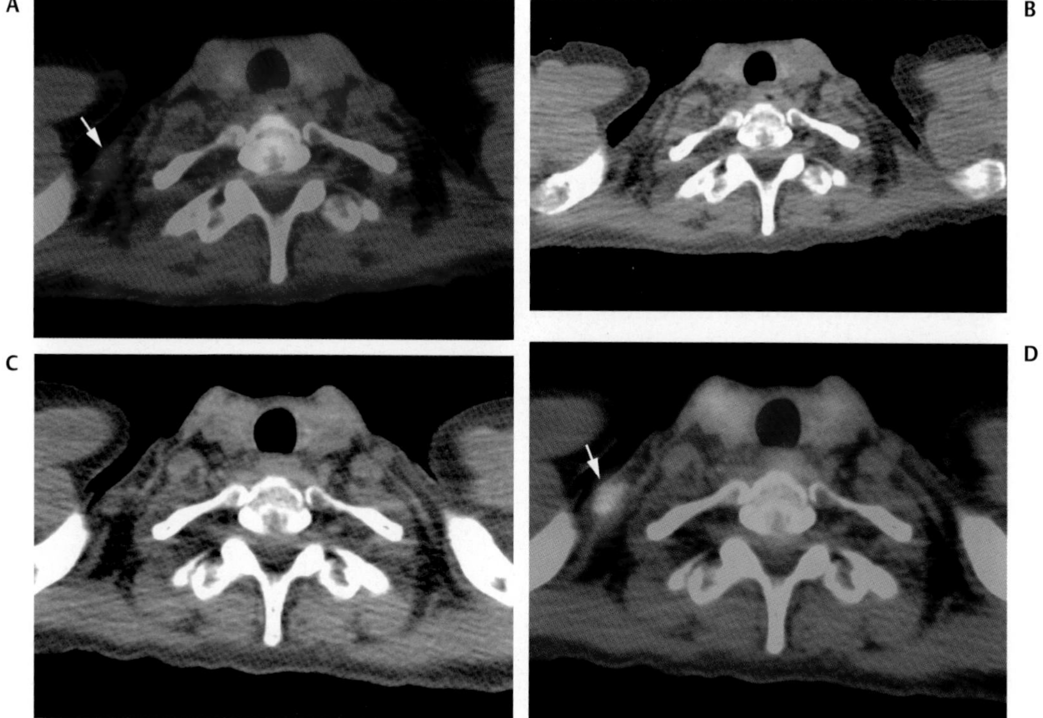

Fig. 7.9 Brown fat pitfall—the value of CT follow-up. **(A)** Axial positron emission tomography/computed tomography (PET/CT) scan demonstrates a mild focus of right supraclavicular uptake (*arrow*). **(B)** Corresponding axial CT scan does not demonstrate a lesion in this location. This was initially thought to represent brown fat uptake. However, no other brown fat uptake was identified. **(C)** Axial PET/CT scan at a later date demonstrates more intense uptake in the previously noted area of right supraclavicular uptake. **(D)** Corresponding axial CT scan demonstrates interval development of a node in this region (*arrow*). This case presents a diagnostic dilemma, as a single focus of supraclavicular brown fat uptake would be very rare, but the initial absence of a corresponding CT abnormality would also be very unusual. In these cases, close interval follow-up with CT is helpful, as positive PET abnormalities initially invisible on CT may manifest on follow-up CT examinations.

References

1. Bleckmann C, Dose J, Bohuslavizki KH, et al. Effect of attenuation correction on lesion detectability in FDG PET of breast cancer. J Nucl Med 1999;40(12):2021–2024
2. Bai C, Kinahan PE, Brasse D, et al. An analytic study of the effects of attenuation on tumor detection in whole-body PET oncology imaging. J Nucl Med 2003; 44(11):1855–1861
3. Reinhardt MJ, Wiethoelter N, Matthies A, et al. PET recognition of pulmonary metastases on PET/CT imaging: impact of attenuation-corrected and non-attenuation-corrected PET images. Eur J Nucl Med Mol Imaging 2006;33(2):134–139
4. Wahl RL. To AC or not to AC: that is the question. J Nucl Med 1999;40(12):2025–2028
5. Pandit-Taskar N, Schoder H, Gonen M, et al. Clinical significance of unexplained abnormal focal FDG uptake in the abdomen during whole-body PET. AJR Am J Roentgenol 2004;183(4):1143–1147
6. Agress H Jr, Cooper BZ. Detection of clinically unexpected malignant and premalignant tumors with whole-body FDG PET: histopathologic comparison. Radiology 2004;230(2):417–422

8

The Value of PET/CT

Eugene C. Lin, Paul E. Kinahan, and Abass Alavi

Positron emission tomography combined with computed tomography (PET/CT) has tremendous potential, as it combines the most sensitive imaging modality (PET) with the highest resolution cross-sectional imaging modality (CT). The addition of fused CT to PET images has numerous advantages over PET alone, but the interpreter should be aware of potential pitfalls introduced by the process of CT fusion and attenuation correction in PET.

◆ Advantages

1. ***Increased accuracy.*** PET/CT adds a substantial incremental benefit compared with using PET alone, and to a lesser extent compared with side-by-side reading of PET and CT. In one study,[1] only 52% of pathologic lesions were accurately characterized (localization and infiltration of adjacent structures) by PET alone. The remaining 48% required either side-by-side CT reading or combined PET/CT. However, many of the cases that may require CT correlation can be accurately interpreted with side-by-side reading of PET and CT. In ~6 to 12%[1,2] of total PET cases, side-by-side reading is not adequate for either accurate lesion localization or characterization, and combined PET/CT may be needed for these purposes. In tumor staging, PET/CT has an incremental 8% increase in accuracy relative to PET and side-by-side CT interpretation and a 20% increase relative to PET interpretation alone.[3]
2. ***Specific advantages.*** PET/CT provides the same advantages that can be achieved by correlating any type of functional and structural imaging techniques (see Chapter 7). PET/CT maximizes these advantages by providing the most accurate correlation. The improved accuracy achieved is noted in
   - ***a.*** Localizing lesions (**Fig. 8.1**)
   - ***b.*** Identifying false-positive findings (**Fig. 8.2**)
   - ***c.*** Determining the nature of subtle or equivocal PET findings and therefore improving the degree of certainty of the results (**Fig. 8.3**)

   PET/CT usually enhances the specificity rather than sensitivity compared with PET alone. Many sources of false-positive findings are easily identified by PET/CT. However, sensitivity can also improve with PET/CT. For example, areas that may be thought to definitely or questionably represent physiologic activity on PET alone can be shown to localize to a pathologic sites on the fused CT scan. The color images used to interpret PET/CT can also make some lesions more conspicuous.
3. ***Contemporaneous correlation.*** Although side-by-side CT correlation is often ad-

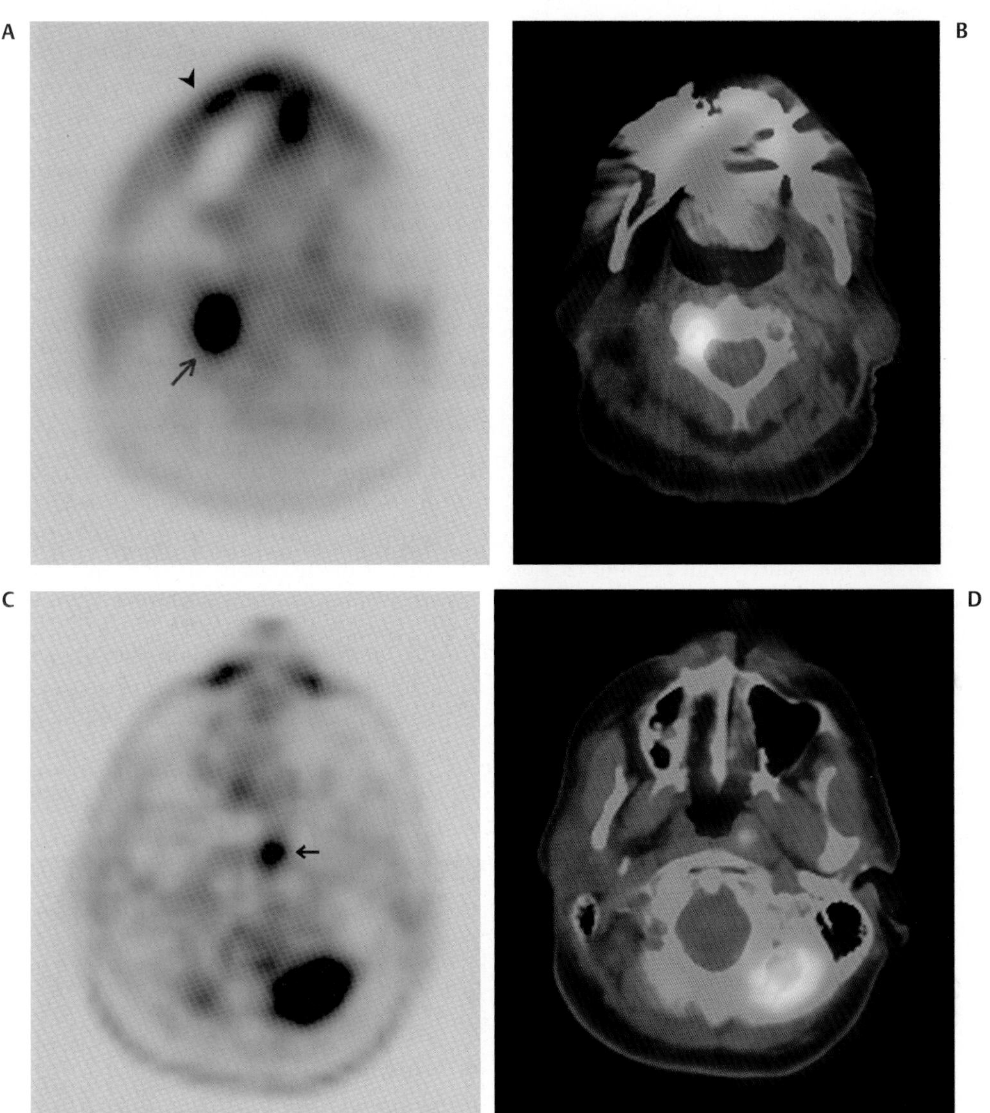

Fig. 8.1 Head and neck localization with positron emission tomography/computed tomography (PET/CT). Localization of fluorodeoxyglucose (FDG) uptake is usually the hardest in the head and neck region due to the lack of anatomical landmarks in this region on PET. **(A)** Axial PET scan demonstrates focal uptake in the right base of the skull region (*arrow*). This cannot be localized on PET. Note the artifact (*arrowhead*) around photopenic dental hardware. **(B)** Axial PET/CT localizes this activity to the cervical spine (bone metastasis). **(C)** Axial PET in a different patient demonstrates focal uptake in the left base of the skull region (*arrow*). This also cannot be localized on PET. **(D)** Axial PET/CT localizes this activity to the nasopharynx (nasopharyngeal carcinoma).

equate, the CT studies are often not contemporaneous. This can result in errors (as seen in **Fig. 7.7**, p. 85) from changes that have taken place during the time interval between acquiring the CT and the PET scan. This issue is obviated with PET/CT.

4. ***CT-based attenuation correction for PET.*** The CT scan can be used for attenuation correction of PET data[4], allowing for decreased scan time, as the CT is completed more quickly than a radionuclide source scan. In addition, PET image noise is reduced due

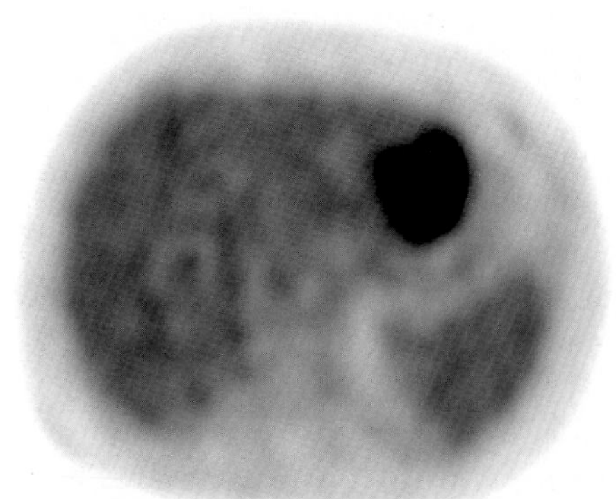

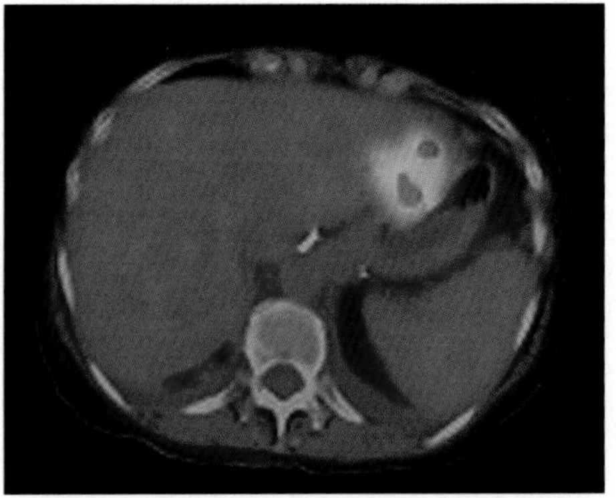

Fig. 8.2 Abscess mimicking gastric cancer. **(A)** Axial positron emission tomography (PET) scan demonstrates intense uptake in the stomach region worrisome for gastric carcinoma. **(B)** Axial PET/computed tomography scan at the same level shows the activity to lie in an abscess medial to the stomach.

to the decreased noise of the CT relative to a radionuclide source scan and the lack of postemission contamination on transmission images.

◆ Disadvantages

1. ***PET/CT artifacts.*** The only disadvantages of combined PET/CT relative to PET alone are the artifacts specific to PET/CT (see Chapter 30 for a discussion of artifacts specific to cardiac PET/CT). These artifacts are primarily related to three factors:[5]
   - Misregistration due to differences in position of structures between PET and CT
   - Artifacts due to differences in attenuation of structures between PET and CT
   - Truncation artifacts related to the CT field of view diameter (typically 50 cm) differ-

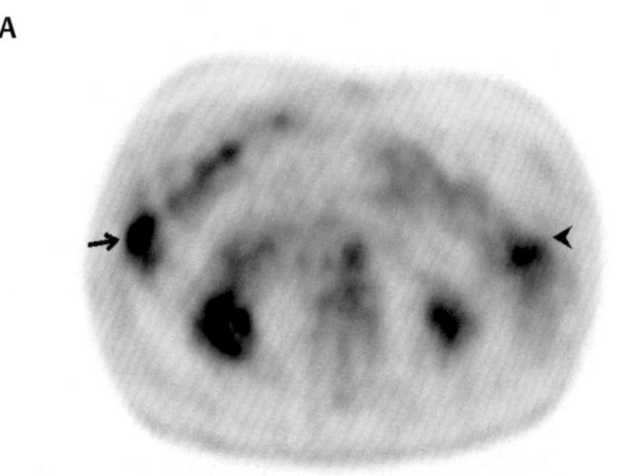

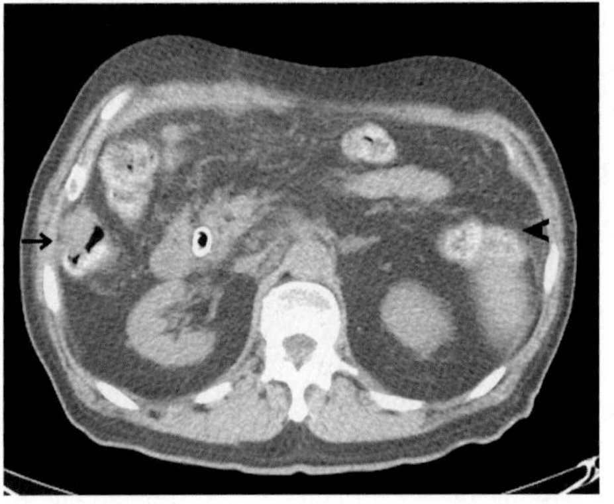

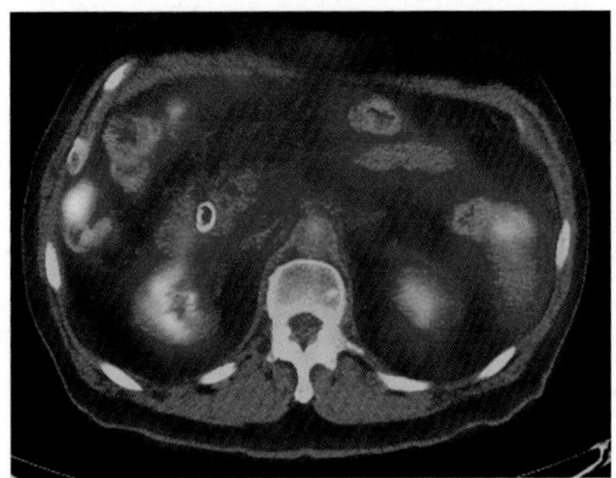

Fig. 8.3 Bowel versus peritoneal disease. **(A)** Axial positron emission tomography (PET) in a patient with cholangiocarcinoma demonstrates focal areas of increased uptake in the right (*arrow*) and left (*arrowhead*) abdomen. It cannot be determined whether these areas represent normal bowel uptake or peritoneal disease on PET alone. Correlation with **(B)** computed tomography (CT) and **(C)** PET/CT demonstrates that the focus of the uptake on the right is a peritoneal lesion (*arrow*), and the focus on the left is bowel activity (*arrowhead*).

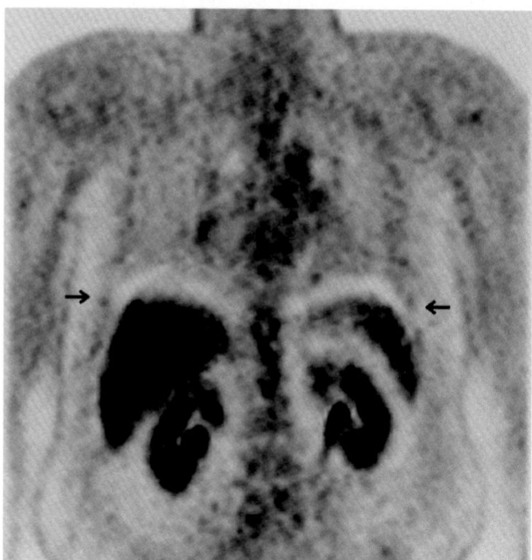

Fig. 8.4 Positron emission tomography/computed tomography (PET/CT) photopenic respiratory artifact. Coronal PET scan done with CT attenuation correction demonstrates curvilinear photopenic artifacts at the lung diaphragm interface bilaterally (*arrows*). This artifact is usually seen if the CT scans this region during inspiration (either during an inspiratory breath-hold or free breathing), resulting in a mismatch with the PET scan, which is primarily in the expiratory phase of the respiratory cycle.

ing from the larger PET field of view diameter (typically 70 cm). All manufacturers are addressing this issue by allowing for reconstruction of an extended CT field of view.

Misregistration

Misregistration artifacts are most prominent in areas of greatest respiratory motion—the lung bases and the diaphragmatic region. Misregistration results in two basic artifacts:

- *Incorrect uptake levels.* Motion between PET and CT results in inaccurate attenuation correction, as the region on CT used for attenuation correction does not correspond exactly to the region on PET. This can result in artifactually decreased or increased visual levels of uptake and inaccurate calculation of standardized uptake value (SUV).
- *Mislocalization.* Lesions can be localized to the wrong location on fused PET/CT images.

1. ***Type of respiration.*** In a combined PET/CT study, the CT scan can be acquired during free (shallow) breathing, maximum inspiration, and normal expiration. The PET scan must be acquired during free breathing due to the length of the scan. The type of breathing during the CT will affect the incidence of artifacts.[6] Mislocalizations from respiration will usually be in the superior to inferior dimension.
   a. *Normal expiration.* This will usually result in the most accurate fusion, as most of the breathing cycle is spent in expiration. This may be the preferred protocol with fast CT scanners. Scanning in normal expiration is preferred, but may not be possible, as some patients may not be able to breath-hold in normal expiration for the duration of the CT.
   b. *Inspiration.* Inspiratory maneuvers, whether a small or regular breath in, will typically result in the most significant misalignment of PET and CT at the diaphragm and heart.[7] Inspiration can cause photopenic curvilinear artifacts at the lung–diaphragm interface (**Fig. 8.4**). This occurs because measured attenuation in this region is too low (there is only lung in this region on the maximum inspiration CT, whereas subdiaphragmatic structures are present in the same region on PET), leading to undercorrection of the detected activity in this region. Photopenic artifact can also be seen at the interface between the heart and the lungs (**Fig. 8.5**).

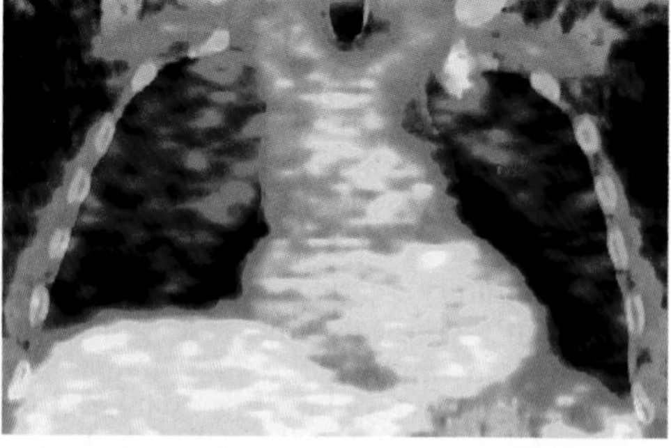

Fig. 8.5 Misregistration artifact. Coronal positron emission tomography/computed tomography scan demonstrates photopenic artifact around the heart.

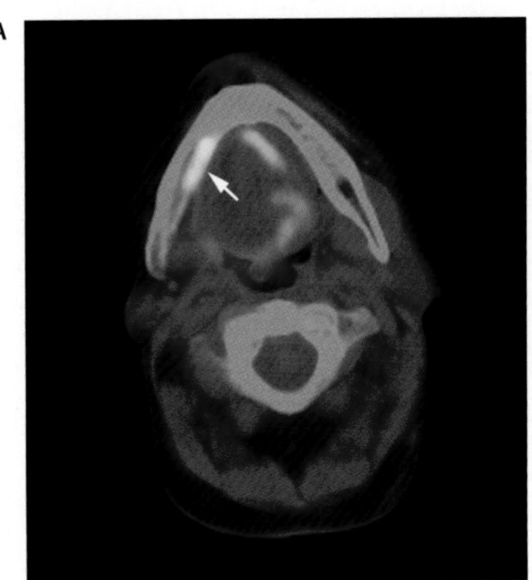
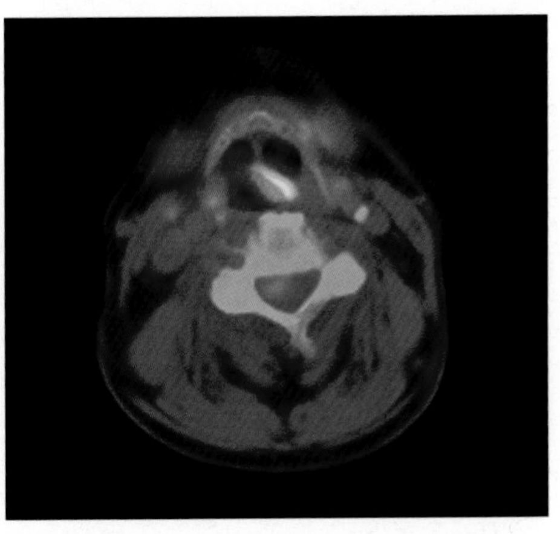

Fig. 8.6 Head and neck mislocalization. Mislocalizations in the head and neck usually result from motion of the head between the computed tomography (CT) and positron emission tomography (PET) studies. Mislocalizations are usually in the medial to lateral direction. **(A)** Axial PET/CT demonstrates mislocalization of linear mylohyoid uptake to the right, with the right mylohyoid uptake (*arrow*) overlapping the mandible. **(B)** More inferior axial PET/CT slice from the same study demonstrates that uptake from a left epiglottic neoplasm appears to be centered medial to the epiglottis, and normal cervical cord activity is in the right spinal canal. Submandibular gland uptake is localized slightly to the right of the submandibular glands. However, the mislocalization did not result in a diagnostic error in this case.

   c. *Free breathing.* Free breathing can also cause photopenic curvilinear artifacts at the lung–diaphragm interface if the peridiaphragmatic area is scanned during inspiration. However, image coregistration with shallow breathing is typically superior to that with inspiration.[7]

2. ***Corrections for respiratory misregistration***
   a. *Respiratory averaged low-dose CT scanning.* For some PET/CT scanners, this method uses cine-CT acquisition to form a respiratory-blurred CT-based attenuation correction image. This potentially reduces the mismatch with the respiratory-blurred PET image.[8] The low-dose respiratory-blurred CT image is not viewed, and care must be taken to use as low CT technique factors as possible to avoid excessive radiation dose to the patient.
   b. *Respiratory gating.* Four-dimensional PET/CT protocols with respiratory gating can improve the spatial matching between PET and CT, but they often require long acquisition and postprocessing times. Other protocols[9] have been developed that might improve registration with minimal acquisition and postprocessing time and effort.

3. ***Nonrespiratory motion.*** This is most commonly seen in the head and neck where motion between the CT and PET scans results in mislocalization mostly in the medial to lateral dimension (**Figs. 8.6** and **8.7**). Another area where this is commonly seen is the breast (**Fig. 8.8**). On some systems this can be corrected (on the scanner console) by realignment tools.

4. ***SUV.*** Areas of artifactually decreased and increased activity and therefore inaccurate SUV measurements have been described in the lung bases and bowel. This can result in both a false-positive and a negative interpretation of the resulting images.
   a. *Lung bases.* The SUV can be altered by up to 30%.
   b. *Bowel.* Differences in bowel motion between PET and CT from peristalsis and respiration can result in areas of falsely increased or decreased activity and SUVs on CT attenuation-corrected imaging. This could result in reduced sensitivity for detecting adjacent malignant peritoneal implants and nodes, or false-positive

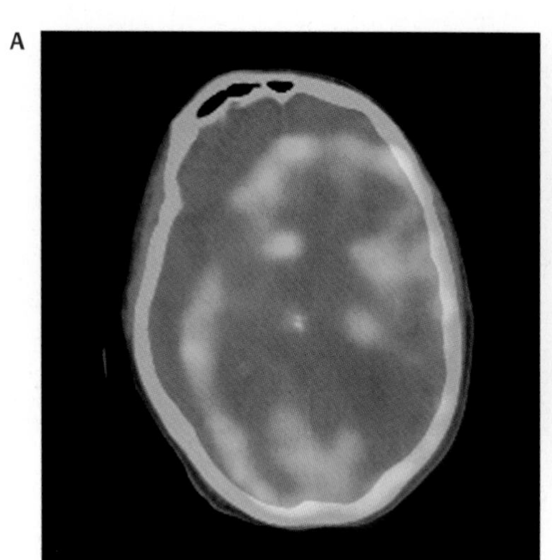

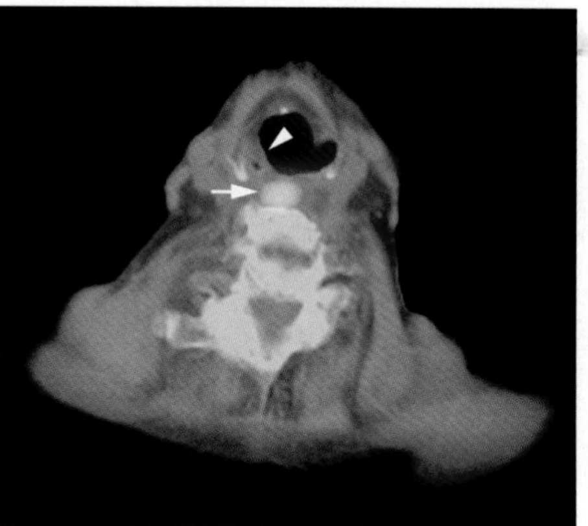

Fig. 8.7 Head and neck mislocalization. Sometimes mislocalizations can result in diagnostic errors. **(A)** Axial positron emission tomography/computed tomography (PET/CT) study demonstrates severe mislocalization at the brain level. Review of this image suggests that mislocalization will cause activity to localize posteriorly and to the left of the actual location. **(B)** Axial PET/CT scan demonstrates a focus of activity localizing to the esophagus (*arrow*). However, mislocalization would occur posteriorly and to the left based on image **(A)**, and the focus of activity is actually in the right piriform sinus (*arrowhead*), which demonstrates abnormal soft tissue thickening on the CT.

findings (**Fig. 8.9**). Areas of artifactually reduced activity are more common than those with increased activity.[10]

5. ***Mislocalizations.*** Significant mislocalizations can occur in the lung bases and the liver dome (e.g., a liver lesion localized to the lung) (**Fig. 8.10**).[11]

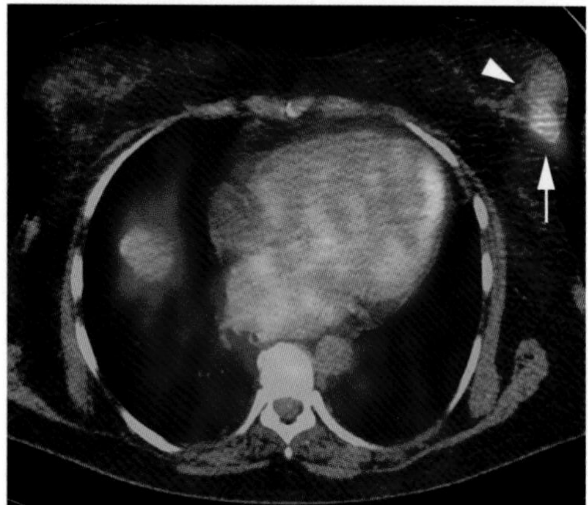

Fig. 8.8 Breast lesion misregistration. Axial positron emission tomography/computed tomography (PET/CT) scan demonstrates a left breast lesion (*arrowhead*). Fluorodeoxyglucose (FDG) uptake (*arrow*) appears posterior to the lesion secondary to misregistration between the PET and CT studies.

   a. *Thorax.* Error in lung nodule location is in the range of 7 to 10 mm on average, and is more pronounced in both the lung bases and the left lung.[12]
   b. *Abdomen.* There is usually < 1 cm discrepancy noted, but discrepancy can be > 2 cm at the upper liver margin and the lower splenic margin.

6. ***Differences between PET and CT.*** The visceral organs may be in different positions and have different sizes on PET compared with CT due to normal physiologic motion.[13]
   a. *Liver.* The liver is slightly larger in size and superior and lateral in position on PET compared with CT.
   b. *Spleen.* The spleen is slightly smaller in size and is positioned superior and posterior on PET compared with CT.
   c. *Kidneys.* The kidneys are slightly smaller in size and superior, posterior, and rightward in position on PET compared with CT.

Attenuation Artifacts Secondary to Dense Material

Due to the method used to scale the CT image for PET attenuation correction, dense or high

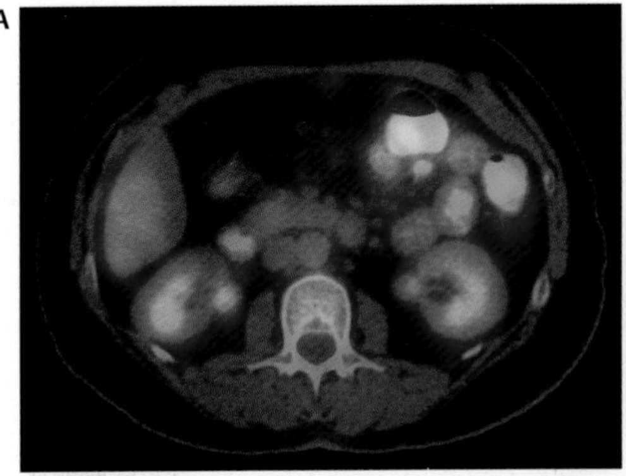

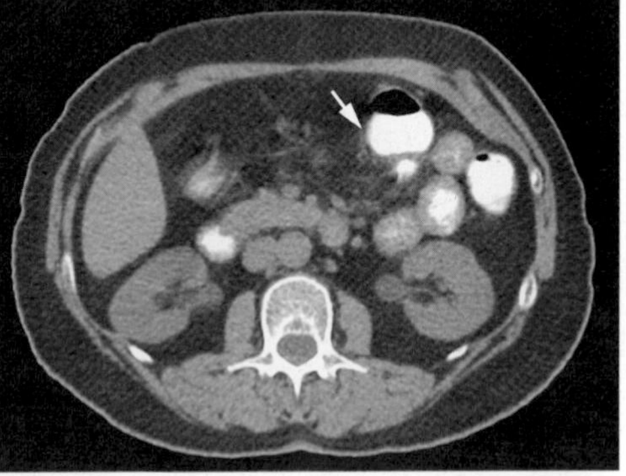

Fig. 8.9 Misregistration. Sagittal positron emission tomography/computed tomography (PET/CT) scan demonstrates misregistration between the PET and CT datasets, best seen at the inferior margin of the liver and kidney. Note that bowel activity (*arrow*) appears to localize to the mesentery.

atomic number materials can cause artifactually increased activity on the PET image. With the 511 keV energy of positron emitters, the attenuation of gamma rays by barium and iodine solutions is not greatly different from that from soft tissues. However, there is a significant difference in attenuation between barium/iodine solutions and soft tissue on CT. As a result, the 511 keV photon attenuation is overestimated in areas containing dense material when CT is used. In these areas the visualized activity and SUVs will be artifactually elevated due to incorrect (too high) attenuation values provided by CT. The activity on the PET image is incorrectly increased to correct for attenuation that is not present. Roughly, the SUV error is ~0.1% per Hounsfield unit (HU). In other words, a contrast enhancement of 100 HU causes a 10% error in PET SUV.[5]

On some PET/CT scanners it is possible to process the attenuation-corrected PET images by assuming that regions on the CT image with high HU value correspond to contrast agents, and not bone. This will lead to PET images with

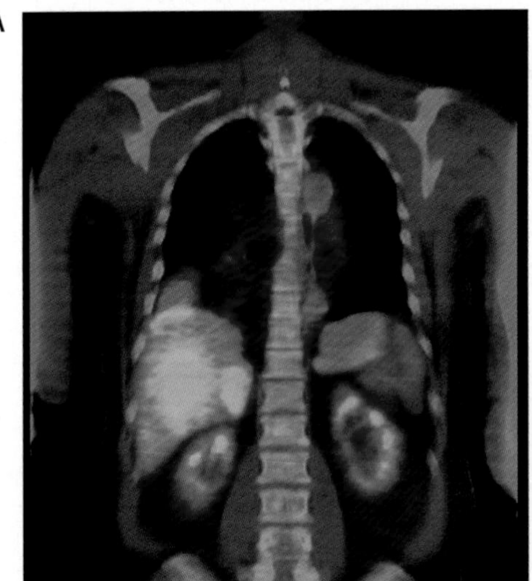

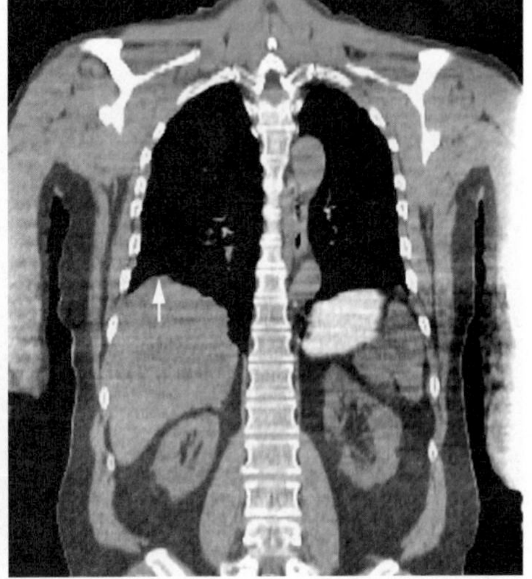

Fig. 8.10 Liver lesion mislocalization. **(A)** Coronal positron emission tomography/computed tomography (PET/CT) scan demonstrates an apparent lesion in the base of the right lung. **(B)** Coronal CT scan at the same level does not demonstrate a lung lesion in this location. The apparent lung uptake is secondary to mislocalization of the lesion in the liver dome. A bulge in the contour of the liver dome (*arrow*) is seen secondary to this lesion (which is not otherwise seen on this noncontrast study).

correct SUVs in soft tissue, even if significant contrast enhancement is present in the CT image. It should be noted, however, that any fluorodeoxyglucose (FDG) uptake in bone may be incorrect because of this type of processing, and the original PET image should be used for the bone uptake values.

1. ***Oral contrast.*** The amount of artifactually increased activity will depend upon the density of contrast used. Although high-density barium can cause substantial artifactual increased values (**Fig. 8.11**), the degree of artifactual increase from the low-density barium used in CT is minimal.[14]
   a. On average, the SUV error will be < 5%, and at the most slightly > 10%.
   b. Negative oral contrast (e.g., water with 2.5% mannitol and 0.2% locust bean gum) can be used to avoid artifacts.[15]
2. ***Intravenous contrast.*** Intravenous contrast can also cause artifactually increased activity. As for oral contrast agents, the higher the density of intravenous contrast material, the greater the artifactually increased activity.[16]
   a. *Thoracic veins.* Artifact is most prominent in the thoracic veins containing undiluted contrast from injection (**Fig. 8.12**).[17]
   b. *Urinary tract.* Artifact from urinary contrast excretion is also prominent in the kidneys, ureters, and bladder, where the percentage error can be > 25%.
   c. *Arterial phase imaging.* Artifacts from dense vessels will be more pronounced on CT arterial phase imaging compared with the portal venous phase.
   d. *Normal tissue.* The amount of increase in normal tissue is minimal and most prominent in the liver, spleen, and aorta, where the maximum SUV increases 5 to 7%.[18]
   e. *Pathologic tissue.* Pathologic tissue usually enhances due to neovascularity and/or increased perfusion. Increases in maximum SUV are variable but are usually minimal (4% average increase).[18]
   f. *CT protocol.* Artifact from contrast in the thoracic veins can be minimized by scanning caudocranially with a biphasic contrast injection.[19]
3. ***Calcified lesions.*** Calcified lesions usually are not dense enough to result in artifactually increased activity. However, nonattenuation-corrected images should always be reviewed if activity is noted in a calcified lesion (see Chapter 25) to determine that the activity is not artifactual.

A

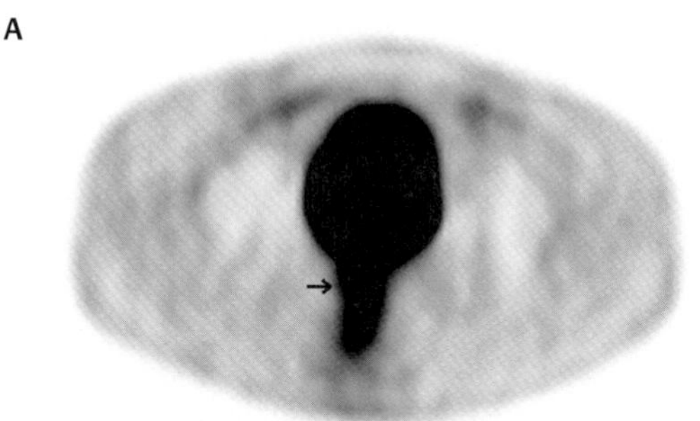

B

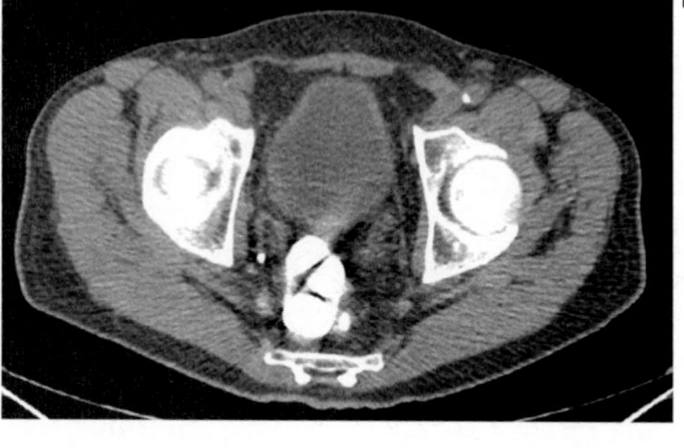

C

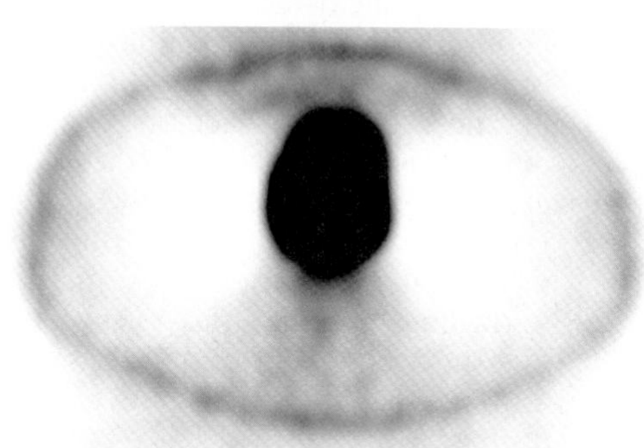

Fig. 8.11 Barium artifact. **(A)** Attenuation-corrected axial positron emission tomography (PET) scan demonstrates intense activity in the rectum (*arrow*). **(B)** Corresponding axial computed tomography scan demonstrates dense barium in this region. **(C)** Nonattenuation corrected axial PET scan does not demonstrate increased activity in this region.

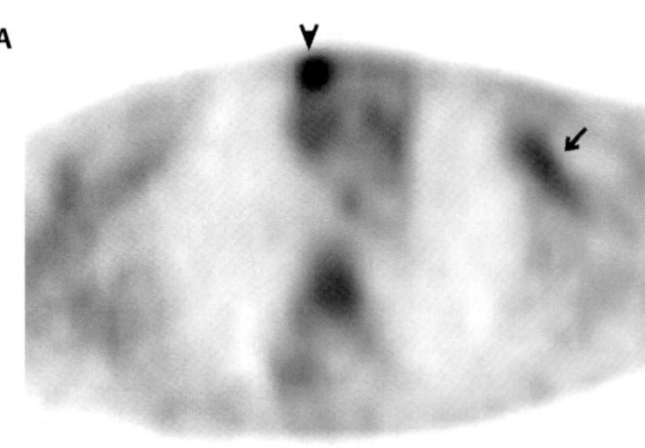

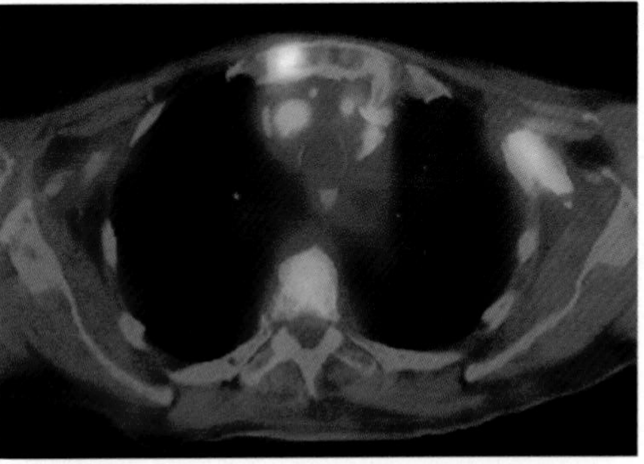

Fig. 8.12 Intravenous contrast artifact. **(A)** Axial positron emission tomography (PET) with computed tomography (CT) attenuation correction demonstrates increased activity in the left axilla (*arrow*) and right parasternal region (*arrowhead*). The right parasternal activity could represent sternal or internal thoracic nodal uptake on PET. **(B)** Axial PET/CT scan demonstrates that the activity on PET in the left axilla is artifactual from dense intravenous contrast and that the parasternal uptake is in the bone. (Courtesy of Carolyn Meltzer, MD, Atlanta, GA.)

4. ***Metallic/dense material artifact.*** Metallic and dense foreign material can cause artifactually increased activity. Examples include
   a. Metallic dental prostheses, orthopedic implants, and cement (see Variants section)
   b. Cardiac leads and central venous line reservoirs.[20]
      - In cardiac PET/CT, there are often significant artifacts seen with implantable cardioverter defibrillator leads, but pacemaker leads usually do not cause noticeable artifact.[21]

Truncation Artifact

Truncation artifact occurs due to differences in the field of view (FOV) between PET and CT. Obese patients may have part of their anatomy outside the FOV of the CT scan. This truncated portion does not provide data for attenuation correction, resulting in artifactually low SUVs. Some PET/CT scanners provide methods for estimating the truncated regions of the CT images. Although these enlarged FOV CT images may not always be suitable for diagnostic CT interpretation, they provide accurate attenuation correction for the PET images.

◆ Interpretation

Interpretation of PET/CT is similar to that of PET alone with CT correlation (see Chapter 7), but the interpreter must be aware of the potential artifacts associated with combined PET/CT imaging. Some issues specific to PET/CT interpretation are

1. ***Registration.*** Before review of fused PET/CT images, it should be first determined whether the fused images are accurately registered.
2. ***Nonattenuation-corrected (NAC) images.*** Review of NAC images is more essential in interpretation of combined PET/CT than in PET alone. Most of the PET/CT-specific artifacts are related to the use of CT-based attenuation correction. Therefore, the absence of a PET/CT abnormality on the NAC images would suggest the possibility of a PET/CT artifact.
3. ***Lungs***
   a. *Lung nodules.* If PET/CT is performed in shallow breathing, small lung nodules are often not detected.[22] Thus, PET/CT performed in shallow breathing cannot completely replace breath-hold chest CT in cancer staging. The addition of an additional low-dose chest CT to the PET/CT examination may be helpful.[23]
   b. *Lung bases.* Caution must be employed in the interpretation of potential abnormalities in the lung bases, given the high incidence of PET/CT misregistration artifacts in this region. In particular, the degree of uptake in distal esophageal

and lung base lesions may be artifactually decreased if misregistration artifact is present.

4. ***SUV***
   a. SUVs can be artifactually decreased or increased secondary to motion, as described in the Disadvantages section.
   b. One study suggests that SUVs may be slightly higher on CT/attenuation-corrected PET compared with SUVs generated by germanium-corrected PET (see Chapter 5),[24] but another study suggests there is no difference.[25] Caution should be used when comparing PET/CT and PET SUV values.

◆ Patient Preparation

Patient preparation for PET/CT is the same as for PET. However, factors specific to PET/CT are

1. ***Patient position.*** For standard PET scans, patients may be scanned with their arms at the sides for comfort. For PET/CT, it is preferable to scan the patient with the arms above the head if tolerated to avoid beam-hardening artifacts, which will degrade images of the upper abdomen. The exception is the head and neck, where the arms should be down. The increased speed of PET/CT makes arms-up scanning tolerable for most patients.
2. ***Oral contrast.*** The choice of whether to use oral contrast may depend upon the indication. For tumors that are unlikely to have peritoneal/mesenteric spread (e.g., lung cancer), oral contrast is unlikely to be helpful. Oral contrast may be very helpful for tumors with a propensity for peritoneal and/or mesenteric nodal spread. However, although oral contrast may allow differentiation between bowel and adjacent peritoneal disease, the increased density of the contrast could accentuate areas of artifactually increased and decreased activity due to bowel motion (see Disadvantages section). The key is to minimize the density of the contrast used. In addition, the physiologic effects of oral contrast may increase bowel activity independent of the effects of increased density.
3. ***Intravenous contrast.*** Intravenous contrast will improve the diagnostic quality of the CT, but it may introduce artifacts (see Disadvantages section). Below are factors to consider in deciding whether to employ intravenous contrast.
   a. Contrast enhancement of visceral organs will slightly increase the measured physiologic activity. This could potentially decrease visualization of pathologic lesions in these organs.
   b. Pathologic lesions that enhance may have artifactually increased SUV values.
   c. More intense activity in the thoracic veins and urinary tract from undiluted or concentrated contrast may obscure adjacent pathologic lesions.
      - This can be minimized by scanning before renal contrast excretion and scanning caudocranially to minimize thoracic vein activity.
   d. The patient may have contrast-enhanced CT studies before or after the PET exam. In many cases, review of the fused PET/noncontrast CT and the separate contrast-enhanced CT in conjunction can be comparable to review of a PET/contrast CT study, but without the possible artifacts.
4. ***Respiration.*** The phase of respiration during the CT scan may affect the type and incidence of artifacts (see Disadvantages section). The choice is often dependent upon the degree of patient cooperation.

References

1. Reinartz P, Wieres FJ, Schneider W, et al. Side-by-side reading of PET and CT scans in oncology: which patients might profit from integrated PET/CT? Eur J Nucl Med Mol Imaging 2004;31(11):1456–1461
2. Pelosi E, Messa C, Sironi S, et al. Value of integrated PET/CT for lesion localisation in cancer patients: a comparative study. Eur J Nucl Med Mol Imaging 2004;31(7):932–939
3. Antoch G, Saoudi N, Kuehl H, et al. Accuracy of whole-body dual-modality fluorine-18-2-fluoro-2-deoxy-D-glucose positron emission tomography and computed tomography (FDG-PET/CT) for tumor staging in solid tumors: comparison with CT and PET. J Clin Oncol 2004;22(21):4357–4368
4. Kinahan PE, Townsend DW, Beyer T, Sashin D. Attenuation correction for a combined 3D PET/CT scanner. Med Phys 1998;25(10):2046–2053
5. Kinahan PE, Hasegawa BH, Beyer T. X-ray-based attenuation correction for positron emission tomography/computed tomography scanners. Semin Nucl Med 2003;33(3):166–179
6. Goerres GW, Burger C, Kamel E, et al. Respiration-induced attenuation artifact at PET/CT: technical considerations. Radiology 2003;226(3):906–910

7. Gilman MD, Fischman AJ, Krishnasetty V, et al. Optimal CT breathing protocol for combined thoracic PET/CT. AJR Am J Roentgenol 2006;187(5):1357–1360
8. Pan T, Mawlawi O, Nehmeh SA, et al. Attenuation correction of PET images with respiration-averaged CT images in PET/CT. J Nucl Med 2005;46(9):1481–1487
9. Nehmeh SA, Erdi YE, Meirelles GS, et al. Deep-inspiration breath-hold PET/CT of the thorax. J Nucl Med 2007;48(1):22–26
10. Nakamoto Y, Chin BB, Cohade C, et al. PET/CT: artifacts caused by bowel motion. Nucl Med Commun 2004;25(3):221–225
11. Osman MM, Cohade C, Nakamoto Y, et al. Clinically significant inaccurate localization of lesions with PET/CT: frequency in 300 patients. J Nucl Med 2003;44(2):240–243
12. Cohade C, Osman M, Marshall LN, Wahl RN. PET-CT: accuracy of PET and CT spatial registration of lung lesions. Eur J Nucl Med Mol Imaging 2003;30(5):721–726
13. Nakamoto Y, Tatsumi M, Cohade C, et al. Accuracy of image fusion of normal upper abdominal organs visualized with PET/CT. Eur J Nucl Med Mol Imaging 2003;30(4):597–602
14. Dizendorf E, Hany TF, Buck A, et al. Cause and magnitude of the error induced by oral CT contrast agent in CT-based attenuation correction of PET emission studies. J Nucl Med 2003;44(5):732–738
15. Antoch G, Kuehl H, Kanja J, et al. Dual-modality PET/CT scanning with negative oral contrast agent to avoid artifacts: introduction and evaluation. Radiology 2004;230(3):879–885
16. Nakamoto Y, Chin BB, Kraitchman DL, et al. Effects of nonionic intravenous contrast agents at PET/CT imaging: phantom and canine studies. Radiology 2003;227(3):817–824
17. Antoch G, Freudenberg LS, Egelhof T, et al. Focal tracer uptake: a potential artifact in contrast-enhanced dual-modality PET/CT scans. J Nucl Med 2002;43(10):1339–1342
18. Yau YY, Chan WS, Tam YM, et al. Application of intravenous contrast in PET/CT: does it really introduce significant attenuation correction error? J Nucl Med 2005;46(2):283–291
19. Beyer T, Antoch G, Bockisch A, Stattaus J. Optimized intravenous contrast administration for diagnostic whole-body ^{18}F-FDG PET/CT. J Nucl Med 2005;46(3):429–435
20. Halpern BS, Dahlbom M, Waldherr C, et al. Cardiac pacemakers and central venous lines can induce focal artifacts on CT-corrected PET images. J Nucl Med 2004;45(2):290–293
21. DiFilippo FP, Brunken RC. Do implanted pacemaker leads and ICD leads cause metal-related artifact in cardiac PET/CT? J Nucl Med 2005;46(3):436–443
22. Allen-Auerbach M, Yeom K, Park J, et al. Standard PET/CT of the chest during shallow breathing is inadequate for comprehensive staging of lung cancer. J Nucl Med 2006;47(2):298–301
23. Juergens KU, Weckesser M, Stegger L, et al. Tumor staging using whole-body high-resolution 16-channel PET-CT: does additional low-dose chest CT in inspiration improve the detection of solitary pulmonary nodules? Eur Radiol 2006;16(5):1131–1137
24. Nakamoto Y, Osman M, Cohade C, et al. PET/CT: comparison of quantitative tracer uptake between germanium and CT transmission attenuation-corrected images. J Nucl Med 2002;43(9):1137–1143
25. Souvatzoglou M, Ziegler SI, Martinez MJ, et al. Standardised uptake values from PET/CT images: comparison with conventional attenuation-corrected PET. Eur J Nucl Med Mol Imaging 2007;34(3):405–412

9

Levels of Evidence for Clinical Indications of FDG PET

Eugene C. Lin

Fluorodeoxyglucose positron emission tomography (FDG PET) has a wide range of clinical applications in oncology and to a lesser extent in neurology and cardiology. These clinical applications vary substantially in the amount of clinical experience and literature available.

The chapters on clinical topics will contain Clinical Indication sections, where a general assessment is made as to the level of evidence for specific clinical applications of FDG PET.

For quick reference, letters have been assigned for each clinical indication according to the following:

A. The use of FDG PET for this clinical indication is well established. Its value is supported by a large amount of clinical experience and literature.

B. FDG PET is useful for this clinical indication. However, compared with the A-level applications, the clinical experience and literature supporting the use of FDG PET for this clinical indication are less available or substantial. This may mean that more experience and research are needed to fully define the value of FDG PET in this clinical setting, or that FDG PET is useful but has a lesser degree of incremental benefit over conventional imaging techniques than the A-level applications.

C. FDG PET is potentially useful for this clinical indication. There is a minimal amount of clinical experience and literature supporting the use of FDG PET for this clinical indication. A substantially greater amount of experience and research is needed to fully define the value of FDG PET.

D. FDG PET has limited value and is not recommended as a standard imaging technique for this clinical indication. This may be because of limited accuracy, lack of cost-effectiveness, or lack of impact on clinical management. However, there may be specific situations where FDG PET can provide valuable information.

These levels are intended only as general guidelines. Practitioners may find FDG PET more or less valuable for each clinical indication based on their specific experience and patient populations. As clinical experience and research accumulate, it is likely that many of the C- and B-level applications will become A-level applications.

III

Oncologic Applications

10

Oncologic PET by Anatomical Region

Eugene C. Lin and Abass Alavi

◆ General Principles

The primary attribute of positron emission tomography (PET) imaging is its great contrast resolution compared with anatomical imaging techniques. Because of this contrast resolution, in oncologic imaging PET has substantial advantages over anatomical techniques in the early detection of disease in staging and recurrence and the accurate evaluation of therapy response. In general, the disadvantages of PET are related to its relatively poor resolution relative to anatomical imaging techniques and the numerous sources of nonneoplastic uptake of fluorodeoxyglucose (FDG). However, many of the disadvantages of PET are greatly mitigated with the use of combined PET/computed tomography (CT) imaging (see Chapter 8).

1. ***Advantages.*** The advantages of PET over conventional imaging techniques in assessing cancer are found in two areas:
   a. PET can detect early disease before gross anatomical changes (**Fig. 10.1**). PET can detect disease in areas that would be interpreted as normal on anatomical imaging techniques due to the lack of structural changes.
   b. There is a greater contrast-to-noise ratio of abnormal to normal structures on PET compared with that of the anatomical modalities (**Fig. 10.2**). Because of this, abnormalities clearly seen on PET are often not prospectively detected on anatomical imaging techniques. In many cases, these abnormalities can be retrospectively detected after attention is specifically directed to the abnormal area by PET.
2. ***Disadvantages***
   a. Limited sensitivity for small lesions. In general, the sensitivity of PET is low for lesions < 1 cm. PET (or any other gross imaging modality) cannot detect micrometastases.
   b. False-positives. Potential false-positive results can be seen from a wide range of inflammatory/infectious processes or other benign etiologies.
   c. Anatomical localization. Occasionally, it is difficult to localize lesions to their exact anatomical sites based on PET, particularly in the head, neck, and pelvic sites. This is largely remedied by combined PET/CT, although misregistration is sometimes encountered with this approach.
   d. Low sensitivity in specific areas. PET has poor sensitivity for brain and lung metastases and sclerotic bone lesions.

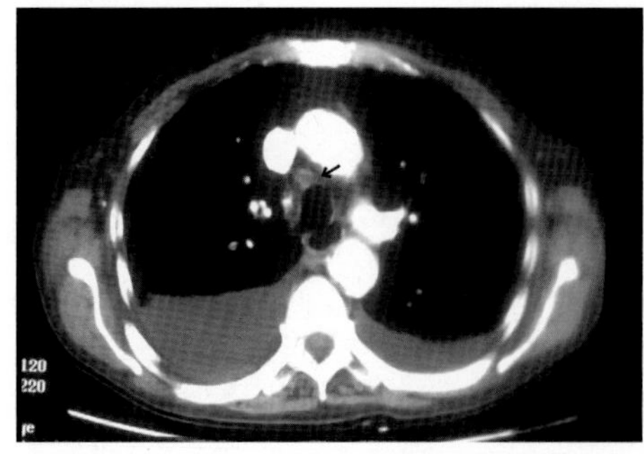

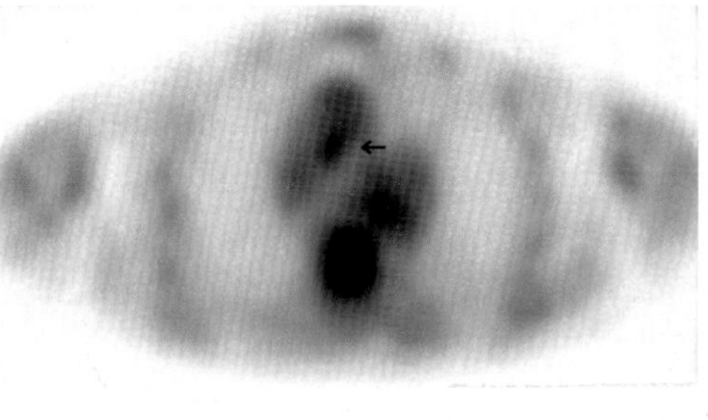

Fig. 10.1 Fluorodeoxyglucose (FDG) uptake in a benign-appearing but malignant node. **(A)** Computed tomography (CT) scan in a lung cancer patient demonstrates a nonenlarged mediastinal node with fatty hilum (*arrow*). This is a sign of a benign node on CT. **(B)** There is increased uptake (*arrow*) on axial positron emission tomography scan corresponding to this node, consistent with malignancy.

e. *Decreased sensitivity for specific tumors.* PET has poor sensitivity for specific tumors, such as prostate cancer, bronchoalveolar carcinoma, and mucinous adenocarcinoma.

3. Metastatic disease demonstrated by PET will often alter patient management. Given the possibility of false-positive findings, confirmation with anatomical imaging techniques or biopsy should be strongly considered for PET findings that will alter patient management. This is particularly true if there is a solitary lesion demonstrated on PET that will potentially alter patient management.

◆ Liver

1. ***Liver metastases.*** PET is very sensitive for detecting liver metastases that are > 1 cm in size. In general, PET is more specific than CT or magnetic resonance imaging (MRI).[1] Some studies have suggested that PET is more sensitive than CT or MRI,[2] but other studies suggest that PET is less sensitive.[1] Note that liver MRI performed with specific liver imaging agents such as superparamagnetic iron oxide[1] or mangafodipir trisodium[3] is more sensitive than PET.
2. ***Differentiation of benign from malignant lesions.*** Focal uptake in a liver lesion is very

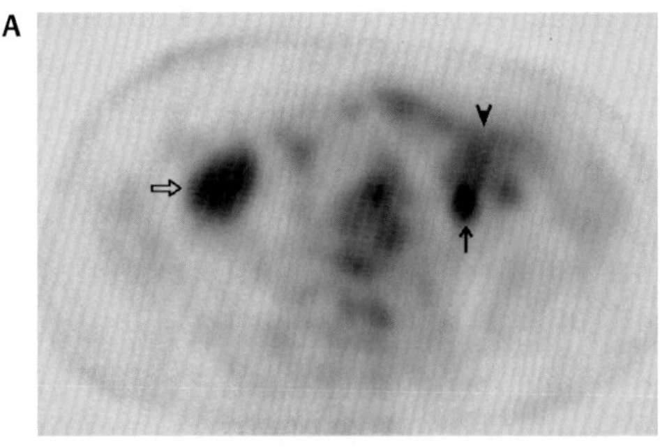

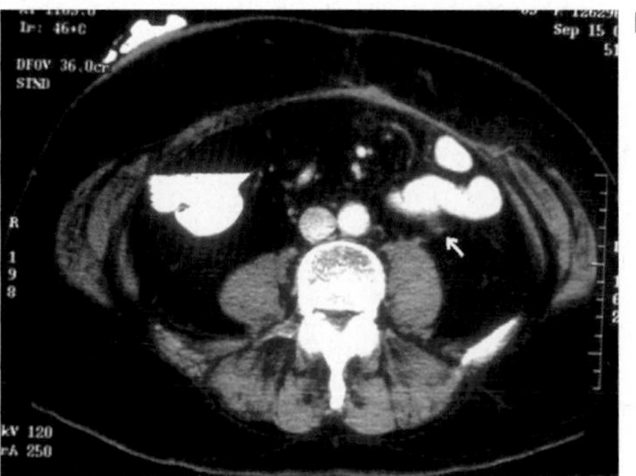

Fig. 10.2 Peritoneal metastasis from colon cancer. **(A)** Axial positron emission tomography (PET) scan shows focal uptake (*arrow*) adjacent to small bowel (*arrowhead*). Although mild diffuse small bowel uptake is usually normal, focal areas of uptake greater than the surrounding small bowel are usually not normal. It is normal to have substantially greater uptake in the right colon (*open arrow*) than the small bowel. **(B)** Computed tomography (CT) scan at the same level demonstrates a small focus of abnormal soft tissue (*arrow*) adjacent to small bowel. This was not seen prospectively on the CT and was present only on one slice. The contrast-to-noise ratio of the abnormality on PET is much greater than on CT.

specific for malignancy and may represent metastases, hepatocellular carcinoma (HCC), or cholangiocarcinoma.[4]

a. Benign lesions such as hemangiomas, focal nodular hyperplasia, and hepatic adenomas typically do not have increased FDG uptake.
   - There is a single report of a focal nodular hyperplasia with increased uptake.[5]

b. *False-positives.* Hepatic abscess, nodular lymphoid hyperplasia (pseudolymphoma), inflammatory pseudotumor, sarcoidosis[6,7]

c. *False-negative.* Low-grade HCC (see Chapter 20)

3. ***Evaluation of small liver lesions.*** Although FDG PET has a limited sensitivity for liver lesions < 1 cm in size, it still has a high specificity. This is particularly useful when CT detects liver lesions < 1 cm but cannot further characterize the nature of these lesions. Statistically, these lesions most likely represent small cysts or hemangiomas, but in the setting of primary malignancy elsewhere, it is not possible to determine noninvasively the true nature of these lesions. Given the low sensitivity, PET should not be used primarily for evaluating these small liver lesions, but PET is indicated for assessing for disease activity elsewhere. If focal FDG uptake is noted in these small lesions, they are almost certainly metastatic (**Fig. 10.3**). However, even when there is no increased uptake seen on PET, these lesions cannot be diagnosed as benign, as they could be malignant and not detected on PET due to their small size.
4. ***Artifacts.*** The liver is often heterogeneous due to image noise on attenuation-corrected images. Image noise is more prominent in the liver than in any other organ. Due to the normal heterogeneity of the liver, caution must be exercised before interpreting subtle findings as liver metastases (**Fig. 10.4**).
5. ***How should one interpret subtle foci of uptake in the liver?*** Most metastases in the liver will demonstrate greatly increased

A

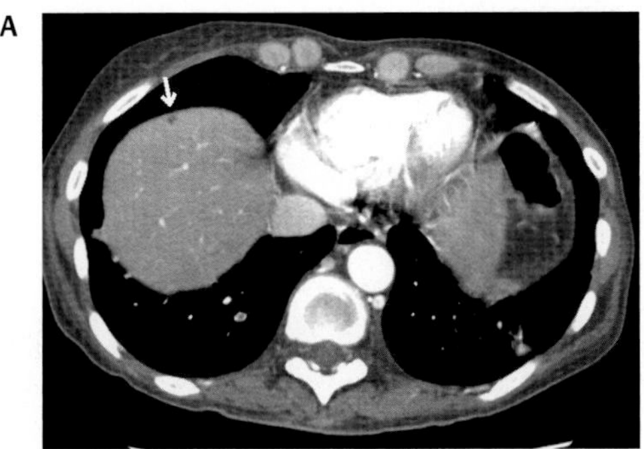

B

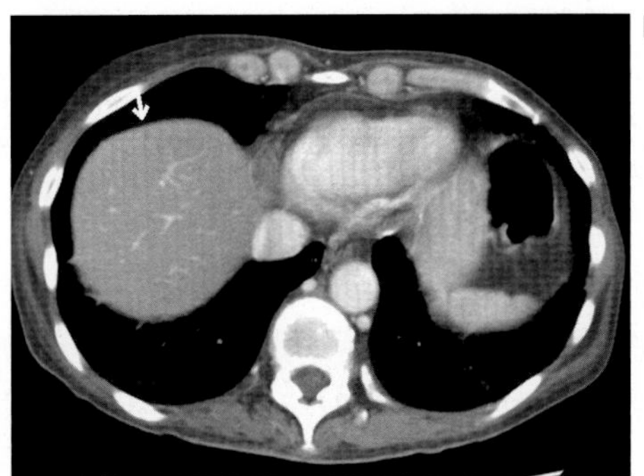

C

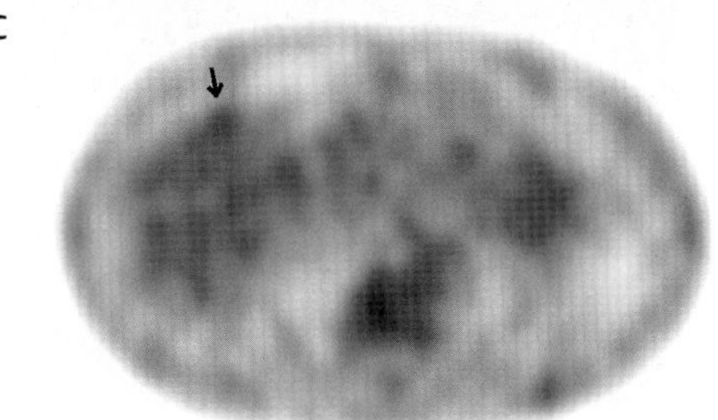

Fig. 10.3 Subtle liver metastasis. A metastasis in the dome of the liver (*arrow*) is much better seen on **(A)** an arterial-phase axial computed tomography (CT) scan than on **(B)** a portal phase scan. **(C)** This lesion has mild FDG uptake on an axial PET scan. This lesion might be interpreted as artifactual secondary to image noise on the positron emission tomography scan alone, or if correlated with the portal phase CT. Correlation with arterial phase CT was necessary. The lesion itself is nonspecific in appearance on CT, but the presence of visible fluorodeoxyglucose uptake in this small lesion is consistent with metastatic disease.

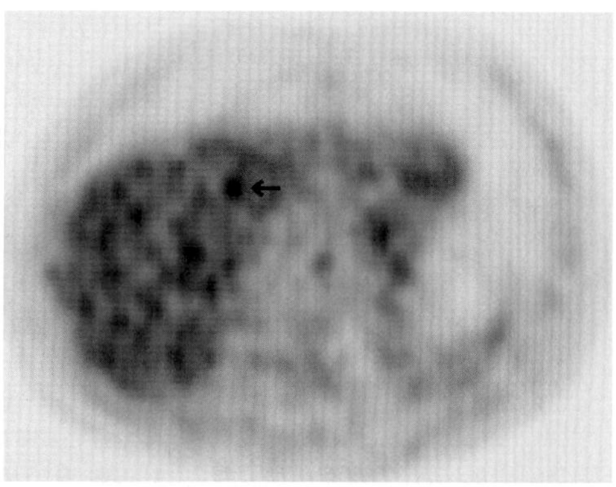

Fig. 10.4 Liver noise mimicking a lesion. Multiple foci of increased activity in the liver are present. It is difficult to differentiate whether these are secondary to lesions or image noise. One focus (*arrow*) is slightly more intense and was suspicious for a possible lesion. Note that this does not appear substantially different from the true-positive liver lesion in **Fig. 10.3**. However, this was a false-positive finding, as no lesion was identified by either computed tomography or magnetic resonance imaging in this region.

activity relative to normal liver. A subtle focus of activity in the liver on attenuation-corrected images may be due to image noise rather than a lesion. Before interpreting a subtle focus as a lesion:

a. Review the nonattenuation-corrected (NAC) images. If the focus is seen on the less noisy NAC images, the level of confidence for a lesion is greatly increased. If the focus is not detected on NAC images, it may be artifactual secondary to image noise. Note that this method may be less helpful for central lesions, which may not be seen on NAC images due to attenuation.

b. Correlation with CT must be performed. CT is very sensitive for detecting small liver lesions, but it often cannot characterize these lesions. It is likely that if a focus seen on PET is a true lesion, it will be recognized on a contrast-enhanced CT, often in retrospect. Rarely, true-positive lesions may not be seen on CT, particularly if the liver is fatty infiltrated and/or imaged in only one phase of enhancement (**Figs. 10.3** and **10.5**). However, if a noncontrast CT is obtained as part of a PET/CT exam, many true-positive liver lesions identified on PET will not be detected on the noncontrast CT.

◆ Spleen

There are limited data on PET/CT imaging for the evaluation of solid splenic masses.[8]

A

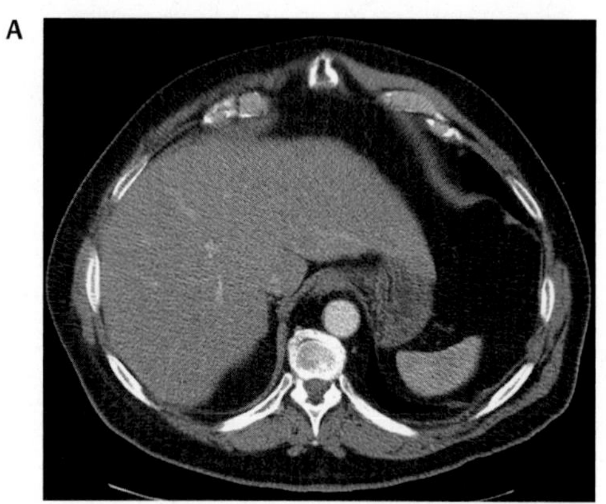

B

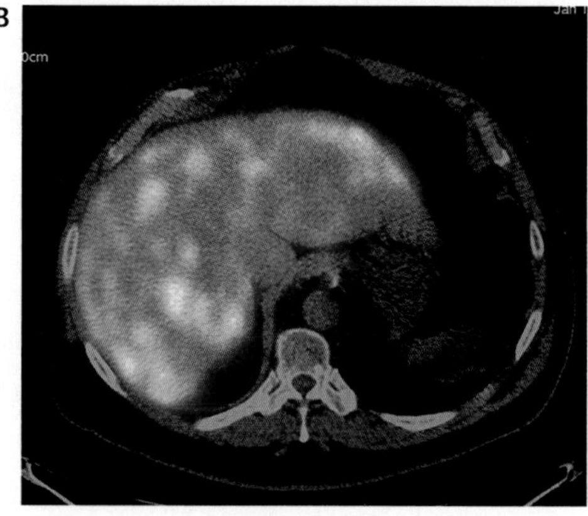

Fig. 10.5 Liver metastases seen by positron emission tomography (PET) only. **(A)** Axial computed tomography (CT) scan does not demonstrate any liver lesions. **(B)** Corresponding PET/CT scan demonstrates multiple hepatic metastases. This is a rare finding, as the majority of liver metastases seen on PET can be visualized by contrast-enhanced CT. However, liver metastases are occasionally not visualized on portal-phase CT scans. The fatty infiltration of the liver in this case may contribute to the lack of visualization of the metastases. An arterial-phase CT was not done in this case, so it is unclear whether the metastases would have been visualized in a different phase of contrast enhancement.

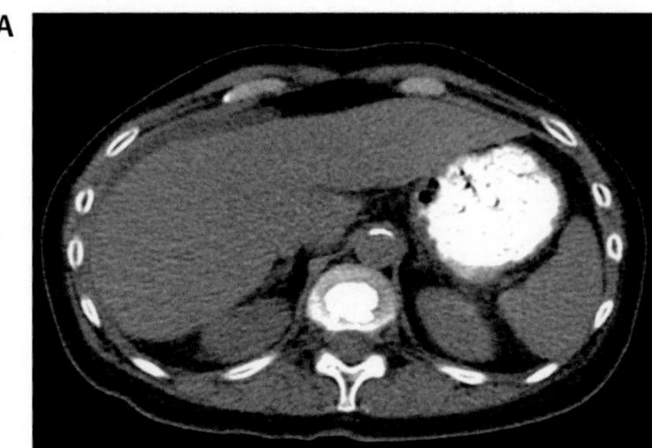

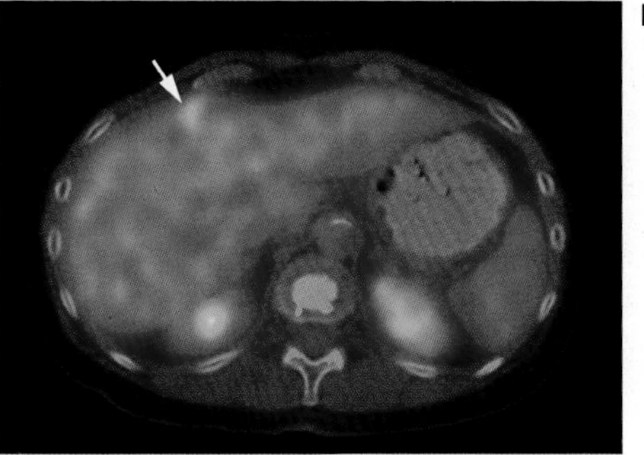

Fig. 10.6 Ascites and solid serosal implant. **(A)** Axial computed tomography (CT) demonstrates free fluid over the liver. **(B)** A solid serosal implant (*arrow*) is identified in this free fluid on the corresponding positron emission tomography/CT.

1. ***Known FDG-avid malignancy***
   a. *PET/CT.* Sensitivity 100%, specificity 100%
   b. *Standardized uptake value (SUV).* An SUV of 2.3 is useful for differentiating benign from malignant lesions.
2. ***No known malignancy***
   a. *PET/CT.* Sensitivity 100%, specificity 83%
   b. PET has a high negative predictive value in this setting.
      - However, a non-FDG-avid primary tumor should be excluded before diagnosing the splenic mass as a benign process.

   c. An FDG-avid splenic mass is likely (80%) to be malignant even without a known primary.
      - Possible false-positives include infection, sarcoidosis, and hyalinized nodules.[9]

◆ Peritoneum

1. ***Peritoneal metastases.*** Peritoneal metastases are most common in ovarian and gastrointestinal cancers. PET is more accurate than CT in detecting peritoneal metastases, but it will not detect very small implants (thus, it will not replace second-look laparotomy). PET is particularly helpful when intraperitoneal fluid is present—it can detect malignant ascites or small solid implants (**Fig. 10.6**).
2. ***Patterns of spread.*** It is important to understand the classic patterns of peritoneal spread. Specific attention should be directed to these areas (**Fig. 10.7**):
   a. Serosal surfaces of the liver and spleen (note that when correlating with CT, splenic serosal metastases can appear cystic)
   b. Omentum
   c. Paracolic gutters, particularly on the right
   d. Medial to the cecum (this must be differentiated from normal physiologic cecal uptake) (**Fig. 10.8**)

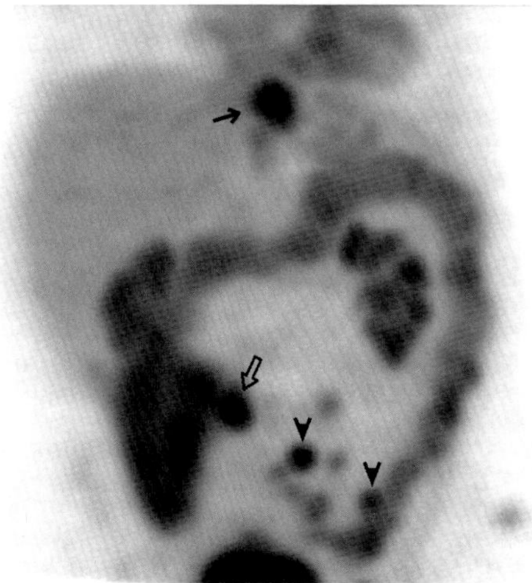

Fig. 10.7 Peritoneal seeding pattern. Coronal positron emission tomography scan demonstrates multiple foci of peritoneal seeding medial to the cecum (*open arrow*) and on the sigmoid mesocolon (arrowheads) from a gastroesophageal carcinoma (*arrow*). This is a classic pattern of peritoneal spread. (From Lin EC, Lear J, Quaife RA. Metastatic peritoneal seeding patterns demonstrated by FDG positron emission tomographic imaging. Clin Nucl Med 2001;26(3):249–250. Reprinted with permission.)

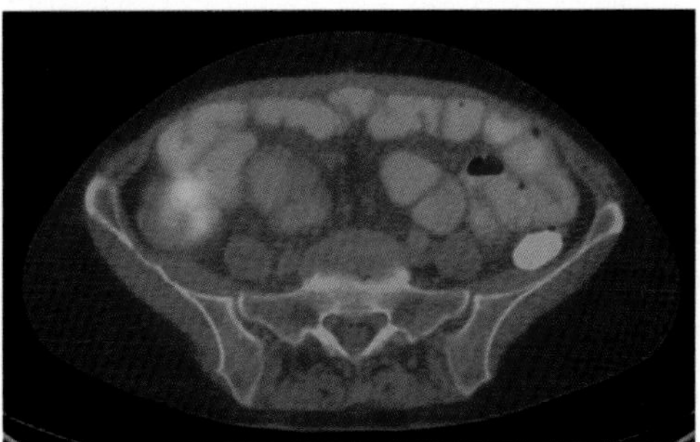

Fig. 10.8 Peritoneal implant. Axial positron emission tomography/computed tomography scan demonstrates focal uptake in a peritoneal implant on the surface of the medial cecum. This is difficult to distinguish from physiologic cecal activity. The eccentric location of the uptake is helpful in differentiating this from physiologic uptake.

e. Sigmoid mesocolon

f. Pelvis—particularly between the bladder and uterus and between the uterus and rectum

3. ***Distinguishing peritoneal metastasis from bowel activity.*** It is sometimes difficult to differentiate peritoneal metastasis from bowel activity without PET/CT.
   a. The focus should be reviewed in all three planes, with an attempt to link the activity to a segment of bowel in at least one plane. Often foci that appear outside the bowel in one plane are clearly visualized in the bowel on another plane.
   b. Outside the right colon, cecum, and rectosigmoid where normal intense areas of uptake are often noted, it is unusual to see foci of bowel activity, which are substantially more intense than the surrounding structures; this is particularly true in the small bowel (**Fig. 10.2**).
   c. CT correlation is very helpful, as peritoneal metastases are often identified retrospectively with this modality after attention is directed to the area of abnormality by PET.
   d. *SUV*. An SUV cutoff of 5.1[10] may be helpful for the diagnosis of peritoneal carcinomatosis.
   e. *PET/CT*. Although PET/CT can often allow for differentiation of bowel activity from peritoneal disease, PET/CT has the potential disadvantage of causing areas of artifactually increased and decreased uptake in the bowel (see Chapter 8). Potential peritoneal disease should be interpreted with caution on PET/CT, as bowel motion between the CT and PET scans can result in both false-positive and false-negative findings. NAC images should always be reviewed in conjunction with the corrected scans.
4. ***Diffuse peritoneal carcinomatosis.*** Diffuse peritoneal carcinomatosis can result in diffuse peritoneal uptake, which may be difficult to clearly define, as no focal lesions are seen in this setting.[11] Clues to identifying diffuse disease are (**Fig. 10.9**)[12]
   a. *Liver border*. The liver border is poorly visualized, as peritoneal activity is close in intensity to that of liver.
   b. *Straight-line sign*. On sagittal and axial images, the retroperitoneum is less intense than the peritoneum in peritoneal carcinomatosis (normally, the peritoneum and retroperitoneum are of comparable intensity). This results in a straight line demarcating the peritoneum and retroperitoneum on sagittal images.

◆ Lymph Nodes

1. ***Lymph node metastases.*** PET is more sensitive than CT in detecting lymph node metastases. Malignant nodes can be detected by PET before nodal enlargement (> 1 cm) on CT.
2. ***Size.*** The sensitivity of PET for metastatic deposits in nodes measuring 6 to 10 mm is 83%; it drops to 23% for those ≤ 5 mm.[13] Because PET will not detect micrometastases, it is not a substitute for sentinel node imaging procedures. Thus, PET is not a substitute for sentinel node imaging for axillary nodal staging in breast cancer and local nodal staging in melanoma.
3. ***Inflammatory versus malignant lymph nodes.*** A common problem is differentiating benign from malignant nodal uptake.
   a. *SUV*. As a general rule, malignant nodes have higher SUV values (usually > 2.5) compared with inflammatory nodes. However, small nodes with metastases, due to partial volume effects, may have a low SUV and low uptake by visual interpretation.

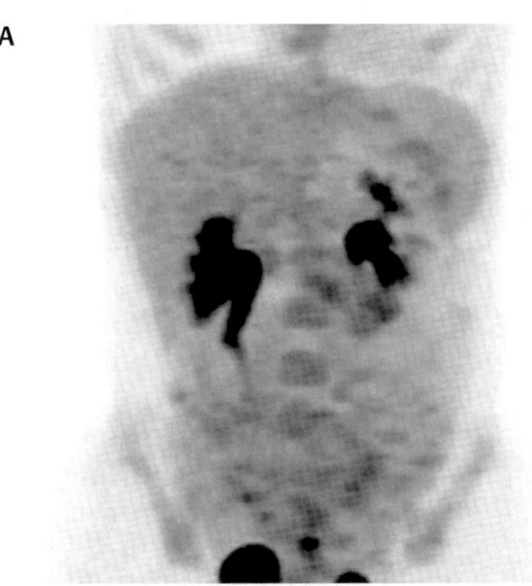

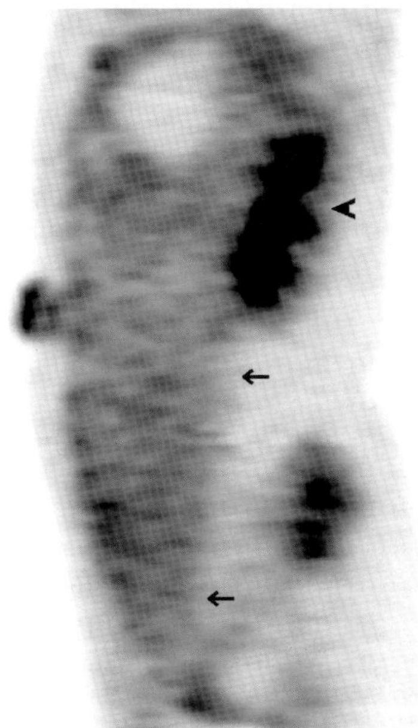

Fig. 10.9 Diffuse peritoneal carcinomatosis. **(A)** Coronal positron emission tomography (PET) scan in a patient with ovarian cancer demonstrates diffuse increased peritoneal uptake (note that the inferior border of the liver is not visualized). **(B)** On sagittal PET, there is a straight line (*arrows*) caused by increased intensity of the peritoneum relative to the retroperitoneum. Normally, there is no demarcation between the peritoneum and retroperitoneum. Kidney activity (*arrowhead*) lies in the retroperitoneum. An umbilical nodule or "Sister Mary Joseph node" is also noted.

b. *CT correlation.* Theoretically, there should be a detectable node by CT in any region of FDG uptake. The lack of a detectable node on CT suggests that the uptake may be related to a nonnodal structure. Although PET commonly detects metastases in normal-appearing nodes on CT, it is unlikely that a metastatic node would not be seen at all on CT. Note that this does not apply to areas where small nodes may be difficult to visualize (e.g., the hila). In addition, mediastinal nodes can sometimes be "flat" in shape and may be difficult to detect on CT (**Fig. 10.10**).

- Substantial uptake in a normal-size node is very specific for malignancy, as

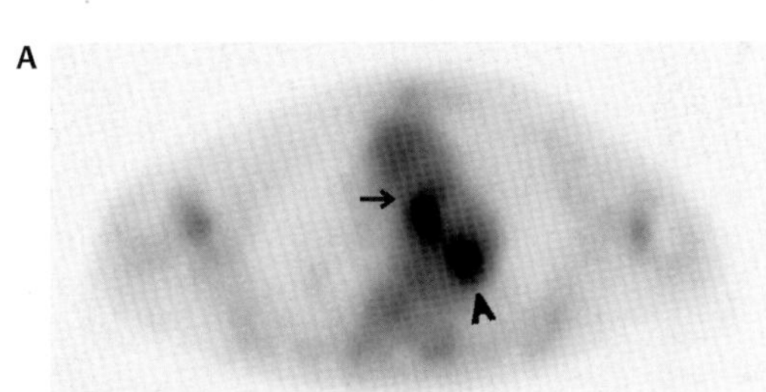

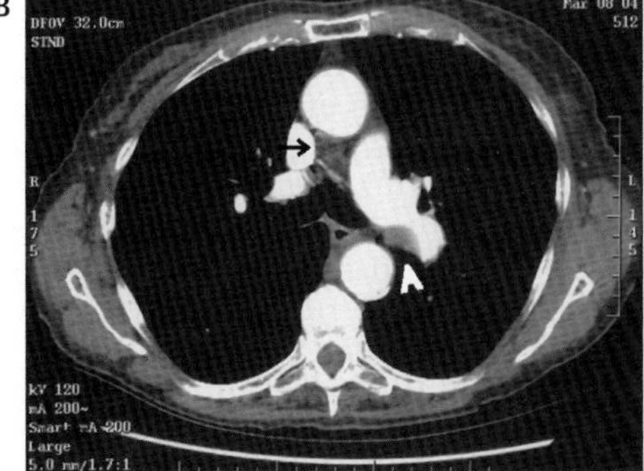

Fig. 10.10 Flat node missed by computed tomography (CT) but detected on positron emission tomography (PET). **(A)** Axial PET scan in a patient with lung cancer demonstrates uptake in central mediastinal (*arrow*) and left hilar (*arrowhead*) nodes. **(B)** CT scan at the same level demonstrates the left hilar node (*arrowhead*). A less dense node (*arrow*) is seen corresponding to the central mediastinal uptake seen on PET. This is a "flat" node and was seen only on one slice of the CT. This was not prospectively called abnormal on CT because it resembles the superior pericardial recess, which is a normal variant.

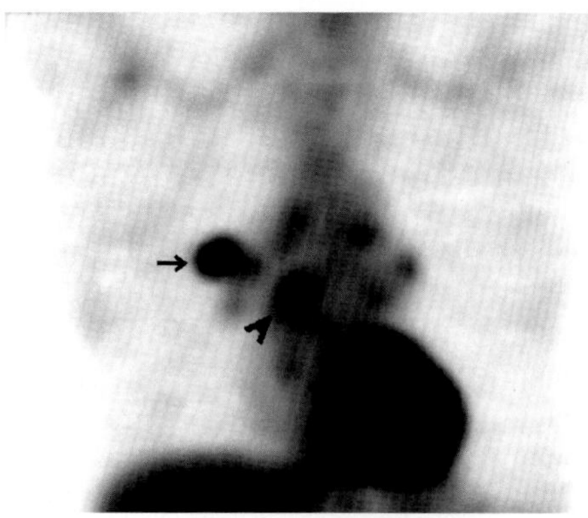

Fig. 10.11 Malignant drainage pattern. Coronal positron emission tomography (PET) scan in a patient with a right upper lobe lung cancer (*arrow*) demonstrates activity in multiple nodes, with the most intense uptake in the first nodal basin (*arrowhead*). This is a typical drainage pattern for a right upper lobe carcinoma, which spreads first to lymph nodes along the medial surface of the right mainstem bronchus (seen as a linear photopenic area between the node and tumor). These nodes are known as the lymphatic sump of Borrie.

inflammatory nodes would most likely be enlarged with the same amount of uptake. For example, definite positive uptake in a 5 mm mediastinal node in lung cancer is highly likely a true-positive finding for metastasis.

- Nodes are typically considered benign if a fatty hilum is seen on CT. However, if the node has substantial FDG uptake, malignancy should be suspected, as PET may detect disease before the fatty hilum is fully replaced by tumor (**Fig. 10.1**).
- FDG uptake in a mediastinal or hilar node can be suspected as false-positive if[14]
  - o The nodes are calcified.
  - o The nodes have attenuation greater than the surrounding vessels on noncontrast CT.

c. Location and pattern. The location and pattern of nodal uptake are often useful in differentiating between benign and malignant processes.

- For example, a left upper lobe lung carcinoma will spread first to the aortopulmonary window; thus, a lack of aortopulmonary window uptake with nodal uptake elsewhere suggests a benign etiology.
- If multiple nodes are seen, the node in the first drainage area is usually the most intense if the etiology is metastatic disease (**Fig. 10.11**).
- Symmetric low-grade uptake (e.g., bilateral hilar) is usually benign (**Fig. 10.12**).

d. Pelvic lymph nodes

- If pelvic lymph nodes are of clinical concern, it is important to reduce urinary activity (see Chapter 4).
- Ovarian activity is a common mimic of iliac nodal disease, as the ovaries are usually close to the iliac nodes. If the ureters are visualized on PET, they can be helpful in distinguishing ovarian from pelvic nodal activity.[15] The pelvic ureters are at the boundary of the intraperitoneal space medially and extraperitoneal space laterally. Ovaries are intraperitoneal and will be medial to the ureters (**Fig. 10.13**). Iliac nodes are extraperitoneal and will be lateral to the ureters.

◆ Lungs

1. ***Lung metastases.*** The primary value of PET in the lung parenchyma is in evaluating

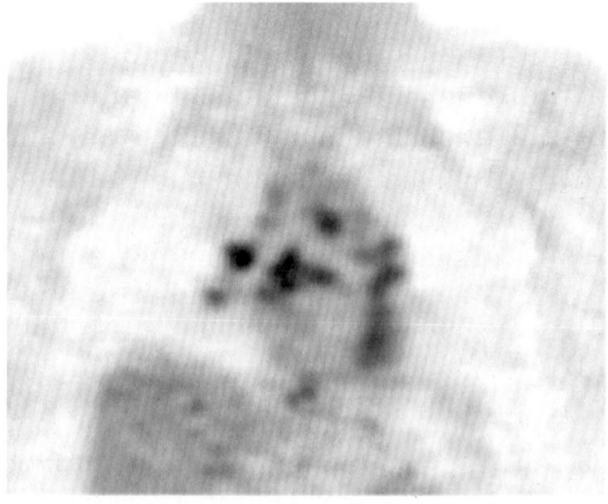

Fig. 10.12 Sarcoidosis. Coronal positron emission tomography scan demonstrates a symmetric pattern of hilar and mediastinal uptake in sarcoidosis. (Courtesy of Bruce Higginbotham, Little Rock, AR.)

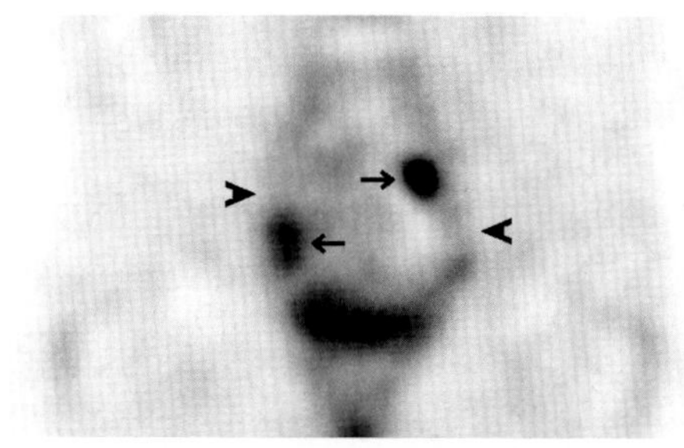
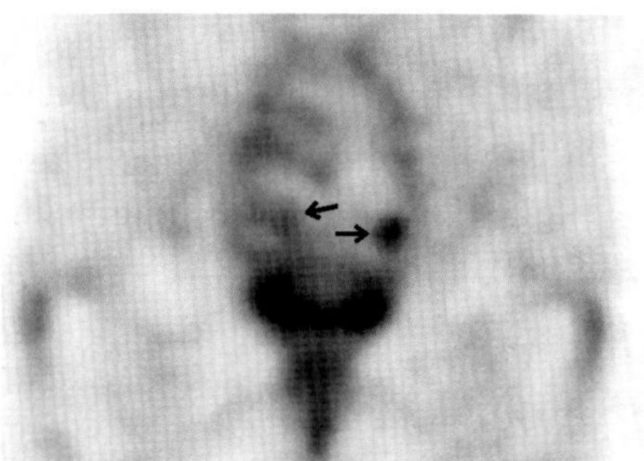

Fig. 10.13 Ovarian fluorodeoxyglucose (FDG) uptake diagnosed using ureteral landmarks. **(A)** Coronal positron emission tomography (PET) scan in a patient with lymphoma demonstrated two foci of pelvic uptake (*arrows*). Although iliac lymphadenopathy is a concern, the iliac nodes are extraperitoneal and should lie lateral to the ureters (*arrowheads*). The intraperitoneal ovaries lie medial to the ureters. Although ureteral activity is typically a confounding factor, the ureters can be used as a landmark to differentiate ovarian uptake from iliac nodal uptake. Computed tomography (CT) did not demonstrate any nodes in the region. **(B)** The patient had a follow-up PET that demonstrates the two foci (*arrows*) to have moved and decreased in intensity, consistent with ovarian uptake. (From Lin EC, Siegal J. Pelvic anatomic localization using ureteral activity on FDG positron emission tomography. Clin Nucl Med 2003;28(10):836–7. Reprinted with permission.)

solitary pulmonary nodules rather than detecting lung metastases. Sensitivity for lung metastases < 1 cm is poor. Thus, PET does not replace CT in the detection of lung metastases.

a. PET/CT versus CT. PET/CT, if performed with shallow breathing, does not replace a breath-hold chest CT for detection of lung metastases. PET/CT performed in shallow breathing often does not detect small lung nodules.[16] The addition of a low-dose breath-hold chest CT to the PET/CT examination may be helpful.[17]

b. Small nodules with minimal or no uptake. In patients with nonthoracic malignancies, small lung nodules (≤ 1 cm) with minimal or no FDG uptake turn out to be malignant approximately one fifth of the time.[18]

- These small nodules are more likely to be malignant when no other benign pulmonary lesions can be identified.
- Small nodules with no visible uptake are not less likely to be malignant than those with minimal uptake.

2. If there are known lung lesions in a cancer patient, PET can be helpful in differentiating these lesions from benign etiologies if the lesions are > 1 cm. The interpretation of FDG PET in small subcentimeter pulmonary nodules is similar to the interpretation of subcentimeter liver lesions. A positive result is very useful, indicating that metastatic disease is likely, but a negative result is less helpful, as the nodule could be malignant and not detectable by PET.
3. ***SUV.*** SUV values should be used with caution in evaluation of potential pulmonary metastases. An SUV cutoff of 2.5 may have value in this setting,[19] but this is not well established (as is the case for solitary pulmonary nodules).

◆ Bone Marrow Metastases

1. ***Bone marrow metastases.*** The mechanism of uptake in bone marrow metastases is different on FDG PET than on bone scan. The bone marrow metastasis is positive on PET because the tumor itself has increased FDG uptake, whereas the metastasis will be positive on bone scan due to increased reactive uptake around the tumor (**Fig. 10.14**).
2. ***Lytic versus sclerotic metastasis.*** FDG PET is sensitive for lytic bone metastases (**Fig. 10.14**) but less sensitive for sclerotic metastasis (**Fig. 10.15**).[20] Thus, the sensitivity of PET for bone metastases depends on the primary tumor. However, many sclerotic metastases without FDG uptake may represent treated

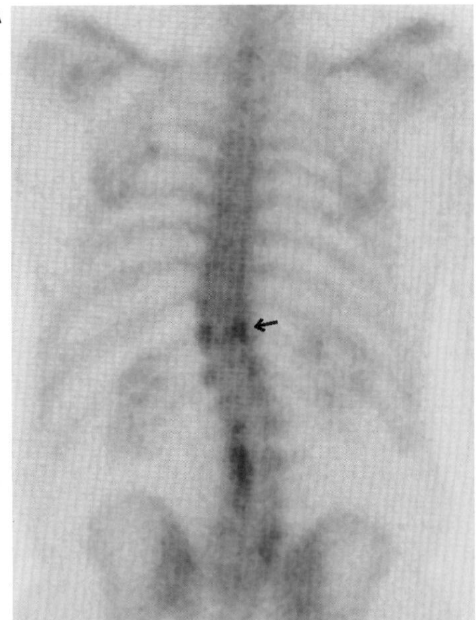

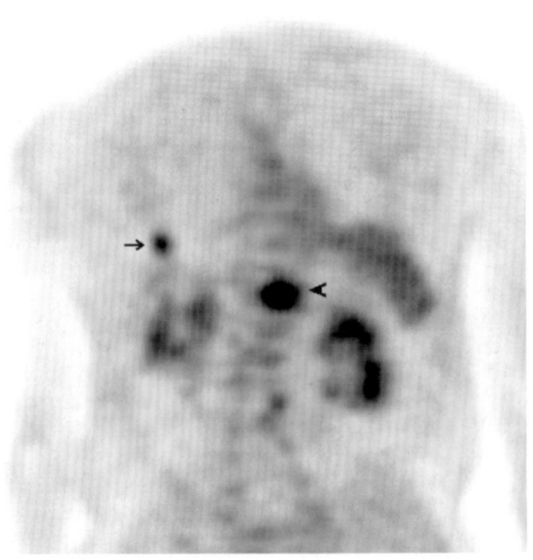

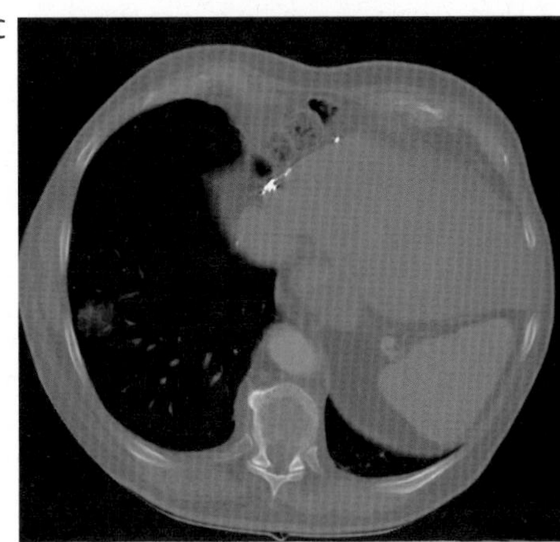

Fig. 10.14 Lytic bone metastases from lung cancer detected by positron emission tomography (PET) only. **(A)** Whole-body bone scan in a lung cancer patient demonstrates peripheral uptake at the T11 vertebral body (*arrow*). This appearance is not typical for metastasis. This was initially interpreted as negative for metastasis. **(B)** Coronal PET scan demonstrates intense uptake in the T11 vertebral body (*arrowhead*). Uptake is also seen in the primary right lower lobe lung cancer (*arrow*). This case illustrates the difference in uptake between PET and a bone scan: uptake on PET is in the lesion itself, whereas bone scan uptake is in reactive bone around the lesion. The minimal peripheral bone scan uptake is in reactive bone around the central fluorodeoxyglucose (FDG), avid lesion. **(C)** Computed tomography scan demonstrates a central lytic vertebral body metastasis. Note that there is still intact bone seen around the lesion, which accounts for the peripheral uptake seen on bone scan.

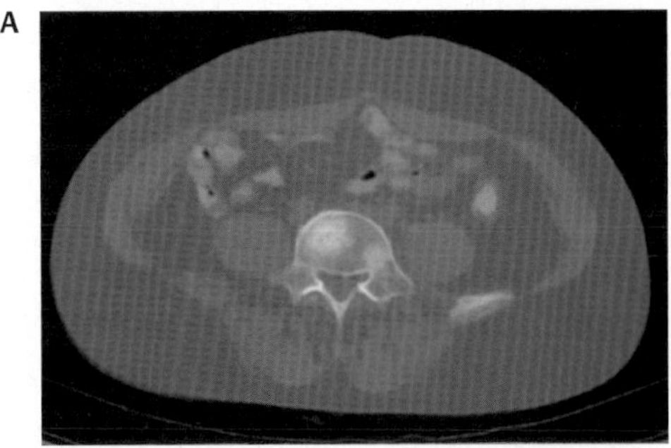

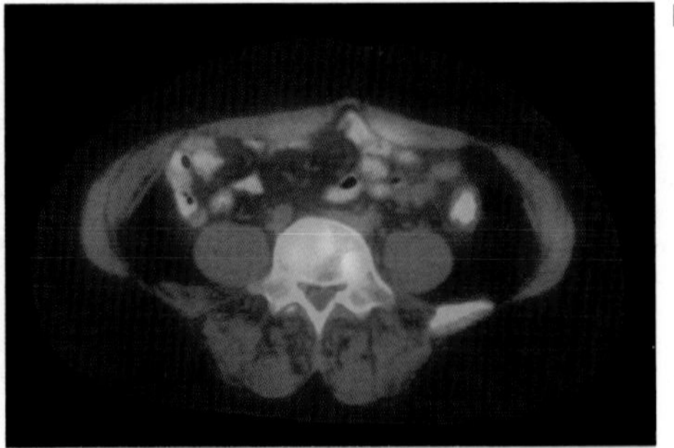

Fig. 10.15 Sclerotic bone metastases. **(A)** Computed tomography (CT) scan demonstrates sclerotic lumbar vertebral body metastases. **(B)** Axial positron emission tomography (PET)/CT does not demonstrate increased uptake in the large right anterior vertebral body metastasis. There is minimal peripheral uptake in the smaller left posterior vertebral body metastasis.

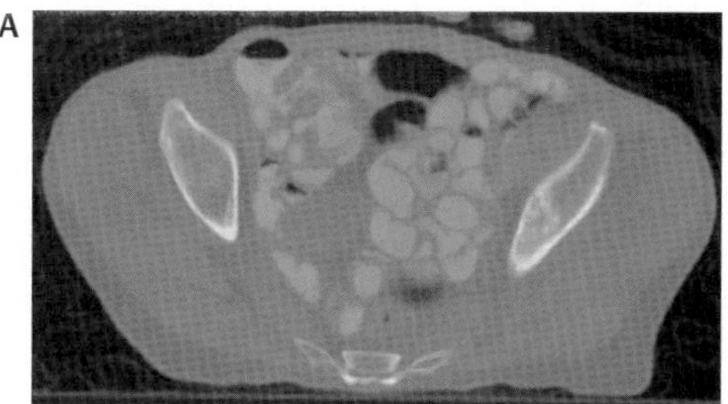
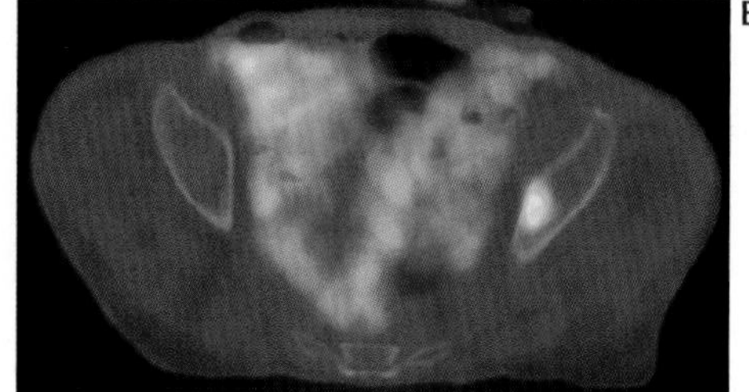
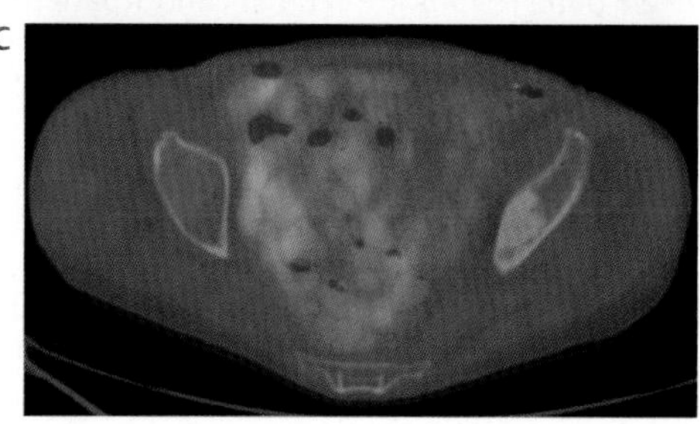

Fig. 10.16 Treated bone metastasis. **(A)** Axial computed tomography (CT) demonstrates a mixed lytic and sclerotic lesion in the left pelvis with fluorodeoxyglucose (FDG) uptake on positron emission tomography (PET)/CT **(B)** After treatment, a follow-up PET/CT study (C) shows no uptake in the lesion, which is now slightly more sclerotic. PET is more accurate than CT in assessing bone metastases after therapy, as there may be minimal or no change in appearance on CT in bone metastases that respond to therapy.

metastases (**Fig. 10.16**); in these cases, the lack of FDG uptake in the sclerotic treated metastasis is an accurate finding. Osteoblastic lesions that are FDG avid may be more resistant to treatment.

3. ***PET versus bone scan.*** Although the CT portion of a PET/CT study may detect some bone metastases missed on PET, it is unclear at this time whether the combination of the PET and CT data can replace a bone scan.
   a. *Lung cancer.* PET is likely superior to a bone scan.
   b. *Esophageal cancer.* Limited data suggest PET is superior to a bone scan.[21]
   c. *Nasopharyngeal cancer.* Limited data suggest PET is superior to a bone scan.[22]
   d. *Breast cancer.* PET is complementary to a bone scan, but it cannot replace a bone scan. PET detects some metastases that bone scan does not and vice versa.
   e. *Prostate cancer.* PET is much less sensitive than a bone scan.
   f. *Thyroid cancer.* One study suggests that PET is more specific and accurate than a bone scan,[23] but another suggests that a bone scan can identify metastases that are PET negative.[24]
4. ***PET and CT correlation***
   a. There will be no correlative finding on CT in ~50% of bone metastases detected by PET (**Fig. 10.17**).[25] Thus, the absence of a correlative CT finding in the presence of

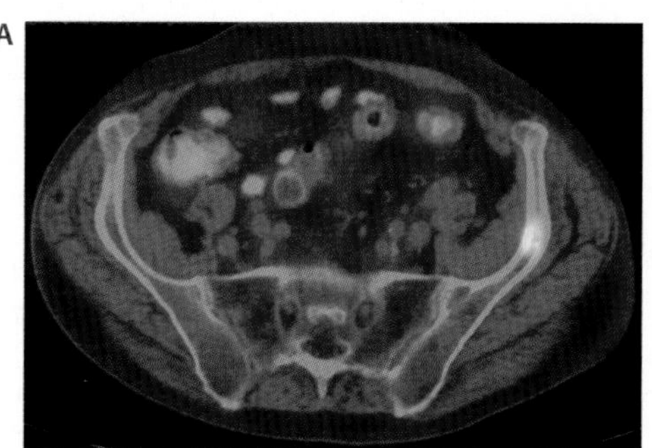
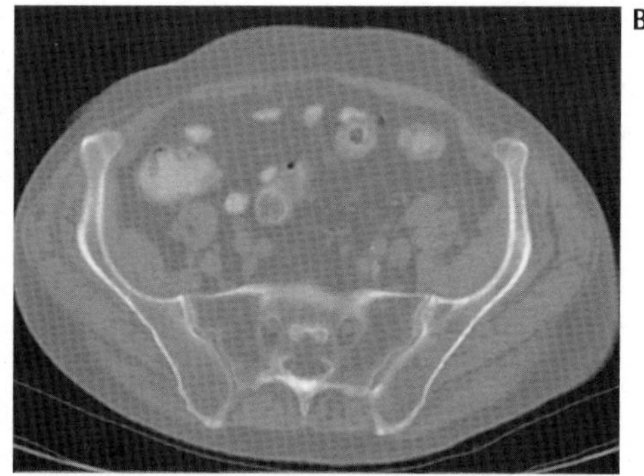

Fig. 10.17 Invisible metastasis. **(A)** A left iliac bone metastasis seen on axial positron emission tomography/computed tomography (PET/CT) scan is not visualized on **(B)** the corresponding CT scan.

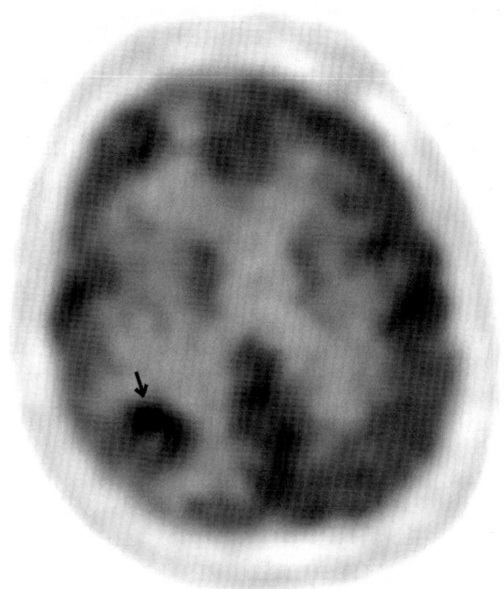

Fig. 10.18 Brain metastasis. Axial positron emission tomography scan demonstrates a right parietal metastasis at the gray–white junction (*arrow*).

osseous FDG uptake does not exclude a lesion.

b. The positive predictive value (PPV) of PET/CT for bone malignancy is 98% when the results of PET and CT are concordant. However, if PET is positive and CT is negative, the PPV is 61%. If the lesion is solitary in this scenario, the PPV is 43%.[26] Therefore, confirmation with additional tests such as MRI is often necessary for bone lesions identified by PET but not by CT, particularly if solitary.

c. Bone lesions that are positive on CT but negative on PET have a PPV of 17% for malignancy.[26]

d. The sensitivity of PET is substantially superior to a bone scan for lesions that are invisible on CT.[27]

e. FDG PET better reflects tumor activity of bone metastases than does CT. Radiographic changes vary widely after treatment and do not correlate well with the presence of active tumor.[28] Prior chemotherapy does not affect the PPV of PET, but it decreases the PPV of CT.[26] Treated bone metastases tend to be blastic on CT and PET negative (**Fig. 10.16**).[29]

5. PET is more specific than bone scan, as degenerative joint disease typically does not have substantial uptake (although there can be substantial uptake with an inflammatory component).
6. Although standard PET protocols image only from the face to upper thighs, this is not a major drawback, given the low risk of solitary bone metastases to the skull and lower extremities.[30]
7. Radiographic correlation is necessary if single bone lesions are seen in cancer patients, as benign primary bone lesions can often have increased uptake (see Chapter 25).

◆ Brain

1. ***Brain tumors and metastases.*** The primary value of PET is in primary brain tumors rather than brain metastases. The overall sensitivity of PET for brain metastases is ~60%. Because most metastases are at the gray–white matter junction, detection is limited by high normal cortical brain activity (**Fig. 10.18**). Smaller metastases are less well detected, with sensitivity for 1 cm lesions of ~40%.[31]
2. If brain imaging is added to the imaging protocol for patients with non–central nervous system malignancies, management is changed in < 1% of patients.[32]

◆ Adrenals

1. ***Adrenal metastases and tumors.*** FDG PET is useful in
   a. Detecting unsuspected adrenal metastases (**Fig. 10.19**)
   b. Evaluating equivocal adrenal masses seen on CT or MRI
2. ***Accuracy***
   a. Detection of adrenal metastases (lung cancer). Sensitivity 100%, specificity 80%[33]
   b. Characterizing adrenal lesions in patients with known malignancy. Sensitivity 98%, specificity 92%[34]
   - Combining CT data (Hounsfield unit measurement) with PET data improves specificity to 98%.[34]
   - An SUV cutoff of 3.1[34] or adrenal uptake more than twice that of the liver[35] can be used to differentiate metastases from adenomas. However,

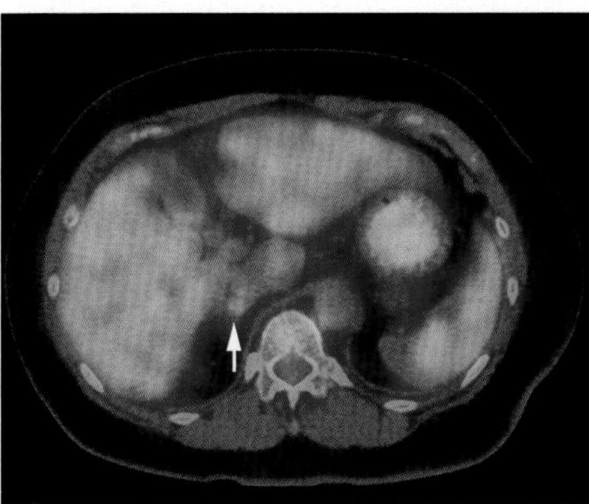

Fig. 10.19 Adrenal metastasis. Axial positron emission tomography/computed tomography scan demonstrates a small right adrenal metastasis (*arrow*).

visual interpretation is as accurate as SUV.[36]

- Most benign adrenal lesions have uptake less than liver.[35]
- FDG uptake does not differ between lipid-rich and lipid-poor adenomas.[34] Thus, PET is accurate in cases where noncontrast CT is equivocal.[36]
- The sensitivity of PET is equal to MRI and superior to CT.[37]

3. ***Nonmetastatic causes of adrenal uptake***
   a. Adrenal hyperplasia can have FDG uptake, mimicking bilateral adrenal metastases (see **Fig. 6.34**, p. 61).
   b. Adrenal neoplasms other than metastases have FDG uptake (see Chapter 6), but these can usually be differentiated from metastasis by CT or MRI.
   c. Adrenal hemorrhage and histoplasmosis can have FDG uptake.[38,39]
   d. Approximately 5% of adrenal adenomas will have substantial FDG uptake.[40]
4. ***False-negative results.*** False-negative results can be seen in lesions < 1 cm, metastases from primary tumors with low FDG avidity (e.g., carcinoid), and lesions with hemorrhage and necrosis.[36,40]

References

1. Rappeport ED, Loft A, Berthelsen AK, et al. Contrast-enhanced FDG-PET/CT vs. SPIO-enhanced MRI vs. FDG-PET vs. CT in patients with liver metastases from colorectal cancer: a prospective study with intraoperative confirmation. Acta Radiol 2007;48(4):369–378
2. Kinkel K, Lu Y, Both M, et al. Detection of hepatic metastases from cancers of the gastrointestinal tract by using noninvasive imaging methods (US, CT, MR imaging, PET): a meta-analysis. Radiology 2002;224(3):748–756
3. Sahani DV, Kalva SP, Fischman AJ, et al. Detection of liver metastases from adenocarcinoma of the colon and pancreas: comparison of mangafodipir trisodium-enhanced liver MRI and whole-body FDG PET. AJR Am J Roentgenol 2005;185(1):239–246
4. Delbeke D, Martin WH, Sandler MP, et al. Evaluation of benign vs malignant hepatic lesions with positron emission tomography. Arch Surg 1998;133(5):510–515
5. Aznar DL, Ojeda R, Garcia EU, et al. Focal nodular hyperplasia (FNH): a potential cause of false-positive positron emission tomography. Clin Nucl Med 2005;30(9):636–637
6. Kawamura E, Habu D, Tsushima H, et al. A case of hepatic inflammatory pseudotumor identified by FDG-PET. Ann Nucl Med 2006;20(4):321–323
7. Guglielmi AN, Kim BY, Bybel B, Slifkin N. False-positive uptake of FDG in hepatic sarcoidosis. Clin Nucl Med 2006;31(3):175
8. Metser U, Miller E, Kessler A, et al. Solid splenic masses: evaluation with ^{18}F-FDG PET/CT. J Nucl Med 2005;46(1):52–59
9. Choi AY, Wax BN, Yung E. Focal F-18 fluorodeoxyglucose positron emission tomography uptake in a hyalinized nodule as a false-positive splenic metastasis in a patient with breast cancer and metastatic thyroid cancer. Clin Nucl Med 2005;30(12):799–800
10. Suzuki A, Kawano T, Takahashi N, et al. Value of ^{18}F-FDG PET in the detection of peritoneal carcinomatosis. Eur J Nucl Med Mol Imaging 2004;31(10):1413–1420
11. Turlakow A, Yeung HW, Salmon AS, et al. Peritoneal carcinomatosis: role of (18)F-FDG PET. J Nucl Med 2003;44(9):1407–1412
12. Lin EC. "Straight line" sign of diffuse peritoneal carcinomatosis on sagittal FDG positron emission tomographic images. Clin Nucl Med 2002;27(10):735–736
13. Crippa F, Leutner M, Belli F, et al. Which kinds of lymph node metastases can FDG PET detect? A clinical study in melanoma. J Nucl Med 2000;41(9):1491–1494
14. Shim SS, Lee KS, Kim BT, et al. Non-small cell lung cancer: prospective comparison of integrated FDG PET/CT and CT alone for preoperative staging. Radiology 2005;236(3):1011–1019
15. Lin EC, Siegal J. Pelvic anatomic localization using ureteral activity on FDG positron emission tomography. Clin Nucl Med 2003;28(10):836–837
16. Allen-Auerbach M, Yeom K, Park J, et al. Standard PET/CT of the chest during shallow breathing is inadequate for comprehensive staging of lung cancer. J Nucl Med 2006;47(2):298–301
17. Juergens KU, Weckesser M, Stegger L, et al. Tumor staging using whole-body high-resolution 16-channel PET-CT: does additional low-dose chest CT in inspiration improve the detection of solitary pulmonary nodules? Eur Radiol 2006;16(5):1131–1137
18. O JH, Yoo I, Kim SH, et al. Clinical significance of small pulmonary nodules with little or no ^{18}F-FDG uptake on PET/CT images of patients with nonthoracic malignancies. J Nucl Med 2007;48(1):15–21
19. Hsu WH, Hsu NY, Shen YY, et al. Differentiating solitary pulmonary metastases in patients with extrapulmonary neoplasms using FDG-PET. Cancer Invest 2003;21(1):47–52

20. Cook GJ, Fogelman I. The role of positron emission tomography in skeletal disease. Semin Nucl Med 2001;31(1):50–61

21. Kato H, Miyazaki T, Nakajima M, et al. Comparison between whole-body positron emission tomography and bone scintigraphy in evaluating bony metastases of esophageal carcinomas. Anticancer Res 2005;25(6C):4439–4444

22. Liu FY, Chang JT, Wang HM, et al. [18F]fluorodeoxyglucose positron emission tomography is more sensitive than skeletal scintigraphy for detecting bone metastasis in endemic nasopharyngeal carcinoma at initial staging. J Clin Oncol 2006;24(4):599–604

23. Ito S, Kato K, Ikeda M, et al. Comparison of 18F-FDG PET and bone scintigraphy in detection of bone metastases of thyroid cancer. J Nucl Med 2007;48(6):889–895

24. Phan HT, Jager PL, Plukker JT, Wolffenbuttel BH, Dierckx RA, Links TP. Detection of bone metastases in thyroid cancer patients: bone scintigraphy or ^{18}F-FDG PET? Nucl Med Commun 2007;28(8):597–602

25. Nakamoto Y, Cohade C, Tatsumi M, et al. CT appearance of bone metastases detected with FDG PET as part of the same PET/CT examination. Radiology 2005; 237(2):627–634

26. Taira AV, Herfkens RJ, Gambhir SS, Quon A. Detection of bone metastases: assessment of integrated FDG PET/CT imaging. Radiology 2007;243(1):204–211

27. Nakai T, Okuyama C, Kubota T, et al. Pitfalls of FDG-PET for the diagnosis of osteoblastic bone metastases in patients with breast cancer. Eur J Nucl Med Mol Imaging 2005;32(11):1253–1258

28. Tann M, Sandrasegaran K, Jennings SG, Skandarajah A, McHenry L, Schmidt CM. Positron-emission tomography and computed tomography of cystic pancreatic masses. Clin Radiol 2007;62(8):745–751

29. Israel O, Goldberg A, Nachtigal A, et al. FDG-PET and CT patterns of bone metastases and their relationship to previously administered anti-cancer therapy. Eur J Nucl Med Mol Imaging 2006;33(11):1280–1284

30. Fujimoto R, Higashi T, Nakamoto Y, et al. Diagnostic accuracy of bone metastases detection in cancer patients: comparison between bone scintigraphy and whole-body FDG-PET. Ann Nucl Med 2006;20(6):399–408

31. Rohren EM, Provenzale JM, Barboriak DP, Coleman RE. Screening for cerebral metastases with FDG PET in patients undergoing whole-body staging of non-central nervous system malignancy. Radiology 2003;226(1):181–187

32. Larcos G, Maisey MN. FDG-PET screening for cerebral metastases in patients with suspected malignancy. Nucl Med Commun 1996;17(3):197–198

33. Marom EM, McAdams HP, Erasmus JJ, et al. Staging non-small cell lung cancer with whole-body PET. Radiology 1999;212(3):803–809

34. Metser U, Miller E, Lerman H, et al. ^{18}F-FDG PET/CT in the evaluation of adrenal masses. J Nucl Med 2006; 47(1):32–37

35. Blake MA, Slattery JM, Kalra MK, et al. Adrenal lesions: characterization with fused PET/CT image in patients with proved or suspected malignancy—initial experience. Radiology 2006;238(3):970–977

36. Jana S, Zhang T, Milstein DM, et al. FDG-PET and CT characterization of adrenal lesions in cancer patients. Eur J Nucl Med Mol Imaging 2006;33(1):29–35

37. Frilling A, Tecklenborg K, Weber F, et al. Importance of adrenal incidentaloma in patients with a history of malignancy. Surgery 2004;136(6):1289–1296

38. Umeoka S, Koyama T, Saga T, et al. High ^{18}F-fluorodeoxyglucose uptake in adrenal histoplasmosis; a case report. Eur Radiol 2005;15(12):2483–2486

39. Votrubova J, Belohlavek O, Jaruskova M, et al. The role of FDG-PET/CT in the detection of recurrent colorectal cancer. Eur J Nucl Med Mol Imaging 2006;33(7): 779–784

40. Chong S, Lee KS, Kim HY, et al. Integrated PET-CT for the characterization of adrenal gland lesions in cancer patients: diagnostic efficacy and interpretation pitfalls. Radiographics 2006;26(6):1811–1824

11

Therapy Response

Eugene C. Lin and Abass Alavi

This is a general overview of positron emission tomography (PET) for therapy response. Information about the role of PET in relation to specific tumors is found in the following chapters.

General Principles

Therapy response imaging can be divided into two categories: early and late prediction.

1. ***Early prediction.*** The goal of imaging is to predict response early during therapy. In this case, the cancer should be one in which viable alternative therapies are available if the first-line therapy is ineffective. If there is a lack of response, the initial therapy can be changed early during the course of therapy. PET is particularly valuable, as an early response to therapy often does not result in change on conventional imaging modalities.
2. ***Late prediction.*** The goals of imaging are to evaluate response after the completion of therapy and to predict future outcome. PET is particularly valuable, as conventional imaging techniques are often not able to differentiate tumor from scar tissue.

Pearls

1. ***Definition of response***
   a. There are no accepted general criteria for defining response that are applicable to all tumors. Proposed general criteria are[1]
      - *Progressive metabolic disease:* > 25% increase in standardized uptake value (SUV), or new lesions
      - *Stable metabolic disease:* between < 25% SUV increase and < 15% SUV decrease
      - *Partial metabolic response:* 15 to 25% SUV decrease after one cycle of chemotherapy, or > 25% SUV decrease after more than one treatment cycle
      - *Complete metabolic response:* complete resolution of fluorodeoxyglucose (FDG) uptake. This is usually associated with a good prognosis, even though microscopic disease cannot be excluded.

   b. However, the definition of response may be specific to the particular tumor and the specific point in therapy. Published thresholds (amount of decrease in activity) to define response are usually specific to particular tumors, time intervals, and treatment methods. These are likely applicable only in those scenarios. If published thresholds are used, the method of SUV determination used and the time intervals of imaging after therapy should be duplicated as closely as possible.

c. *What is a significant change in SUV?*
   - The mean difference in serial SUV measurements is around 10%.[2–4]
   - For most lesions, changes in SUV > 20% are outside the 95% range for spontaneous fluctuation and can be considered to reflect true changes in glucose metabolism.[3]
   - However, the range of spontaneous fluctuation depends upon the initial SUV. The higher the SUV, the less the range of fluctuation.[3]
   - In practice, report SUV differences of 20 to 25% as significant unless the initial SUV is very high, in which case report 10 to 15% changes as significant.

2. ***Measurement of response.***[5] SUV measurements are feasible for the measurement of tumor response in the majority of cases and are the easiest method to implement in a busy clinical practice.
   a. Discussion of tracer kinetic approaches is beyond the scope of this chapter. However, patients with diabetes mellitus in particular may benefit from tracer kinetic approaches, as clearance and distribution of FDG may be altered.
   b. It is very important to standardize the imaging protocol in patients being followed for therapy response. Patients should ideally be scanned at the same institution on the same equipment. SUV values between institutions and between PET and PET/computed tomography (CT) may be poorly reproducible.

3. ***Midtreatment versus posttreatment results.***[6] A given treatment dose of radiation or chemotherapy will typically kill the same fraction rather than the same number of cells, regardless of the size of the tumor. Therefore, small tumors may still require multiple cycles of therapy to cure. This has implications for the interpretation of PET results in therapy response. As the resolution of PET is limited for small tumor volumes, PET can likely detect only the first few log units (90% reduction in tumor mass) of tumor cell killing. Thus, a tumor that is PET negative after therapy may still require multiple cycles of therapy to eliminate. Midtreatment and posttreatment PET results often have different implications.
   a. *Midtreatment.* Midtreatment PET scans provide information on the rate of tumor cell killing. A negative PET scan after a few cycles of therapy implies that the rate of tumor cell killing is sufficient to produce cure if the therapy is completed. Although the negative PET scan could be seen with a few or many log units of tumor cell killing, even a few log units of response early in the therapy cycle implies a rapid rate of response. A positive PET scan implies that the rate of tumor cell killing may be inadequate to produce cure if the entire cycle is completed.
   b. *Posttreatment.* A positive PET scan after completion of therapy usually indicates a slow rate of tumor cell killing and a resistant cancer, as many cycles of therapy have not resulted in even a few log units of tumor cell killing. However, a negative posttreatment PET scan could have two possible implications. Due to limited resolution, a negative posttreatment PET scan cannot differentiate between a few log units and many log units of tumor cell killing (i.e., between minimal residual disease and complete response). Thus, a negative posttreatment PET scan typically has a lower predictive value than a negative midtreatment scan.
   c. High sensitivity is usually preferred to specificity in the posttherapy setting, as false-negative results are usually less desirable than false-positive results.
   d. Variable response in different lesions in the same patient (**Fig. 11.1**) indicates tumor heterogeneity, which may contribute to tumor treatment resistance.
   - However, if there is a lack of response in one region and response in all other regions, a nonneoplastic etiology in the nonresponding region should be considered (**Fig. 11.2**).

4. ***Normal tissue response.*** Increased inflammatory uptake in normal tissue postradiation positively correlates with tumor response. Normal tissue radiosensitivity may correlate with tumor radiosensitivity.[7]

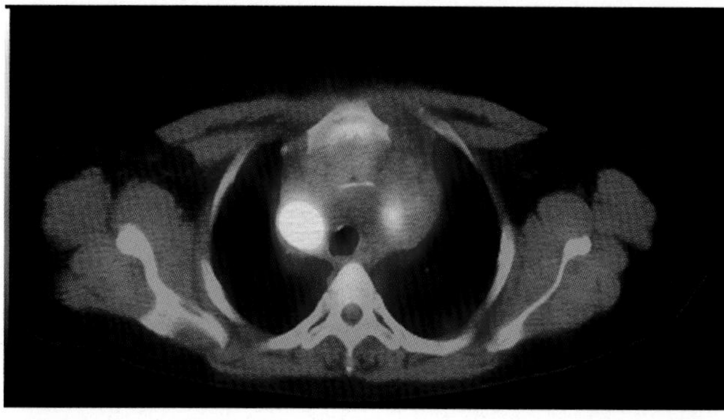

Fig. 11.1 Mixed tumor response. Axial positron emission tomography/computed tomography scan demonstrates extensive superior and anterior mediastinal adenopathy in a lymphoma patient posttherapy. Most of the nodes do not have increased fluorodeoxyglucose uptake, but two of the nodes have intense increased uptake. This finding often indicates increased tumor resistance to treatment.

Pitfalls

1. ***Treatment effects.*** See Chapter 4 for recommended minimum scan times after therapy. Chemotherapy and radiotherapy can cause false-positive and false-negative results.
   a. *False-positive results*
      - False-positive results are usually seen early after therapy.
      - A false-positive flare phenomenon has been described in responders to tamoxifen,[8] in patients undergoing chemotherapy for liver metastases in the first 2 weeks,[9] and in patients with glioblastoma treated with chemotherapy.[10] In some cases, this may be associated with an improved response to therapy.[8,10]
      - However, flare phenomenon seen on other modalities such as a bone scan may not result in a similar flare phenomenon on PET.[11]
      - After radiation, uptake around the periphery of a tumor may be secondary to a fibrous pseudocapsule.[12]
   b. *False-negative results*
      - False-negative results from presumed tumor "stunning" are usually seen for

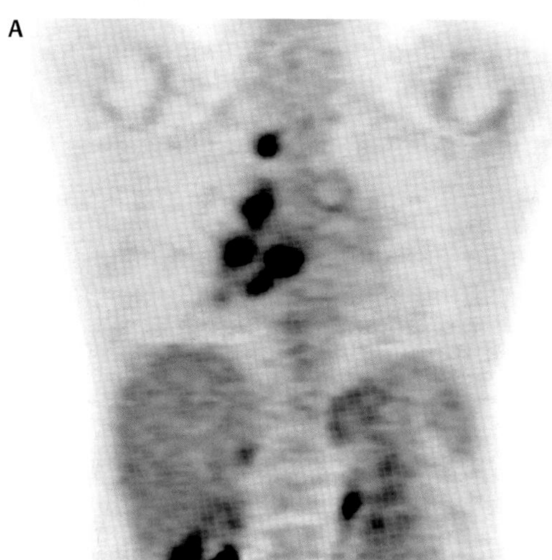

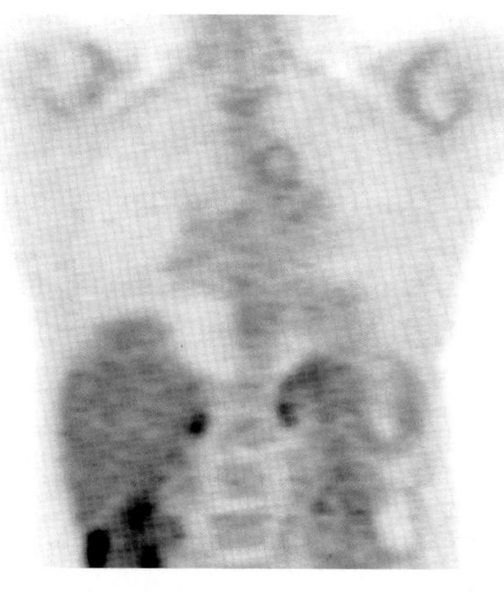

Fig. 11.2 False-positive uptake or mixed response? **(A)** Coronal positron emission tomography (PET) scan demonstrates extensive right lung and mediastinal disease along with bilateral adrenal uptake in a patient with small cell lung cancer. The adrenal uptake was initially interpreted as adrenal metastasis. **(B)** Coronal PET scan after therapy demonstrates complete resolution of the lung and mediastinal uptake. The bilateral adrenal uptake is slightly increased. This lack of concordance in a single region suggests that the adrenal uptake is nonneoplastic. The uptake was secondary to adrenal hyperplasia.

a much longer time frame than false-positive results.

2. ***SUV measurement error.*** There are numerous potential sources of error in SUV measurement discussed in Chapters 5 and 8. Some sources of measurement error specific to therapy response are
   a. Decreases in the size of the tumor will artifactually decrease SUVs due to partial volume effects.
   b. Changes in the surrounding background activity between exams can affect the degree of "spill in" of background activity and thus the SUV.[13]
3. ***Infection.*** Infection is always a potential cause of false-positive PET results; however, it should be more strongly considered in patients who have received bone marrow suppressing therapies.
4. ***Lack of baseline PET study.*** The lack of a baseline PET exam can result in both false-positives and false-negatives.
   a. False-positives. High levels of FDG uptake after therapy may not indicate therapy failure if the level of uptake prior to therapy was even greater. In this case, the response may have been partial.
   b. False-negatives. Minimal FDG uptake after therapy may not indicate therapy response if there was minimal uptake prior to therapy.
5. ***Low pretherapy FDG uptake.*** Lesions with low initial FDG uptake (SUV < 3 or tumor-to-background ratio < 5) may have a lower maximum detectable percentage change in SUV.[14,15] This may be secondary to a background of unmetabolized FDG included in SUV measurements.[15] This suggests that SUV measurements are less sensitive in detecting response in lesions with low initial FDG uptake. Measurements of the metabolic rate of FDG may be more helpful in lesions with low initial uptake.
6. ***Hepatic and splenic lesions.*** If hepatic and splenic involvement is demonstrated by initial staging, these lesions should usually be followed by contrast-enhanced CT or contrast-enhanced PET/CT. These lesions may be difficult to detect by PET and noncontrast PET/CT if they decrease in size after therapy.[16]

References

1. Young H, Baum R, Cremerius U, et al. Measurement of clinical and subclinical tumour response using [^{18}F]-fluorodeoxyglucose and positron emission tomography: review and 1999 EORTC recommendations. European Organization for Research and Treatment of Cancer (EORTC) PET Study Group. Eur J Cancer 1999;35(13):1773–1782
2. Minn H, Zasadny KR, Quint LE, Wahl RL. Lung cancer: reproducibility of quantitative measurements for evaluating 2-[F-18]-fluoro-2-deoxy-D-glucose uptake at PET. Radiology 1995;196(1):167–173
3. Weber WA, Ziegler SI, Thodtmann R, et al. Reproducibility of metabolic measurements in malignant tumors using FDG PET. J Nucl Med 1999;40(11):1771–1777
4. Nakamoto Y, Zasadny KR, Minn H, Wahl RL. Reproducibility of common semi-quantitative parameters for evaluating lung cancer glucose metabolism with positron emission tomography using 2-deoxy-2-[^{18}F] fluoro-D-glucose. Mol Imaging Biol 2002;4(2):171–178
5. Avril NE, Weber WA. Monitoring response to treatment in patients utilizing PET. Radiol Clin North Am 2005;43(1):189–204
6. Kasamon YL, Jones RJ, Wahl RL. Integrating PET and PET/CT into the risk-adapted therapy of lymphoma. J Nucl Med 2007;48(1, Suppl)19S–27S
7. Hicks RJ, MacManus MP, Matthews JP, et al. Early FDG-PET imaging after radical radiotherapy for non-small-cell lung cancer: inflammatory changes in normal tissues correlate with tumor response and do not confound therapeutic response evaluation. Int J Radiat Oncol Biol Phys 2004;60(2):412–418
8. Mortimer JE, Dehdashti F, Siegel BA, et al. Metabolic flare: indicator of hormone responsiveness in advanced breast cancer. J Clin Oncol 2001;19(11):2797–2803
9. Findlay M, Young H, Cunningham D, et al. Noninvasive monitoring of tumor metabolism using fluorodeoxyglucose and positron emission tomography in colorectal cancer liver metastases: correlation with tumor response to fluorouracil. J Clin Oncol 1996;14(3):700–708
10. De Witte O, Hildebrand J, Luxen A, Goldman S. Acute effect of carmustine on glucose metabolism in brain and glioblastoma. Cancer 1994;74(10):2836–2842
11. Shimizu N, Masuda H, Yamanaka H, et al. Fluorodeoxyglucose positron emission tomography scan of prostate cancer bone metastases with flare reaction after endocrine therapy. J Urol 1999;161(2):608–609
12. Aoki J, Endo K, Watanabe H, et al. FDG-PET for evaluating musculoskeletal tumors: a review. J Orthop Sci 2003;8(3):435–441
13. Soret M, Bacharach SL, Buvat I. Partial-volume effect in PET tumor imaging. J Nucl Med 2007;48(6):932–945
14. McDermott GM, Welch A, Staff RT, et al. Monitoring primary breast cancer throughout chemotherapy using FDG-PET. Breast Cancer Res Treat 2007;102(1):75–84
15. Doot RK, Dunnwald LK, Schubert EK, et al. Dynamic and static approaches to quantifying ^{18}F-FDG uptake for measuring cancer response to therapy, including the effect of granulocyte CSF. J Nucl Med 2007;48(6):920–925
16. Juweid ME, Stroobants S, Hoekstra OS, et al. Use of positron emission tomography for response assessment of lymphoma: consensus of the Imaging Subcommittee of International Harmonization Project in Lymphoma. J Clin Oncol 2007;25(5):571–578

12

Brain Neoplasms

Eugene C. Lin and Abass Alavi

◆ Primary Brain Tumors[1]

Clinical Indication: C

Although positron emission tomography (PET) imaging may not be indicated in the majority of newly diagnosed brain tumors, it is useful in specific situations:

1. Determining the best biopsy site for optimal grading of the tumor
2. Metabolic grading of the tumor: the degree of glucose metabolism correlates with prognosis and outcome in these patients (**Fig. 12.1**).
3. Evaluating possible transformation of a low-grade glioma to a high-grade tumor

Pearls

1. ***Factors affecting fluorodeoxyglucose (FDG) uptake***
   - ***a.*** *Corticosteroids.* Corticosteroids decrease glucose metabolism in normal brain tissue but do not affect metabolism within brain tumors. However, corticosteroid administration will limit evaluation of brain tumors, as overall image quality and anatomical detail are adversely affected.[2,3] Many of the effects of corticosteroids may be due to increased blood glucose levels.
   - ***b.*** *Cushing disease.* Patients with Cushing disease have decreased brain glucose metabolism.
   - ***c.*** *Sedatives and anticonvulsants.* Sedatives and anticonvulsants can also reduce glucose metabolism.
   - ***d.*** *Brain edema.* Uptake of FDG is substantially reduced in any area of the brain that is adjacent to white matter edema seen on magnetic resonance imaging (MRI) or computed tomography (CT) images. This is probably a reversible process and should disappear with reduction in the degree of edema.[3] The decreased gray matter uptake secondary to edema may improve the contrast between the tumor and adjacent structures.
   - ***e.*** *Glucose level.* High blood glucose decreases FDG uptake in both the tumor and the cortex, but there is a greater decrease in cortical activity; thus, a higher tumor-to-background ratio is often noted in hyperglycemic states.
   - ***f.*** *Hyperglycemia.* Although most patients should not be scanned in a hyperglycemic state, high blood glucose may potentially be advantageous in the detection of tumors near or in the cortex.[4]

A

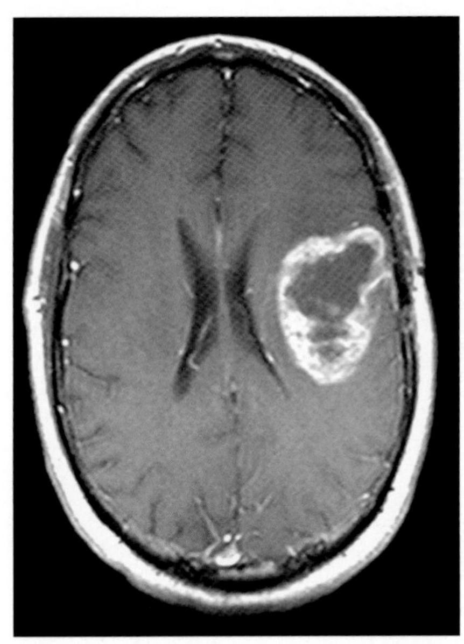

B

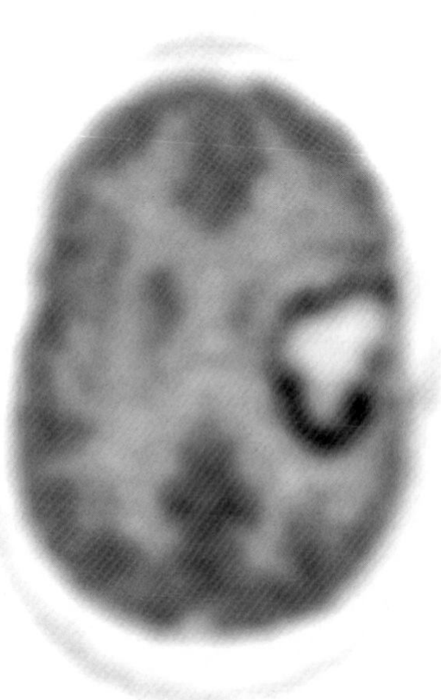

Fig. 12.1 High-grade glioma. **(A)** Axial magnetic resonance imaging (MRI) scan demonstrates peripheral enhancement of a left frontal high-grade glioma. **(B)** Axial positron emission tomography scan demonstrates intense uptake greater than gray matter corresponding to the enhancement seen on MRI.

g. Delayed imaging. Delayed imaging (3 to 8 hours after injection) increases uptake in the tumor relative to normal brain. This is most helpful in tumors near the gray matter.[5]

2. ***Standardized uptake value (SUV).*** SUV may not be as useful in the brain, as it may not correlate well with regional glucose metabolism. Tumor-to-white matter or tumor-to-cortex ratios may be preferable.[6]

Pitfalls

1. ***False-negatives.*** Small low-grade neoplasms are often undetectable on PET. A minority of high-grade tumors are also undetectable on PET.
2. ***False-positives***
   a. Low-grade neoplasms such as pilocytic astrocytoma, pleomorphic xanthoastrocytoma, ganglioglioma, and oligodendroglioma can be hypermetabolic.[6,7]
   b. Benign lesions such as meningioma (**Fig. 12.2**), pituitary adenoma (**Fig. 12.3**), and histiocytosis X can be hypermetabolic.
   c. Seizures at the time of FDG administration can cause false-positive results due to activated cortex adjacent to the tumor site.
   d. A hypermetabolic flare phenomenon may be seen in glioblastoma treated with chemotherapy if PET is performed 24 hours after the first dose.[8] This may predict longer survival.

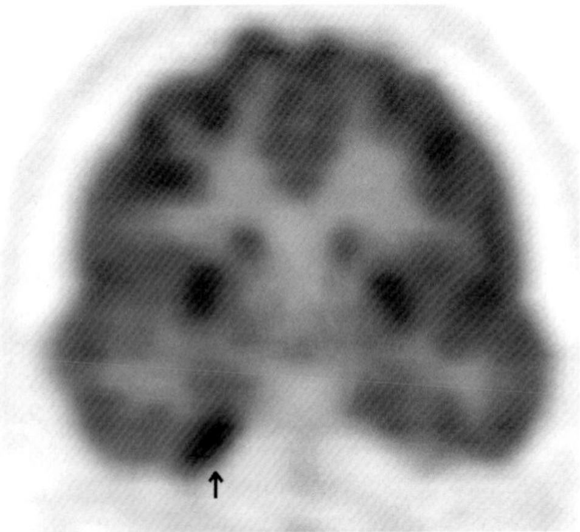

Fig. 12.2 Meningioma. Coronal positron emission tomography scan demonstrates focal uptake (*arrow*) along the medial surface of the right temporal lobe corresponding to a meningioma.

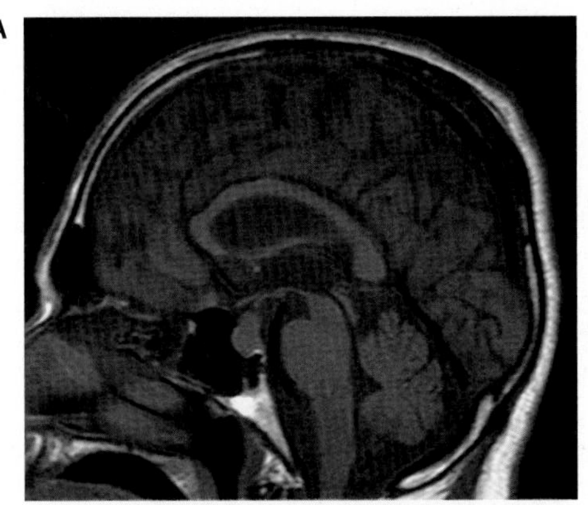

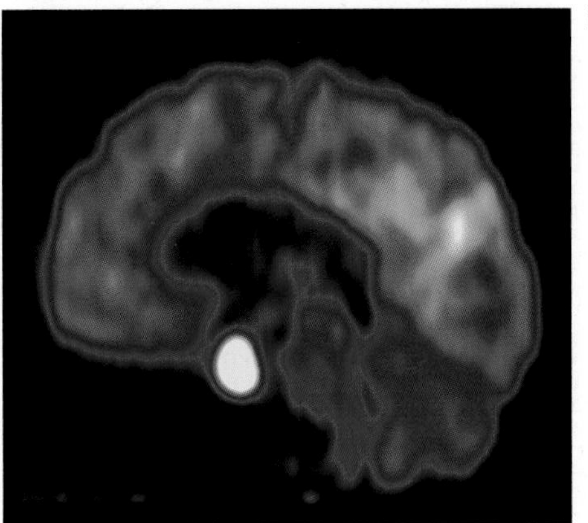

Fig. 12.3 Pituitary adenoma. **(A)** Sagittal T1-weighted magnetic resonance imaging scan demonstrates a pituitary macroadenoma. **(B)** Sagittal positron emission tomography scan demonstrates intense uptake in this adenoma.

◆ Tumor versus Radiation Necrosis[9]

Clinical Indication: B

It is often difficult to differentiate tumor recurrence versus radiation necrosis on CT or MRI, as both entities demonstrate contrast enhancement. PET is valuable in this situation (**Figs. 12.4** and **12.5**). This is the main indication for performing FDG PET imaging in patients with brain tumors.

Accuracy/Comparison to Other Modalities

1. Reported accuracies in larger series vary from 68 to 84%.
   - Specificity (40 to 92%) varies more than sensitivity (81 to 86%).
2. MRI coregistration may increase sensitivity for tumor recurrence.[10] The sensitivity is 65% without MRI coregistration compared with 86% with coregistration.
3. Competing modalities are thallium single photon emission tomography and MR spectroscopy (MRS). PET and thallium imaging may be of comparable accuracy. PET has not been directly compared with MRS in a large series.

Pearls

1. ***Imaging correlation.*** Correlation with MRI and CT scans is extremely helpful. Without such correlation, the findings from PET will often be misinterpreted.
2. ***Postsurgical changes.*** Postsurgical changes usually do not cause significant increased uptake and will not interfere with PET imaging for tumor recurrence.[7]
3. ***Radiation effects***
   a. In most cases a hypometabolic area will be seen following radiation adjacent to and distant from the primary tumor. This finding could be secondary to edema.[9]
   b. Occasionally, there can be increased uptake in the tumor after radiation, likely related to migration of macrophages to the radiated site. This uptake is usually diffuse and moderate (between white and gray matter). In rare cases, the uptake is nodular and greater than gray matter and cannot be differentiated from recurrent tumor.[7]
   c. Intracavitary radioimmunotherapy can cause increased FDG accumulation (rim of increased uptake). The peripheral increased activity in this case is usually not secondary to tumor. However, if the activity is nodular, tumor recurrence is likely.[7]
4. ***Interpretation criteria***
   a. The main criterion for diagnosing recurrence of tumor on PET is relatively increased uptake compared with the adjacent or contralateral white matter.
   b. The ipsilateral white matter may be less suitable as a reference because[11]

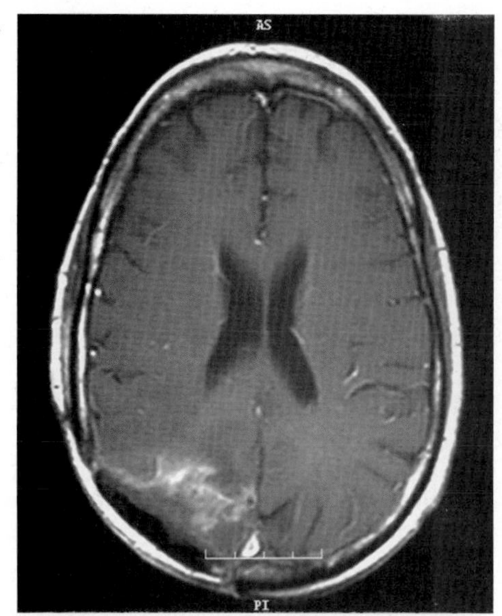

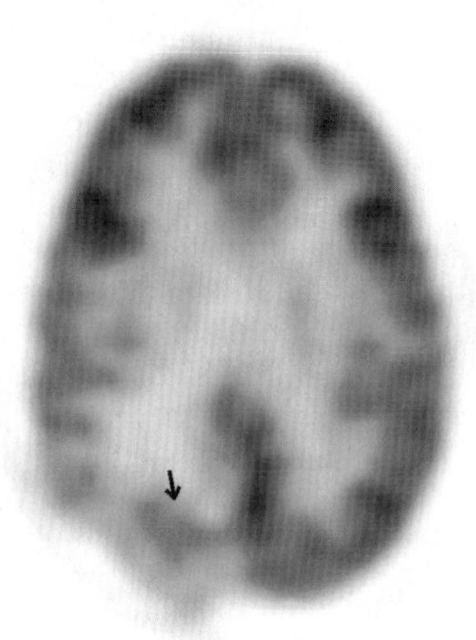

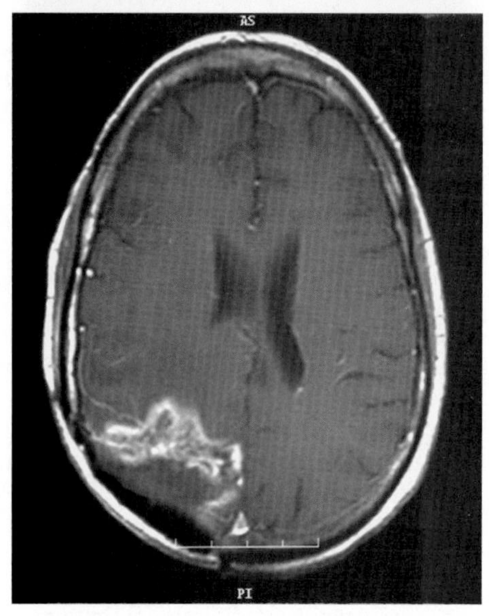

Fig. 12.4 Tumor recurrence. **(A)** Axial magnetic resonance imaging (MRI) scan demonstrates enhancement at the margin of a right parietal glioma resection site postradiation, equivocal for radiation necrosis versus tumor. **(B)** Axial positron emission tomography (PET) scan demonstrates increased uptake (*arrow*) in the area of enhancement seen on MRI, consistent with tumor recurrence. Note that it is important to differentiate this activity from normal gray matter activity decreased in intensity postradiation. There was no gray matter in this region by MRI correlation. **(C)** Follow-up axial MRI done several months after the PET scan demonstrates further increased enhancement in this region, which now has the exact configuration as the uptake seen on PET.

- Tumor cells may infiltrate around a focal lesion, causing diffuse increased white matter uptake ipsilaterally.
- Areas of encephalomalacia from prior surgery can cause apparent decreased white matter uptake. However, this will be apparent when PET and MRI images are compared.

c. Uptake greater than contralateral gray matter can also be used as a criterion for a positive study (**Fig. 12.5**): this increases specificity but decreases sensitivity.[11] We do not advocate this as an optimal criterion, as the majority of recurrences will be false-negative. The degree of uptake does reflect the aggressiveness of the recurrent tumor.

5. Low-grade brain tumors are usually hypometabolic; therefore, it might be thought that differentiation of radiation necrosis versus tumor may pose a challenge in these patients. However, in most cases recurrence is typically of the high-grade type and is hypermetabolic on PET.

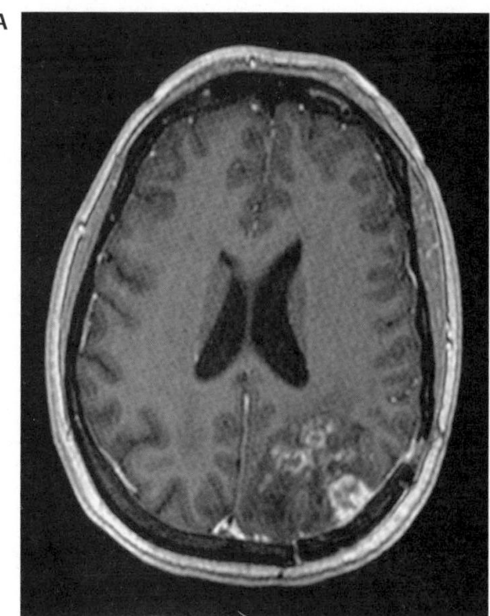

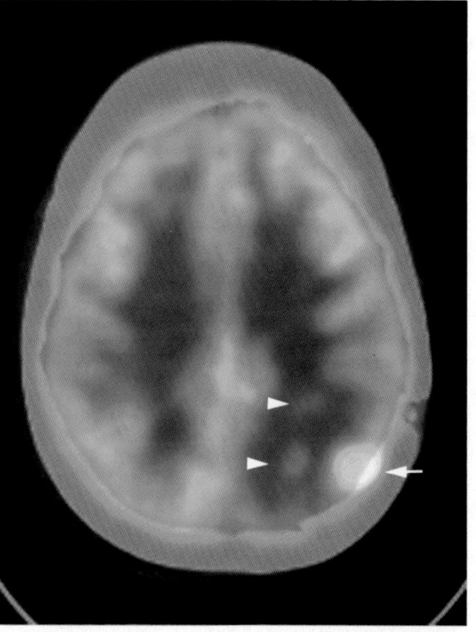

Fig. 12.5 Different levels of uptake in tumor recurrence. **(A)** Three foci of enhancement in the left parietal lobe are seen on a contrast-enhanced magnetic resonance imaging (MRI) scan in a patient after resection of a left parietal glioma and radiation. **(B)** The two medial foci (*arrowheads*) demonstrate mild uptake greater than white matter on axial positron emission tomography/computed tomography (PET/CT). Using this level of uptake as a criterion for tumor recurrence would increase sensitivity but decrease specificity. The larger peripheral focus (*arrow*) demonstrates intense uptake greater than gray matter. Using this level of uptake as a criterion for tumor recurrence would decrease sensitivity but increase specificity.

6. Typically, a PET scan is ordered because enhancement is seen on MRI that is nondiagnostic for tumor versus radiation necrosis. It is important to determine the exact location of the area of enhancement seen on MRI on the PET scan, either by visual comparison or with coregistration of the two image sets.
   - Any area of increased activity on PET should correspond to an area of enhancement on MRI before it is interpreted as tumor activity. However, the area of PET uptake may be slightly larger than the area of MRI enhancement (**Fig. 12.4**). Areas of increased uptake definitely outside the enhancement area on MRI could represent other etiologies as a seizure focus in the cortex at the margin of the lesion.

Pitfalls

1. A seizure at the time of FDG administration can cause a false-positive result.
   - Seizure foci are often seen in the cortex adjacent to the original tumor site.
2. If the recurrent tumor has a thin rim of tissue, PET may appear negative for tumor activity secondary to partial volume effects.
3. Active small lesions near the cortex may be difficult to detect due to the high normal gray matter activity. Often, this does not pose a problem, as adjacent edema or prior radiation usually results in decreased normal gray matter activity and therefore improves lesion contrast. Fusion imaging with MRI is very helpful and should be employed to minimize errors related to such circumstances.

◆ Lymphoma versus Toxoplasmosis

Clinical Indication: C

PET has been effective in differentiating lymphoma from toxoplasmosis in small series.

1. Toxoplasmosis is hypometabolic; lymphomas usually are active.
2. However, progressive multifocal leukocephalopathy can be hypermetabolic and cause a false-positive result.[12]

References

1. Fulham MJ. Central nervous system. In: R Wahl, ed. Principles and Practice of Positron Emission Tomography. Philadelphia, PA: Lippincott Williams & Wilkins; 2002:276–297
2. Fulham MJ, Brunetti A, Aloj L, Raman R, Dwyer AJ, Di CG. Decreased cerebral glucose metabolism in patients with brain tumors: an effect of corticosteroids. J Neurosurg 1995;83(4):657–664
3. Roelcke U, Blasberg RG, von Ammon K, et al. Dexamethasone treatment and plasma glucose levels: relevance for fluorine-18-fluorodeoxyglucose uptake measurements in gliomas. J Nucl Med 1998;39(5): 879–884
4. Ishizu K, Nishizawa S, Yonekura Y, et al. Effects of hyperglycemia on FDG uptake in human brain and glioma. J Nucl Med 1994;35(7):1104–1109
5. Spence AM, Muzi M, Mankoff DA, et al. ^{18}F-FDG PET of gliomas at delayed intervals: improved distinction between tumor and normal gray matter. J Nucl Med 2004;45(10):1653–1659
6. Benard F, Romsa J, Hustinx R. Imaging gliomas with positron emission tomography and single-photon emission computed tomography. Semin Nucl Med 2003;33(2):148–162
7. Wong TZ, van der Westhuizen GJ, Coleman RE. Positron emission tomography imaging of brain tumors. Neuroimaging Clin N Am 2002;12(4):615–626
8. De Witte O, Hildebrand J, Luxen A, Goldman S. Acute effect of carmustine on glucose metabolism in brain and glioblastoma. Cancer 1994;74(10):2836–2842
9. Hustinx R, Pourdehnad M, Kaschten B, Alavi A. PET imaging for differentiating recurrent brain tumor from radiation necrosis. Radiol Clin North Am 2005; 43(1):35–47
10. Chao ST, Suh JH, Raja S, Lee SY, Barnett G. The sensitivity and specificity of FDG PET in distinguishing recurrent brain tumor from radionecrosis in patients treated with stereotactic radiosurgery. Int J Cancer 2001;96(3):191–197
11. Ricci PE, Karis JP, Heiserman JE, Fram EK, Bice AN, Drayer BP. Differentiating recurrent tumor from radiation necrosis: time for re-evaluation of positron emission tomography? AJNR Am J Neuroradiol 1998;19(3):407–413
12. Pierce MA, Johnson MD, Maciunas RJ, et al. Evaluating contrast-enhancing brain lesions in patients with AIDS by using positron emission tomography. Ann Intern Med 1995;123(8):594–598

13

Head and Neck Cancer

Eugene C. Lin and Abass Alavi

◆ Cervical Metastasis, Unknown Primary

Clinical Indication: B

1. Although reported sensitivities vary, positron emission tomography (PET) can be useful for identifying the primary tumor in patients presenting with metastasis to cervical nodes (**Figs. 13.1, 13.2,** and **13.3**).
2. In addition, PET can identify unsuspected distant metastases and define regional disease in N2 (nodes > 3 cm but < 6 cm) patients.
3. It is best to perform PET after physical examination and panendoscopy are negative. In one study the risk of subsequent primary tumor was < 6% if both PET and panendoscopy were negative.[1]

Accuracy/Comparison to Other Modalities

1. The reported sensitivities of PET are variable (8 to 46%),[2,3] and a substantial incidence of false-positive results has been reported. The results may be improved with PET/computed tomography (CT), which identified the primary site in 68% of patients in one study.[4]
   - PET may have poor sensitivity for occult tonsillar cancer.[5]
2. However, PET overall is more accurate than conventional imaging.[3]

Pearls/Pitfalls

1. The main areas to search for primary tumors are the nasopharynx, base of tongue (**Fig. 13.1**), tonsils (**Fig. 13.2**), and pyriform sinuses (**Fig. 13.3**).
2. Primary tumors that are not identified by PET are generally superficial with a depth < 4 mm.[6]

◆ Staging

Clinical Indication: B

1. Although PET is more accurate than CT or magnetic resonance imaging (MRI) for nodal staging, it cannot replace these modalities for tumor (T) staging. Although clinically proven primary tumors are visualized by PET in the majority of cases, PET does not have the resolution to evaluate local spread.
2. ***Specific uses of PET***
   - ***a.*** *N0 neck.* Nodal staging in the N0 (clinically node negative) neck, particularly in patients with oral or oropharyngeal cancer where the probability of occult nodal metastases is higher

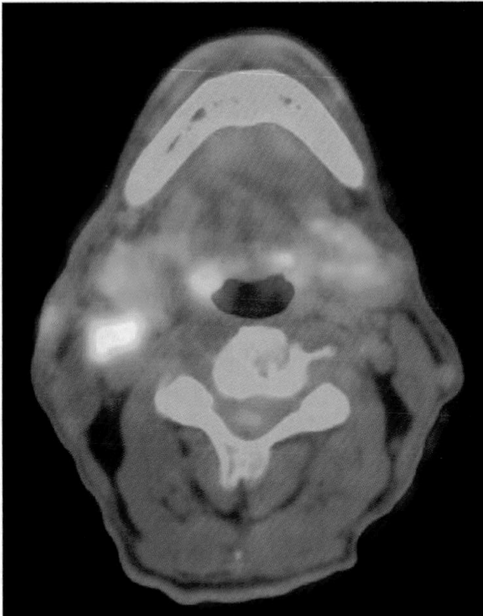

Fig. 13.1 Primary tumor localization: tongue base. Axial positron emission tomography/computed tomography scan in a patient with a malignant right neck node demonstrates uptake in the primary tumor in the right tongue base (*arrow*).

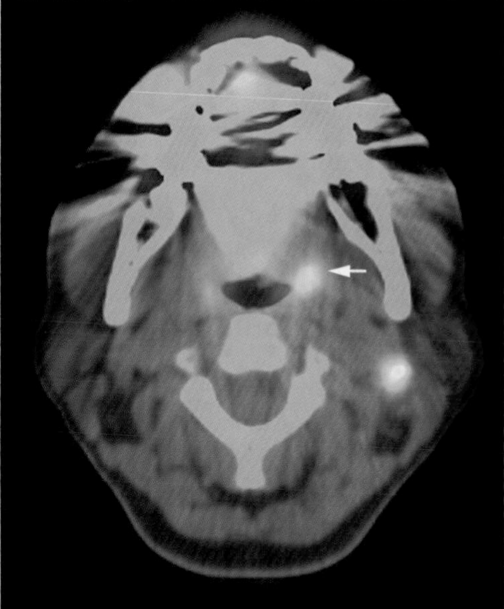

Fig. 13.2 Primary tumor localization: tonsil. Axial positron emission tomography/computed tomography scan in a patient with a malignant left neck node demonstrates uptake in the primary tumor in the left tonsil (*arrow*).

- The sensitivity of PET in this setting is variable, ranging from 33 to 67%.[7–9]
- In patients with T4 (stage 2 of tumor growth) disease, false-negative results are more likely, and PET is less helpful.
- PET is more helpful in patients with T1 to T3 disease. The use of PET in this population can reduce the probability of occult neck metastases to < 15%.
- PET is insensitive compared with sentinel node biopsy, but specificity is high.
- One potential use of PET is to perform sentinel node biopsy if PET is negative and neck dissection if PET is positive. This may reduce the number of unnecessary neck dissections.[10]

b. *Detecting distant metastases*

- PET can detect distant metastases, particularly in the mediastinum, bone marrow, and liver (**Fig. 13.4**).
- PET is particularly useful for detecting mediastinal disease in stage III and IV cancer.

c. *Detection of synchronous lesions.*[11,12] PET can detect additional tumors in the lung (**Fig. 13.5**) and aerodigestive tract (**Fig. 13.6**). The overall incidence of coincidental secondary primary tumors is 3 to 8%.

- *Coincidental lung lesions.* PET has an accuracy of 80% for such lung lesions.

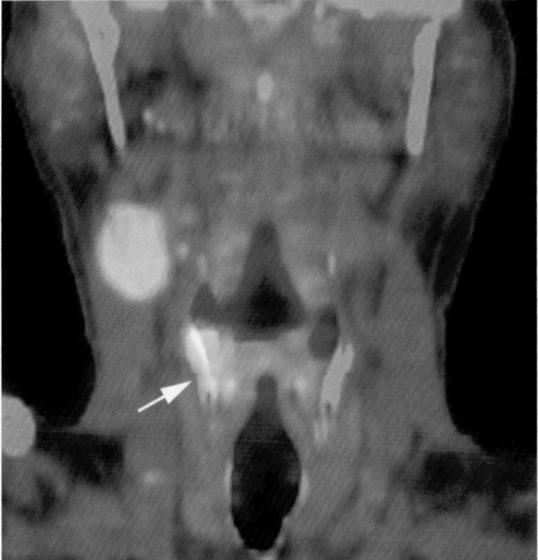

Fig. 13.3 Primary tumor localization: pyriform sinus. Coronal positron emission tomography computed tomography scan in a patient with a malignant right neck node demonstrates uptake in the primary tumor in the right pyriform sinus (*arrow*).

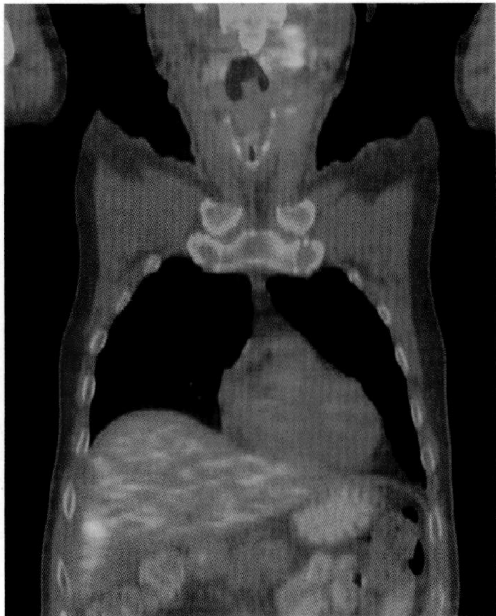

Fig. 13.4 Metastastic head and neck cancer. Coronal positron emission tomography/computed tomography scan in a patient with head and neck cancer demonstrates metastases to the left neck nodes and the liver.

A PET scan, which includes the thorax, will detect lung lesions not seen on chest x-ray. However, in general, CT is more sensitive than PET for lung lesions.

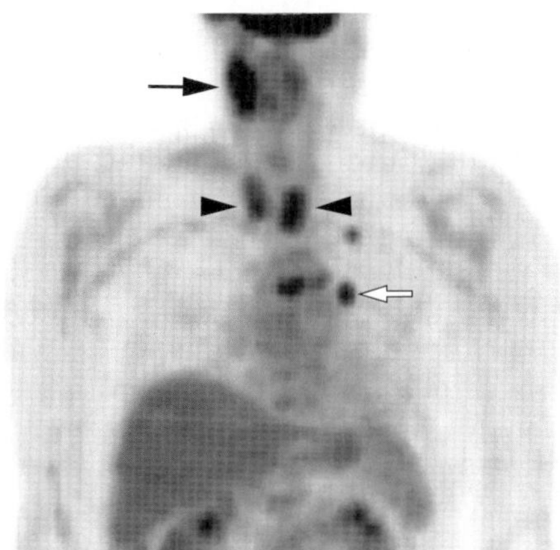

Fig. 13.5 Synchronrous lung cancer. Coronal positron emission tomography scan in a patient with a right parotid malignancy (*arrow*) demonstrates a synchronous left upper lobe lung cancer (*open arrow*) with mediastinal metastases and another nodule in the left apex. Uptake in the thyroid (*arrowheads*) is nonspecific but related to thyroiditis in this patient.

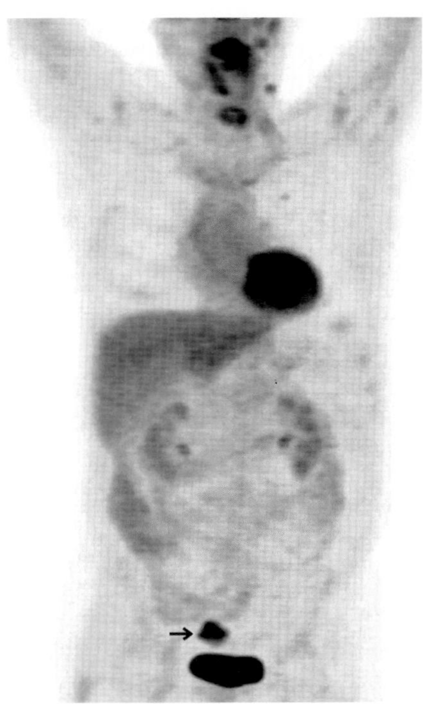

Fig. 13.6 Synchronous colon cancer. Coronal positron emission tomography scan in a patient with head and neck cancer with metastatic cervical nodes also demonstrates a synchronous sigmoid carcinoma (*arrow*).

d. *Prognosis*. Pretreatment tumor standardized uptake value (SUV) is an independent prognostic factor.[13]

Accuracy/Comparison with Other Modalities

1. ***PET versus CT/MRI.***[14] See **Table 13.1**.
2. PET is more sensitive than CT and MRI and more specific than CT, MRI, and ultrasound (US).[11]
3. ***Bone metastases.*** PET may be more sensitive than a bone scan for bone metastases in endemic nasopharyngeal carcinoma.[16]

Pearls/Pitfalls

1. Knowledge of the common sites and incidence of cervical metastases for different primary tumors is helpful in interpretation of PET scans.[17]

Table 13.1 Sensitivity and Specificity of Positron Emission Tomography Compared with Other Imaging Modalities in the Staging of Head and Neck Cancer

	Sensitivity %	Specificity %
PET	87–90	80–93
CT/MRI	61–97	21–100

Abbreviations: CT, computed tomography; MRI, magnetic resonance imaging; PET, positron emission tomography.

a. Oral cavity tumors have high incidence of metastases despite being clinically node negative.
b. Laryngeal tumors have a low incidence of metastases even in advanced stages of disease.
c. Supraglottic larynx tumors often spread to nodes bilaterally (**Fig. 13.7**).
d. Nasopharyngeal tumors often spread to nodes bilaterally and to the posterior triangle (**Fig. 13.8**).

2. ***Scan volume.*** It is helpful to include the abdomen and pelvis in the scan volume because of the possibility of coincidental tumors and distant metastases.

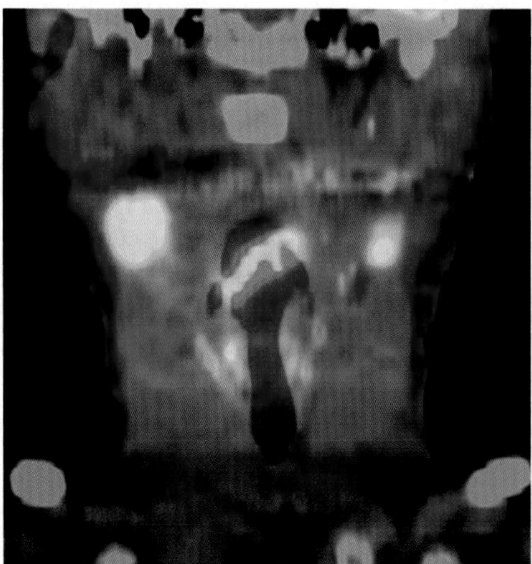

Fig. 13.7 Metastastic supraglottic cancer. Coronal positron emission tomography/computed tomography scan demonstrates a supraglottic cancer with metastases to bilateral neck nodes. Supraglottic cancers have a propensity for bilateral nodal metastases.

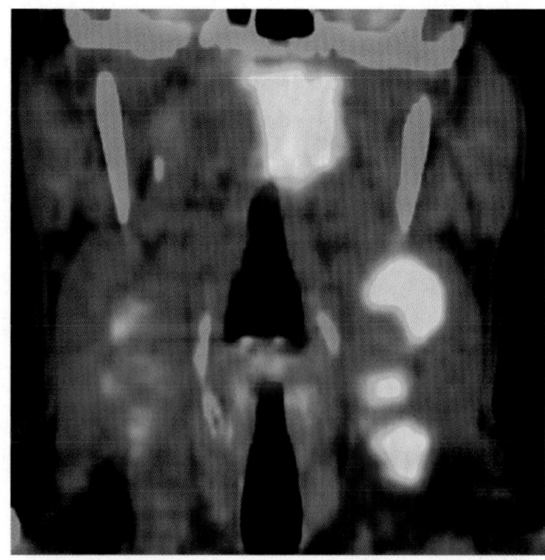

Fig. 13.8 Metastatic nasopharyngeal cancer. Coronal positron emission tomography/computed tomography scan demonstrates a large left nasopharyngeal cancer with metastases to bilateral neck nodes. Nasopharyngeal cancers have a propensity for bilateral nodal metastases.

3. ***Bone invasion.*** In patients with oral cancer, PET does not improve identification of bone infiltration compared with CT.[18]
4. ***SUV.*** The use of size-based SUV cutoffs may be helpful for nodal staging. In one study, SUV cutoffs of 1.9, 2.5, and 3.0 for lymph nodes < 10 mm, 10 to 15 mm, and > 15 mm yielded a 79% sensitivity and 99% specificity for nodal staging.[19]
5. ***Dedicated head and neck protocol.*** The use of a dedicated head and neck PET protocol (longer acquisition, higher count study reconstructed with smaller pixels) improves detection of disease in small nodes.[20] However, SUVs with a dedicated protocol are significantly higher than with a standard protocol. Thus, SUVs from a dedicated PET study cannot be compared with those from a standard PET.

◆ Recurrence

Clinical Indication: A

PET is very valuable for detecting recurrent disease, as CT and MRI are limited in the postoperative/posttherapy neck.

Table 13.2 Sensitivity and Specificity of Positron Emission Tomography Compared after Radionuclides in the Detection of Recurrent Disease

	Sensitivity %	Specificity %
PET	100	96
Tc-99m sestamibi	73	96
Tc-99m tetrofosmin	64	96

Abbreviations: PET, positron emission tomography; Tc, technetium.

Accuracy

1. ***Overall.*** Sensitivity 84 to 100%, specificity 61 to 93%[21]
2. ***By region***[22]
   a. *Local.* Sensitivity 97%, specificity 79%
   b. *Regional.* Sensitivity 92%, specificity 95%
   c. *Distant.* Sensitivity 94%, specificity 96%[22]
3. PET is sensitive and specific for disease at regional and distant sites. Specificity is lower in the head and neck region due to false-positive results from inflammation related to infection or other processes.[22] The primary value of PET is its high negative predictive value.[23]
4. If PET is negative, no biopsy is needed.
5. If PET is positive and biopsy is negative, a follow-up scan should be performed. Decreased activity on the follow-up scan indicates that the initial result was likely false-positive due to an inflammatory process.[24]

Comparison with Other Modalities[25]

1. ***Other radionuclides.*** PET is more sensitive than sestamibi, tetrofosmin, or thallium; specificity is comparable. However, sestamibi or tetrofosmin combined with CT is comparable to PET (**Table 13.2**).[25,26]
2. ***MRI.***[27] See **Table 13.3**.

Pearls

1. ***SUV.*** SUV cutoffs of 3.0 to 3.2 have been used to detect recurrence.[22,28] However, an increasing SUV on dual time point PET imaging is of greater value than a single SUV measurement.
2. Radiation has minimal effect on FDG uptake in normal structures. There is mildly increased uptake, mostly in muscle, in the early postradiation period, which is related to inflammation.

Pitfalls

1. ***Tumor stunning.*** A delay in PET imaging for at least 4 months after radiation can be helpful in avoiding false-negative results from presumed tumor "stunning."[29]
2. ***Laryngeal uptake.*** Laryngeal uptake of FDG can be noted normally, particularly in the posterior portion (see Chapter 6).
   a. It is better to use asymmetry of uptake rather than absolute uptake in the larynx as a criterion of abnormality.
   b. Anterior uptake is more suggestive of a malignant process than uptake in posterior structures.
   c. However, laryngeal uptake may be asymmetric due to postoperative changes or vocal cord paralysis.
3. ***Postoperative.*** False-positive results are particularly unavoidable when evaluating for recurrence. Besides the typical physiologic areas of uptake, abnormal patterns of uptake can be seen from postoperative distortion of normal anatomy or as a result of postsurgical or therapeutic inflammation. However, reconstruction hardware typically does not interfere with interpretability. Osteotomy sites do have slightly greater (25% on average) uptake, but less than that seen in tumor.[30] PET/CT can be used in free flap cases with acceptable levels of accuracy.

Table 13.3 Sensitivity and Specificity of Positron Emission Tomography (PET) Compared with Magnetic Resonance Imaging (MRI) in the Detection of Recurrent Disease

	Sensitivity %	Specificity %
PET	100	93
MRI	62	43

◆ Therapy Response/Prognosis[31]

Clinical Indication: B

Potential applications of PET in therapy response are

1. ***Evaluation of residual disease following radiotherapy or chemoradiotherapy.*** PET is useful in evaluating therapy response in preoperative induction chemoradiotherapy, chemoradiotherapy protocols that are aimed at organ preservation, and definitive radiotherapy.[11,12]
   - ***a.*** *Postchemoradiotherapy*. In patients with head and neck squamous cell cancer, chemoradiotherapy regimens that attempt to preserve organ function (e.g., larynx and tongue) often achieve regional control at the primary site. However, residual tumor is more likely if cervical nodal disease (particularly N2 or N3) is present, even if there is a clinical complete response. In patients with advanced nodal disease, posttreatment neck dissection can often reduce regional recurrence. The role of PET in predicting the need for posttreatment neck dissection is controversial. PET/CT does appear to be superior to contrast-enhanced CT for predicting persistent disease in the neck.[32] Some data suggest that PET is a reliable predictor of the absence of residual tumor after chemoradiotherapy in the N positive neck,[33] but this is not supported by some studies.[34]
   - ***b.*** *Postradiotherapy*. There is controversy over the role of neck dissection after definitive radiation therapy for advanced neck disease. One study suggests that PET/CT is more accurate than CT in assessing therapy response in this setting.[35] Limited data suggest that if there is no residual lymphadenopathy and a negative PET, neck dissection can be withheld.[36] However, if there is substantial residual lymphadenopathy (> 2 cm) and a negative PET, further studies are required before withholding neck dissection.[37]
2. ***Prognosis.*** PET is helpful for both early and late prediction of outcome.
   - ***a.*** *Primary tumor*. High SUV (> 10) in the primary tumor is correlated with poor prognosis.[38]
   - ***b.*** *Nodes*. Nodal SUV does not predict prognosis.[39]
   - ***c.*** *Early prediction*. Low levels of tumor metabolic activity after 1 cycle of chemotherapy or radiation predict complete remission and longer survival.
   - ***d.*** *Late prediction*. High SUV after treatment predicts local recurrence and decreased survival.

Table 13.4 Sensitivity and Specificity of Positron Emission Tomography Compared with Other Imaging Modalities in the Evaluation of Therapy Response

	Sensitivity %	Specificity %
PET/CT	77	93
CT	92	47

Abbreviations: CT, computed tomography; PET, positron emission tomography.

Accuracy/Comparison with Other Modalities

Postradiotherapy.[35] See **Table 13.4**.

Pitfalls

1. PET has a limited clinical value in assessing response to postoperative adjuvant chemoradiotherapy.
   - ***a.*** Postsurgical inflammatory reactions can cause false-positive results and therefore render subsequent response assessment inaccurate.
   - ***b.*** Microscopic residual disease cannot be detected.
2. As in all settings, there should be a substantial time interval between radiotherapy and PET imaging. Typically, false-negative results are more commonly seen if imaging is performed early after radiation. Some studies suggest that a 4- or 8-week delay is adequate[35,36] for evaluating therapy response, but other studies suggest 12 weeks or longer.[37] If postradiotherapy neck dissection is

being considered, PET may be more valuable if it can be accurately performed earlier after therapy (within 12 weeks), as fibrosis can increase the technical difficulty and morbidity of delayed neck dissection.[40]

3. Osteoradionecrosis can cause false-positive results.[41]

◆ Radiotherapy Planning

Clinical Indication: B

Potential applications of PET in radiotherapy planning are[42]

1. Coregistration of PET and treatment planning CT
2. Detection of additional/distant disease by PET
3. Gross tumor volume assessment: gross tumor volume assessment by PET is closer to the surgical specimen than CT or MRI, although all imaging modalities overestimate tumor extension.

◆ Characterization of Head and Neck Tumors

Clinical Indication: D

1. **Parotid lesions.** PET cannot distinguish between benign and malignant parotid tumors.[43] Warthin tumors and pleomorphic adenomas can have fluorodeoxyglucose (FDG) uptake. High-grade salivary gland tumors tend to have more uptake than lower grade tumors, but there is substantial overlap.[44] PET and PET/CT may be superior to CT for staging patients' known salivary gland malignancies.[44–46]
2. **Cystic neck masses.** PET/CT may not be accurate in identifying malignancy in adults with cystic neck masses.[47]

◆ PET/CT

PET/CT is of particular value in head and neck evaluations, given the complex anatomy and relative lack of anatomical landmarks on PET.

1. The use of PET/CT compared with PET alone will decrease the fraction of equivocal lesions by 53%, greatly improve lesion localization (see **Fig. 8.1**, p. 89), slightly improve accuracy, and change management in 18% of cases.[11,12]
2. Particular attention must be paid to the possibility of mislocalization on PET/CT studies due to movement of the head between the CT and PET studies (see **Figs. 8.6**, p. 92 and **8.7**, p. 93).
3. If PET/CT or fusion with CT or MRI is not available, potential anatomical landmarks that can be used to aid in localization include the tonsils, palate, tongue, floor of mouth, salivary glands, mandible, and cervical spine.

References

1. Miller FR, Karnad AB, Eng T, Hussey DH, Stan MH, Otto RA. Management of the unknown primary carcinoma: long-term follow-up on a negative PET scan and negative panendoscopy. Head Neck 2008;30(1):28–34
2. Kole AC, Nieweg OE, Pruim J, et al. Detection of unknown occult primary tumors using positron emission tomography. Cancer 1998;82(6):1160–1166
3. Greven KM, Keyes JW Jr, Williams DW III, et al. Occult primary tumors of the head and neck: lack of benefit from positron emission tomography imaging with 2-[F-18]fluoro-2-deoxy-D-glucose. Cancer 1999;86(1):114–118
4. Wartski M, Le Stanc E, Gontier E, et al. In search of an unknown primary tumour presenting with cervical metastases: performance of hybrid FDG-PET-CT. Nucl Med Commun 2007;28(5):365–371
5. Nabili V, Zaia B, Blackwell KE, Head CS, Grabski K, Sercarz JA. Positron emission tomography: poor sensitivity for occult tonsillar cancer. Am J Otolaryngol 2007;28(3):153–157
6. Hannah A, Scott AM, Tochon-Danguy H, et al. Evaluation of ^{18}F-fluorodeoxyglucose positron emission tomography and computed tomography with histopathologic correlation in the initial staging of head and neck cancer. Ann Surg 2002;236(2):208–217
7. Ng SH, Yen TC, Chang JT, et al. Prospective study of [^{18}F]fluorodeoxyglucose positron emission tomography and computed tomography and magnetic resonance imaging in oral cavity squamous cell carcinoma with palpably negative neck. J Clin Oncol 2006;24(27):4371–4376
8. Schoder H, Carlson DL, Kraus DH, et al. ^{18}F-FDG PET/CT for detecting nodal metastases in patients with oral cancer staged N0 by clinical examination and CT/MRI. J Nucl Med 2006;47(5):755–762
9. Wensing BM, Vogel WV, Marres HA, et al. FDG-PET in the clinically negative neck in oral squamous cell carcinoma. Laryngoscope 2006;116(5):809–813
10. Kovacs AF, Dobert N, Gaa J, et al. Positron emission tomography in combination with sentinel node bi-

opsy reduces the rate of elective neck dissections in the treatment of oral and oropharyngeal cancer. J Clin Oncol 2004;22(19):3973–3980

11. Schoder H, Yeung HW. Positron emission imaging of head and neck cancer, including thyroid carcinoma. Semin Nucl Med 2004;34(3):180–197

12. Schoder H, Yeung HW, Gonen M, et al. Head and neck cancer: clinical usefulness and accuracy of PET/CT image fusion. Radiology 2004;231(1):65–72

13. Kim SY, Roh JL, Kim MR, et al. Use of ^{18}F-FDG PET for primary treatment strategy in patients with squamous cell carcinoma of the oropharynx. J Nucl Med 2007;48(5):752–757

14. Schoder H, Yeung HW. Positron emission imaging of head and neck cancer, including thyroid carcinoma. Semin Nucl Med 2004;34(3):180–197

15. Stuckensen T, Kovacs AF, Adams S, Baum RP. Staging of the neck in patients with oral cavity squamous cell carcinomas: a prospective comparison of PET, ultrasound, CT and MRI. J Craniomaxillofac Surg 2000;28(6):319–324

16. LiuFY,ChangJT,WangHM,etal.[^{18}F]fluorodeoxyglucose positron emission tomography is more sensitive than skeletal scintigraphy for detecting bone metastasis in endemic nasopharyngeal carcinoma at initial staging. J Clin Oncol 2006;24(4):599–604

17. Lowe VJ, Stack BC Jr. Esophageal cancer and head and neck cancer. Semin Roentgenol 2002;37(2):140–150

18. Goerres GW, Schmid DT, Schuknecht B, Eyrich GK. Bone invasion in patients with oral cavity cancer: comparison of conventional CT with PET/CT and SPECT/CT. Radiology 2005;237(1):281–287

19. Murakami R, Uozumi H, Hirai T, et al. Impact of FDG-PET/CT imaging on nodal staging for head-and-neck squamous cell carcinoma. Int J Radiat Oncol Biol Phys 2007;68(2):377–382

20. Yamamoto Y, Wong TZ, Turkington TG, Hawk TC, Coleman RE. Head and neck cancer: dedicated FDG PET/CT protocol for detection–phantom and initial clinical studies. Radiology 2007;244(1):263–272

21. Kutler DI, Wong RJ, Schoder H, Kraus DH. The current status of positron-emission tomography scanning in the evaluation and follow-up of patients with head and neck cancer. Curr Opin Otolaryngol Head Neck Surg 2006;14(2):73–81

22. Wong RJ, Lin DT, Schoder H, et al. Diagnostic and prognostic value of [(18)F]fluorodeoxyglucose positron emission tomography for recurrent head and neck squamous cell carcinoma. J Clin Oncol 2002;20(20): 4199–4208

23. Ryan WR, Fee WE Jr, Le QT, Pinto HA. Positron-emission tomography for surveillance of head and neck cancer. Laryngoscope 2005;115(4):645–650

24. Terhaard CH, Bongers V, van Rijk PP, Hordijk GJ. F-18-fluoro-deoxy-glucose positron-emission tomography scanning in detection of local recurrence after radiotherapy for laryngeal/ pharyngeal cancer. Head Neck 2001;23(11):933–941

25. Kao CH, Shiau YC, Shen YY, Yen RF. Detection of recurrent or persistent nasopharyngeal carcinomas after radiotherapy with technetium-99m methoxyisobutylisonitrile single photon emission computed tomography and computed tomography: comparison with 18-fluoro-2-deoxyglucose positron emission tomography. Cancer 2002;94(7):1981–1986

26. Kao CH, Tsai SC, Wang JJ, et al. Comparing 18-fluoro-2-deoxyglucose positron emission tomography with a combination of technetium 99m tetrofosmin single photon emission computed tomography and computed tomography to detect recurrent or persistent nasopharyngeal carcinomas after radiotherapy. Cancer 2001;92(2):434–439

27. Yen RF, Hung RL, Pan MH, et al. 18-fluoro-2-deoxyglucose positron emission tomography in detecting residual/recurrent nasopharyngeal carcinomas and comparison with magnetic resonance imaging. Cancer 2003;98(2):283–287

28. Yao M, Luo P, Hoffman HT, et al. Pathology and FDG PET correlation of residual lymph nodes in head and neck cancer after radiation treatment. Am J Clin Oncol 2007;30(3):264–270

29. Keyes JW Jr, Watson NE Jr, Williams DW III, et al. FDG PET in head and neck cancer. AJR Am J Roentgenol 1997;169(6):1663–1669

30. Oliver C, Muthukrishnan A, Mountz J, Deeb E, Johnson J, Deleyiannis F. Interpretability of PET/CT imaging in head and neck cancer patients following composite mandibular resection and osteocutaneous free flap reconstruction. Head Neck 2008;30(2):187–193

31. Kostakoglu L, Goldsmith SJ. PET in the assessment of therapy response in patients with carcinoma of the head and neck and of the esophagus. J Nucl Med 2004;45(1):56–68

32. Chen AY, Vilaseca I, Hudgins PA, et al. PET-CT vs contrast-enhanced CT: what is the role for each after chemoradiation for advanced oropharyngeal cancer? Head Neck 2006;28(6):487–495

33. Brkovich VS, Miller FR, Karnad AB, et al. The role of positron emission tomography scans in the management of the N-positive neck in head and neck squamous cell carcinoma after chemoradiotherapy. Laryngoscope 2006;116(6):855–858

34. Gourin CG, Williams HT, Seabolt WN, et al. Utility of positron emission tomography-computed tomography in identification of residual nodal disease after chemoradiation for advanced head and neck cancer. Laryngoscope 2006;116(5):705–710

35. Andrade RS, Heron DE, Degirmenci B, et al. Posttreatment assessment of response using FDG-PET/CT for patients treated with definitive radiation therapy for head and neck cancers. Int J Radiat Oncol Biol Phys 2006;65(5):1315–1322

36. Kim SY, Lee SW, Nam SY, et al. The feasibility of ^{18}F-FDG PET scans 1 month after completing radiotherapy of squamous cell carcinoma of the head and neck. J Nucl Med 2007;48(3):373–378

37. Yao M, Smith RB, Graham MM, et al. The role of FDG PET in management of neck metastasis from head-and-neck cancer after definitive radiation treatment. Int J Radiat Oncol Biol Phys 2005;63(4): 991–999

38. Halfpenny W, Hain SF, Biassoni L, et al. FDG-PET. A possible prognostic factor in head and neck cancer. Br J Cancer 2002;86(4):512–516

39. Schwartz DL, Rajendran J, Yueh B, et al. FDG-PET prediction of head and neck squamous cell cancer outcomes. Arch Otolaryngol Head Neck Surg 2004;130(12):1361–1367

40. Frank SJ, Chao KS, Schwartz DL, et al. Technology insight: PET and PET/CT in head and neck tumor staging and radiation therapy planning. Nat Clin Pract Oncol 2005;2(10):526–533

41. Liu SH, Chang JT, Ng SH, Chan SC, Yen TC. False positive fluorine-18 fluorodeoxy-D-glucose positron emission tomography finding caused by osteoradionecrosis in a nasopharyngeal carcinoma patient. Br J Radiol 2004; 77(915):257–260

42. Daisne JF, Duprez T, Weynand B, et al. Tumor volume in pharyngolaryngeal squamous cell carcinoma: comparison at CT, MR imaging, and FDG PET and validation with surgical specimen. Radiology 2004; 233(1):93–100
43. Rubello D, Nanni C, Castellucci P, et al. Does ^{18}F-FDG PET/CT play a role in the differential diagnosis of parotid masses. Panminerva Med 2005;47(3):187–189
44. Roh JL, Ryu CH, Choi SH, et al. Clinical utility of ^{18}F-FDG PET for patients with salivary gland malignancies. J Nucl Med 2007;48(2):240–246
45. Otsuka H, Graham MM, Kogame M, Nishitani H. The impact of FDG-PET in the management of patients with salivary gland malignancy. Ann Nucl Med 2005;19(8):691–694
46. Jeong HS, Chung MK, Son YI, et al. Role of ^{18}F-FDG PET/CT in management of high-grade salivary gland malignancies. J Nucl Med 2007;48(8):1237–1244
47. Ferris RL, Branstetter BF, Nayak JV. Diagnostic utility of positron emission tomography-computed tomography for predicting malignancy in cystic neck masses in adults. Laryngoscope 2005;115(11):1979–1982

14

Thyroid Cancer

Eugene C. Lin and Abass Alavi

◆ Thyroid Nodules

Clinical Indication: C

Positron emission tomography (PET) has a limited role in primary evaluation of thyroid nodules. However, uptake in thyroid nodules is often seen as an incidental finding (**Fig. 14.1**).

Accuracy: Differentiating Benign from Malignant Nodules

1. ***PET.*** 100% sensitivity, 63% specificity[1]
   - These results were obtained using a standardized uptake value (SUV) cutoff of 2.0.
2. ***SUV.*** There have been numerous SUV cutoffs suggested for distinguishing benign from malignant thyroid nodules. These should be used with caution, as published cutoffs vary greatly (from 2.0 to 8.5).[2] In one study,[3] SUVs were unable to distinguish benign from malignant nodules. For practical purposes, focal uptake in the thyroid requires further work-up, as malignancy cannot be excluded based on SUV alone.

Pearls

1. Both benign and malignant thyroid nodules can have increased fluorodeoxyglucose

A

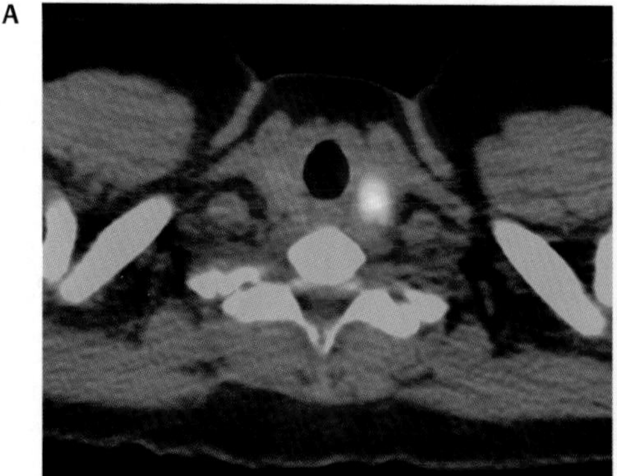

B

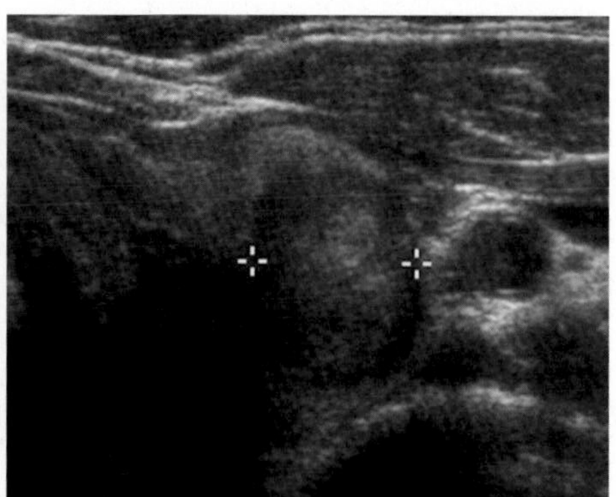

Fig. 14.1 Thyroid nodule. **(A)** Axial positron emission tomography/computed tomography scan demonstrates focal uptake in the left thyroid. **(B)** Ultrasound confirms the presence of a left thyroid nodule.

(FDG) uptake, but malignant nodules are usually more metabolically active than those without cancer.

a. Most malignant thyroid nodules > 1 cm will have FDG uptake.

b. Approximately one third of benign thyroid nodules have FDG uptake.[4]

c. Hürthle cell adenomas often have increased uptake.[4,5]

d. SUVs overlap between follicular neoplasms and benign thyroid nodules.[6]

2. Fourteen to 50% of incidentally detected thyroid nodules on PET will be malignant.[7,8]

3. ***CT correlation.*** Correlation with computed tomography (CT) images can be helpful in determining whether thyroid FDG uptake is benign or malignant. The following features suggest benign FDG uptake:[9]

   a. The FDG uptake corresponds to a very low attenuation lesion (< 25 Hounsfield units [HU] on CT).

   b. There is no nodule on CT that corresponds to the FDG uptake.

   c. The FDG uptake is diffuse.

4. ***Known thyroid nodules.*** PET may be helpful in the work-up of patients with known thyroid nodules. The absence of FDG uptake in a thyroid nodule > 1 cm has a high negative predictive value for malignancy.[4] However, PET will often miss carcinomas < 1 cm in size.[5] The overall positive and negative predictive values are 75 and 83%, respectively.[5]

Pitfalls

1. ***Thyroid nodule mimics.*** Structures adjacent to the thyroid can mimic thyroid nodules. Before thyroid nodules are diagnosed by PET, anatomical correlation is necessary.

   a. Nodes. Medial neck lymph nodes can be adjacent to the thyroid (**Fig. 14.2**).

   b. Vocal cord. Asymmetric vocal cord uptake secondary to vocal cord paralysis can mimic thyroid uptake (as seen in **Fig. 6.14**, p. 49).

   c. Parathyroid adenomas can have uptake.

2. ***Diffuse uptake.*** Diffuse uptake (e.g., secondary to thyroiditis) can obscure thyroid nodule uptake.

◆ Recurrent Thyroid Cancer[10–12]

Clinical Indication: B

Localizing metastatic disease in patients with an elevated thyroglobulin and negative radioiodine whole-body scan is the primary clinical

A

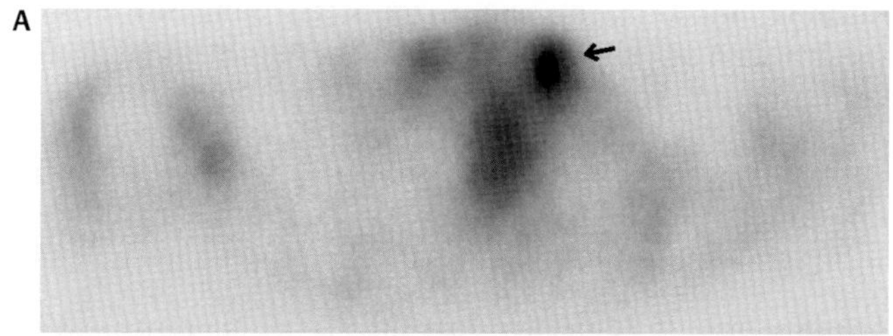

B

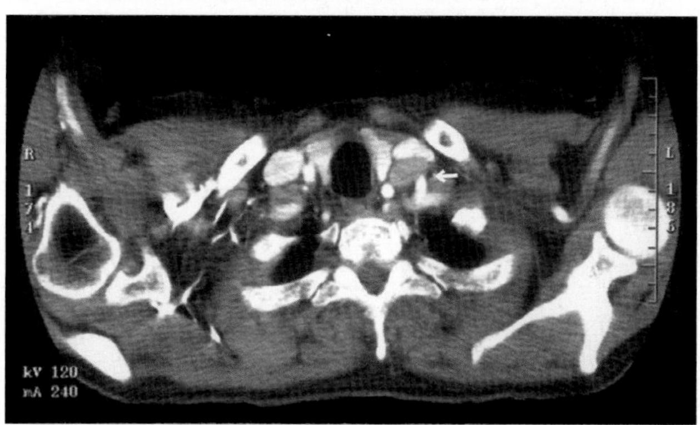

Fig. 14.2 Medial neck node mimicking a thyroid nodule. **(A)** Focal uptake in the left neck (*arrow*) on axial positron emission tomography scan is suspicious for a thyroid nodule. **(B)** Computed tomography scan demonstrates a medial node (*arrow*) immediately lateral to the left thyroid lobe, corresponding to the area of fluorodeoxyglucose uptake. Conversely, a thyroid nodule can mimic a medial neck node.

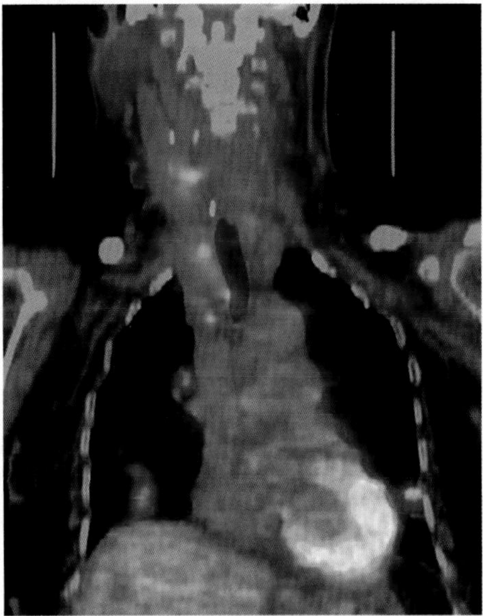

Fig. 14.3 Recurrent thyroid cancer. Coronal positron emission tomography/computed tomography scan demonstrates metastatic disease to the right neck nodes, superior mediastinal nodes, and lungs.

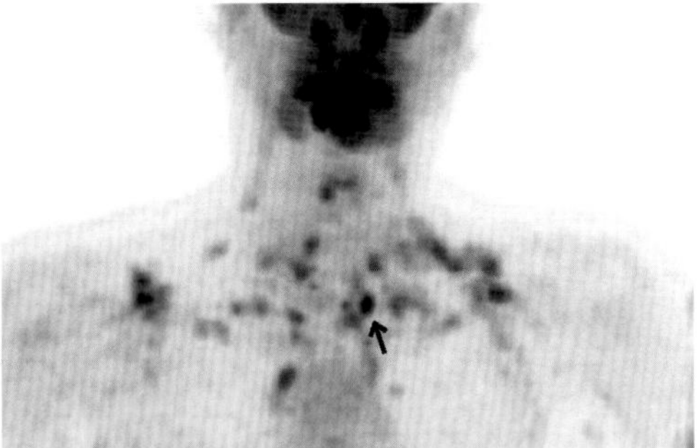

Fig. 14.5 Brown fat uptake and nodal metastases. Extensive brown fat uptake in the neck, supraclavicular regions, and superior mediastinum on a coronal positron emission tomography (PET) scan severely limits evaluation in a patient with suspected metastatic thyroid cancer. A single superior mediastinal nodal metastasis (*arrow*) was present. This is slightly more intense than the brown fat uptake but otherwise similar in appearance. PET/computed tomography was necessary to identify this node.

indication for PET in thyroid cancer (**Figs. 14.3, 14.4,** and **14.5**).

1. ***Work-up.***[10] In patients with elevated thyroglobulin and negative whole-body radioiodine scans, the following issues should be considered in determining whether PET will be helpful:
   a. *Surgical candidate.* If surgical intervention is contemplated, PET can be very useful in localizing the sites of the disease. If surgery is not a consideration, then localization of disease is less significant, and high-dose radioiodine therapy without further imaging work-up should be considered.
   b. *Anatomical imaging.* Because metastases are often confined to the neck and chest region, anatomical imaging modalities such as ultrasound and chest CT might be considered first before PET is performed.
   c. *Prior radioiodine exposure.* PET should be strongly considered in cases where high cumulative radioiodine exposure precludes or limits further radioiodine therapy.
2. ***Histology.*** In addition to papillary and follicular carcinoma, PET is useful in
   a. Hürthle cell subtype of follicular cancer[13]
   b. Insular cell subtype of follicular cancer[14]

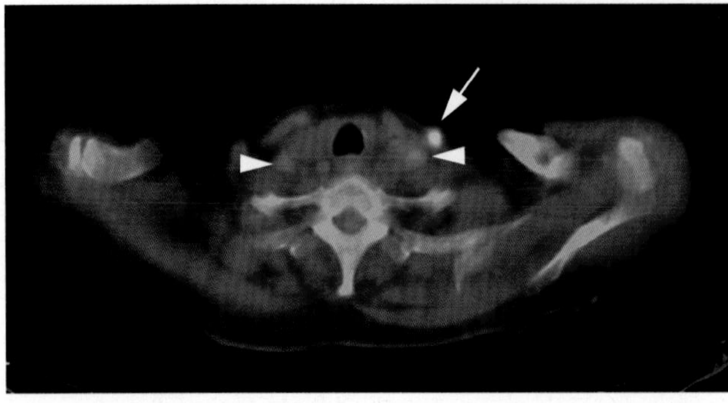

Fig. 14.4 Muscle uptake and nodal metastases. Axial positron emission tomography/computed tomography scan demonstrates increased uptake in a left neck node (*arrow*) secondary to metastatic thyroid cancer. Note the proximity of the node to muscle uptake (*arrowheads*).

c. Medullary thyroid carcinoma with rising calcitonin[15]

3. ***Prognosis.*** A large volume of metabolically active diseased sites and high SUVs (> 10) are strong negative predictors of survival.[16]
4. Other potential indications of PET are
   a. As a complement to conventional work-up in patients with known neoplastic sites
   b. Patients with negative radioiodine scan and normal levels of serum markers in whom clinical suspicion of relapse is high
   c. Posttreatment response assessment

Accuracy

1. ***Papillary/follicular carcinoma***
   a. *PET.* Sensitivity 75%, specificity 90%[17]
   b. *PET/CT.* Sensitivity 95%, specificity 91%[18]
   c. The diagnostic accuracy for PET/CT is 93% compared with 78% for PET alone.[18]
   d. PET is most useful when the thyroglobulin is > 10 ng/mL and the radioiodine scan is negative.
   e. The sensitivity is higher (85%) in patients with a negative radioiodine scan.[17]
2. ***Hürthle cell carcinoma: PET.*** Sensitivity 96%, specificity 95%[13]
3. ***Medullary thyroid carcinoma: PET.*** Sensitivity 78%, specificity 79%[15]
4. ***Anatomical region***
   a. PET is most valuable for the detection of cervical lymph node metastases.[19] However, for initial staging, ultrasound and contrast-enhanced CT are comparable in accuracy to PET for the detection of cervical lymph node metastases.[20]
   b. In medullary thyroid cancer, PET is most valuable for detecting cervical, supraclavicular, and mediastinal metastases.
   c. *Bone metastases.* Sensitivity 85%, specificity 100% in differentiated thyroid cancer[21]

Comparison with Other Modalities

1. ***Papillary/follicular cancer.***[17] See **Table 14.1.**
   a. *Relationship between FDG and radioiodine uptake.* There is usually an inverse relation between FDG and radioiodine uptake in thyroid metastases (flip-flop phenomenon). Poorly differentiated metastases have FDG uptake but no or minimal radioiodine uptake, and the reverse is true in well-differentiated metastatic lesions. Somatostatin receptor scintigraphy with technetium (Tc) 99m depreotide is also able to detect disease in the setting of detectable thyroglobulin and negative radioiodine scan. There may also be a flip-flop phenomenon between FDG and Tc-99m depreotide; for example, poorly differentiated lesions may have FDG uptake but no or minimal depreotide uptake.[22]
   b. FDG-positive lesions are resistant to high-dose iodine 131 treatment.[23] Thyroglobulin levels are much more likely to normalize in PET-negative patients than in PET-positive patients after radioiodine therapy.[24]
   c. FDG uptake correlates with thallium and sestamibi uptake.[17,25] However, FDG is preferred to thallium or sestamibi due to its superior resolution and higher sensitivity.
   d. *Bone metastases.* One study suggests that PET is comparable in sensitivity but superior in specificity and accuracy to a bone scan.[21] However, another study[26] suggests that a bone scan may identify metastases that are PET negative.
2. ***Medullary thyroid cancer.***[15] One study[14] suggests there is no correlation between calcitonin levels and lesion detection (the less-differentiated lesions with FDG uptake may secrete less calcitonin). In contrast, another study[27] suggests that PET is most useful if the calcitonin level is > 1000 ng/mL and of limited use if the calcitonin level is < 500 ng/mL (**Table 14.2**).

Table 14.1 Sensitivity and Specificity of Positron Emission Tomography (PET) Compared to Other Radionuclides in Papillary/Follicular Cancer

	Sensitivity %	Specificity %
PET	75	90
Iodine 131	50	99
Sestamibi/thallium	53	92

Pearls

1. ***Thyroglobulin level.*** In patients with a negative radioiodine whole-body scan and el-

Table 14.2 Sensitivity and Specificity of Positron Emission Tomography Compared with Other Modalities in Medullary Thyroid Cancer

	Sensitivity %	Specificity %
PET	78	79
Somatostatin receptor Scintigraphy	25	92
Dimercaptosuccinic acid	33	78
Sestamibi	25	100
CT	50	20
MRI	82	67

Abbreviations: CT, computed tomography; MRI, magnetic resonance imaging; PET, positron emission tomography.

evated thyroglobulin, PET is most useful at thyroglobulin levels > 10 ng/mL.[28]

2. ***Thyroid hormone withdrawal/recombinant thyroid-stimulating hormone (TSH).*** Although radioiodine imaging is most helpful when performed in patients with elevated TSH levels (thyroid hormone withdrawal or recombinant TSH administration), there are several other factors to consider with FDG PET imaging:
   - *a.* Although thyroid carcinomas may increase their metabolic demand after TSH stimulation, the tumors that have FDG uptake are usually poorly differentiated and may be less dependent upon TSH.
   - *b.* A TSH-stimulated hypothyroid state can decrease metabolic organ activity and may decrease metabolic activity in tumor cells.
3. ***Thyroid hormone withdrawal.*** Conflicting studies indicate both increased and decreased sensitivity with an elevated TSH after thyroid hormone withdrawal.[17,29,30]
   - The discrepant results may represent the conflicting effects of increased tumor metabolism from TSH stimulation and decreased metabolism from hypothyroidism.
4. ***Recombinant TSH.*** Lesion detectability is greater with recombinant TSH compared with TSH suppression.[31] Using recombinant TSH has two advantages over thyroid hormone withdrawal: patients are spared a prolonged hypothyroid state, and the possible negative effects of hypothyroidism on tumor FDG uptake are avoided. However, given the substantial cost of recombinant TSH, it is unclear whether this is cost-effective in most clinical settings.
5. ***Thyroglobulin and TSH.*** In patients with a thyroglobulin > 100 ng/mL, TSH stimulation is probably not necessary due to the high sensitivity of PET in this subpopulation.[32]

Pitfalls

1. ***Pulmonary metastases.*** PET has poor sensitivity for pulmonary metastases from thyroid cancer < 1 cm. If pulmonary metastases are of clinical concern, a chest CT should be performed.
2. ***Muscle/brown fat.*** Neck muscle or brown fat uptake can be mistaken for cervical or mediastinal nodal disease (**Figs. 14.4** and **14.5**). Anatomical correlation is necessary to avoid such errors; this is particularly important in thyroid cancer, where the prevalence of cervical node disease is high.
3. ***Vocal cord.*** Unilateral vocal cord activity can cause false-positive results (as seen in **Fig. 6.14**, p. 49).

References

1. Kresnik E, Gallowitsch HJ, Mikosch P, et al. Fluorine-18-fluorodeoxyglucose positron emission tomography in the preoperative assessment of thyroid nodules in an endemic goiter area. Surgery 2003;133(3):294–299
2. Bloom AD, Adler LP, Shuck JM. Determination of malignancy of thyroid nodules with positron emission tomography. Surgery 1993;114(4):728–734
3. Bogsrud TV, Karantanis D, Nathan MA, et al. The value of quantifying ^{18}F-FDG uptake in thyroid nodules found incidentally on whole-body PET-CT. Nucl Med Commun 2007;28(5):373–381
4. de Geus-Oei LF, Pieters GF, Bonenkamp JJ, et al. ^{18}F-FDG PET reduces unnecessary hemithyroidectomies for thyroid nodules with inconclusive cytologic results. J Nucl Med 2006;47(5):770–775
5. Mitchell JC, Grant F, Evenson AR, et al. Preoperative evaluation of thyroid nodules with 18FDG-PET/CT. Surgery 2005;138(6):1166–1174
6. Kim JM, Ryu JS, Kim TY, et al. ^{18}F-fluorodeoxyglucose positron emission tomography does not predict malignancy in thyroid nodules cytologically diagnosed as follicular neoplasm. J Clin Endocrinol Metab 2007;92(5):1630–1634
7. Chen YK, Ding HJ, Chen KT, et al. Prevalence and risk of cancer of focal thyroid incidentaloma identified by ^{18}F-fluorodeoxyglucose positron emission tomography

for cancer screening in healthy subjects. Anticancer Res 2005;25(2B):1421–1426

8. Kang KW, Kim SK, Kang HS, et al. Prevalence and risk of cancer of focal thyroid incidentaloma identified by ^{18}F-fluorodeoxyglucose positron emission tomography for metastasis evaluation and cancer screening in healthy subjects. J Clin Endocrinol Metab 2003;88(9):4100–4104
9. Choi JY, Lee KS, Kim HJ, et al. Focal thyroid lesions incidentally identified by integrated ^{18}F-FDG PET/CT: clinical significance and improved characterization. J Nucl Med 2006;47(4):609–615
10. Haugen BR, Lin EC. Isotope imaging for metastatic thyroid cancer. Endocrinol Metab Clin North Am 2001;30(2):469–492
11. Larson SM, Robbins R. Positron emission tomography in thyroid cancer management. Semin Roentgenol 2002;37(2):169–174
12. Zhuang H, Kumar R, Mandel S, Alavi A. Investigation of thyroid, head, and neck cancers with PET. Radiol Clin North Am 2004;42(6):1101–1111 viii.
13. Pryma DA, Schoder H, Gonen M, et al. Diagnostic accuracy and prognostic value of ^{18}F-FDG PET in Hürthle cell thyroid cancer patients. J Nucl Med 2006;47(8):1260–1266
14. Diehl M, Graichen S, Menzel C, et al. F-18 FDG PET in insular thyroid cancer. Clin Nucl Med 2003;28(9):728–731
15. Diehl M, Risse JH, Brandt-Mainz K, et al. Fluorine-18 fluorodeoxyglucose positron emission tomography in medullary thyroid cancer: results of a multicentre study. Eur J Nucl Med 2001;28(11):1671–1676
16. Wang W, Larson SM, Fazzari M, et al. Prognostic value of [^{18}F]fluorodeoxyglucose positron emission tomographic scanning in patients with thyroid cancer. J Clin Endocrinol Metab 2000;85(3):1107–1113
17. Grunwald F, Kalicke T, Feine U, et al. Fluorine-18 fluorodeoxyglucose positron emission tomography in thyroid cancer: results of a multicentre study. Eur J Nucl Med 1999;26(12):1547–1552
18. Palmedo H, Bucerius J, Joe A, et al. Integrated PET/CT in differentiated thyroid cancer: diagnostic accuracy and impact on patient management. J Nucl Med 2006;47(4):616–624
19. Chung JK, So Y, Lee JS, et al. Value of FDG PET in papillary thyroid carcinoma with negative 131I whole-body scan. J Nucl Med 1999;40(6):986–992
20. Jeong HS, Baek CH, Son YI, et al. Integrated ^{18}F-FDG PET/CT for the initial evaluation of cervical node level of patients with papillary thyroid carcinoma: comparison with ultrasound and contrast-enhanced CT. Clin Endocrinol (Oxf) 2006;65(3):402–407
21. Ito S, Kato K, Ikeda M, et al. Comparison of ^{18}F-FDG PET and bone scintigraphy in detection of bone metastases of thyroid cancer. J Nucl Med 2007;48(6):889–895
22. Rodrigues M, Li S, Gabriel M, et al. 99mTc-depreotide scintigraphy versus ^{18}F-FDG-PET in the diagnosis of radioiodine-negative thyroid cancer. J Clin Endocrinol Metab 2006;91(10):3997–4000
23. Wang W, Larson SM, Tuttle RM, et al. Resistance of [^{18}F]-fluorodeoxyglucose-avid metastatic thyroid cancer lesions to treatment with high-dose radioactive iodine. Thyroid 2001;11(12):1169–1175
24. Salvatore B, Paone G, Klain M, et al. Fluorodeoxyglucose PET/CT in patients with differentiated thyroid cancer and elevated thyroglobulin after total thyroidectomy and (131)I ablation. Q J Nucl Med Mol Imaging 2008;52(1):2–8
25. Shiga T, Tsukamoto E, Nakada K, et al. Comparison of (18)F-FDG, (131)I-Na, and (201)Tl in diagnosis of recurrent or metastatic thyroid carcinoma. J Nucl Med 2001;42(3):414–419
26. Phan HT, Jager PL, Plukker JT, Wolffenbuttel BH, Dierckx RA, Links TP. Detection of bone metastases in thyroid cancer patients: bone scintigraphy or ^{18}F-FDG PET? Nucl Med Commun 2007;28(8):597–602
27. Ong SC, Schoder H, Patel SG, et al. Diagnostic accuracy of ^{18}F-FDG PET in restaging patients with medullary thyroid carcinoma and elevated calcitonin levels. J Nucl Med 2007;48(4):501–507
28. Schluter B, Bohuslavizki KH, Beyer W, et al. Impact of FDG PET on patients with differentiated thyroid cancer who present with elevated thyroglobulin and negative ^{131}I scan. J Nucl Med 2001;42(1):71–76
29. Grunwald F, Biersack HJ. FDG PET in thyroid cancer: thyroxine or not? J Nucl Med 2000;41(12):1996–1998
30. van Tol KM, Jager PL, Piers DA, et al. Better yield of (18)fluorodeoxyglucose-positron emission tomography in patients with metastatic differentiated thyroid carcinoma during thyrotropin stimulation. Thyroid 2002;12(5):381–387
31. Chin BB, Patel P, Cohade C, et al. Recombinant human thyrotropin stimulation of fluoro-D-glucose positron emission tomography uptake in well-differentiated thyroid carcinoma. J Clin Endocrinol Metab 2004; 89(1):91–95
32. Stokkel MP, Duchateau CS, Dragoiescu C. The value of FDG-PET in the follow-up of differentiated thyroid cancer: a review of the literature. Q J Nucl Med Mol Imaging 2006;50(1):78–87

15

Thoracic Neoplasms

Eugene C. Lin and Abass Alavi

◆ Solitary Pulmonary Nodule

Clinical Indication: A

Positron emission tomography (PET) is a well-established modality for evaluating indeterminate solitary pulmonary nodules. It is most cost-effective when used in nodules with a pretest probability of malignancy between 12 and 69%.[1]

1. If the pretest probability of malignancy is very low, observation alone is considered acceptable in most circumstances.
2. If the pretest probability is high, biopsy/resection should be considered instead. With a pretest probability of 80%, the probability of malignancy is still 14% with a negative PET.
3. A negative PET scan indicates that a nodule is highly likely to be benign, but follow-up is still necessary, as a small number of nodules will be malignant and have low fluorodeoxyglucose (FDG) uptake.
   - It is important to take the pretest probability of malignancy into account with a negative PET scan result.
4. A positive result indicates that the nodule is most likely malignant.
   - Although false-positive results are noted with PET, PET has higher specificity than competing modalities.
5. A negative PET result is usually more accurate than a positive result, as false-negative findings are less common than false-positive lesions for malignancy.

Accuracy

1. ***PET.*** Sensitivity 97%, specificity 78%[2]
2. ***PET/CT.*** Sensitivity 97%, specificity 85%[3]
   - By incorporating the computed tomography (CT) findings into the PET/CT interpretation (e.g., a highly suspicious nodule on CT would be interpreted as positive even if PET is negative), the sensitivity of CT and specificity of PET are synergistic. This approach results in a higher accuracy compared with PET alone[3] and may be particularly helpful for nodules < 1 cm.

Comparison with Other Modalities

1. ***Dynamic contrast-enhanced CT.*** Sensitivity 98%, specificity 58%[4]
   - In two studies comparing PET and contrast-enhanced CT, PET had a slightly lower sensitivity and much higher specificity in one[5] and a greater sensitivity and comparable specificity in another.[6] Overall, PET is more accurate than contrast-enhanced CT for pulmonary nodule evaluation. CT should primarily be used in nodules < 1 cm, if PET is not available, or in low-risk patients.

2. ***Technetium 99m depreotide (somatostatin analogue).*** PET is more sensitive than technetium 99m depreotide, and specificity is comparable.[7,8]
3. PET scan can be useful after a positive dynamic contrast CT examination if biopsy is not desirable.
   - Over half of false-positive lesions on contrast CT can be shown to be true-negative on PET.[9]
4. An additional benefit of PET over other modalities is that if a PET scan is performed to evaluate a solitary pulmonary nodule and is positive for malignancy, PET is the most accurate modality for staging.

Pearls

1. ***Interpretation.***[10] A nodule is positive for malignancy if
   a. *Standardized uptake value (SUV).* SUV > 2.5
   b. *Visual analysis.* Intensity is greater than that of the mediastinum (**Fig. 15.1**).
      - Visual and SUV analyses are comparable in accuracy.
   c. Lower thresholds (SUV > 2.0 and intensity equal or greater than mediastinum) have also been used successfully.[3]
   d. *Small nodules.* Use caution when evaluating small nodules. For nodules < 1 cm, SUV values will be substantially lower due to partial volume effects. Visual analysis threshold should also be lowered.
      - If a nodule < 1 cm demonstrates any FDG uptake, it should be considered potentially malignant.[11]
2. ***What size pulmonary nodule should be evaluated?***
   a. Detection of malignancy in nodules as small as 5 mm[12] has been reported. As a practical consideration, PET is best used in nodules > 1 cm in size (dynamic contrast-enhanced CT is an alternative method for nodules < 1 cm).
      - However, there is limited evidence that PET may be accurate in nodules ≤ 1 cm.[13]
   b. Small nodules in the upper and anterior lungs are more optimal sites for assessment by PET than other sites because
      - There is less respiratory motion in the upper lungs.
      - Significant scatter from the liver in the lower lungs obscures small lesions.
      - There is normal background activity in the posterior and lower lungs, particularly if the PET is acquired primarily in expiration, which may decrease the contrast between the lesion and the adjacent tissues and therefore limit detectability.
      - Respiratory misregistration artifact (seen on PET/CT but not PET) can artifactually decrease uptake in lung nodules near the hemidiaphragms.
   c. PET could be considered in nodules < 1 cm in intermediate-risk patients if negative nodules are closely observed.[14–16]

A

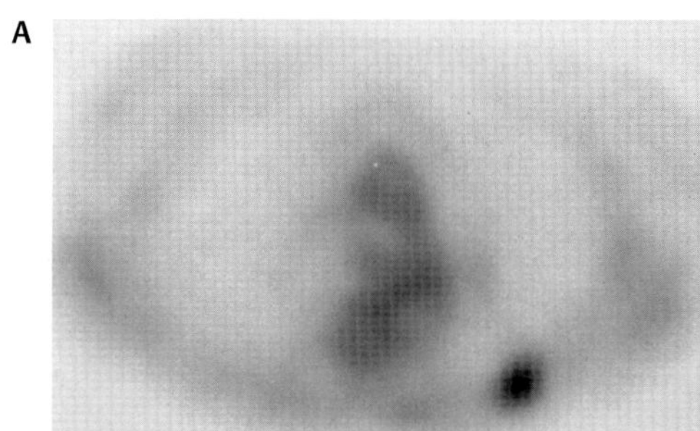

B

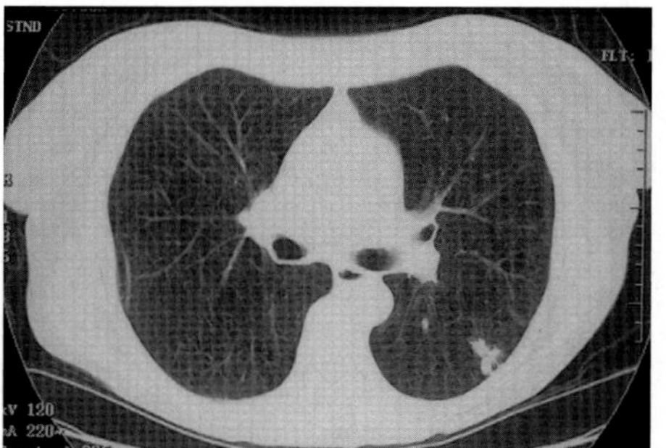

Fig. 15.1 Peripheral lung nodule. **(A)** Axial positron emission tomography (PET) scan demonstrates focal uptake in the peripheral left thorax. PET often has difficulty localizing peripheral lesions, and it cannot be determined whether this is in the lung or chest wall. **(B)** Axial computed tomography scan at the same level demonstrates an irregular lung nodule corresponding to the fluorodeoxyglucose (FDG) uptake. The degree of FDG uptake in this nodule is consistent with malignancy.

3. ***Scan time.*** Scanning should begin ~50 minutes after FDG injection to best separate malignant from benign lesions.[17]
4. ***Dual point imaging.*** Imaging at 1 and 3 hours (using a threshold of 10% SUV increase for malignancy) improves accuracy.[18] Malignant lesions show increased uptake on delayed images, whereas benign inflammatory lesions are stable or less active on the second scan.
   a. This technique may be particularly helpful for equivocal lesions with SUVs ~2.5.
   b. Benign lesions (in particular, granulomas) can sometimes demonstrate increasing uptake, but this is typically less than seen in malignancies. However, uptake in malignant lesions should not decrease.[19]
5. ***Histology.*** Squamous cell carcinomas have greater FDG uptake than adenocarcinomas or large cell carcinomas.[20]
6. ***Round atelectasis.*** Round atelectasis usually does not have FDG uptake (**Fig. 15.2**). PET can be used to differentiate atypical round atelectasis from malignant tumors.[21]

Pitfalls

1. ***False-positives.*** Active granulomatous/inflammatory process (tuberculosis, fungal infection, rheumatoid nodule, sarcoid, lipoid pneumonia, talc granulomata, inflammatory pseudotumor), benign tumors (sclerosing hemangioma, leiomyoma)[22]
2. ***False-negatives.*** Bronchioalveolar carcinoma (particularly in lesions without an invasive component) (**Fig. 15.3**), differentiated adenocarcinoma, carcinoid, mucoepidermoid carcinoma,[22] small lesions
   a. Most false-negative malignant pulmonary nodules on PET imaging are differentiated adenocarcinoma.[23]
   b. The sensitivity of PET for the multifocal form of bronchioalveolar carcinoma is substantially higher than for the solitary form.[24]
   c. The average SUV in a pulmonary carcinoid tumor is 3.0.[25]
   d. The false-negative rate may be higher if PET is used to evaluate nodules detected during screening chest CT, as these nodules, if malignant, tend to be small and/or low-grade.[26]
3. ***Ground glass opacities.*** PET should not be used to evaluate ground glass opacities seen on CT (sensitivity 10%, specificity 20%).[27]
   a. False-negative results are common due to bronchoalveolar carcinoma.
   b. False-positive results are common due to pneumonia.
4. ***Lack of CT correlate.*** A focus of FDG uptake in the lung should not be considered to represent a nodule if there is no CT correlate, as the latter can detect almost any nodule in the lung. This may not be true if a CT performed during respiration (as part of a PET/CT) is used for correlation, as small lung nodules may not be detected. If there is no corresponding CT lesion, consider these possibilities:

A

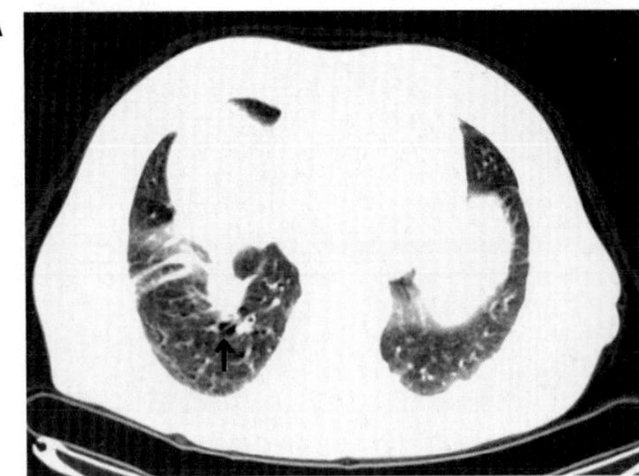

B

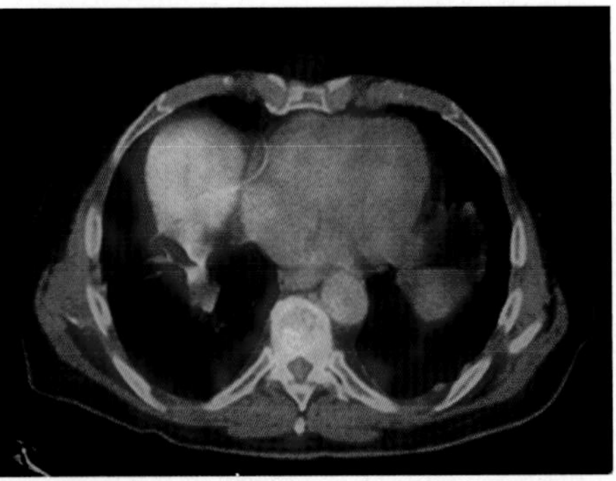

Fig. 15.2 Round atelectasis. **(A)** Axial computed tomography (CT) scan demonstrates round atelectasis in the right lung base (*arrow*). **(B)** Corresponding positron emission tomography/CT scan does not demonstrate uptake in the area of round atelectasis.

A

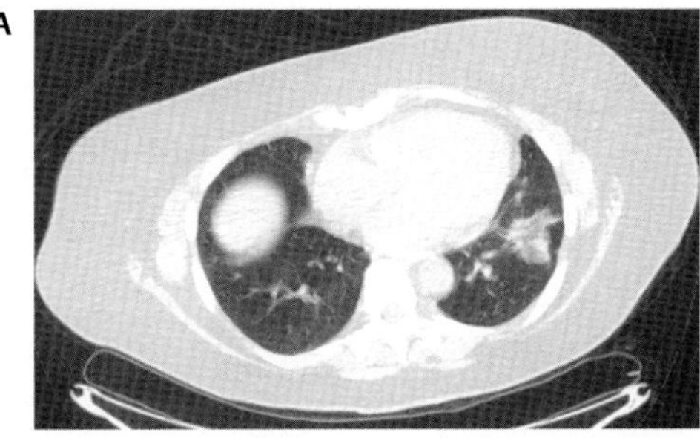

B

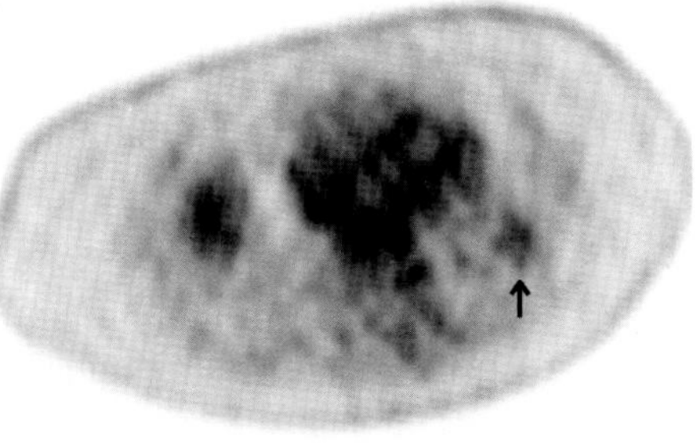

Fig. 15.3 Bronchoalveolar carcinoma. **(A)** Axial computed tomography scan demonstrates ground glass opacity in the left lower lobe secondary to bronchoalveolar carcinoma. **(B)** Axial positron emission tomography scan demonstrates mild fluorodeoxyglucose uptake (*arrow*) in this lesion.

   a. *Misregistration on PET/CT* (see Chapter 7). If the study is a PET/CT, the PET uptake and lung nodule may be misregistered and appear to be in different sites from each other. In addition, a liver dome lesion could appear to be in the lung base due to misregistration (see **Fig. 8.10**).
   b. *Injected clot.* Injection of radioactive clot (following blood draw) in the syringe can result in pulmonary hot spots without a CT correlate (see **Fig. 6.22**, p. 54). A similar phenomenon is seen on pulmonary perfusion images during ventilation perfusion scans.

5. ***Lesions with FDG uptake and SUV < 2.5.*** There is some evidence that lesions with SUV < 2.5 should be further stratified by level of visual uptake. In one study,[23] lesions with faint or no visible uptake had a very low probability of malignancy, whereas lesions that were visually evident had a probability of malignancy of 60%, even if SUV was < 2.5. An SUV cutoff of 1.6 was proposed by the authors of this study. Another study suggests using an SUV cutoff of 2.0 for nodules < 1 cm.[28] In practice, we recommend reporting discordant visual and SUV findings (e.g., visual uptake greater than mediastinum, but SUV < 2.5) as suspicious for malignancy. This is particularly true for small nodules where SUV may be artifactually low due to partial volume effects. If a nodule is not small (> 2 cm) and there is uptake less than the mediastinum and SUV < 2.5, we would report this as probably benign. Small nodules (between 1 and 2 cm) with definite uptake less than mediastinum and SUV < 2.5 are the most problematic. If the SUV is > 1.6 for these nodules, we will at least recommend very close follow-up. In addition, we would give greater weight to the CT characteristics in these nodules. Nodules < 1 cm cannot be diagnosed as benign by PET even if there is no FDG uptake.[29]
6. ***Lung base nodules.*** PET/CT should be used with caution in nodules near the hemidiaphragms. Due to photopenic respiratory misregistration artifact (see Chapter 8), SUVs can be artifactually decreased in these nodules.

◆ Pulmonary Metastasis versus Benign Nodule

Clinical Indication: C

PET can be used to evaluate an indeterminate pulmonary lesion in a patient with a known primary tumor. Minimal data exist for this application of PET. Note that in this setting, a metastasis cannot be distinguished from other causes of uptake, including bronchogenic carcinoma.

Accuracy

Using a cutoff SUV of 2.5 or lesion-to-background ratio of 3.0, PET can distinguish a pulmonary metastasis from a benign nodule with an accuracy of 91%.[30]

◆ Staging of Non–Small Cell Lung Cancer

Clinical Indication: A

1. PET is a standard modality for staging non–small cell lung cancer (NSCLC).
2. The addition of PET to the conventional work-up will prevent unnecessary surgery in one out of five patients[31] and results in changing stage from that determined by conventional modalities in over half of patients.[32]
3. PET is valuable in both mediastinal and distant staging.
4. ***Mediastinal staging***[16]
   a. PET is most useful in patients without enlarged mediastinal nodes on CT and no clinical evidence of systemic metastases.
   b. In patients with enlarged mediastinal nodes, PET is usually less valuable, as a negative PET may not preclude mediastinoscopy due to possible false-negative results.
   c. PET has a limited role in clinical stage I (peripheral) tumors, as the incidence of mediastinal metastases is low.
5. ***Distant staging***[16]
   a. PET is most useful in patients with a positive clinical evaluation suggesting systemic metastasis (clinical stage IV) or radiographic evidence of mediastinal lymph node enlargement (clinical stage III).
   - In these situations, PET should be performed in conjunction with a head CT or MRI.

   b. PET may also be useful to detect distant metastases in patients with clinical stage II tumors (particularly central tumors or adenocarcinoma).
   c. PET has a limited role in clinical stage I (peripheral) tumors, as the incidence of unsuspected distant metastases is low.

Accuracy and Comparison with Other Modalities

1. ***Mediastinal staging***[33]
   a. *PET*
   - PET is superior to CT for N0, N2, and N3 disease, but not N1 disease.
   - PET has a lower frequency of false-positive findings in the upper mediastinal nodes.
   - PET has a lower frequency of false-negative findings in adenocarcinoma and false-positive findings in squamous cell carcinoma.

   b. PET vs. CT[34] **Table 15.1**
   c. PET/CT. PET/CT has superior accuracy to that of CT, PET alone, or visual correlation of CT and PET for tumor and nodal staging.[35]
   - *Tumor stage.* PET/CT is superior to PET for T (tumor) staging. The CT component allows for determination of tumor size and extension in adjacent soft tissues. PET/CT is ideally suited for assessing chest wall and mediastinal invasion (**Fig. 15.4**). The advantages of PET/CT compared with PET are probably greater for T staging than nodal staging.[36]
   - *Nodal stage.* PET/CT increases confidence in diagnosing nodal disease and decreases equivocal results substantially.
     - o PET/CT has superior sensitivity to PET alone for left hilar, subaortic, and right paratracheal nodes and higher accuracy for subcarinal and interlobar nodes.[37]
2. ***Distant staging***[16]
   a. PET. PET will detect unsuspected distant metastases in ~10% of patients.[32]
   b. PET/CT. For distant metastases, PET/CT is primarily useful in determining the exact location of abnormalities noted on the FDG study.[35]
3. ***Bone marrow metastases***
   a. PET. Sensitivity 92%, specificity 99%[38]
   b. Compared with bone scintigraphy, PET is equal or greater in sensitivity and more

Table 15.1 Sensitivity and Specificity of Positron Emission Tomography (PET) versus Computed Tomography (CT) in the Mediastinal Staging of Non–Small Cell Lung Cancer

	Sensitivity %	Specificity %
PET	83	87
CT	68	76

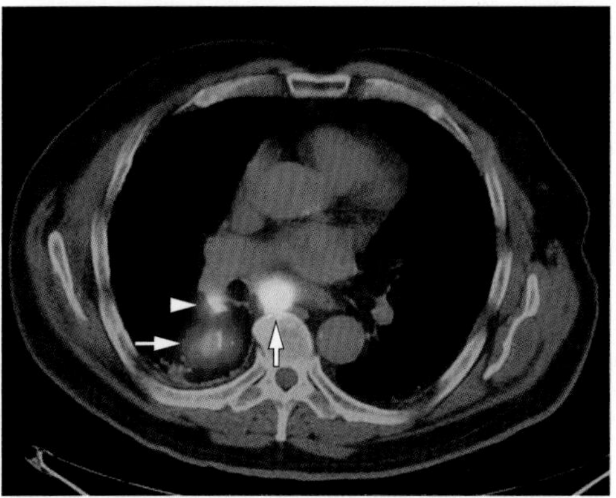

Fig. 15.4 Mediastinal and hilar metastases. Axial positron emission tomography/computed tomography scan demonstrates a right lower lobe carcinoma (*arrow*) with right hilar (*arrowhead*) and subcarinal (*open arrow*) nodal metastases.

specific for the diagnosis of bone marrow metastases from lung carcinoma (**Fig. 15.5**).

c. PET is more valuable for detecting bone marrow metastases in lung carcinoma than in other primary neoplasms because the bone lesions are often lytic with this malignancy.

4. ***Adrenal metastases*** (**Fig. 15.6**): ***PET.*** Sensitivity 100%, specificity 80%[38]
5. ***Brain metastases***
   a. *PET.* Sensitivity 60%[38]
   b. Cannot substitute for CT or MRI
6. ***Malignant versus benign pleural disease.*** PET can be used to differentiate malignant from benign pleural disease. It can evaluate both effusions (**Fig. 15.7**) and pleural thickening.
   a. *PET.* Sensitivity 97%, specificity 89%[39]
   b. *Degree of uptake.* Intense uptake is highly predictive of malignancy; however, moderate uptake should be interpreted with caution because it also can be seen in infection and other inflammatory disorders.
   - An SUV cutoff of 2.2 has an accuracy of 82% for distinguishing between benign and malignant pleural processes.[40]
   - Pleural metastases from thoracic primaries tend to have more uptake than

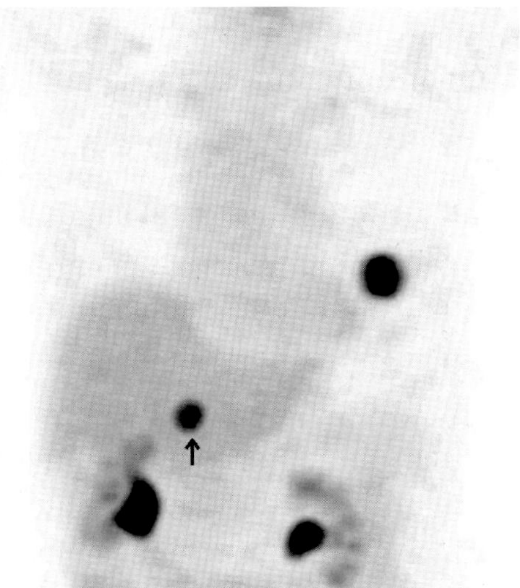

Fig. 15.6 Adrenal metastasis. Coronal positron emission tomography scan demonstrates a left lung cancer metastatic to the right adrenal (*arrow*).

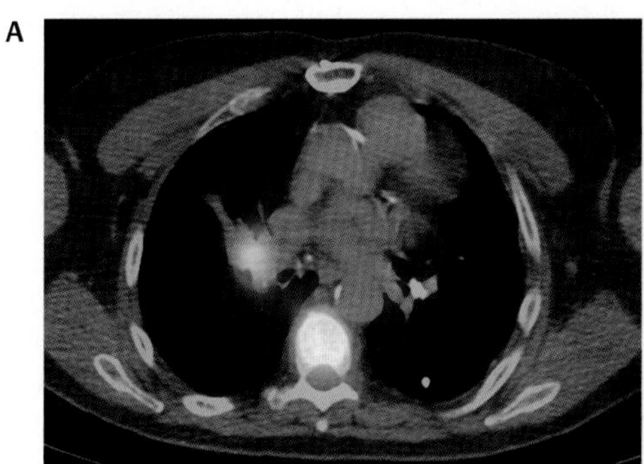

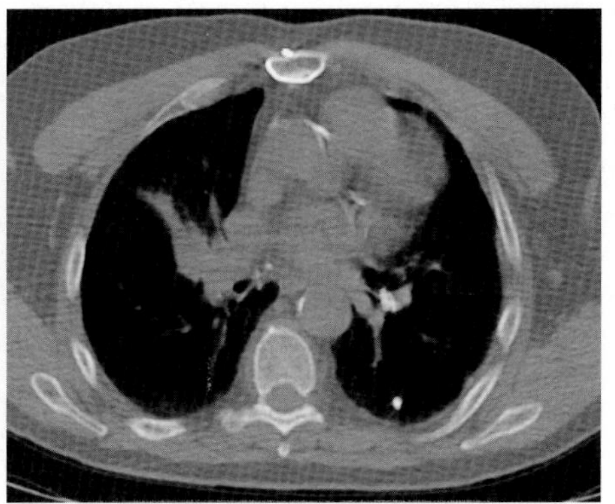

Fig. 15.5 Bone metastasis. **(A)** Axial positron emission tomography/computed tomography (PET/CT) scan demonstrates a right lung cancer metastatic to a vertebral body. **(B)** The metastasis is not visible on CT.

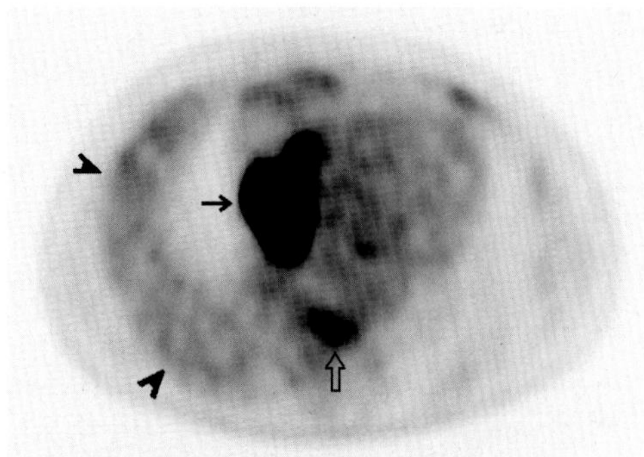

Fig. 15.7 Malignant effusion. Axial positron emission tomography scan demonstrates uptake in a malignant right effusion (*arrowheads*) in a patient with a large central right lung carcinoma (*arrow*). A bone metastasis is also noted (*open arrow*).

metastases from extrathoracic primaries.

c. Correlation with anatomical imaging is necessary to discover false-positive results due to peripheral but nonpleural (e.g., rib) uptake (see **Fig. 6.41**, p. 70).

Pearls

1. ***Do positive PET scans in the mediastinum require mediastinoscopy?*** Positive results on PET scan should be confirmed by mediastinoscopy or lymph node sampling before excluding surgery as an option. The false-positive rate of PET in the mediastinum is 13 to 22%.[16] However, PET is useful in guiding more invasive methods of mediastinal node sampling.
2. Confirmation may not be avoided if the pretest probability of metastasis is very high (> 85 to 90%), for example, if there is diffuse mediastinal infiltration on CT.
3. ***Do negative PET scans in the mediastinum obviate the need for mediastinoscopy?*** Mediastinoscopy can potentially be avoided before thoracotomy if PET is negative. The false-negative rate of PET in the mediastinum is 5 to 8% compared with an average false-negative rate for mediastinoscopy of 9%.[16] However, mediastinoscopy can detect microscopic disease, which will be missed on PET. It is important to consider the following factors:

   a. Pretest probability. Mediastinoscopy is usually indicated if the pretest probability of mediastinal nodal involvement is high (e.g., central tumor, adenocarcinoma, hilar involvement). The negative predictive value of PET is much lower in the presence of PET-positive N1 nodes and/or a centrally located primary tumor.[41] Patients who are clinical stage 1 (N0) after PET/CT and CT may not require mediastinoscopy. However, this is not supported by one study in which the sensitivity of PET/CT for mediastinal nodal metastases in stage T1 NSCLC was only 42%.[42] The following cases may benefit from mediastinoscopy:[43,44]
   - Patients clinically staged as N1 with PET/CT
   - Adenocarcinoma
   - Upper lobe (particularly right upper lobe) or central tumors
   - Tumors with SUV ≥ 10
   - Lymph nodes > 15 mm in short axis on CT

   b. Lymph node enlargement. If enlarged lymph nodes seen on CT and PET appear negative, mediastinoscopy should be considered. This applies more to moderately enlarged nodes. However, if lymph node enlargement is substantial, it may be less likely that PET is false-negative. Tumor burdens large enough to cause large degrees of nodal enlargement commonly demonstrate high FDG uptake. The sensitivity of PET/CT is higher in nodes > 1 cm, but specificity and accuracy are lower.[45]

   c. Uptake in the primary tumor. The relation between uptake in the primary tumor and that in the mediastinum is unclear. Low uptake in the primary tumor may be associated with hypometabolic metastatic sites. However, in some cases, low uptake in the primary tumor may be predictive of a lower propensity for lymph node metastasis.[46]
4. ***Pattern of uptake.*** Understanding the standard pattern of lymphatic spread of lung lesions by location is helpful in avoiding false-positive results. For example, left upper lobe malignancies will usually first metastasize to the aortopulmonary window nodes. The first level of nodal drainage is usually the most intense if multiple nodes are involved (see **Fig. 10.11**, p. 110). This can help distinguish metastatic disease from benign

causes of adenopathy, such as sarcoidosis, in which the nodes usually appear with similar intensity (see **Fig. 10.12**, p. 110).

5. Patients with other pulmonary pathologies (e.g., interstitial pneumonitis, tuberculosis) are more likely to have false-positive results, even if the disease is inactive.
6. ***SUVs and visual analysis mediastinal nodes.***
   a. *SUV cutoff.* SUV cutoffs of 2.5 to 5.3 have been used to distinguish between benign and malignant adenopathy.[47,48] One study[49] suggests using an SUV of 2.5, as the resulting high negative predictive value of 96% may allow the omission of mediastinoscopy in PET-negative cases. However, the highest diagnostic accuracy was achieved with an SUV of 4.5 in this study. As uptake from granulomatous disease is common in mediastinal nodes, relatively high SUV cutoffs will minimize false-positive results and achieve the highest accuracy. However, it can be argued that lower SUV cutoffs, while less accurate, are preferred as the goal of PET imaging is a low false-negative rate which will obviate mediastinoscopy in PET-negative cases.
   b. It is not clear whether using SUVs is superior to visual interpretation (using uptake greater than mediastinum as positive); in one study there was no difference,[47] whereas in another, use of visual criteria resulted in overdiagnosis.[50]

Pitfalls

1. Mild bilateral hilar nodal uptake from inflammatory etiologies is often seen in the lung cancer population as well as in patients without any known underlying disease.
2. False-positive mediastinal and hilar nodes often have histologic findings of follicular hyperplasia, anthracotic pigmentation, and macrophage infiltration.[51] FDG uptake in a mediastinal or hilar node can be suspected as false-positive if
   a. The nodes are calcified.
   b. The nodes have attenuation greater than the surrounding vessels on noncontrast CT.
3. Inaccurate mediastinal nodal staging is more often seen in patients with rheumatoid arthritis, diabetes, tuberculosis, and pneumonia.[52]
4. The highest rate of inaccuracy is nodal station 4 (lower paratracheal), followed by station 7 (inferior mediastinal) and station 9 (pulmonary ligament).[52]
5. Adrenal hyperplasia may have increased uptake. In patients with carcinoid or small cell tumors, adrenal hyperplasia can mimic bilateral adrenal metastases (see **Fig. 6.34**, p. 61).
6. Prior talc pleurodesis can cause increased pleural uptake, likely secondary to inflammation.
7. Pleural dissemination without an effusion from peripheral lung adenocarcinomas often presents as small pleural nodules and uneven pleural thickening. This is often beyond the resolution of PET, and in a patient with peripheral lung adenocarcinoma these findings on the CT portion of a PET/CT exam should be reported as suspicious for pleural dissemination even in the absence of FDG uptake.[53]
8. As false-positive results can result in incorrect M1 staging, metastatic disease identified by PET requires additional confirmation, particularly if there is a single site.[54]

◆ Prognosis and Therapy Response for Non–Small Cell Lung Cancer[55,56]

Clinical Indication: B

PET has several potential applications for therapy response and prognosis in NSCLC: prognosis of newly diagnosed tumors, restaging after neoadjuvant therapy, early assessment of therapy response, and restaging after therapy completion.[57] For restaging, PET is primarily useful in stage III disease and stage IV disease with solitary metastasis. In these cases PET should ideally be performed 2 to 3 months after therapy. PET may not be helpful in restaging patients with stage I and II disease.[58]

1. ***Prognosis.*** PET may be a useful tool for identifying patients at a high risk of recurrence; this may help guide therapy in resected stage I and II NSCLC.[59] The majority of the evidence suggests that the amount of uptake in the primary tumor and the tumor stage

determined by PET[60,61] are independent predictors of survival, although in one study tumor FDG uptake did not provide additional prognostic information.[62] In contrast to the primary tumor, the prognostic ability of regional nodal SUV is less certain.[63] PET also provides prognostic information for tumors that tend to have less FDG uptake, such as bronchioalveolar carcinoma and stage I adenocarcinomas. For these tumors, even relatively low levels of FDG uptake (SUV ≥ 2.5 in bronchioalveolar carcinoma and 3.3 in stage I adenocarcinoma) are associated with poor prognosis.[64,65] In recurrent lung cancer, the SUV in the recurrent tumor is also an independent prognostic factor in survival.[66] PET may also have prognostic value after neoadjuvant therapy for stage III NSCLC.[67]

2. ***Early prediction.*** Preliminary data indicate that early changes in FDG uptake during radiotherapy and/or chemotherapy may predict response to these interventions. In one study,[68] PET studies performed at 1 and 3 weeks after the initiation of chemotherapy predicted survival.
3. ***Late prediction.*** PET may have a potential role in restaging and response prediction after induction therapy for locally advanced disease (**Fig. 15.8**). In patients receiving neoadjuvant therapy before planned surgical resection, assessment of clearance of tumor from mediastinal lymph nodes is very important. Survival is substantially higher in patients with mediastinal clearance and complete resection of disease, and surgical resection is often avoided if there is residual tumor in the mediastinal nodes after induction therapy. Parameters that can be assessed include residual tumor viability, persistent mediastinal disease, and distant disease. However, the data on restaging with PET (primarily in stage IIIA-N2 disease) after neoadjuvant therapy are conflicting. Although PET or PET/CT may be more accurate in assessing response than CT[69] or repeat mediastinoscopy,[70] the published accuracy ranges from 50 to 95%.[15,71] In general, PET is less accurate for assessing the mediastinum after induction therapy than in untreated patients. PET/CT has superior sensitivity to PET for this application without compromising the specificity.[72] Histologic confirmation is still necessary in most cases, but PET may be useful in guiding mediastinoscopy or endoscopic procedures, or in detecting extrathoracic metastatic disease.
   a. *Primary tumor.* PET is sensitive but nonspecific for detection of residual disease in the primary tumor.[73]
   b. *Mediastinal nodes.* PET is specific but has limited sensitivity for restaging of mediastinal nodes.[73]
   c. *Hilar nodes.* After neoadjuvant chemotherapy, PET is more accurate than CT in detecting residual tumor, except in N1 nodes, where PET and CT are comparable.
4. ***Radiotherapy planning.*** PET is useful in determining the size of the radiation field,

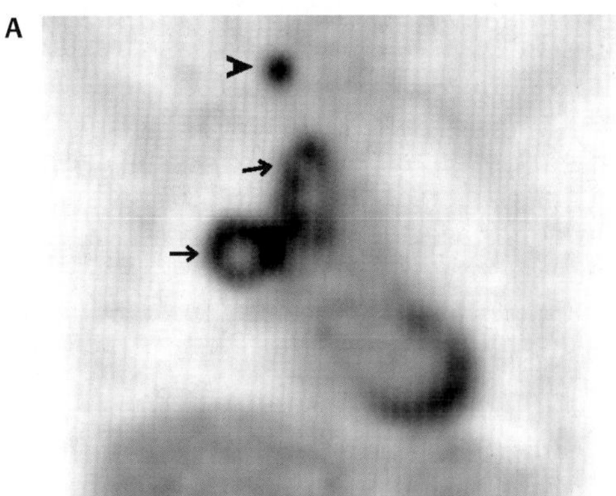

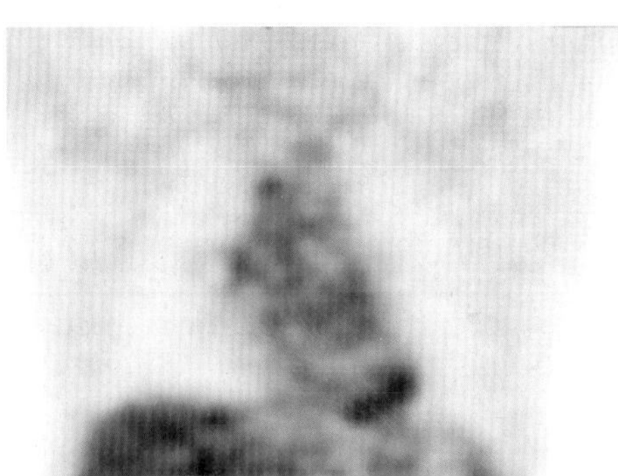

Fig. 15.8 Therapy follow-up for lung cancer. **(A)** Coronal positron emission tomography (PET) scan demonstrates uptake in necrotic right hilar and mediastinal nodes (*arrows*) and a right supraclavicular node (*arrowhead*). **(B)** Posttherapy coronal PET scan demonstrates that the supraclavicular activity has resolved and that the hilar and mediastinal activity has decreased.

particularly if postobstructive atelectasis is present on CT images.

Pearls and Pitfalls

1. PET is particularly useful when posttreatment scarring and pleural thickening limit the role of CT for assessing disease.
2. Radiation pneumonitis has a characteristic linear border and diffuse intense uptake (see **Fig. 6.23**, p. 55). Uptake on PET can be seen before radiographic findings. Tumor recurrence has more focal uptake and can usually be differentiated from radiation pneumonitis. However, radiation pneumonitis can occasionally have heterogeneous uptake in the early stages; thus, PET imaging should be delayed for 3 to 6 months after radiotherapy if possible.[74]

◆ Recurrence of Non–Small Cell Lung Cancer[55,75]

Clinical Indication: B

PET is useful in evaluation of local recurrence following treatment.

1. Residual thoracic abnormalities on CT are common as a result of treatment. PET can differentiate between local recurrence and posttreatment changes (**Fig. 15.9**) with a sensitivity of 97 to 100% and a specificity of 62 to 100%. Specificity is lower due to false-positive results from inflammatory reactions following therapy.
2. PET is more accurate than CT for the detection of local disease recurrence.
3. PET/CT has comparable sensitivity to PET for recurrence but has substantially higher specificity.[76]
4. The SUV in the recurrent tumor is an independent survival factor.[66]

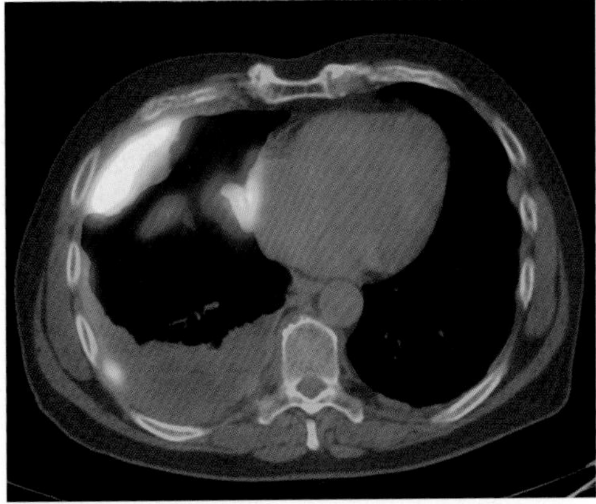

Fig. 15.10 Mesothelioma. Axial positron emission tomography/computed tomography scan demonstrates medial and lateral pleural uptake in a patient with mesothelioma.

◆ Small Cell Lung Cancer

Clinical Indication: C

Limited data indicate that PET and PET/CT are more accurate than conventional imaging in

A

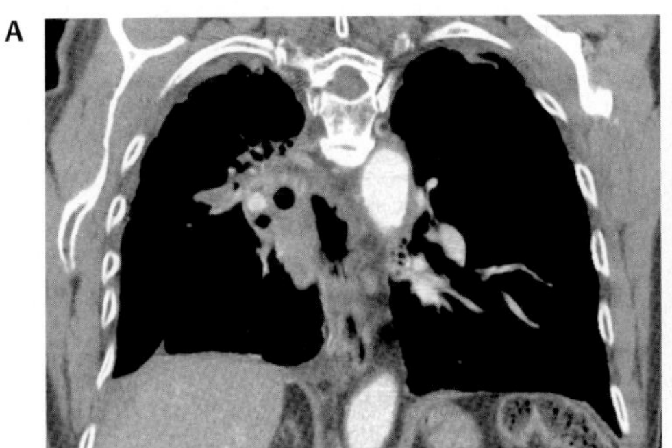

B

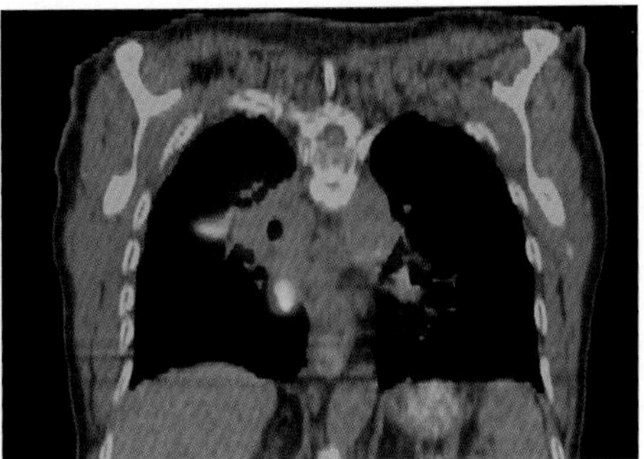

Fig. 15.9 Recurrent lung cancer. **(A)** Coronal contrast-enhanced computed tomography (CT) scan in a patient with lung cancer (status: postradiotherapy) demonstrates extensive soft tissue in the right hilar region. Tumor cannot be differentiated from fibrosis in this case. **(B)** Coronal positron emission tomography/CT scan at the same level demonstrates two small foci of tumor in the hilar soft tissue.

the staging and follow-up of small cell lung cancer, with superior accuracy for mediastinal, hilar, and extrathoracic lymph nodes, distant metastases, and bone marrow metastases. Compared with conventional imaging, PET or PET/CT can result in a change in stage in 10 to 17% of patients.[77–79]

◆ Mesothelioma

Clinical Indication: C

1. PET may have limited sensitivity for determining the extent of the local tumor (**Fig. 15.10**) (subtle transdiaphragmatic extension is particularly hard to detect) and mediastinal nodal metastases. The primary value of PET is in identifying extrathoracic metastases, obviating thoracotomy.[80]
2. A high level of uptake in the primary tumor is associated with the presence of N2 disease and with poor survival.
3. SUV > 10 is associated with poor survival.[81]
4. Localized fibrous tumor of the pleura (benign mesothelioma) typically has low (< 2.5 SUV) uptake.[82]
5. Most benign pleural processes have an SUV < 2.2.[37]

References

1. Gambhir SS, Shepherd JE, Shah BD, et al. Analytical decision model for the cost-effective management of solitary pulmonary nodules. J Clin Oncol 1998;16(6):2113–2125
2. Gould MK, Maclean CC, Kuschner WG, et al. Accuracy of positron emission tomography for diagnosis of pulmonary nodules and mass lesions: a meta-analysis. JAMA 2001;285(7):914–924
3. Kim SK, Allen-Auerbach M, Goldin J, et al. Accuracy of PET/CT in characterization of solitary pulmonary lesions. J Nucl Med 2007;48(2):214–220
4. Swensen SJ, Viggiano RW, Midthun DE, et al. Lung nodule enhancement at CT: multicenter study. Radiology 2000;214(1):73–80
5. Christensen JA, Nathan MA, Mullan BP, et al. Characterization of the solitary pulmonary nodule: ^{18}F-FDG PET versus nodule-enhancement CT. AJR Am J Roentgenol 2006;187(5):1361–1367
6. Yi CA, Lee KS, Kim BT, et al. Tissue characterization of solitary pulmonary nodule: comparative study between helical dynamic CT and integrated PET/CT. J Nucl Med 2006;47(3):443–450
7. Blum J, Handmaker H, Lister-James J, Rinne N. A multicenter trial with a somatostatin analog (99m)Tc depreotide in the evaluation of solitary pulmonary nodules. Chest 2000;117(5):1232–1238
8. Ferran N, Ricart Y, Lopez M, et al. Characterization of radiologically indeterminate lung lesions: 99mTc-depreotide SPECT versus ^{18}F-FDG PET. Nucl Med Commun 2006;27(6):507–514
9. Rohren EM, Lowe VJ. Update in PET imaging of nonsmall cell lung cancer. Semin Nucl Med 2004;34(2):134–153
10. Lowe VJ, Fletcher JW, Gobar L, et al. Prospective investigation of positron emission tomography in lung nodules. J Clin Oncol 1998;16(3):1075–1084
11. Hagge RJ, Coleman RE. Positron emission tomography: lung cancer. Semin Roentgenol 2002;37(2):110–117
12. Marom EM, Sarvis S, Herndon JE, Patz EF Jr. T1 lung cancers: sensitivity of diagnosis with fluorodeoxyglucose PET. Radiology 2002;223(2):453–459
13. Herder GJ, Golding RP, Hoekstra OS, et al. The performance of (18)F-fluorodeoxyglucose positron emission tomography in small solitary pulmonary nodules. Eur J Nucl Med Mol Imaging 2004;31(9):1231–1236
14. Detterbeck FC, Falen S, Rivera MP, et al. Seeking a home for a PET, part 1: Defining the appropriate place for positron emission tomography imaging in the diagnosis of pulmonary nodules or masses. Chest 2004;125(6):2294–2299
15. Detterbeck FC, Vansteenkiste JF, Morris DE, et al. Seeking a home for a PET, part 3: Emerging applications of positron emission tomography imaging in the management of patients with lung cancer. Chest 2004;126(5):1656–1666
16. Detterbeck FC, Falen S, Rivera MP, et al. Seeking a home for a PET, part 2: Defining the appropriate place for positron emission tomography imaging in the staging of patients with suspected lung cancer. Chest 2004;125(6):2300–2308
17. Lowe VJ, DeLong DM, Hoffman JM, Coleman RE. Optimum scanning protocol for FDG-PET evaluation of pulmonary malignancy. J Nucl Med 1995;36(5):883–887
18. Demura Y, Tsuchida T, Ishizaki T, et al. 18F-FDG accumulation with PET for differentiation between benign and malignant lesions in the thorax. J Nucl Med 2003;44(4):540–548
19. Nunez R, Kalapparambath A, Varela J. Improvement in sensitivity with delayed imaging of pulmonary lesions with FDG-PET. Rev Esp Med Nucl 2007;26(4):196–207
20. de Geus-Oei LF, Krieken JH, Aliredjo RP, et al. Biological correlates of FDG uptake in non-small cell lung cancer. Lung Cancer 2007;55(1):79–87
21. McAdams HP, Erasums JJ, Patz EF, et al. Evaluation of patients with round atelectasis using 2-[^{18}F]-fluoro-2-deoxy-D-glucose PET. J Comput Assist Tomogr 1998; 22(4):601–604
22. Shim SS, Lee KS, Kim BT, et al. Focal parenchymal lung lesions showing a potential of false-positive and false-negative interpretations on integrated PET/CT. AJR Am J Roentgenol 2006;186(3):639–648
23. Hashimoto Y, Tsujikawa T, Kondo C, et al. Accuracy of PET for diagnosis of solid pulmonary lesions with ^{18}F-FDG uptake below the standardized uptake value of 2.5. J Nucl Med 2006;47(3):426–431
24. Heyneman LE, Patz EF. PET imaging in patients with bronchioloalveolar cell carcinoma. Lung Cancer 2002;38(3):261–266
25. Kruger S, Buck AK, Blumstein NM, et al. Use of integrated FDG PET/CT imaging in pulmonary carcinoid tumours. J Intern Med 2006;260(6):545–550

26. Lindell RM, Hartman TE, Swensen SJ, et al. Lung cancer screening experience: a retrospective review of PET in 22 non-small cell lung carcinomas detected on screening chest CT in a high-risk population. AJR Am J Roentgenol 2005;185(1):126–131
27. Nomori H, Watanabe K, Ohtsuka T, et al. Evaluation of F-18 fluorodeoxyglucose (FDG) PET scanning for pulmonary nodules less than 3 cm in diameter, with special reference to the CT images. Lung Cancer 2004;45(1):19–27
28. Veronesi G, Bellomi M, Veronesi U, et al. Role of positron emission tomography scanning in the management of lung nodules detected at baseline computed tomography screening. Ann Thorac Surg 2007;84(3):959–965
29. O JH, Yoo IR, Kim SH, et al. Clinical significance of small pulmonary nodules with little or no ^{18}F-FDG uptake on PET/CT images of patients with nonthoracic malignancies. J Nucl Med 2007;48(1):15–21
30. Hsu WH, Hsu NY, Shen YY, et al. Differentiating solitary pulmonary metastases in patients with extrapulmonary neoplasms using FDG-PET. Cancer Invest 2003;21(1):47–52
31. van Tinteren H, Hoekstra OS, Smit EF, et al. Effectiveness of positron emission tomography in the preoperative assessment of patients with suspected non-small-cell lung cancer: the PLUS multicentre randomised trial. Lancet 2002;359(9315):1388–1393
32. Pieterman RM, van Putten JW, Meuzelaar JJ, et al. Preoperative staging of non-small-cell lung cancer with positron-emission tomography. N Engl J Med 2000;343(4):254–261
33. Alongi F, Ragusa P, Montemaggi P, Bona CM. Combining independent studies of diagnostic fluorodeoxyglucose positron-emission tomography and computed tomography in mediastinal lymph node staging for non-small cell lung cancer. Tumori 2006;92(4):327–333
34. Ebihara A, Nomori H, Watanabe K, et al. Characteristics of advantages of positron emission tomography over computed tomography for N-staging in lung cancer patients. Jpn J Clin Oncol 2006;36(11):694–698
35. Lardinois D, Weder W, Hany TF, et al. Staging of non-small-cell lung cancer with integrated positron-emission tomography and computed tomography. N Engl J Med 2003;348(25):2500–2507
36. Czernin J, Allen-Auerbach M, Schelbert HR. Improvements in cancer staging with PET/CT: literature-based evidence as of September 2006. J Nucl Med 2007;48(Suppl 1):78S–88S
37. Cerfolio RJ, Ojha B, Bryant AS, et al. The accuracy of integrated PET-CT compared with dedicated PET alone for the staging of patients with nonsmall cell lung cancer. Ann Thorac Surg 2004;78(3):1017–1023
38. Marom EM, McAdams HP, Erasmus JJ, et al. Staging non-small cell lung cancer with whole-body PET. Radiology 1999;212(3):803–809
39. Duysinx B, Nguyen D, Louis R, et al. Evaluation of pleural disease with 18-fluorodeoxyglucose positron emission tomography imaging. Chest 2004;125(2):489–493
40. Duysinx BC, Larock MP, Nguyen D, et al. ^{18}F-FDG PET imaging in assessing exudative pleural effusions. Nucl Med Commun 2006;27(12):971–976
41. Verhagen AF, Bootsma GP, Tjan-Heijnen VC, et al. FDG-PET in staging lung cancer: how does it change the algorithm? Lung Cancer 2004;44(2):175–181
42. Kim BT, Lee KS, Shim SS, et al. Stage T1 non-small cell lung cancer: preoperative mediastinal nodal staging with integrated FDG PET/CT–a prospective study. Radiology 2006;241(2):501–509
43. Cerfolio RJ, Bryant AS, Eloubeidi MA. Routine mediastinoscopy and esophageal ultrasound fine-needle aspiration in patients with non-small cell lung cancer who are clinically N2 negative: a prospective study. Chest 2006;130(6):1791–1795
44. de Langen AJ, Raijmakers P, Riphagen I, et al. The size of mediastinal lymph nodes and its relation with metastatic involvement: a meta-analysis. Eur J Cardiothorac Surg 2006;29(1):26–29
45. Al-Sarraf N, Gately K, Lucey J, Wilson L, McGovern E, Young V. Lymph node staging by means of positron emission tomography is less accurate in non-small cell lung cancer patients with enlarged lymph nodes: Analysis of 1145 lymph nodes. Lung Cancer 2008;60(1):62–68
46. Nomori H, Watanabe K, Ohtsuka T, et al. Fluorine 18-tagged fluorodeoxyglucose positron emission tomographic scanning to predict lymph node metastasis, invasiveness, or both, in clinical T1 N0 M0 lung adenocarcinoma. J Thorac Cardiovasc Surg 2004;128(3):396–401
47. Vansteenkiste JF, Stroobants SG, De Leyn PR, et al. Lymph node staging in non-small-cell lung cancer with FDG-PET scan: a prospective study on 690 lymph node stations from 68 patients. J Clin Oncol 1998;16(6):2142–2149
48. Bryant AS, Cerfolio RJ, Klemm KM, Ojha B. Maximum standard uptake value of mediastinal lymph nodes on integrated FDG-PET-CT predicts pathology in patients with non-small cell lung cancer. Ann Thorac Surg 2006;82(2):417–422
49. Hellwig D, Graeter TP, Ukena D, et al. ^{18}F-FDG PET for mediastinal staging of lung cancer: which SUV threshold makes sense? J Nucl Med 2007;48(11):1761–1766
50. Hara M, Shiraki N, Itoh M, et al. A problem in diagnosing N3 disease using FDG-PET in patients with lung cancer—high false positive rate with visual assessment. Ann Nucl Med 2004;18(6):483–488
51. Shim SS, Lee KS, Kim BT, et al. Non-small cell lung cancer: prospective comparison of integrated FDG PET/CT and CT alone for preoperative staging. Radiology 2005;236(3):1011–1019
52. Al-Sarraf N, Aziz R, Doddakula K, et al. Factors causing inaccurate staging of mediastinal nodal involvement in non-small cell lung cancer patients staged by positron emission tomography. Interact Cardiovasc Thorac Surg 2007;6(3):350–353
53. Shim SS, Lee KS, Kim BT, et al. Integrated PET/CT and the dry pleural dissemination of peripheral adenocarcinoma of the lung: diagnostic implications. J Comput Assist Tomogr 2006;30(1):70–76
54. Reed CE, Harpole DH, Posther KE, et al. Results of the American College of Surgeons Oncology Group Z0050 trial: the utility of positron emission tomography in staging potentially operable non-small cell lung cancer. J Thorac Cardiovasc Surg 2003;126(6):1943–1951
55. Vansteenkiste JF, Stroobants SG. Positron emission tomography in the management of non-small cell lung cancer. Hematol Oncol Clin North Am 2004;18(1):269–288
56. Kostakoglu L, Goldsmith SJ. ^{18}F-FDG PET evaluation of the response to therapy for lymphoma and for breast, lung, and colorectal carcinoma. J Nucl Med 2003;44(2):224–239
57. Bunyaviroch T, Coleman RE. PET evaluation of lung cancer. J Nucl Med 2006;47(3):451–469

58. Podoloff DA, Advani RH, Allred C, et al. NCCN task force report: positron emission tomography (PET)/ computed tomography (CT) scanning in cancer. J Natl Compr Canc Netw 2007;5(Suppl 1):S1–S22
59. Pillot G, Siegel BA, Govindan R. Prognostic value of fluorodeoxyglucose positron emission tomography in non-small cell lung cancer: a review. J Thorac Oncol 2006;1(2):152–159
60. Cerfolio RJ, Bryant AS, Ohja B, Bartolucci AA. The maximum standardized uptake values on positron emission tomography of a non-small cell lung cancer predict stage, recurrence, and survival. J Thorac Cardiovasc Surg 2005;130(1):151–159
61. Kramer H, Post WJ, Pruim J, Groen HJ. The prognostic value of positron emission tomography in non-small cell lung cancer: analysis of 266 cases. Lung Cancer 2006;52(2):213–217
62. Vesselle H, Freeman JD, Wiens L, et al. Fluorodeoxyglucose uptake of primary non-small cell lung cancer at positron emission tomography: new contrary data on prognostic role. Clin Cancer Res 2007;13(11):3255–3263
63. de Geus-Oei LF, van der Heijden HF, Corstens FH, Oyen WJ. Predictive and prognostic value of FDG-PET in nonsmall-cell lung cancer: a systematic review. Cancer 2007;110(8):1654–1664
64. Ohtsuka T, Nomori H, Watanabe K, et al. Prognostic significance of [(18)F]fluorodeoxyglucose uptake on positron emission tomography in patients with pathologic stage I lung adenocarcinoma. Cancer 2006;107(10):2468–2473
65. Raz DJ, Odisho AY, Franc BL, Jablons DM. Tumor fluoro-2-deoxy-D-glucose avidity on positron emission tomographic scan predicts mortality in patients with early-stage pure and mixed bronchioloalveolar carcinoma. J Thorac Cardiovasc Surg 2006;132(5): 1189–1195
66. Hellwig D, Groschel A, Graeter TP, et al. Diagnostic performance and prognostic impact of FDG-PET in suspected recurrence of surgically treated non-small cell lung cancer. Eur J Nucl Med Mol Imaging 2006;33(1):13–21
67. Dooms C, Vansteenkiste J. Positron emission tomography in nonsmall cell lung cancer. Curr Opin Pulm Med 2007;13(4):256–260
68. Nahmias C, Hanna WT, Wahl LM, Long MJ, Hubner KF, Townsend DW. Time course of early response to chemotherapy in non-small cell lung cancer patients with ^{18}F-FDG PET/CT. J Nucl Med 2007;48(5): 744–751
69. Cerfolio RJ, Bryant AS, Ojha B. Restaging patients with N2 (stage IIIa) non-small cell lung cancer after neoadjuvant chemoradiotherapy: a prospective study. J Thorac Cardiovasc Surg 2006;131(6):1229–1235
70. De Leyn P, Stroobants S, De Wever W, et al. Prospective comparative study of integrated positron emission tomography-computed tomography scan compared with remediastinoscopy in the assessment of residual mediastinal lymph node disease after induction chemotherapy for mediastinoscopy-proven stage IIIA-N2 non-small-cell lung cancer: a Leuven Lung Cancer Group Study. J Clin Oncol 2006;24(21): 3333–3339
71. Knoepp UW, Ravenel JG. Computed tomography and PET imaging in non-small cell lung cancer. Crit Rev Oncol Hematol 2006;58(1):15–30
72. Vansteenkiste J, Dooms C. Positron emission tomography in nonsmall cell lung cancer. Curr Opin Oncol 2007;19(2):78–83
73. Ryu JS, Choi NC, Fischman AJ, et al. FDG-PET in staging and restaging non-small cell lung cancer after neoadjuvant chemoradiotherapy: correlation with histopathology. Lung Cancer 2002;35(2):179–187
74. Bruzzi JF, Munden RF. PET/CT imaging of lung cancer. J Thorac Imaging 2006;21(2):123–136
75. Vansteenkiste J, Fischer BM, Dooms C, Mortensen J. Positron-emission tomography in prognostic and therapeutic assessment of lung cancer: systematic review. Lancet Oncol 2004;5(9):531–540
76. Keidar Z, Haim N, Guralnik L, et al. PET/CT using ^{18}F-FDG in suspected lung cancer recurrence: diagnostic value and impact on patient management. J Nucl Med 2004;45(10):1640–1646
77. Bradley JD, Dehdashti F, Mintun MA, et al. Positron emission tomography in limited-stage small-cell lung cancer: a prospective study. J Clin Oncol 2004;22(16):3248–3254
78. Brink I, Schumacher T, Mix M, et al. Impact of [^{18}F]FDG-PET on the primary staging of small-cell lung cancer. Eur J Nucl Med Mol Imaging 2004;31(12):1614–1620
79. Fischer BM, Mortensen J, Langer SW, et al. A prospective study of PET/CT in initial staging of small-cell lung cancer: comparison with CT, bone scintigraphy and bone marrow analysis. Ann Oncol 2007;18(2):338–345 Epub 2006
80. Flores RM, Akhurst T, Gonen M, et al. Positron emission tomography defines metastatic disease but not locoregional disease in patients with malignant pleural mesothelioma. J Thorac Cardiovasc Surg 2003;126(1):11–16
81. Flores RM, Akhurst T, Gonen M, et al. Positron emission tomography predicts survival in malignant pleural mesothelioma. J Thorac Cardiovasc Surg 2006;132(4):763–768
82. Cortes J, Rodriguez J, Garcia-Velloso MJ, et al. [(18)F]-FDG PET and localized fibrous mesothelioma. Lung 2003;181(1):49–54

16

Breast Cancer

Eugene C. Lin, Marie E. Lee, and Abass Alavi

◆ Detection of Breast Masses

Clinical Indication: B

Positron emission tomography (PET) is sensitive for detecting breast lesions that are > 1 cm, but it is not currently used as a screening modality due to cost. PET may be more cost-effective with dedicated breast imaging PET machines. High-resolution positron emission mammography (PEM) is an approved device to perform PET imaging of the breast under gentle compression. Advantages of PEM are higher spatial resolution, shorter imaging time, and reduced soft tissue attenuation. PEM may be of value to define extent of disease for surgical planning, detect multifocal or bilateral disease, and monitor response to therapy. There are ongoing trials to evaluate PEM versus breast magnetic resonance imaging (MRI).

Not infrequently, breast lesions are detected as incidental findings on PET studies performed for other indications and should be reported when discovered.

Accuracy

1. ***PET.*** Sensitivity 89%, specificity 80%[1]
2. ***PEM.*** Sensitivity 90%, specificity 86%[2]
   - PEM was able to identify ductal carcinoma in situ in 10 of 11 cases.
3. ***Tumor size.*** Sensitivity is highly dependent on tumor size[3] and grade.[4]
   a. Detection rate for T1a and b tumors (< 1 cm) is low, and tumors < 0.5 cm (T1a) will likely not be detected.
   b. Sensitivity increases substantially for T2 lesions (2 to 5 cm) and T3 lesions (> 5 cm).

Comparison with Other Modalities

1. ***Technetium (Tc) 99m-sestamibi***
   a. The sensitivity of PET and sestamibi for breast lesions is comparable.[5]
   b. Tumors usually have higher uptake relative to normal tissue on PET than on sestamibi.
2. ***Contrast-enhanced breast MRI***
   a. PET is less sensitive but more specific than MRI for characterizing and detecting breast lesions.[6]
   b. MRI has superior sensitivity for lesions < 1 cm and lobular carcinoma.

Pearls

1. ***Standardized uptake value (SUV).*** An SUV of 2.0 and a tumor-to-background ratio of 2.5 are both potential cutoffs between benign and malignant.[7–9]
   a. However, as there are minimal data on SUV of breast lesions, any focal abnormal uptake of fluorodeoxyglucose (FDG) should undergo further work-up.

b. In general, breast cancer has lower metabolic activity than most other malignancies.

2. ***Incidental breast uptake.*** Focal FDG uptake in the breast is sometimes seen incidentally and is associated with a high likelihood of malignancy.[10] Initial work-up of incidentally detected breast abnormality on PET should include the standard examinations in such settings: physical examination and mammography. Contrast-enhanced breast MRI may be particularly helpful after negative initial work-up due to its high sensitivity for breast lesions. Ultrasound may also be helpful in selected circumstances.
3. ***Delayed/dual time point imaging.*** Delayed imaging increases tumor visualization by PET.[11] Tumors will accumulate FDG over time, whereas normal breast tissue will reveal decreased or unchanged FDG uptake. Dual time point imaging improves the sensitivity and accuracy of PET for primary breast cancer, particularly for noninvasive, small invasive, and invasive lobular and mixed carcinomas.[12]
4. ***Dense breasts.*** Dense breasts have more FDG uptake, but the uptake in dense breasts is not substantial and therefore will not interfere with detectability of breast lesions. Even in dense breasts, the maximum SUV in normal tissue is usually relatively low (< 1).[13]
5. ***Estrogen and progesterone receptors.*** Estrogen receptor (ER)–positive tumors have lower SUVs than ER negative tumors. Progesterone receptor status does not affect FDG uptake.[14]

Pitfalls

1. ***False negatives.*** Small lesions, invasive lobular carcinoma, tubular carcinoma, carcinoma in situ, ER-positive tumors
2. ***False positives***
   a. *Inflammatory.* Abscess, soft tissue inflammation, tuberculosis, sarcoidosis
   b. *Traumatic.* Postbiopsy, hematoma, seroma (**Fig. 16.1**) (often has a ringlike pattern of uptake)
   c. *Benign neoplasms.* Ductal adenoma, fibrous dysplasia, fibroadenomas (rare, the majority of fibroadenomas do not have significant uptake)[3]

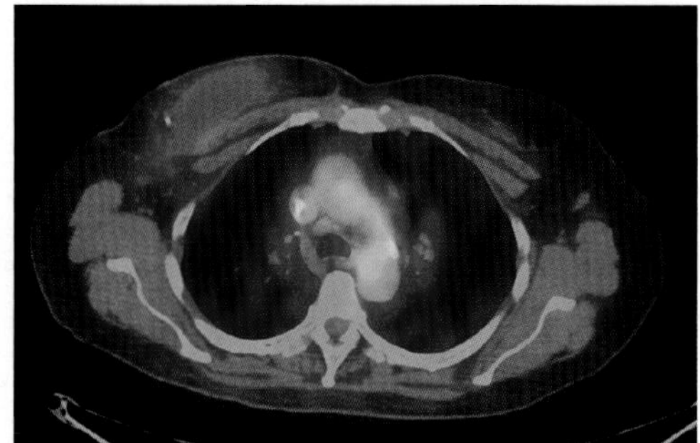

Fig. 16.1 Breast seroma. Axial positron emission tomography/computed tomography scan demonstrates peripheral uptake around a right breast seroma.

◆ Staging of Breast Cancer

Clinical Indication: B

PET is relatively insensitive for axillary nodal metastasis but has a high specificity. Although PET cannot replace sentinel node biopsy, a positive PET scan suggests that axillary nodal dissection could be performed instead of sentinel node biopsy.[15,16] However, in practice most surgeons will want pathological proof and may biopsy abnormal nodes seen on sonography before node dissection. PET is superior to computed tomography (CT) for the detection of mediastinal and internal mammary nodal metastases.[17] PET is also relatively sensitive in detecting distant metastases. PET is most valuable in staging in specific circumstances:[18,19]

1. The primary tumor is T3 or T4.
2. Stage 4 disease
3. Neoadjuvant therapy is planned without axillary dissection or sentinel node sampling.
4. Equivocal findings are seen on CT, ultrasound, or MRI.
5. The primary lesion is medial or superior, which indicates a higher risk for internal mammary metastases or supraclavicular metastases. Patients with inner quadrant breast tumors are 6 times more likely to have isolated extra-axillary metastases identified by PET.[20]

Accuracy and Comparison with Other Modalities

1. ***Multifocal disease: PET.*** Sensitivity 92%, specificity 90%
   a. PET is superior to conventional imaging (mammography and ultrasound combined).
   b. However, contrast-enhanced MRI is more sensitive than PET (**Fig. 16.2**).[6,21]
2. ***Axillary staging***
   a. PET does not substitute for axillary nodal dissection in most patients.
   b. *PET*: Sensitivity 61%, specificity 80%[22]
3. ***Other nodal groups.*** PET is more accurate than CT for the diagnosis of internal mammary (**Fig. 16.3**) and mediastinal nodal metastases (**Fig. 16.4, Table 16.1**).[17,23]
4. ***Distant staging.*** PET has a sensitivity of 84 to 93% and a specificity of 55 to 86% for the detection of distant metastases.[17] In patients with locally advanced breast cancer, the addition of PET to the work-up for staging will result in detection of distant metastases not detected by conventional imaging in 8% of cases.[24]
5. ***Bone marrow metastases***
   a. Overall sensitivity of PET and bone scan is comparable, but PET has superior specificity.[25]

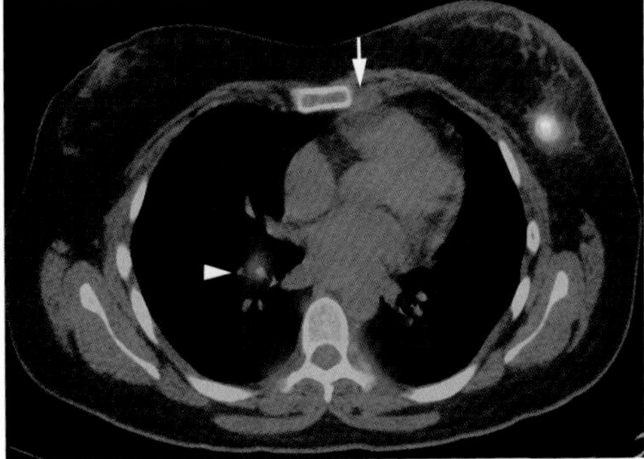

Fig. 16.3 Metastatic breast cancer. Axial positron emission tomography/computed tomography scan demonstrates a primary left breast cancer with internal mammary node (*arrow*) and lung (*arrowhead*) metastases. Paravertebral brown fat uptake is also noted.

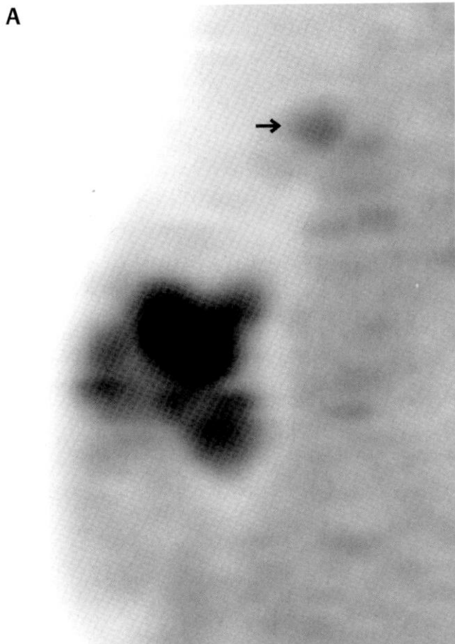

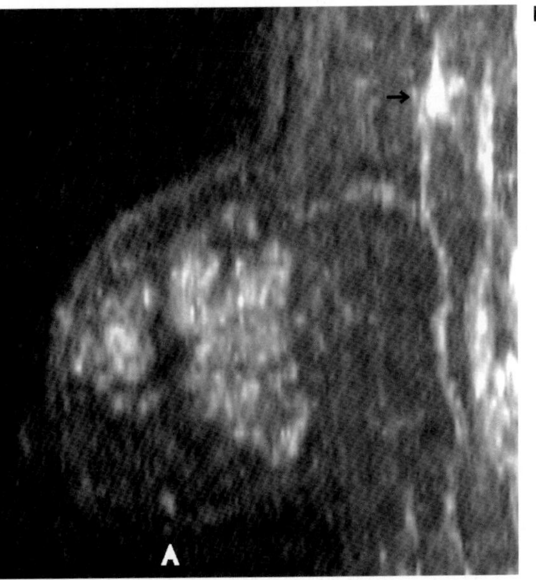

Fig. 16.2 Multifocal breast cancer on positron emission tomography (PET) and magnetic resonance imaging (MRI). **(A)** Sagittal PET scan demonstrates a multifocal breast cancer. Uptake in an axillary node (*arrow*) is also seen. **(B)** Sagittal contrast-enhanced MRI scan in the same patient demonstrates the enhancing lesions corresponding to the areas of increased uptake on PET. Enhancement in the axillary node that had fluorodeoxyglucose uptake (*arrow*) is also seen. However, the MRI identified a small tumor in the inferior breast (*arrowhead*) not seen on PET.

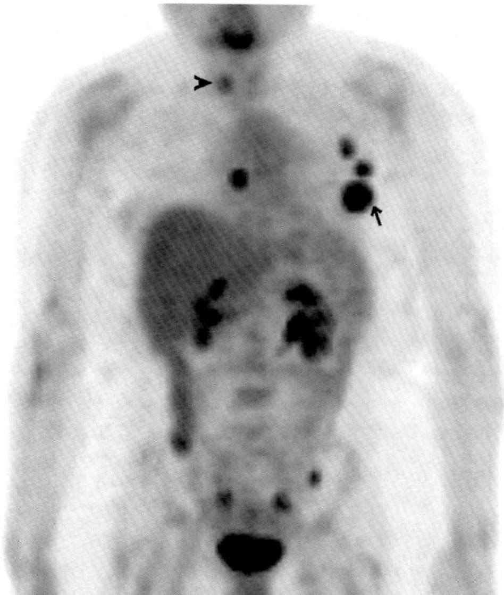

Fig. 16.4 Metastatic disease from breast cancer. Coronal positron emission tomography scan demontrates increased uptake in a left breast cancer (*arrow*). Metastases are present in the left axillary lymph nodes, the mediastinum, and the left iliac bone. Uptake is present in an incidentally noted right thyroid nodule (*arrowhead*).

b. FDG PET is superior to bone scan for detecting osteolytic metastases, but it is inferior for visualizing osteoblastic metastases. PET is more sensitive than bone scan for mixed lytic and sclerotic metastases and substantially more sensitive for invisible (not detected on CT) metastases.[26] Overall, FDG PET cannot replace a bone scan for detection of bone metastases in breast cancer due to relatively low sensitivity (56 to 74%)[26,27] for blastic metastasis. However, many blastic metastases missed on PET could potentially be detected on the CT portion of a PET/CT study.

Table 16.1 Sensitivity and Specificity of Positron Emission Tomography (PET) versus Computed Tomography (CT) in the Diagnosis of Internal Mammary and Mediastinal Nodal Metastases

	Sensitivity %	Specificity %
PET	85	90
CT	54	85

c. Patients with more aggressive tumors may benefit more from PET, given the high likelihood of osteolytic bone metastases with these malignancies.

Pearls

Axillary staging[22]

1. An SUV cutoff of > 2.3 has a sensitivity of 60% and specificity of 100% for axillary nodal metastasis.[28]
2. Multiple foci of axillary uptake are specific but insensitive.
3. PET is more sensitive for detecting lesions in patients with T2 or T3 disease (> 2 cm).
4. Sensitivity increases as the degree of FDG uptake in primary tumor increases and the axillary tumor load increases.[29]
5. Sensitivity increases with large primary tumors, but specificity is the highest for the small lesions.[30]
6. PET has little role in axillary staging for patients with palpable nodes, as these patients will undergo axillary lymph node dissection (ALND) after pathologic confirmation of nodal metastasis. PET has a high sensitivity and low specificity in this group of patients.[30]
7. A negative PET scan should not preclude ALND.
8. A positive PET scan is helpful, as the false-positive rate in the axilla in breast cancer is relatively low, and identification of multiple foci of uptake further increases specificity.
9. Similarly, identifying multiple foci of axillary uptake could potentially obviate ALND in patients receiving neoadjuvant chemotherapy.
10. Patients with a positive axillary PET scan could potentially forgo sentinel node biopsy and proceed to ALND.[31]

Pitfalls

Sternal metastases and internal mammary nodal metastases can be confused on PET due to their possible close proximity. These metastases should be easily differentiated with PET/CT.

◆ Recurrence of Breast Cancer[32,33]

Clinical Indication: B

PET is accurate in detecting both locoregional and distant tumor recurrence, and it is useful in both asymptomatic patients with elevated tumor markers and patients with clinical suspicion for recurrence and negative tumor markers. PET can be used to evaluate suspected recurrence or to identify multifocal or distant disease in locoregional recurrence. Between 16 and 30% of patients with a locoregional recurrence have distant metastases identified by PET.[34] PET is most helpful when aggressive local therapy is planned, as the detection of additional disease often alters management.

Accuracy and Comparison with Other Modalities

1. ***Overall accuracy.*** PET and PET/CT are more accurate than CT (**Table 16.2**).[35,36]
2. ***PET/CT.*** PET/CT has ~10% increase in diagnostic accuracy compared with PET alone.[37]

Pearls and Pitfalls

1. ***Locoregional recurrence***
   - ***a.*** PET is valuable in differentiating locoregional recurrence from postoperative changes. CT/MRI is often limited in this capacity.
     - Areas where PET is particularly useful are the chest wall (**Fig. 16.5**) and brachial plexus (**Fig. 16.6**) region.
     - However, anatomical imaging is often still necessary to depict relationships to adjacent structures (e.g., neurovascular invasion).
   - ***b.*** PET is useful in evaluating the axillary, supraclavicular, mediastinal, and internal mammary nodes.
     - However, if the patient has had an axillary lymph node dissection, sensitivity for axillary lymph node metastases is decreased.[38]
2. ***Distant recurrence***
   - ***a.*** PET detects more lymph node metastases than conventional imaging.
   - ***b.*** PET should be employed in conjunction with a bone scan to detect bone metastases.
3. ***Elevated tumor markers***
   - ***a.*** The sensitivity of PET is > 90% in detecting recurrence in patients with asymptomatically elevated tumor markers.
   - ***b.*** PET should be considered in patients with equivocal conventional imaging results and asymptomatically elevated tumor markers.
   - ***c.*** The likelihood of detecting recurrence is higher if cancer antigen (CA) 15–3 blood level is > 60 U/mL.[39]
   - ***d.*** False-negative results are noted in patients with invasive lobular cancer and elevated CA 15–3.

Table 16.2 Sensitivity and Specificity of Positron Emission Tomography (PET) and PET/CT versus Computed Tomography (CT) in the Detection of Tumor Recurrence of Breast Cancer

	Sensitivity %	Specificity %
PET/CT	85	76
CT	70	47

◆ Therapy Response and Prognosis for Breast Cancer[40,41]

Clinical Indication: B

1. PET is useful in evaluating response during induction therapy for advanced disease and during preoperative chemoradiotherapy (**Fig. 16.7**). In one study, PET altered therapy most frequently in patients with suspected or proven locoregional recurrence under consideration for aggressive therapy, as well as in patients with known metastases being evaluated for therapy response.[42]
2. ***Prognosis.*** SUV ≥ 3.0 in the primary breast tumor is usually associated with poor survival.

Accuracy and Comparison with Other Modalities

1. ***Early prediction.*** Change in FDG uptake after 1 to 3 courses of chemotherapy[43,44] predicts pathological response and survival in locally advanced and metastatic breast tumors.

A

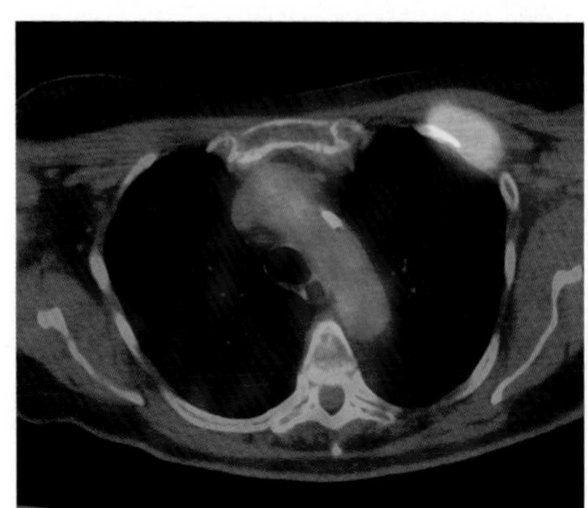

B

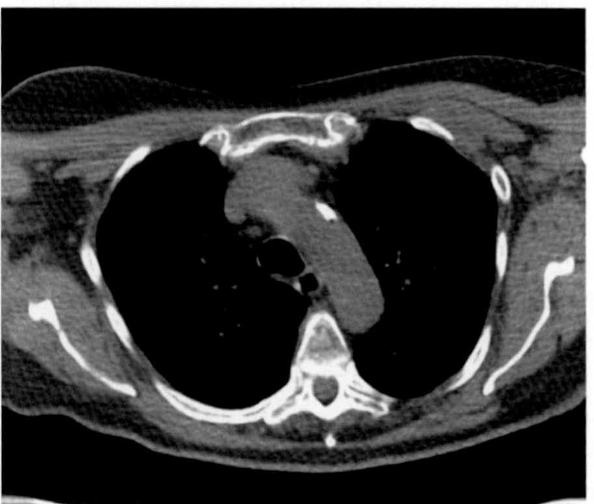

Fig. 16.5 Chest wall metastases. **(A)** Axial positron emission tomography scan in a patient with breast cancer demonstrates a left chest wall metastasis. **(B)** This is difficult to visualize on the corresponding computed tomography scan.

   a. An SUV decrease of > 55% below baseline may distinguish responders from nonresponders, with an accuracy of 88% after the first cycle of chemotherapy.[45]
   b. However, patients with decreased uptake may still have microscopic residual disease.
   c. An additional PET scan after further cycles of chemotherapy may be helpful in confirming initial results.
2. ***Posttherapy response.*** After therapy, PET is more accurate than conventional imaging for predicting outcome.[46]
   a. However, the sensitivity for lymph node disease after completion of therapy is low, and a negative PET scan has a very low predictive value for complete response.[41] This is particularly true for axillary nodal disease.
   b. PET may be particularly helpful in assessing treatment response in bone-dominant breast cancer.[47]

Pearls and Pitfalls

1. PET and MRI are complementary in monitoring response. PET predicts lack of response more accurately than MRI. When PET predicts response, MRI is able to define the extent of residual disease accurately.[48] However, PEM may potentially be superior to PET for monitoring therapy response.
2. PET is less effective in predicting response in tumors with low FDG uptake. In one study, PET could only predict response in tumors with a tumor-to-background ratio > 5.[49]
3. In patients treated with tamoxifen, responders can demonstrate increased activity

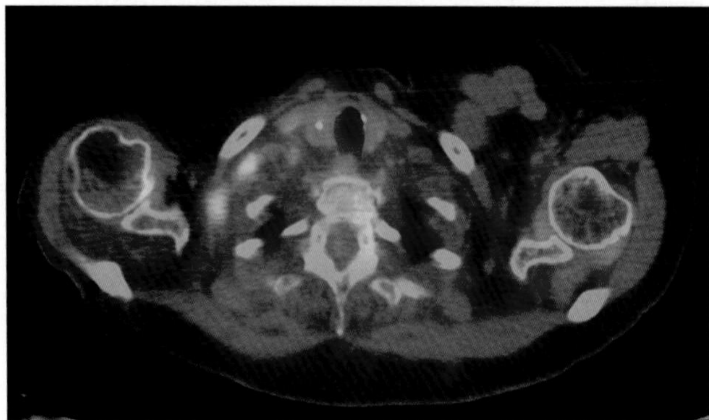

Fig. 16.6 Brachial plexus disease. Axial positron emission tomography/computed tomography scan in a patient with breast cancer demonstrates uptake secondary to recurrence in the right brachial plexus region.

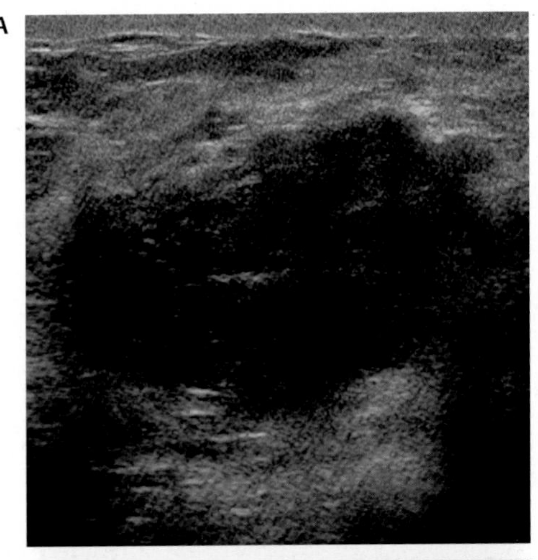

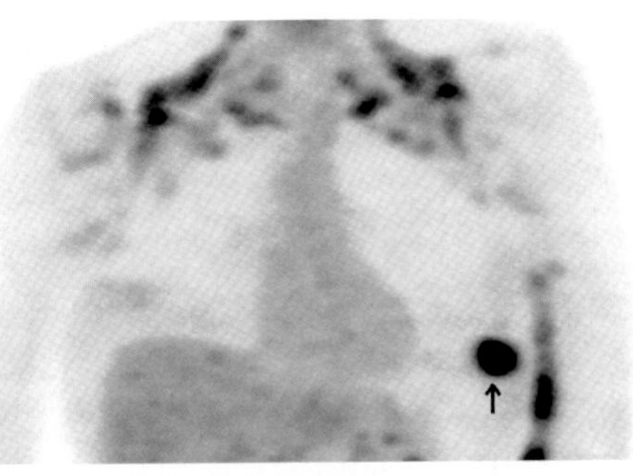

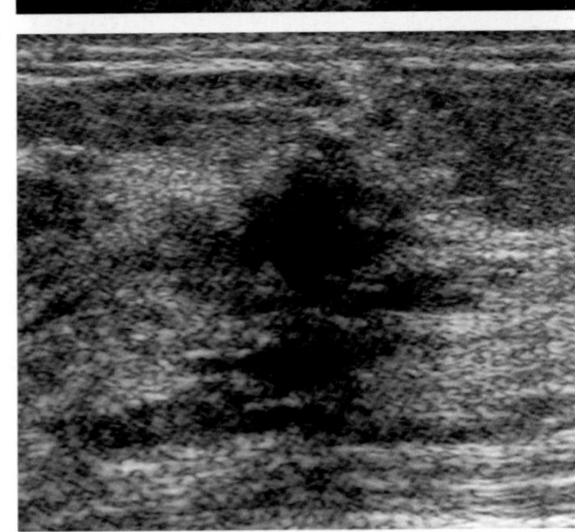

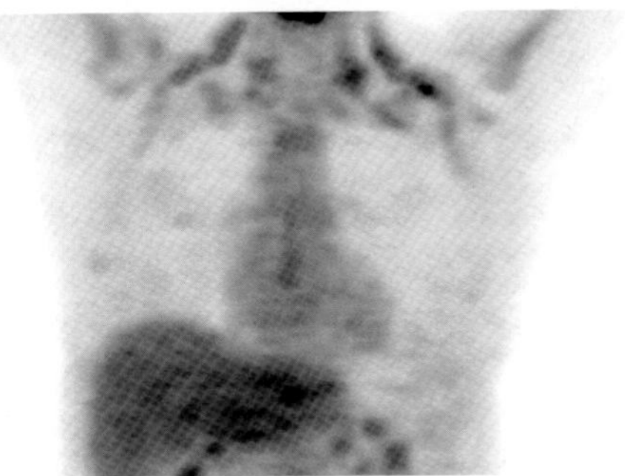

Fig. 16.7 Breast cancer: response to neoadjuvant therapy. **(A)** Ultrasound demonstrates a large left breast cancer, **(B)** with intense uptake (*arrow*) on a coronal positron emission tomography (PET) scan. After neoadjuvant therapy, the mass is much smaller on **(C)** ultrasound and not visualized on **(D)** PET.

initially from metabolic flare, likely due to inflammatory reaction. This is seen 7 to 10 days after therapy, but the time course is unknown and could be variable.[50]

References

1. Samson DJ, Flamm CR, Pisano ED, Aronson N. Should FDG PET be used to decide whether a patient with an abnormal mammogram or breast finding at physical examination should undergo biopsy? Acad Radiol 2002;9(7):773–783
2. Berg WA, Weinberg IN, Narayanan D, et al. High-resolution fluorodeoxyglucose positron emission tomography with compression ("positron emission mammography") is highly accurate in depicting primary breast cancer. Breast J 2006;12(4):309–323
3. Avril N, Rose CA, Schelling M, et al. Breast imaging with positron emission tomography and fluorine-18 fluorodeoxyglucose: use and limitations. J Clin Oncol 2000;18(20):3495–3502
4. Kumar R, Chauhan A, Zhuang H, et al. Clinicopathologic factors associated with false negative FDG-PET in primary breast cancer. Breast Cancer Res Treat 2006;98(3):267–274
5. Yutani K, Shiba E, Kusuoka H, et al. Comparison of FDG-PET with MIBI-SPECT in the detection of breast cancer and axillary lymph node metastasis. J Comput Assist Tomogr 2000;24(2):274–280
6. Heinisch M, Gallowitsch HJ, Mikosch P, et al. Comparison of FDG-PET and dynamic contrast-enhanced MRI in the evaluation of suggestive breast lesions. Breast 2003;12(1):17–22
7. Dehdashti F, Mortimer JE, Siegel BA, et al. Positron tomographic assessment of estrogen receptors in breast cancer: comparison with FDG-PET and in vitro receptor assays. J Nucl Med 1995;36(10):1766–1774
8. Dehdashti F, Siegel BA. Evaluation of breast and gynecologic cancers by positron emission tomography. Semin Roentgenol 2002;37(2):151–168
9. Levine EA, Freimanis RI, Perrier ND, et al. Positron emission mammography: initial clinical results. Ann Surg Oncol 2003;10(1):86–91
10. Korn RL, Yost AM, May CC, et al. Unexpected focal hypermetabolic activity in the breast: significance in patients undergoing ^{18}F-FDG PET/CT. AJR Am J Roentgenol 2006;187(1):81–85
11. Boerner AR, Weckesser M, Herzog H, et al. Optimal scan time for fluorine-18 fluorodeoxyglucose posi-

tron emission tomography in breast cancer. Eur J Nucl Med 1999;26(3):226–230

12. Mavi A, Urhan M, Yu JQ, et al. Dual time point ^{18}F-FDG PET imaging detects breast cancer with high sensitivity and correlates well with histologic subtypes. J Nucl Med 2006;47(9):1440–1446

13. Vranjesevic D, Schiepers C, Silverman DH, et al. Relationship between ^{18}F-FDG uptake and breast density in women with normal breast tissue. J Nucl Med 2003;44(8):1238–1242

14. Mavi A, Cermik TF, Urhan M, et al. The effects of estrogen, progesterone, and C-erbB-2 receptor states on ^{18}F-FDG uptake of primary breast cancer lesions. J Nucl Med 2007;48(8):1266–1272

15. Kumar R, Zhuang H, Schnall M, et al. FDG PET positive lymph nodes are highly predictive of metastasis in breast cancer. Nucl Med Commun 2006;27(3):231–236

16. Veronesi U, De Cicco C, Galimberti VE, et al. A comparative study on the value of FDG-PET and sentinel node biopsy to identify occult axillary metastases. Ann Oncol 2007;18(3):473–478

17. Quon A, Gambhir SS. FDG-PET and beyond: molecular breast cancer imaging. J Clin Oncol 2005;23(8):1664–1673

18. Wahl RL. Current status of PET in breast cancer imaging, staging, and therapy. Semin Roentgenol 2001; 36(3):250–260

19. Wahl RL. PET imaging in breast cancer. In: Valk PE, Bailey DL, Townsend DW, Maisey MN, eds. Positron Emission Tomography: Basic Science and Clinical Practice. London, UK: Springer-Verlag; 2003:595–610

20. Tran A, Pio BS, Khatibi B, et al. ^{18}F-FDG PET for staging breast cancer in patients with inner-quadrant versus outer-quadrant tumors: comparison with long-term clinical outcome. J Nucl Med 2005;46(9):1455–1459

21. Rieber A, Schirrmeister H, Gabelmann A, et al. Preoperative staging of invasive breast cancer with MR mammography and/or PET: boon or bunk? Br J Radiol 2002;75(898):789–798

22. Wahl RL, Siegel BA, Coleman RE, Gatsonis CG. Prospective multicenter study of axillary nodal staging by positron emission tomography in breast cancer: a report of the staging breast cancer with PET Study Group. J Clin Oncol 2004;22(2):277–285

23. Eubank WB, Mankoff DA, Takasugi J, et al. 18fluorodeoxyglucose positron emission tomography to detect mediastinal or internal mammary metastases in breast cancer. J Clin Oncol 2001;19(15):3516–3523

24. van der Hoeven JJ, Krak NC, Hoekstra OS, et al. 18F-2-fluoro-2-deoxy-D-glucose positron emission tomography in staging of locally advanced breast cancer. J Clin Oncol 2004;22(7):1253–1259

25. Ohta M, Tokuda Y, Suzuki Y, et al. Whole body PET for the evaluation of bony metastases in patients with breast cancer: comparison with 99mTc-MDP bone scintigraphy. Nucl Med Commun 2001;22(8):875–879

26. Nakai T, Okuyama C, Kubota T, et al. Pitfalls of FDG-PET for the diagnosis of osteoblastic bone metastases in patients with breast cancer. Eur J Nucl Med Mol Imaging 2005;32(11):1253–1258

27. Abe K, Sasaki M, Kuwabara Y, et al. Comparison of [18]FDG-PET with 99mTc-HMDP scintigraphy for the detection of bone metastases in patients with breast cancer. Ann Nucl Med 2005;19(7):573–579

28. Chung A, Liou D, Karlan S, et al. Preoperative FDG-PET for axillary metastases in patients with breast cancer. Arch Surg 2006;141(8):783–788

29. van der Hoeven JJ, Hoekstra OS, Comans EF, et al. Determinants of diagnostic performance of [F-18]fluorodeoxyglucose positron emission tomography for axillary staging in breast cancer. Ann Surg 2002;236(5):619–624

30. Greco M, Crippa F, Agresti R, et al. Axillary lymph node staging in breast cancer by 2-fluoro-2-deoxy-D-glucose-positron emission tomography: clinical evaluation and alternative management. J Natl Cancer Inst 2001;93(8):630–635

31. Lovrics PJ, Chen V, Coates G, et al. A prospective evaluation of positron emission tomography scanning, sentinel lymph node biopsy, and standard axillary dissection for axillary staging in patients with early stage breast cancer. Ann Surg Oncol 2004;11(9):846–853

32. Eubank WB, Mankoff DA, Vesselle HJ, et al. Detection of locoregional and distant recurrences in breast cancer patients by using FDG PET. Radiographics 2002;22(1):5–17

33. Siggelkow W, Rath W, Buell U, Zimny M. FDG PET and tumour markers in the diagnosis of recurrent and metastatic breast cancer. Eur J Nucl Med Mol Imaging 2004;31(Suppl 1):S118–S124

34. Tafra L. Positron emission tomography (PET) and mammography (PEM) for breast cancer: importance to surgeons. Ann Surg Oncol 2007;14(1):3–13

35. Gallowitsch HJ, Kresnik E, Gasser J, et al. F-18 fluorodeoxyglucose positron-emission tomography in the diagnosis of tumor recurrence and metastases in the follow-up of patients with breast carcinoma: a comparison to conventional imaging. Invest Radiol 2003;38(5):250–256

36. Radan L, Ben-Haim S, Bar-Shalom R, et al. The role of FDG-PET/CT in suspected recurrence of breast cancer. Cancer 2006;107(11):2545–2551

37. Czernin J, Allen-Auerbach M, Schelbert HR. Improvements in cancer staging with PET/CT: literature-based evidence as of September 2006. J Nucl Med 2007;48(Suppl 1):78S–88S

38. Hubner KF, Smith GT, Thie JA, et al. The potential of F-18-FDG PET in breast cancer: detection of primary lesions, axillary lymph node metastases, or distant metastases. Clin Positron Imaging 2000;3(5):197–205

39. Aide N, Huchet V, Switsers O, et al. Influence of CA 15–3 blood level and doubling time on diagnostic performances of ^{18}F-FDG PET in breast cancer patients with occult recurrence. Nucl Med Commun 2007;28(4):267–272

40. Kostakoglu L, Goldsmith SJ. 18F-FDG PET evaluation of the response to therapy for lymphoma and for breast, lung, and colorectal carcinoma. J Nucl Med 2003;44(2):224–239

41. Krak NC, Hoekstra OS, Lammertsma AA. Measuring response to chemotherapy in locally advanced breast cancer: methodological considerations. Eur J Nucl Med Mol Imaging 2004;31(Suppl 1):S103–S111

42. Eubank WB, Mankoff D, Bhattacharya M, et al. Impact of FDG PET on defining the extent of disease and on the treatment of patients with recurrent or metastatic breast cancer. AJR Am J Roentgenol 2004;183(2):479–486

43. Couturier O, Jerusalem G, N'Guyen JM, Hustinx R. Sequential positron emission tomography using [^{18}F]fluorodeoxyglucose for monitoring response to chemotherapy in metastatic breast cancer. Clin Cancer Res 2006;12(21):6437–6443

44. Rousseau C, Devillers A, Sagan C, et al. Monitoring of early response to neoadjuvant chemotherapy in stage II and III breast cancer by [^{18}F]fluorodeoxyglucose positron emission tomography. J Clin Oncol 2006;24(34):5366–5372
45. Schelling M, Avril N, Nahrig J, et al. Positron emission tomography using [(18)F]fluorodeoxyglucose for monitoring primary chemotherapy in breast cancer. J Clin Oncol 2000;18(8):1689–1695
46. Vranjesevic D, Filmont JE, Meta J, et al. Whole-body (18)F-FDG PET and conventional imaging for predicting outcome in previously treated breast cancer patients. J Nucl Med 2002;43(3):325–329
47. Stafford SE, Gralow JR, Schubert EK, et al. Use of serial FDG PET to measure the response of bone-dominant breast cancer to therapy. Acad Radiol 2002;9(8):913–921
48. Chen X, Moore MO, Lehman CD, et al. Combined use of MRI and PET to monitor response and assess residual disease for locally advanced breast cancer treated with neoadjuvant chemotherapy. Acad Radiol 2004;11(10):1115–1124
49. McDermott GM, Welch A, Staff RT, et al. Monitoring primary breast cancer throughout chemotherapy using FDG-PET. Breast Cancer Res Treat 2007;102(1):75–84
50. Mortimer JE, Dehdashti F, Siegel BA, et al. Metabolic flare: indicator of hormone responsiveness in advanced breast cancer. J Clin Oncol 2001;19(11):2797–2803

17

Gastric, Esophageal, and Gastrointestinal Stromal Tumors

Eugene C. Lin and Abass Alavi

◆ Gastric Cancer

Clinical Indication: C

1. Potential uses of positron emission tomography (PET) in patients with gastric cancer are staging, detecting recurrence, determining prognosis, and evaluating therapy response. However, the clinical role is not currently well defined.
2. ***Prognosis***
   a. Survival rate in patients with high fluorodeoxyglucose (FDG) uptake in the primary tumor is significantly lower than in patients with low FDG uptake.[1] However, because mucinous and signet ring cell carcinomas typically have low FDG uptake, low FDG uptake does not necessarily mean a better prognosis.
   b. A negative PET scan after surgical treatment with curative intent is associated with significantly longer survival.[2]
3. ***Therapy response (early prediction).*** PET performed 14 days after initiation of chemotherapy predicts response to therapy.[3]

Accuracy and Comparison with Other Modalities

1. ***PET.*** Sensitivity 71%, specificity 74 (advanced, metastatic, or recurrent gastric cancer)[4]
2. ***Primary tumor.*** PET does not have a role in the detection of primary gastric cancer. Reported detection rates range from 17 (for tumor < 3 cm) to 96%.[5,6]
   a. A greater degree of FDG uptake is associated with greater depth of invasion, size of tumor, and lymph node metastases.[1]
   b. Signet ring cell and mucinous carcinomas have low FDG uptake.[7,8]
3. ***Nodal metastases.*** The reported sensitivities of PET for detection of nodal metastases (**Fig. 17.1**) vary substantially (23 to 78%).[1,4]

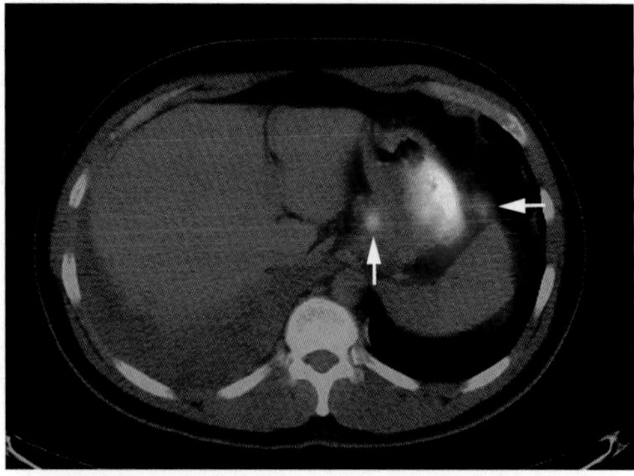

Fig. 17.1 Gastric cancer. Axial positron emission tomography/computed tomography scan demonstrates uptake in a primary gastric cancer with two local nodal metastases (*arrows*).

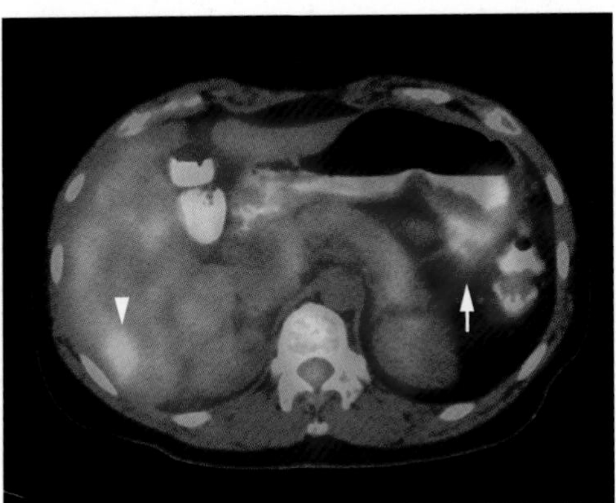

Fig. 17.2 Metastatic gastric cancer. Axial positron emission tomography/computed tomography scan demonstrates uptake in a gastric cancer (*arrow*) that has metastasized to the liver (*arrowhead*).

The primary value of PET in detecting nodal metastases is its specificity (78 to 96%).[4,5,9]

   a. The accuracy of PET and computed tomography (CT) for detecting local and distant nodal metastases is similar.[7]

   b. CT is more sensitive in the detection of lymph node metastases in N1 and N2 disease, but PET is more specific.

4. ***Body region***[7]
   a. Accuracy for the primary lesion and for metastases to the liver (**Fig. 17.2**), lymph nodes, and lung is high.
   b. Accuracy for pleural and peritoneal disease and bone marrow metastases is low. Accuracy for small perigastric nodes can also be low if obscured by uptake in the primary tumor.
5. ***Recurrent gastric cancer.*** Sensitivity 70%, specificity 69%[3]

Pearls and Pitfalls

1. ***Histology.*** Signet ring cell and mucinous carcinomas have low FDG uptake.
2. ***Morphology.*** The amount of uptake in the primary tumor may not correlate with histopathology.
   a. Poorly differentiated tumors may appear to have less uptake due to diffuse infiltration in the gastric wall.
   b. Well-differentiated tumors may appear to have more uptake due to mass formation.
3. ***Other pathologies.*** Increased gastric FDG uptake can be secondary to etiologies other than gastric cancer.
   a. Diffuse increased uptake can be secondary to gastritis or lymphoma.
   b. Focal increased uptake can be secondary to gastric ulcer or lymphoma.
4. ***Gastric remnant.*** Physiologic FDG uptake in a gastric remnant may be difficult to differentiate from recurrent tumor. Ingestion of water may be helpful. Gastric FDG uptake secondary to malignancy will persist after water ingestion.[10]

◆ Detection of Primary Esophageal Cancer

Clinical Indication: D

PET has a limited role in evaluating primary esophageal tumors.

1. ***Detection***
   a. PET can detect primary tumors with depth of invasion of T1b or greater, but in situ and T1a tumors are not detectable.[11]
   b. The overall detection rate of PET for primary esophageal carcinoma is 80%. However, this depends on the T stage. The detection rate for T3 and T4 tumors is close to 100%, but the detection rate for T1 tumors is 43%.[12]
   c. PET cannot determine T stage.
2. ***Level of uptake***[13]
   a. The amount of uptake correlates positively with depth of tumor invasion, presence of lymph node metastases, and lymphatic invasion.
   b. Adenocarcinomas and squamous cell carcinomas overall have similar degrees of FDG uptake, although adenocarcinomas at or near the gastroesophageal junction often have lower uptake secondary to diffuse growth pattern and/or mucinous histopathology.[14,15]
   c. The majority of the evidence suggests that the survival rate with high FDG uptake in the primary tumor is lower, but not all studies support this.[14]

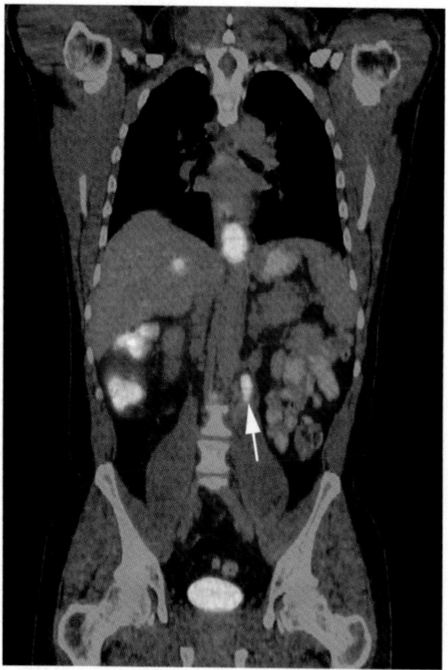

Fig. 17.3 Metastatic esophageal cancer. Coronal positron emission tomography/computed tomography scan in a patient with distal esophageal cancer demonstrates liver and retroperitoneal node (*arrow*) metastases.

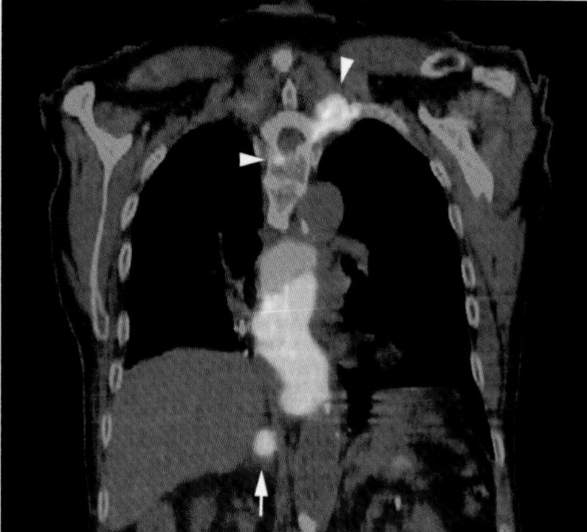

Fig. 17.4 Metastatic esophageal cancer. Coronal positron emission tomography/computed tomography scan in a patient with esophageal carcinoma demonstrates intense uptake in the primary tumor and adrenal (*arrow*) and bone (*arrowheads*) metastases.

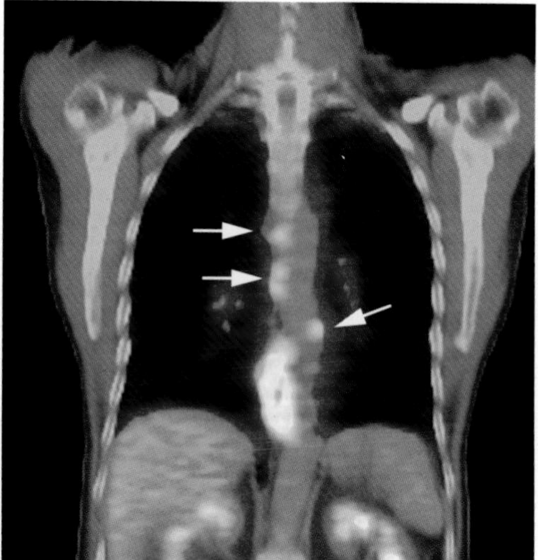

Fig. 17.5 Esophageal cancer with locoregional nodal metastases. Coronal positron emission tomography/computed tomography (PET/CT) scan demonstrates multiple metastases to locoregional paraesophageal nodes (*arrows*) from a distal esophageal cancer. Although endoscopic ultrasound would usually be more sensitive for detection of these nodes, a positive PET study is more specific for metastatic disease.

3. ***Pitfalls***
   a. Mild focal uptake at the gastroesophageal junction could be secondary to esophagitis, or it could be a normal variant (see **Fig. 6.27**, p. 56). An SUV > 4 at the gastroesophageal junction is concerning for malignancy.[16]
   b. Hiatal hernias can cause large areas of uptake at the gastroesophageal junction.
   c. Benign strictures can have substantial FDG uptake after dilatation.
   d. Esophageal leiomyomas can have FDG uptake.[17]

Table 17.1 Sensitivity and Specificity of Positron Emission Tomography (PET) versus Computed Tomography (CT) and Endoscopic Ultrasound (EUS) in the Detection of Locoregional Nodal Disease in Esophageal Cancer

	Sensitivity %	Specificity %
PET	22	91
CT/EUS	83	45

Table 17.2 Sensitivity and Specificity of Positron Emission Tomography (PET) versus Computed Tomography (CT) and Endoscopic Ultrasound (EUS) in the Detection of Distant Nodes in Esophageal Cancer

	Sensitivity %	Specificity %
PET	77	90
CT/EUS	46	69

e. *Respiratory misregistration.* Respiratory misregistration artifact on PET/CT (which is greatest in the peridiaphragmatic region) may result in erroneous SUV measurements of distal esophageal tumors.[18]

◆ Staging of Esophageal Cancer

Clinical Indication: A

1. The combination of PET and endoscopic ultrasound (EUS) can be the most cost-effective method of staging esophageal cancer.[19]
2. The primary value of PET is in[20]
   a. Detecting distant metastases (**Figs. 17.3** and **17.4**)
   b. Improving the specificity of lymph node staging
3. However, PET may not be routinely useful in patients with early-stage esophageal cancer (T ≤ 2), as these patients have a low incidence of lymphatic metastases.[21]
4. The overall incremental benefit in staging accuracy of PET compared with CT is 14%.[12] PET will identify unsuspected distant metastatic disease in 5 to 8%[22] of patients without evidence of metastases after conventional work-up.
5. ***Prognosis.*** Greater tumor length on PET and increased number of PET positive lymph nodes predict low survival rate.[23]

Table 17.3 Sensitivity and Specificity of Positron Emission Tomography (PET) versus Computed Tomography (CT) in the Detection of Distant Metastases (Nodal and Other) in Esophageal Cancer

	Sensitivity %	Specificity %
PET	69	93
CT	46	74

Table 17.4 Sensitivity and Specificity of Positron Emission Tomography (PET) versus Bone Scan in the Detection of Bone Metastases in Esophageal Cancer

	Sensitivity %	Specificity %
PET	92	94
Bone scan	77	84

Accuracy[24]

1. ***PET: locoregional.*** Sensitivity 51%, specificity 94%
2. ***PET: distant metastases.*** Sensitivity 67%, specificity 97%
3. ***PET/CT: locoregional.*** Sensitivity 94%, specificity 92%[25]
   • Significantly more accurate than PET alone

Comparison with Other Modalities

1. ***Locoregional nodes.***[21] PET is insensitive for locoregional disease and cannot replace CT/EUS for locoregional staging, but a positive result is more specific than CT/EUS for nodal disease (**Fig. 17.5**). A large percent-

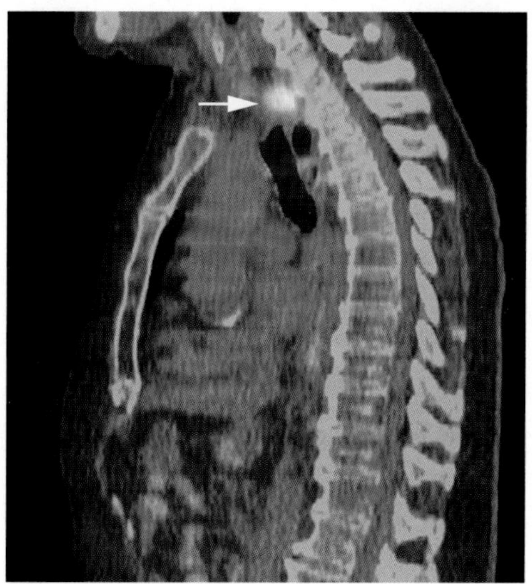

Fig. 17.6 Esophageal cancer recurrence. Sagittal positron emission tomography/computed tomography (PET/CT) in an esophageal cancer patient status postesophagectomy and gastric pull-through demonstrates recurrence at the proximal anastomosis (*arrow*).

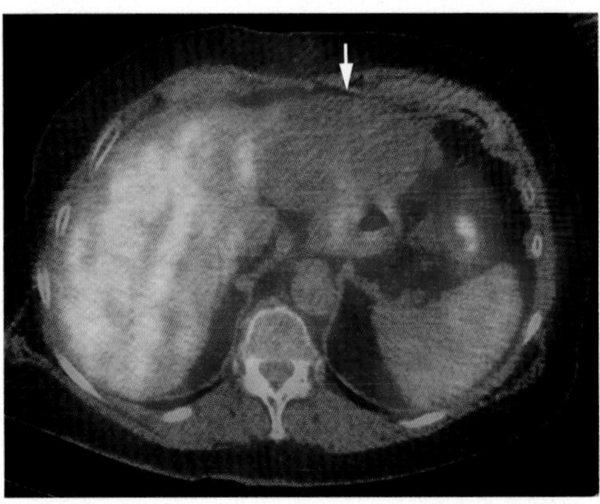

Fig. 17.7 Gastrointestinal stromal tumor (GIST): positron emission tomography (PET) negative. Axial PET/computed tomography demonstrates a large GIST tumor (*arrow*) without substantial fluorodeoxyglucose uptake.

age of false-negative nodal groups on PET are in the immediate vicinity of the primary tumor.[12] EUS will detect more pathologic periesophageal and celiac axis nodes than PET or CT (**Table 17.1**).[26]

2. ***Distant nodes*** **(Table 17.2)**[21]
3. ***Distant metastases (nodal and other)*** **(Table 17.3)**[27]
4. ***Bone metastases.*** PET may be more accurate than bone scintigraphy for bone metastases (**Table 17.4**).[28]
5. ***Anatomical region.*** PET has the highest accuracy in the neck, upper thoracic, and abdominal regions but low sensitivity in the mid- and lower thoracic regions.[13]

Pitfalls

1. Hilar uptake must be interpreted with caution, as it is the most common area of false-positive nodal uptake, particularly in smokers and in geographic locations where granulomatous disease is endemic.[25,29]
2. Small intracapsular locoregional metastases have a high false-negative rate.[27]
3. Uptake in the primary tumor may obscure the abnormal nodes adjacent to it.
4. ***Gastrohepatic versus celiac nodes.*** Resectable gastrohepatic lymph nodes should be distinguished from nonregional celiac

A

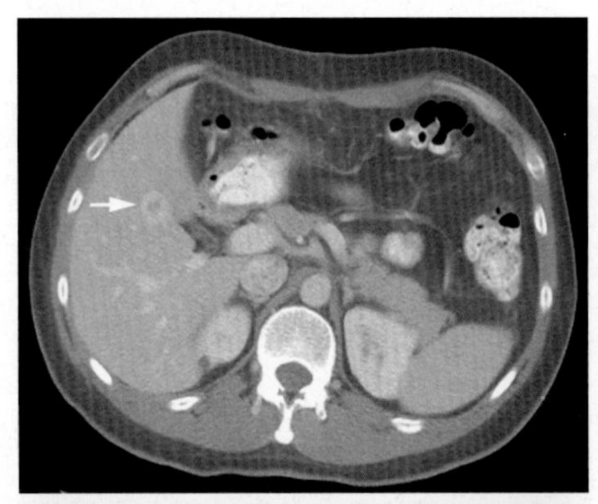

B

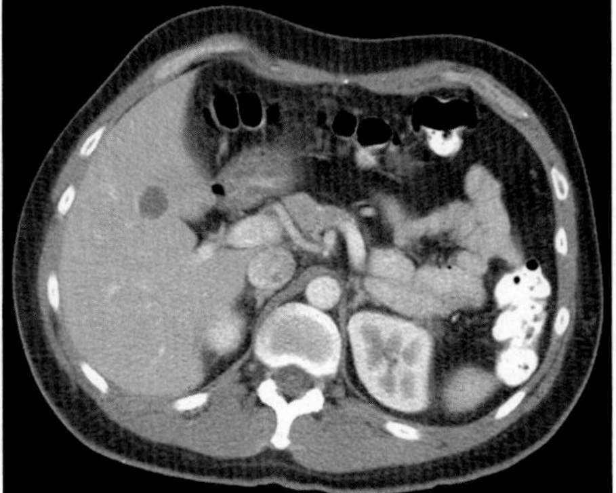

C

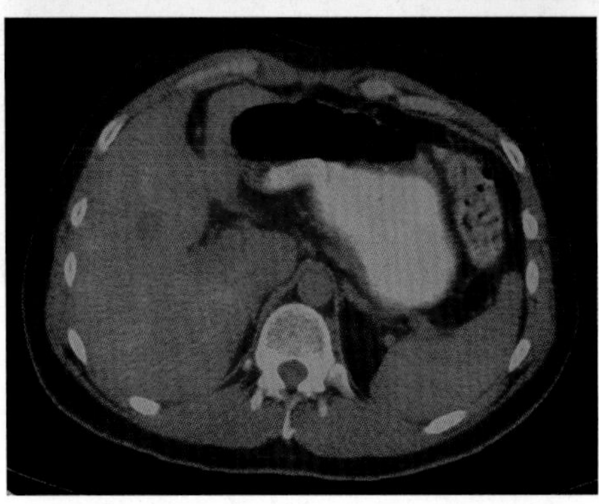

Fig. 17.8 Gastrointestinal stromal tumor (GIST): therapy response. **(A)** Axial computed tomography (CT) demonstrates an enhancing liver metastasis (*arrow*) from a GIST. **(B)** After imatinib mesylate treatment, the metastases are now completely hypodense and appear slightly larger. GIST metastases are difficult to follow by CT, as they change primarily in density rather than size after treatment, and may actually increase in size early after treatment. **(C)** Positron emission tomography scan done after therapy demonstrates lack of uptake in the liver metastasis.

nodes, which are typically nonresectable. This may be difficult, as lower gastrohepatic nodes may appear close to the celiac axis.[18]

5. ***Synchronous neoplasms.*** PET will detect unexpected synchronous primary neoplasms in 5.5% of patients with esophageal cancer.[30] Sites of pathologic uptake should be confirmed by other methods before being ascribed to metastases.

◆ Recurrence of Esophageal Cancer

Clinical Indication: C

PET is accurate for detection of recurrent esophageal cancer (**Fig. 17.6**), but it is not clearly superior to conventional imaging. In patients with recurrence, SUV and disease status on PET/CT predict survival.[31]

Accuracy

- **PET.** Sensitivity 94%, specificity 82%[32]

Pitfalls

PET is not accurate for the diagnosis of perianastomotic recurrence, as inflammation often causes false-positive results. At local sites, the specificity of PET/CT is only 50%, although sensitivity is high.[31]

◆ Therapy Response of Esophageal Cancer[33]

Clinical Indication: B

PET is useful in the evaluation of response to neoadjuvant chemoradiotherapy. It can be used for both early and late prediction of outcome.

1. PET can be helpful for prognosis after both chemotherapy and chemoradiotherapy, including after definitive chemoradiotherapy.[34] Change in FDG uptake after therapy correlates with histopathological response and survival. This can be assessed only 2 weeks after therapy. Relative changes in FDG uptake are a better predictor of treatment outcome than absolute SUV.[35] There are conflicting data on whether pretherapeutic SUV is associated with response and prognosis.[36]
2. However, PET cannot differentiate between minimal residual disease and complete response (local recurrence still occurs after a significant decline in FDG activity). In one study,[34] two thirds of patients with a post-chemoradiotherapy SUV < 2.5 had tumor in the surgical specimen, and two thirds of patients had positive lymph nodes at surgery not detected by PET. Therefore, esophagectomy should remain an option even if PET is normal after therapy.
3. ***Interval metastases.*** There is conflicting evidence as to the effectiveness of PET in detecting interval metastases (which may preclude surgical resection) after neoadjuvant therapy for esophageal carcinoma. In one study, unexpected interval metastases were detected in 8% of patients,[37] but in another study PET was not sensitive for interval metastases.[38]

Accuracy and Comparison with Other Modalities

1. ***Assessment of response to neoadjuvant therapy.*** The accuracy rates of PET and EUS are similar, but EUS is sometimes not feasible after chemotherapy and radiation. The accuracy of CT is significantly lower than PET and EUS.[39]
2. A wide range of cutoff values (30 to 80%) for SUV reduction has been reported as discriminating between responders and nonresponders.[40]
3. ***Early prediction.*** A 35% decrease in FDG uptake (14 days after start of chemotherapy) predicts response with 93% sensitivity and 95% specificity.[41]
4. ***Late prediction***
   a. A 52% decrease in FDG uptake (3 weeks after completion of treatment) detects response with 100% sensitivity and 55% specificity.[42]
   b. A posttherapy SUV ≥ 4 is the best predictor of poor outcome and short survival,[43] superior to EUS mass size or CT wall thickness.

Pitfalls

1. ***Esophagitis.*** After neoadjuvant radiotherapy radiation, esophagitis can interfere with optimal assessment of response to treatment.[44] Unlike the lung, the esophagus may react early to radiation, and elevations in activity can be seen during the course of radiotherapy.[45] The delay in imaging after therapy necessary to avoid uptake from radiation esophagitis is not well established. Delays of 2 to 12 weeks after radiotherapy have been proposed.[46] Another possible approach is to image very early (< 2 weeks) after radiotherapy, before esophagitis has had time to develop.[18]
2. ***Esophageal ulceration.*** Chemoradiotherapy-induced esophageal ulceration can result in false-positive findings of residual malignancy. Endoscopy is very helpful in increasing accuracy in these cases. If ulceration is absent at endoscopy, an SUV ≥ 4 is highly predictive of residual disease.[47]

◆ Gastrointestinal Stromal Tumors

Clinical Indication: A

CT is the standard imaging modality for primary gastrointestinal stromal tumor (GIST). PET may be helpful in imaging in primary GIST when early detection of response to imatinib treatment is needed (e.g., for consideration of surgery after imatinib treatment for rectal tumors). PET may also be helpful in evaluating equivocal metastatic lesions.[48] In addition, PET may be helpful in predicting the malignant potential of GIST prior to surgery.[49] However, PET is less sensitive than CT prior to treatment. Approximately 20% of lesions detected by CT have no FDG uptake (**Fig. 17.7**).[50] In particular, PET is less sensitive for liver metastases.[51]

The primary value of PET in GIST is for evaluation of response to imatinib mesylate treatment (**Fig. 17.8**). Change in tumor size (particularly of hepatic metastases) on CT is often not apparent until late in therapy. Instead, tumors will decrease in attenuation on CT studies.[48] There is a rapid reduction in FDG uptake after imatinib therapy. PET may be more useful than CT for predicting response to therapy, but CT detects more lesions.[52] Reduction in SUV 1 week after treatment predicts progression-free survival.[53]

Pearls

1. PET criteria to define a good response include a decrease in SUV < 70% and a decrease to an absolute SUV < 2.5.[54]
2. Tumors may become larger within the first 6 months of treatment (possibly secondary to hemorrhage, edema, or myxoid degeneration) despite regression clinically and on PET.
3. Lesions without FDG uptake (~20%) could be followed by CT with evaluation of change in attenuation.
4. Recurrence after partial response to imatinib appears as a focal area of FDG uptake within a larger mass. This correlates with an enhancing nodule on CT.[55]

References

1. Mochiki E, Kuwano H, Katoh H, et al. Evaluation of ^{18}F-2-deoxy-2-fluoro-D-glucose positron emission tomography for gastric cancer. World J Surg 2004;28(3):247–253
2. De Potter T, Flamen P, Van CE, et al. Whole-body PET with FDG for the diagnosis of recurrent gastric cancer. Eur J Nucl Med Mol Imaging 2002;29(4):525–529
3. Ott K, Fink U, Becker K, et al. Prediction of response to preoperative chemotherapy in gastric carcinoma by metabolic imaging: results of a prospective trial. J Clin Oncol 2003;21(24):4604–4610
4. Yoshioka T, Yamaguchi K, Kubota K, et al. Evaluation of ^{18}F-FDG PET in patients with a metastatic, or recurrent gastric cancer. J Nucl Med 2003;44(5):690–699
5. Kim SK, Kang KW, Lee JS, et al. Assessment of lymph node metastases using ^{18}F-FDG PET in patients with advanced gastric cancer. Eur J Nucl Med Mol Imaging 2006;33(2):148–155
6. Mukai K, Ishida Y, Okajima K, et al. Usefulness of preoperative FDG-PET for detection of gastric cancer. Gastric Cancer 2006;9(3):192–196
7. Chen J, Cheong JH, Yun MJ, et al. Improvement in preoperative staging of gastric adenocarcinoma with positron emission tomography. Cancer 2005;103(11):2383–2390
8. Stahl A, Ott K, Weber WA, et al. FDG PET imaging of locally advanced gastric carcinomas: correlation with endoscopic and histopathological findings. Eur J Nucl Med Mol Imaging 2003;30(2):288–295
9. Yun M, Lim JS, Noh SH, et al. Lymph node staging of gastric cancer using (18)F-FDG PET: a comparison study with CT. J Nucl Med 2005;46(10):1582–1588
10. Yun M, Choi HS, Yoo E, et al. The role of gastric distention in differentiating recurrent tumor from physi-

ologic uptake in the remnant stomach on ^{18}F-FDG PET. J Nucl Med 2005;46(6):953–957

11. Himeno S, Yasuda S, Shimada H, et al. Evaluation of esophageal cancer by positron emission tomography. Jpn J Clin Oncol 2002;32(9):340–346

12. Kato H, Miyazaki T, Nakajima M, et al. The incremental effect of positron emission tomography on diagnostic accuracy in the initial staging of esophageal carcinoma. Cancer 2005;103(1):148–156

13. Kato H, Kuwano H, Nakajima M, et al. Comparison between positron emission tomography and computed tomography in the use of the assessment of esophageal carcinoma. Cancer 2002;94(4):921–928

14. Dam HQ, Manzone TM, Sagar VV. Evolving role of (18)F-fluorodeoxyglucose positron emission tomography in the management of esophageal carcinoma. Surg Oncol Clin N Am 2006;15(4):733–749

15. Esteves FP, Schuster DM, Halkar RK. Gastrointestinal tract malignancies and positron emission tomography: an overview. Semin Nucl Med 2006;36(2):169–181

16. Salaun PY, Grewal RK, Dodamane I, et al. An analysis of the ^{18}F-FDG uptake pattern in the stomach. J Nucl Med 2005;46(1):48–51

17. Meirelles GS, Ravizzini G, Yeung HW, Akhurst T. Esophageal leiomyoma: a rare cause of false-positive FDG scans. Clin Nucl Med 2006;31(6):342–344

18. Bruzzi JF, Munden RF, Truong MT, et al. PET/CT of esophageal cancer: its role in clinical management. Radiographics 2007;27(6):1635–1652

19. Wallace MB, Nietert PJ, Earle C, et al. An analysis of multiple staging management strategies for carcinoma of the esophagus: computed tomography, endoscopic ultrasound, positron emission tomography, and thoracoscopy/laparoscopy. Ann Thorac Surg 2002;74(4):1026–1032

20. Flamen P, Lerut A, Van CE, et al. Utility of positron emission tomography for the staging of patients with potentially operable esophageal carcinoma. J Clin Oncol 2000;18(18):3202–3210

21. Lerut T, Flamen P, Ectors N, et al. Histopathologic validation of lymph node staging with FDG-PET scan in cancer of the esophagus and gastroesophageal junction: a prospective study based on primary surgery with extensive lymphadenectomy. Ann Surg 2000;232(6):743–752

22. Meyers BF, Downey RJ, Decker PA, et al. The utility of positron emission tomography in staging of potentially operable carcinoma of the thoracic esophagus: results of the American College of Surgeons Oncology Group Z0060 trial. J Thorac Cardiovasc Surg 2007;133(3):738–745

23. Choi JY, Jang HJ, Shim YM, et al. 18F-FDG PET in patients with esophageal squamous cell carcinoma undergoing curative surgery: prognostic implications. J Nucl Med 2004;45(11):1843–1850

24. van Westreenen HL, Westerterp M, Bossuyt PM, et al. Systematic review of the staging performance of ^{18}F-fluorodeoxyglucose positron emission tomography in esophageal cancer. J Clin Oncol 2004;22(18):3805–3812

25. Yuan S, Yu Y, Chao KS, et al. Additional value of PET/CT over PET in assessment of locoregional lymph nodes in thoracic esophageal squamous cell cancer. J Nucl Med 2006;47(8):1255–1259

26. Konski A, Doss M, Milestone B, et al. The integration of 18-fluoro-deoxy-glucose positron emission tomography and endoscopic ultrasound in the treatment-planning process for esophageal carcinoma. Int J Radiat Oncol Biol Phys 2005;61(4):1123–1128

27. Luketich JD, Friedman DM, Weigel TL, et al. Evaluation of distant metastases in esophageal cancer: 100 consecutive positron emission tomography scans. Ann Thorac Surg 1999;68(4):1133–1136

28. Kato H, Miyazaki T, Nakajima M, et al. Comparison between whole-body positron emission tomography and bone scintigraphy in evaluating bony metastases of esophageal carcinomas. Anticancer Res 2005;25(6C):4439–4444

29. Yoon YC, Lee KS, Shim YM, et al. Metastasis to regional lymph nodes in patients with esophageal squamous cell carcinoma: CT versus FDG PET for presurgical detection prospective study. Radiology 2003;227(3):764–770

30. van Westreenen HL, Westerterp M, Jager PL, et al. Synchronous primary neoplasms detected on ^{18}F-FDG PET in staging of patients with esophageal cancer. J Nucl Med 2005;46(8):1321–1325

31. Guo H, Zhu H, Xi Y, et al. Diagnostic and prognostic value of ^{18}F-FDG PET/CT for patients with suspected recurrence from squamous cell carcinoma of the esophagus. J Nucl Med 2007;48(8):1251–1258

32. Flamen P, Lerut A, Van Cutsem E, et al. The utility of positron emission tomography for the diagnosis and staging of recurrent esophageal cancer. J Thorac Cardiovasc Surg 2000;120(6):1085–1092

33. Kostakoglu L, Goldsmith SJ. PET in the assessment of therapy response in patients with carcinoma of the head and neck and of the esophagus. J Nucl Med 2004;45(1):56–68

34. Konski AA, Cheng JD, Goldberg M, et al. Correlation of molecular response as measured by 18-FDG positron emission tomography with outcome after chemoradiotherapy in patients with esophageal carcinoma. Int J Radiat Oncol Biol Phys 2007;69(2):358–363

35. Wieder HA, Ott K, Lordick F, et al. Prediction of tumor response by FDG-PET: comparison of the accuracy of single and sequential studies in patients with adenocarcinomas of the esophagogastric junction. Eur J Nucl Med Mol Imaging 2007;34(12):1925–1932

36. Ott K, Weber W, Siewert JR. The importance of PET in the diagnosis and response evaluation of esophageal cancer. Dis Esophagus 2006;19(6):433–442

37. Bruzzi JF, Swisher SG, Truong MT, et al. Detection of interval distant metastases: clinical utility of integrated CT-PET imaging in patients with esophageal carcinoma after neoadjuvant therapy. Cancer 2007;109(1):125–134

38. Downey RJ, Akhurst T, Ilson D, et al. Whole body 18FDG-PET and the response of esophageal cancer to induction therapy: results of a prospective trial. J Clin Oncol 2003;21(3):428–432

39. Westerterp M, van Westreenen HL, Reitsma JB, et al. Esophageal cancer: CT, endoscopic US, and FDG PET for assessment of response to neoadjuvant therapy–systematic review. Radiology 2005;236(3):841–851

40. Sloof GW. Response monitoring of neoadjuvant therapy using CT, EUS, and FDG-PET. Best Pract Res Clin Gastroenterol 2006;20(5):941–957

41. Weber WA, Ott K, Becker K, et al. Prediction of response to preoperative chemotherapy in adenocarcinomas of the esophagogastric junction by metabolic imaging. J Clin Oncol 2001;19(12):3058–3065

42. Brucher BL, Weber W, Bauer M, et al. Neoadjuvant therapy of esophageal squamous cell carcinoma: response evaluation by positron emission tomography. Ann Surg 2001;233(3):300–309

43. Swisher SG, Maish M, Erasmus JJ, et al. Utility of PET, CT, and EUS to identify pathologic responders in esophageal cancer. Ann Thorac Surg 2004;78(4):1152–1160
44. Gillham CM, Lucey JA, Keogan M, et al. (18)FDG uptake during induction chemoradiation for oesophageal cancer fails to predict histomorphological tumour response. Br J Cancer 2006;95(9):1174–1179
45. Kong FM, Frey KA, Quint LE, et al. A pilot study of [^{18}F]fluorodeoxyglucose positron emission tomography scans during and after radiation-based therapy in patients with non small-cell lung cancer. J Clin Oncol 2007;25(21):3116–3123
46. Wieder HA, Brucher BL, Zimmermann F, et al. Time course of tumor metabolic activity during chemoradiotherapy of esophageal squamous cell carcinoma and response to treatment. J Clin Oncol 2004;22(5):900–908
47. Erasmus JJ, Munden RF, Truong MT, et al. Preoperative chemo-radiation-induced ulceration in patients with esophageal cancer: a confounding factor in tumor response assessment in integrated computed tomographic-positron emission tomographic imaging. J Thorac Oncol 2006;1(5):478–486
48. Blay JY, Bonvalot S, Casali P, et al. Consensus meeting for the management of gastrointestinal stromal tumors. Report of the GIST Consensus Conference of 20–21 March 2004, under the auspices of ESMO. Ann Oncol 2005;16(4):566–578
49. Kamiyama Y, Aihara R, Nakabayashi T, et al. ^{18}F-fluorodeoxyglucose positron emission tomography: useful technique for predicting malignant potential of gastrointestinal stromal tumors. World J Surg 2005;29(11):1429–1435
50. Choi H, Charnsangavej C, de Castro Faria S, et al. CT evaluation of the response of gastrointestinal stromal tumors after imatinib mesylate treatment: a quantitative analysis correlated with FDG PET findings. AJR Am J Roentgenol 2004;183(6):1619–1628
51. Goldstein D, Tan BS, Rossleigh M, Haindl W, Walker B, Dixon J. Gastrointestinal stromal tumours: correlation of F-FDG gamma camera-based coincidence positron emission tomography with CT for the assessment of treatment response—an AGITG study. Oncology 2005;69(4):326–332
52. Goerres GW, Stupp R, Barghouth G, et al. The value of PET, CT and in-line PET/CT in patients with gastrointestinal stromal tumours: long-term outcome of treatment with imatinib mesylate. Eur J Nucl Med Mol Imaging 2005;32(2):153–162
53. Schuetze SM. Utility of positron emission tomography in sarcomas. Curr Opin Oncol 2006;18(4):369–373
54. Choi H, Charnsangavej C, Faria SC, et al. Correlation of computed tomography and positron emission tomography in patients with metastatic gastrointestinal stromal tumor treated at a single institution with imatinib mesylate: proposal of new computed tomography response criteria. J Clin Oncol 2007; 25(13):1753–1759
55. Shankar S, vanSonnenberg E, Desai J, Dipiro PJ, Van Den Abbeele A, Demetri GD. Gastrointestinal stromal tumor: new nodule-within-a-mass pattern of recurrence after partial response to imatinib mesylate. Radiology 2005;235(3):892–898

18

Lymphoma

Eugene C. Lin and Abass Alavi

◆ Staging

Clinical Indication: A1

Positron emission tomography (PET) is a standard modality for staging both Hodgkin disease (HD) and non-Hodgkin lymphoma (NHL) (**Figs. 18.1, 18.2,** and **18.3**).

1. ***Hodgkin disease.*** In HD, PET can be of value in any stage, but it is most useful in stage I and II disease, where a change in stage will alter disease management. Overall, PET changes management in a median of 14% of patients.[2]
2. ***NHL.*** In NHL, PET can be of value in any stage, but it is most useful in staging aggressive disease. It is very helpful as a baseline test if PET is to be used to monitor response to treatment.
   - ***a.*** *Stage.* PET may be more useful in stage I disease (some centers use the same therapy for all stages of aggressive NHL except stage I).
   - ***b.*** *Histology.* PET may have a role in the staging of low-grade follicular NHL. PET is of questionable value in other subtypes of low-grade NHL, such as small lymphocytic and mucosa-associated lymphoid-type (MALT) lymphoma.[3] PET may be of potential value in mantle cell lymphoma.

Accuracy

1. ***PET.*** Sensitivity 90%, specificity 91%[4]
   - ***a.*** *HD.* Sensitivity 93%, specificity 88%
   - ***b.*** *NHL.* Sensitivity 87%, specificity 94%

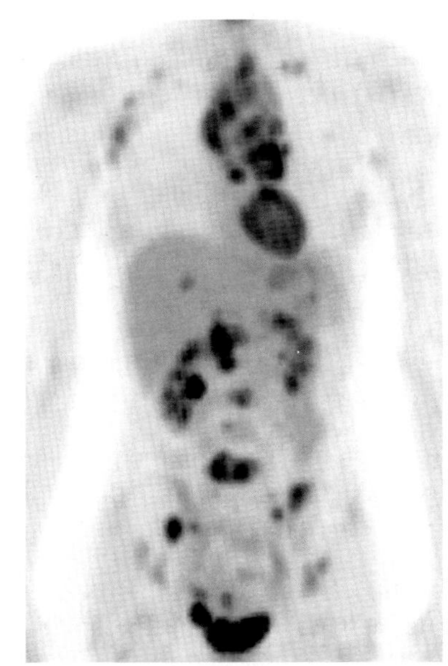

Fig. 18.1 Extensive lymphoma. Coronal positron emission tomography scan in a patient with non-Hodgkin lymphoma demonstrates uptake in mediastinal, supraclavicular, axillary, and retroperitoneal nodes, liver, and bone marrow (pelvis and lumbar spine).

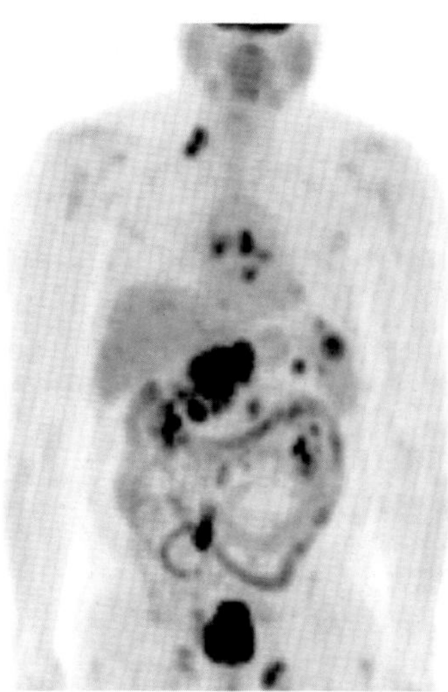

Fig. 18.2 Extensive lymphoma. Coronal positron emission tomography scan in a patient with non-Hodgkin lymphoma demonstrates uptake in mediastinal, supraclavicular, abdominal, pelvic, and groin nodes and the spleen.

2. ***PET/computed tomography (CT).*** Improved staging accuracy by 9%[5]
3. ***Histological subtype.*** PET has variable sensitivity depending on the histological subtype of lymphoma.[6] In general, PET has high sensitivity in the three major classes of this malignancy in clinical practice—diffuse large B cell and follicular lymphomas and Hodgkin disease.
   a. *Hodgkin disease.* The different histological subtypes of Hodgkin disease all have substantial FDG uptake, although the difference in degree of uptake is significant among the subtypes. Mixed cellularity has the most uptake, followed by nodular sclerosis and nodular lymphocytic predominant type.[7] However, the fluorodeoxyglucose (FDG) uptake in the least FDG-avid subtype (lymphocytic predominance) is very high.
   b. *Non-Hodgkin lymphoma.* The sensitivity of PET in low-grade NHL depends on histology. Sensitivity is excellent in follicular lymphoma, moderate in marginal zone lymphoma, and poor in small cell lymphocytic lymphoma.[8] The higher grade lymphomas are in general more FDG avid, but sensitivity in peripheral T cell lymphoma is moderate.[6] Patients with NHL and standardized uptake value (SUV) > 10 have a high likelihood of aggressive disease.[9]
   - *Follicular lymphoma.* PET is accurate in both indolent and aggressive nodal follicular lymphoma.[10] Low-grade follicular lymphomas of the gastrointestinal tract usually have substantial FDG uptake,[11] but the degree of uptake is still less than that in high-grade NHL. However, sensitivity for bone marrow involvement in follicular lymphoma is limited.[12]
   - *Marginal zone lymphoma (MZL).* PET has good sensitivity for nodal MZL but has poor sensitivity for extranodal MZL (in particular, splenic MZL).[13,14]
   - *Mucosa-associated lymphoid tissue lymphoma.* PET has variable sensitivity for MALT lymphoma. The sensitivity in patients with advanced disease is much higher than that in early-stage disease.[15] The sensitivity of PET in typical MALT lymphomas is low, but MALT lymphomas with plasmacytic features usually have substantial FDG uptake.[16] MALT lymphomas of the gastrointestinal tract typically have low FDG uptake.[11]
   - *Peripheral T cell lymphoma.* PET has high sensitivity at nodal and noncutaneous nodal sites but poor sensitivity at cutaneous sites[17] and for bone marrow involvement.[18] FDG uptake in cutaneous T cell lymphoma is much more likely in stage IV disease.[2]
4. ***Anatomical region.*** PET is more sensitive in the thorax than the abdomen/pelvis.[19]
5. ***Bone marrow involvement.*** PET is able to detect sites of bone marrow involvement not sampled with iliac crest biopsy. Initial studies suggested that PET is more sensitive and specific than bone scintigraphy or CT for bone marrow involvement. However, later studies suggest a lower sensitivity for bone marrow involvement, particularly in low-grade NHL.[6] In particular, although PET has good sensitivity in nodal follicular lymphoma,[10] the sensitivity for bone marrow involvement is limited.[12] The overall sensitivity and specificity of PET for bone marrow involvement (compared with bone marrow biopsy) are 51% and 95%, respectively.[20] The sensitivity is higher in HD and high-grade NHL.
6. ***Splenic disease.*** PET is 97% accurate for the diagnosis of splenic involvement in HD.

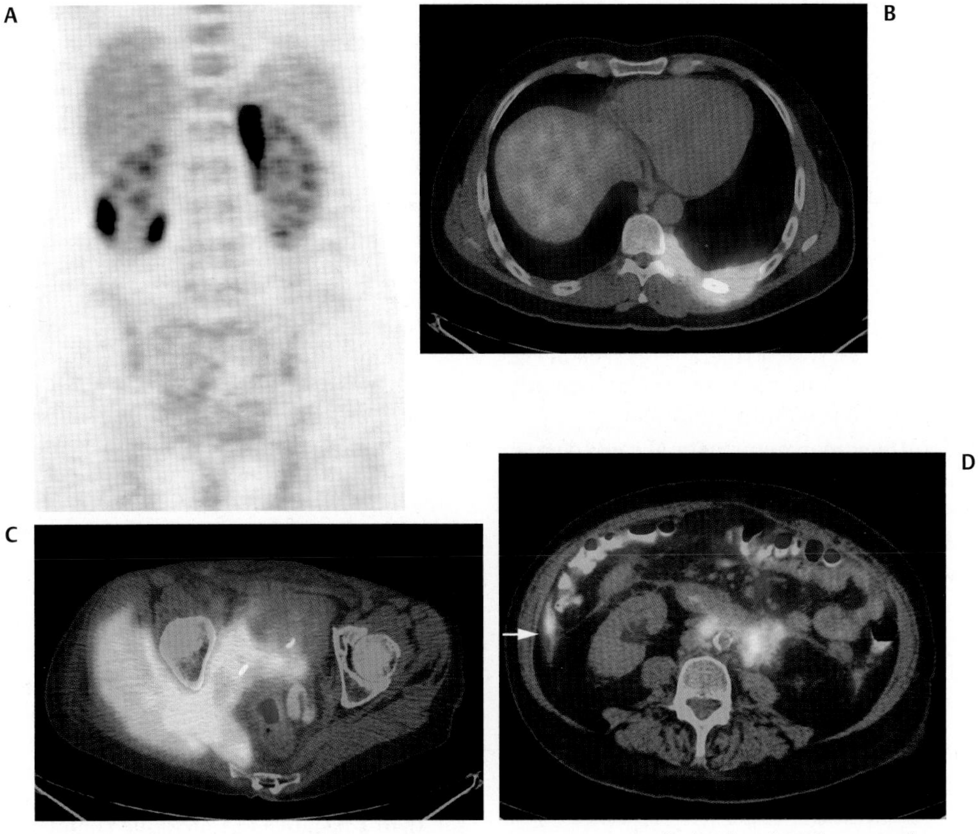

Fig. 18.3 Lymphoma: spectrum of disease. Positron emission tomography (PET) and PET/computed tomography scans in different patients with non-Hodgkin lymphoma demonstrate disease involving the **(A)** perirenal space, **(B)** pleura, **(C)** muscle, and **(D)** peritoneum (*arrow*).

a. This was generated by using a degree of uptake greater than that of the liver as evidence of splenic disease.[21]

b. PET is particularly more accurate for detecting focal splenic involvement than gallium or CT.

Comparison with Other Modalities

1. ***PET versus CT.*** PET and CT have comparable specificity, but PET is ~15% more sensitive.[19]
   a. The primary advantage of PET over CT is in nodal detection in the thorax and periphery; in the abdomen and pelvis, PET and CT provide comparable results.[22,23]
   b. PET and CT are concordant in staging 80 to 90% of patients with diffuse large B cell and follicular lymphoma. In contrast, PET and CT are less likely to be concordant in staging HD (60 to 80%).[24] In both cases, PET discordance usually results in upstaging. However, the higher rate of discordance in HD suggests that both PET and CT need to be performed in staging HD.
2. ***PET/CT versus CT.*** PET/CT (with low-dose nonenhanced CT) is more sensitive and specific than contrast-enhanced CT for both nodal and extranodal disease.
   a. PET/CT is particularly valuable compared with CT in the exclusion of disease.
      - A common problem with CT is false-positive results from lung opacities interpreted as lymphoma; these can be accurately diagnosed by PET.
   b. *Nodal disease* (**Table 18.1**)
   c. *Extranodal disease* (**Table 18.2**)
3. ***PET versus gallium.*** PET is superior to gallium for both initial staging and follow-up of lymphoma.[25]

Pearls and Pitfalls

1. ***Thymus.*** It is important to recognize thymic hyperplasia as a distinct entity in patients with anterior mediastinal uptake. Thymic hyperplasia (as seen in **Figs. 6.19**, p. 52 and **6.20,** p. 53) is a common reaction following chemotherapy and as such is an expected phenomenon.
2. ***Diffuse bone marrow activity.*** Bone marrow uptake postgranulocyte colony-stimulating factor (G-CSF) therapy (as seen in **Fig. 6.30**, p. 58) can mimic or obscure lymphomatous bone marrow infiltration.
3. ***Focal bone marrow activity.*** Always consider a history of prior bone marrow biopsy as a cause of focal uptake in the posterior ilium.
4. ***Spleen***
   a. Splenic uptake post G-CSF therapy can mimic splenic involvement (as seen in **Fig. 6.30**, p. 58).
   b. The spleen is a common site for false-positive findings from infectious/inflammatory etiologies.
5. ***Low-grade lymphomas.*** Certain low-grade lymphomas, such as small-cell lymphocytic lymphoma, typically do not have substantial FDG uptake and may not be detected with high sensitivity by PET. In these cases, a positive scan often demonstrates hazy mild uptake.

◆ Therapy Response[26–28]

Clinical Indication: A

1. PET is increasingly employed as a standard modality for assessing response to therapy in both HD and aggressive NHL (**Fig. 18.4**). It is particularly useful in later stages of the disease, when response to chemotherapy is substantially lower than that in early stages.

Table 18.1 Sensitivity and Specificity of Positron Emission Tomography/Computed Tomography (PET/CT) versus Computed Tomography in the Detection of Nodal Disease

	Sensitivity %	Specificity %
PET/CT	94	100
CT	88	86

Table 18.2 Sensitivity and Specificity of Positron Emission Tomography/Computed Tomography (PET/CT) versus Computed Tomography in the Detection of Extranodal Disease

	Sensitivity %	Specificity %
PET/CT	88	100
CT	50	90

2. ***Early prediction.*** PET is useful as a prognostic indicator after one or a few cycles, or at midtreatment, during first-line chemotherapy of HD and NHL. PET can predict response, progression-free survival, and overall survival. PET may be superior to standard prognostic indicators such as the International Prognostic Score in advanced HD.[29] Lack of response suggests that the treatment regimen should be changed (e.g., second-line chemotherapy with stem cell transplantation). However, even if PET shows a complete response, initial treatment regimen should be completed, as minimal residual disease cannot be excluded.
   - In aggressive lymphomas, a negative PET study after the first chemotherapy cycle predicts progression-free survival better than a negative PET after the completion of chemotherapy.
3. ***Late prediction.*** At the completion of therapy where the presence of a residual mass on CT is a serious challenge, PET can accurately determine the nature of such findings (fibrosis vs residual disease). This is a more common scenario in HD, where there is typically a substantial, but not a complete, response to treatment.
4. ***Low-grade NHL.*** The role of PET for low-grade NHL therapy response is not clear at this time. One study suggests that PET is accurate in the diagnostic assessment of treated grade 1 and 2 follicular lymphomas.[30]

Accuracy

1. ***Early response evaluation***[31]
   a. Sensitivity 79%, specificity 92%
   b. Positive predictive value (PPV) 90%, negative predictive value (NPV) 81%
2. ***Posttreatment evaluation***[32]
   a. *HD.* Sensitivity 84%, specificity 90%
   b. *NHL.* Sensitivity 72%, specificity 100%

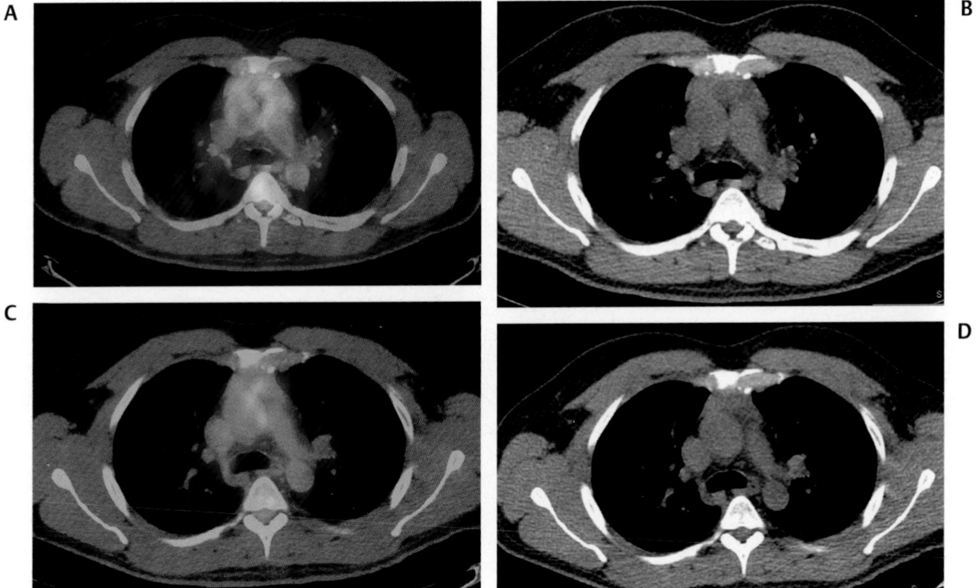

Fig. 18.4 Lymphoma therapy response. **(A)** Axial positron emission tomography (PET)/computed tomography (CT) and **(B)** CT demonstrate an anterior mediastinal mass in a patient with Hodgkin disease posttherapy. This has uptake greater than mediastinum and should be interpreted as residual disease. **(C)** After further therapy, the degree of fluorodeoxyglucose uptake is equal to the mediastinum, and **(D)** the mass is smaller on CT. As the residual mass is still > 2 cm in size, this can be interpreted as negative for disease. If the mass were < 2 cm in size, there should be no visible uptake greater than background activity before interpreting the study as negative.

The predictive value of PET depends upon the type of disease before therapy. HD, particularly in its early stages, usually has a higher response rate than NHL, and thus will have a lower pretest probability of residual disease following therapy. Hence, a negative PET in early stages of HD is predictive of a complete response, but a positive PET has fairly high false-positive rates. The opposite is true of advanced-stage HD and NHL, which has a higher pretest probability of residual disease following therapy. In these cases, a negative PET does not exclude minimal residual disease, but a positive PET is predictive of treatment failure.[3]

Although the bulk of the tumor in NHL is composed of malignant cells, the bulk of the tumor in HD is a benign inflammatory infiltrate. FDG uptake in HD may originate from this inflammatory component as well as the malignant cells.[33] In addition, patients with HD often receive radiation, which may result in inflammatory changes. Along with the lower pretest probability of residual disease in HD, these factors may account for the lower PPV of PET in HD compared with NHL. However, the PPV of PET in HD is still substantially higher than that of CT.

1. ***NHL***
   a. A positive FDG PET study is highly predictive for residual/recurrent disease and disease relapse in high-grade NHL (PPV 92 to 100%).
   b. A negative FDG PET study does not completely exclude minimal residual disease, and late relapse is still a possibility (NPV 83 to 88%).
   c. Follow-up scans are necessary for patients with negative PET and NHL.
2. ***HD*** (See residual posttherapy mass section also).[33]
   a. The NPV of midtreatment PET is high (at least 94%).
   b. However, the PPV is more variable (~62% to 90%).
3. ***Residual posttherapy mass***
   a. *PET.* Sensitivity 71 to 100%, specificity 69 to 100%[26]
   b. *PET.* NPV 80 to 100%, PPV 25 to 100%

c. A negative exam is very helpful in excluding disease, particularly in stage 1 or 2 HD. The NPV is 80 to 100%.
   - Follow-up scans are not necessary in patients with stage I and II HD and negative PET. However, it is unclear whether radiotherapy can be omitted in early-stage HD with a negative PET scan after first-line chemotherapy.[34]
   - Follow-up scans are necessary in patients with stage III and IV HD and negative PET.

d. Given the variable PPV (25 to 100%) and low pretest probability in stage I and II HD, confirmation for positive results should be strongly considered.

Comparison with Other Modalities

1. ***CT.*** PET and CT have comparable sensitivity, but PET is much more specific (69 to 92%) than CT (4 to 31%).
2. ***Bone scintigraphy.*** PET has fewer false-positive results than bone scintigraphy. In particular, PET can often accurately evaluate response in bone lesions when bone scintigraphy is false-positive.

Pearls

1. ***A baseline pretreatment scan is helpful.***
   a. If the disease seen on the pretreatment PET scan is not active, FDG PET should not be used for therapy monitoring. False-negative results will increase if baseline PET scans are not obtained on a routine basis.
   b. Acquiring baseline scans will also decrease false-positive results. As relapses typically occur in the region of previous disease seen on the baseline study, abnormalities on follow-up PET scans outside areas of previous disease should be interpreted with caution (e.g., inflammatory etiologies should be considered).
   c. Baseline scans are helpful but not mandatory in patients with subtypes of lymphomas that are routinely FDG avid, such as HD and diffuse B cell lymphoma. Baseline scans are mandatory in patients with subtypes of lymphoma with variable FDG avidity, such as MALT lymphomas.[35]
2. ***SUV.*** In evaluating posttherapy residual masses, use of SUVs is not superior to visual analysis.
3. Recommendations for interpretation of PET at the conclusion of therapy (per the Imaging Subcommittee of International Harmonization Project in Lymphoma):[35]
   a. Residual masses ≥ 2 cm: uptake greater than mediastinal blood pool should be interpreted as disease.
   b. Residual masses < 2 cm: any uptake greater than background should be interpreted as disease.
   c. Lung nodules ≥ 1.5 cm: uptake greater than mediastinal blood pool should be interpreted as disease. The absence of FDG uptake in nodules < 1.5 cm does not exclude disease; however, new nodules in the presence of complete response at all previously known disease sites are highly likely to be infectious/inflammatory.
   d. Hepatic or splenic lesions ≥ 1.5 cm: uptake greater than or equal to liver or spleen, respectively, should be interpreted as disease.
   e. Hepatic of splenic lesions < 1.5 cm: uptake greater than liver or spleen, respectively, should be considered as disease.
   f. Diffuse splenic uptake: diffuse splenic uptake greater than liver should be considered as secondary to lymphoma unless there has been recent cytokine administration.
   g. Bone marrow: focal or multifocal marrow uptake is usually secondary to lymphoma. Diffuse marrow uptake is usually secondary to marrow hyperplasia.
      - In HD patients, diffuse marrow uptake is often secondary to reactive myeloid hyperplasia.[36]
      - In patients with diffuse B cell lymphoma, isolated residual positivity involving bone marrow usually does not predict subsequent treatment failure.[37]
4. ***Minimal residual uptake.*** Minimal residual uptake in a focus of previously noted disease can be difficult to interpret. In HD, the highest predictive value is achieved when interim scans with minimal residual uptake are counted as negative scans. In NHL, patients with minimal residual uptake behave like patients with a negative PET in the early

stages and patients with a positive PET in the later stages.[2]

Pitfalls

1. Posttreatment uptake outside the sites of initial disease may present false-positive findings.
2. Infectious etiologies should always be considered in immunocompromised patients.
3. In general, PET imaging early after radiotherapy is not recommended. However, if patients are scanned early after radiotherapy for lymphoma, typical findings are mild and nonfocal uptake in the radiation field, which is usually distinguishable from sites with malignancy.[38]

◆ Pretransplantation of Autologous Stem Cells31

Clinical Indication: C

High-dose chemotherapy (HCT) and autologous stem cell transplantation (ASCT) are employed in patients who relapse from NHL or HD after conventional chemotherapy. However, patients must remain chemosensitive. PET is helpful in predicting which patients will benefit from transplantation. Limited data suggest that a positive PET scan prior to HCT and ASCT is predictive of poor prognosis. The risk of treatment failure is further increased if the PET is still positive after ASCT.[39] However, not all patients with a positive PET after induction chemotherapy will relapse, and often there are few therapeutic options besides HCT and ASCT. Thus, a positive PET scan after induction chemotherapy should not exclude patients from transplantation, but modified approaches still including HCT and ASCT or experimental therapies might be considered. Serial PET scans prior to transplantation may predict outcome better than a single scan.[40]

Pearls

1. Superior PPVs are obtained if PET is performed just prior to transplantation compared with early during salvage therapy.[2] After salvage therapy, resistant clones will become apparent when disease sites with sensitive histologies are destroyed.
2. The prognostic value of PET is higher prior to transplantation than after transplantation, because glucose metabolism may be transiently decreased after intense therapy.
3. Patients with negative PET studies prior to ASCT can be managed without post-ASCT PET imaging.[39]

Accuracy

- ***PET***. PPV 84%, NPV 83%[31]

◆ Relapse

Clinical Indication: C

Limited data suggest that PET may be useful in detection of subclinical relapse in both HD and NHL.

References

1. Burton C, Ell P, Linch D. The role of PET imaging in lymphoma. Br J Haematol 2004;126(6):772–784
2. Kirby AM, Mikhaeel NG. The role of FDG PET in the management of lymphoma: what is the evidence base? Nucl Med Commun 2007;28(5):335–354
3. Israel O, Keidar Z, Bar-Shalom R. Positron emission tomography in the evaluation of lymphoma. Semin Nucl Med 2004;34(3):166–179
4. Isasi CR, Lu P, Blaufox MD. A metaanalysis of ^{18}F-2-deoxy-2-fluoro-D-glucose positron emission tomography in the staging and restaging of patients with lymphoma. Cancer 2005;104(5):1066–1074
5. Allen-Auerbach M, Quon A, Weber WA, et al. Comparison between 2-deoxy-2-[^{18}F]fluoro-D-glucose positron emission tomography and positron emission tomography/computed tomography hardware fusion for staging of patients with lymphoma. Mol Imaging Biol 2004;6(6):411–416
6. Elstrom R, Guan L, Baker G, et al. Utility of FDG-PET scanning in lymphoma by WHO classification. Blood 2003;101(10):3875–3876
7. Hutchings M, Loft A, Hansen M, et al. Different histopathological subtypes of Hodgkin lymphoma show significantly different levels of FDG uptake. Hematol Oncol 2006;24(3):146–150
8. Karam M, Novak L, Cyriac J, et al. Role of fluorine-18 fluoro-deoxyglucose positron emission tomography scan in the evaluation and follow-up of patients with low-grade lymphomas. Cancer 2006;107(1):175–183
9. Schoder H, Noy A, Gonen M, et al. Intensity of 18fluoro deoxyglucose uptake in positron emission tomog-

raphy distinguishes between indolent and aggressive non-Hodgkin's lymphoma. J Clin Oncol 2005;23(21):4643–4651

10. Wohrer S, Jaeger U, Kletter K, et al. ^{18}F-fluoro-deoxyglucose positron emission tomography (^{18}F-FDG-PET) visualizes follicular lymphoma irrespective of grading. Ann Oncol 2006;17(5):780–784

11. Phongkitkarun S, Varavithya V, Kazama T, et al. Lymphomatous involvement of gastrointestinal tract: evaluation by positron emission tomography with (18)F-fluorodeoxyglucose. World J Gastroenterol 2005;11(46):7284–7289

12. Fuster D, Chiang S, Andreadis C, et al. Can [^{18}F]fluorodeoxyglucose positron emission tomography imaging complement biopsy results from the iliac crest for the detection of bone marrow involvement in patients with malignant lymphoma? Nucl Med Commun 2006;27(1):11–15

13. Hoffmann M, Kletter K, Becherer A, et al. ^{18}F-fluorodeoxyglucose positron emission tomography (^{18}F-FDG-PET) for staging and follow-up of marginal zone B-cell lymphoma. Oncology 2003;64(4):336–340

14. Tsukamoto N, Kojima M, Hasegawa M, et al. The usefulness of (18)F-fluorodeoxyglucose positron emission tomography ((18)F-FDG-PET) and a comparison of (18)F-FDG-PET with (67)gallium scintigraphy in the evaluation of lymphoma: relation to histologic subtypes based on the World Health Organization classification. Cancer 2007;110(3):652–659

15. Perry C, Herishanu Y, Metzer U, et al. Diagnostic accuracy of PET/CT in patients with extranodal marginal zone MALT lymphoma. Eur J Haematol 2007; 79(3):205–209

16. Hoffmann M, Wohrer S, Becherer A, et al. ^{18}F-fluoro-deoxy-glucose positron emission tomography in lymphoma of mucosa-associated lymphoid tissue: histology makes the difference. Ann Oncol 2006;17(12):1761–1765

17. Bishu S, Quigley JM, Bishu SR, et al. Predictive value and diagnostic accuracy of F-18-fluoro-deoxy-glucose positron emission tomography treated grade 1 and 2 follicular lymphoma. Leuk Lymphoma 2007;48(8): 1548–1555

18. Kako S, Izutsu K, Ota Y, et al. FDG-PET in T-cell and NK-cell neoplasms. Ann Oncol 2007;18(10):1685–1690

19. Schiepers C, Filmont JE, Czernin J. PET for staging of Hodgkin's disease and non-Hodgkin's lymphoma. Eur J Nucl Med Mol Imaging 2003;30(Suppl 1):S82–S88

20. Pakos EE, Fotopoulos AD, Ioannidis JP. ^{18}F-FDG PET for evaluation of bone marrow infiltration in staging of lymphoma: a meta-analysis. J Nucl Med 2005;46(6):958–963

21. Rini JN, Manalili EY, Hoffman MA, et al. F-18 FDG versus Ga-67 for detecting splenic involvement in Hodgkin's disease. Clin Nucl Med 2002;27(8):572–577

22. Jerusalem G, Beguin Y, Najjar F, et al. Positron emission tomography (PET) with ^{18}F-fluorodeoxyglucose (^{18}F-FDG) for the staging of low-grade non-Hodgkin's lymphoma (NHL). Ann Oncol 2001;12(6): 825–830

23. Buchmann I, Reinhardt M, Elsner K, et al. 2-(fluorine-18)fluoro-2-deoxy-D-glucose positron emission tomography in the detection and staging of malignant lymphoma: a bicenter trial. Cancer 2001;91(5):889–899

24. Seam P, Juweid ME, Cheson BD. The role of FDG-PET scans in patients with lymphoma. Blood 2007; 110(10):3507–3516

25. Jhanwar YS, Straus DJ. The role of PET in lymphoma. J Nucl Med 2006;47(8):1326–1334

26. Reske SN. PET and restaging of malignant lymphoma including residual masses and relapse. Eur J Nucl Med Mol Imaging 2003;30(Suppl 1):S89–S96

27. Spaepen K, Stroobants S, Verhoef G, Mortelmans L. Positron emission tomography with [(18)F]FDG for therapy response monitoring in lymphoma patients. Eur J Nucl Med Mol Imaging 2003;30(Suppl 1):S97–S105

28. Kostakoglu L, Goldsmith SJ. ^{18}F-FDG PET evaluation of the response to therapy for lymphoma and for breast, lung, and colorectal carcinoma. J Nucl Med 2003;44(2):224–239

29. Gallamini A, Hutchings M, Rigacci L, et al. Early interim 2-[^{18}F]fluoro-2-deoxy-D-glucose positron emission tomography is prognostically superior to international prognostic score in advanced-stage Hodgkin's lymphoma: a report from a joint Italian-Danish study. J Clin Oncol 2007;25(24):3746–3752

30. Bishu S, Quigley JM, Schmitz J, et al. F-18-fluoro-deoxy-glucose positron emission tomography in the assessment of peripheral T-cell lymphomas. Leuk Lymphoma 2007;48(8):1531–1538

31. Jerusalem G, Hustinx R, Beguin Y, Fillet G. Evaluation of therapy for lymphoma. Semin Nucl Med 2005;35(3):186–196

32. Zijlstra JM, Lindauer-van der Werf G, Hoekstra OS, et al. ^{18}F-fluoro-deoxyglucose positron emission tomography for post-treatment evaluation of malignant lymphoma: a systematic review. Haematologica 2006;91(4):522–529

33. Kasamon YL, Jones RJ, Wahl RL. Integrating PET and PET/CT into the risk-adapted therapy of lymphoma. J Nucl Med 2007; 48(1, suppl)19S–27S

34. Brepoels L, Stroobants S, Verhoef G. PET and PET/CT for response evaluation in lymphoma: current practice and developments. Leuk Lymphoma 2007;48(2):270–282

35. Juweid ME, Stroobants S, Hoekstra OS, et al. Use of positron emission tomography for response assessment of lymphoma: consensus of the Imaging Subcommittee of International Harmonization Project in Lymphoma. J Clin Oncol 2007;25(5):571–578

36. Elstrom RL, Tsai DE, Vergilio JA, Downs LH, Alavi A, Schuster SJ. Enhanced marrow [^{18}F]fluorodeoxyglucose uptake related to myeloid hyperplasia in Hodgkin's lymphoma can simulate lymphoma involvement in marrow. Clin Lymphoma 2004;5(1):62–64

37. Ng AP, Wirth A, Seymour JF, et al. Early therapeutic response assessment by (18)FDG-positron emission tomography during chemotherapy in patients with diffuse large B-cell lymphoma: isolated residual positivity involving bone is not usually a predictor of subsequent treatment failure. Leuk Lymphoma 2007;48(3):596–600

38. Castellucci P, Zinzani P, Nanni C, et al. ^{18}F-FDG PET early after radiotherapy in lymphoma patients. Cancer Biother Radiopharm 2004;19(5):606–612

39. Filmont JE, Gisselbrecht C, Cuenca X, et al. The impact of pre- and post-transplantation positron emission tomography using 18-fluorodeoxyglucose on poor-prognosis lymphoma patients undergoing autologous stem cell transplantation. Cancer 2007;110(6):1361–1369

40. Schot BW, Pruim J, van Imhoff GW, et al. The role of serial pre-transplantation positron emission tomography in predicting progressive disease in relapsed lymphoma. Haematologica 2006;91(4):490–495

19

Melanoma

Eugene C. Lin and Abass Alavi

◆ Initial Staging and Recurrence

Clinical Indication: A

Positron emission tomography (PET) is most useful in staging high-risk disease at diagnosis and evaluation for recurrent disease if surgery is planned. It has a potential role in assessing response and surveillance for recurrence, but the exact value of PET in these settings is not well defined.

1. ***Initial staging***[1,2]
   a. PET is a useful modality for regional and distant staging of high-risk melanoma at initial diagnosis (**Figs. 19.1, 19.2, 19.3,** and **19.4**).
   b. The value of PET for initial staging depends upon the disease stage.
      - PET is most valuable in stage III disease with regional lymph node metastases.
         - o Detection of distant disease will likely influence prognosis and management.
         - o Twenty-two percent of patients will be upstaged by PET.[3]
      - PET has minimal if any role in stage I and II disease.
         - o In these stages, the prevalence of nodal disease is small, and sentinel node biopsy has a much higher negative predictive value (NPV) than PET. The sensitivity of PET for regional lymph node metastases in melanoma is only 17% relative to sentinel lymphadenectomy.[4]
         - o PET may have potential value with a higher pretest likelihood of distant metastases, for example, in melanomas located in the trunk and upper arms, a Breslow thickness > 4 mm, ulceration, or high mitotic rate.[4] However, note that in stage I and II

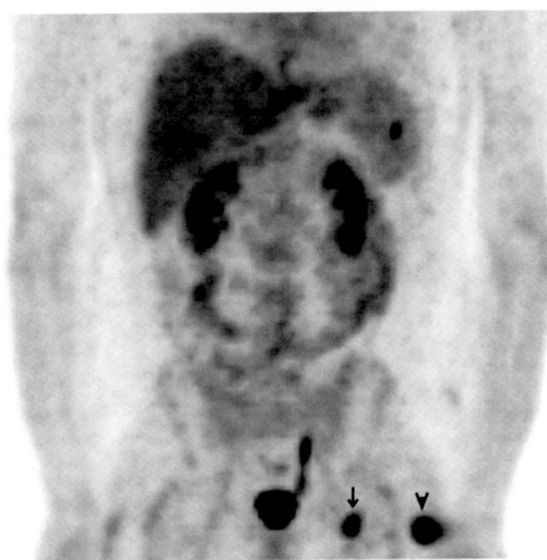

Fig. 19.1 Primary melanoma and metastases. Coronal positron emission tomography scan demonstrates uptake in a primary left thigh melanoma (*arrowhead*), a left groin nodal metastasis (*arrow*), and a splenic metastasis.

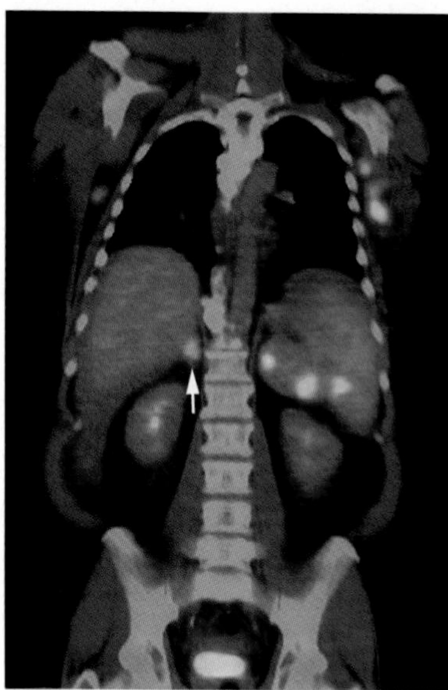

Fig. 19.2 Melanoma metastases. Coronal positron emission tomography/computed tomography scan demonstrates melanoma metastases to the right adrenal (*arrow*), spleen, and axillary nodes.

disease, possible distant disease identified by PET has a high false-positive rate.[5]

- PET may occasionally be of value in stage IV disease.
  - o PET is usually not helpful if metastases are multiple, as demonstration of additional metastases usually will not alter management. However, PET could be useful in this situation to determine response if experimental therapies are employed.
  - In patients with potentially surgically remediable disease (solitary or limited distant metastases), PET is helpful in detecting additional disease, which may obviate plans for surgery.

c. PET is more useful in identifying distant disease than regional metastases, given the established role of sentinel node imaging and biopsy. PET and any other gross imaging technique cannot replace sentinel node biopsy because these techniques will not detect micrometastases.[6]
- However, if used in intermediate- and high-risk lesions, a positive PET study can guide biopsy of appropriate regional nodes.[7]
- A sentinel node biopsy must be performed if PET is negative, as micrometastases can be missed.
- In general, there is a distinct and appropriate role for both PET and sentinel node biopsy, and either or both should be employed accordingly.

2. *Recurrent disease*[1,2]

a. PET is a standard modality in evaluation of recurrent melanoma. It is useful for
- Diagnosis of recurrent or metastatic disease
- Pretreatment staging of recurrent disease

b. The primary indication for PET in recurrence is when surgery is planned.
- Detection of additional sites of disease will avoid unnecessary surgery.
- Equivocal findings on conventional imaging can be characterized.

A

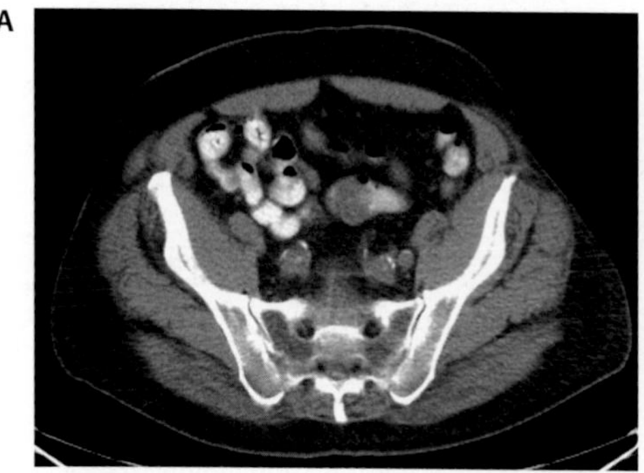

B

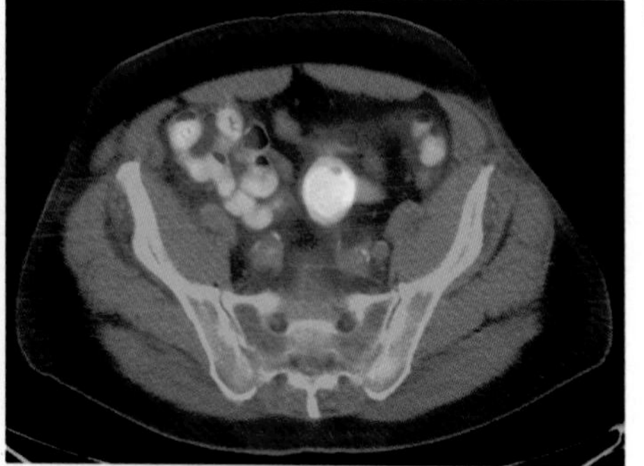

Fig. 19.3 Bowel metastasis. **(A)** Axial computed tomography (CT) and **(B)** positron emission tomography (PET)/CT demonstrate a bowel metastasis from melanoma. There is intense uptake in this metastatic lesion, which is much more easily identified by PET than CT.

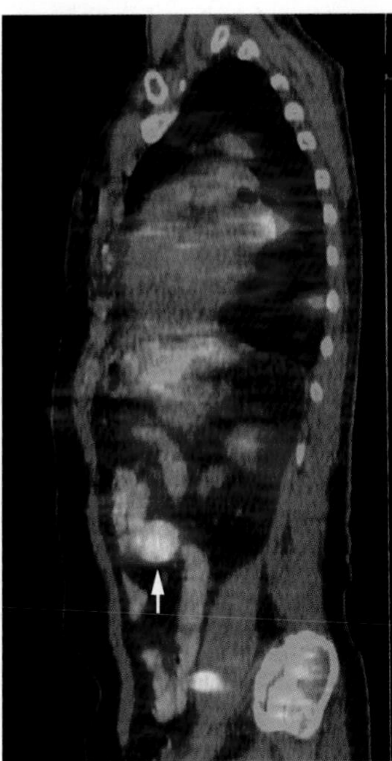

Fig. 19.4 Metastastic melanoma. Sagittal positron emission tomography/computed tomography image demonstrates metastases to the hilum, lung base, psoas muscle, and a mesenteric node (*arrow*).

3. ***Prognosis***
    - High standardized uptake value (SUV) in lymph node metastases is an independent negative prognostic factor for disease-free survival.[8] However, there is no impact on overall survival.

Accuracy and Comparison with Other Modalities

1. ***PET.*** Sensitivity 79%, specificity 86% (including both initial staging and recurrence)[9]
    a. PET is more accurate for systemic staging than regional staging.
    b. The accuracy is poor in thinner lesions < 1.5 mm.[10]
2. ***PET/CT***[11]
    a. PET/computed tomography (CT) has an overall accuracy for N and M staging of 97% compared with 93% for PET and 79% for CT.
    b. The primary value of PET/CT over PET is increased accuracy in M staging. The sensitivity of PET is comparable to PET/CT for all areas except the lungs, but PET/CT is more specific.
3. ***Distant metastases.*** PET is more sensitive than CT with comparable specificity.[12]
    a. *Body region*
        - PET is more sensitive than CT for skin lesions, lymph node, soft tissue, liver, bone marrow, and bowel metastases (**Fig. 19.3**).[12,13] However, magnetic resonance imaging (MRI) is more sensitive than PET for liver metastases.[14]
        - CT is more sensitive for lung and brain metastases.
    b. In patients with advanced stage IV disease being considered for surgical resection, combined PET and conventional imaging is recommended, as it has higher sensitivity and specificity than either PET or conventional imaging alone.[15]

Pearls and Pitfalls

1. In melanoma, PET is limited in the brain, lungs, and liver. If there is concern for brain and lung metastases, PET must be supplemented with CT or MRI of the brain and chest CT. Lung metastases in melanoma are often very small and undetectable by PET. Liver MRI is substantially more sensitive than PET for liver metastases from melanoma.[14]
2. ***Melanin content.*** Melanin content does not influence lesion detectability by PET.[14]
3. ***Lung metastases.*** Although PET has limited sensitivity for lung metastases, it is still useful for assessment of the lungs. The higher specificity (92% vs 70%)[13] of PET versus CT is useful to evaluate indeterminate lung lesions seen on CT.
4. ***Peripheral lesions.*** Skin or subcutaneous lesions may be missed on nonattenuation-corrected images due to the high skin activity on these images. However, it is also possible that peripheral subcutaneous lesions could also be better seen on nonattenuation-corrected images due to the lack of attenuation relative to central structures.
5. Given that melanoma has the potential to metastasize to a wider range of anatomical sites than most neoplasms, false-positive results are often more of an issue in this cancer than in others. The full range of normal/

benign variants and artifacts in PET imaging can cause false-positive findings. Because of this, close clinical and radiographic correlation is necessary to avoid such errors. Confirmation of assumed disease sites should be obtained if possible for optimal management.

6. ***Interpretation.*** The diagnostic accuracy of PET/CT in melanoma may be improved by using a high threshold approach to interpretation (i.e., subtle findings are interpreted as negative).[16]
7. ***Scan volume.*** One study[17] suggests that scanning the lower extremities and skull in melanoma patients is of low yield.

References

1. Friedman KP, Wahl RL. Clinical use of positron emission tomography in the management of cutaneous melanoma. Semin Nucl Med 2004;34(4):242–253
2. Kumar R, Alavi A. Clinical applications of fluorodeoxyglucose–positron emission tomography in the management of malignant melanoma. Curr Opin Oncol 2005;17(2):154–159
3. Bastiaannet E, Oyen WJ, Meijer S, et al. Impact of [18F]fluorodeoxyglucose positron emission tomography on surgical management of melanoma patients. Br J Surg 2006;93(2):243–249
4. Belhocine TZ, Scott AM, Even-Sapir E, et al. Role of nuclear medicine in the management of cutaneous malignant melanoma. J Nucl Med 2006;47(6):957–967
5. Wagner JD. Fluorodeoxyglucose positron emission tomography for melanoma staging: refining the indications. Ann Surg Oncol 2006;13(4):444–446
6. Wagner JD, Schauwecker D, Davidson D, et al. Prospective study of fluorodeoxyglucose-positron emission tomography imaging of lymph node basins in melanoma patients undergoing sentinel node biopsy. J Clin Oncol 1999;17(5):1508–1515
7. Abella-Columna E, Valk PE. Positron emission tomography imaging in melanoma and lymphoma. Semin Roentgenol 2002;37(2):129–139
8. Bastiaannet E, Hoekstra OS, Oyen WJ, et al. Level of fluorodeoxyglucose uptake predicts risk for recurrence in melanoma patients presenting with lymph node metastases. Ann Surg Oncol 2006;13(7):919–926
9. Mijnhout GS, Hoekstra OS, van Tulder MW, et al. Systematic review of the diagnostic accuracy of (18)F-fluorodeoxyglucose positron emission tomography in melanoma patients. Cancer 2001;91(8):1530–1542
10. Prichard RS, Hill AD, Skehan SJ, O'Higgins NJ. Positron emission tomography for staging and management of malignant melanoma. Br J Surg 2002;89(4):389–396
11. Reinhardt MJ, Joe AY, Jaeger U, et al. Diagnostic performance of whole body dual modality ^{18}F-FDG PET/CT imaging for N- and M-staging of malignant melanoma: experience with 250 consecutive patients. J Clin Oncol 2006;24(7):1178–1187
12. Holder WD Jr, White RL Jr, Zuger JH, et al. Effectiveness of positron emission tomography for the detection of melanoma metastases. Ann Surg 1998;227(5):764–769
13. Fuster D, Chiang S, Johnson G, et al. Is ^{18}F-FDG PET more accurate than standard diagnostic procedures in the detection of suspected recurrent melanoma? J Nucl Med 2004;45(8):1323–1327
14. Ghanem N, Altehoefer C, Hogerle S, et al. Detectability of liver metastases in malignant melanoma: prospective comparison of magnetic resonance imaging and positron emission tomography. Eur J Radiol 2005;54(2):264–270
15. Finkelstein SE, Carrasquillo JA, Hoffman JM, et al. A prospective analysis of positron emission tomography and conventional imaging for detection of stage IV metastatic melanoma in patients undergoing metastasectomy. Ann Surg Oncol 2004;11(8):731–738
16. Falk MS, Truitt AK, Coakley FV, et al. Interpretation, accuracy and management implications of FDG PET/CT in cutaneous malignant melanoma. Nucl Med Commun 2007;28(4):273–280
17. Niederkohr RD, Rosenberg J, Shabo G, Quon A. Clinical value of including the head and lower extremities in ^{18}F-FDG PET/CT imaging for patients with malignant melanoma. Nucl Med Commun 2007;28(9):688–695

20

Hepatobiliary Tumors

Eugene C. Lin and Abass Alavi

◆ Hepatocellular Carcinoma[1,2]

Clinical Indication: C

The primary value of positron emission tomography (PET) is in detection of extrahepatic disease and monitoring treatment.

1. ***Primary tumor detection***
   a. PET has limited sensitivity for well-differentiated hepatocellular carcinoma (HCC) (**Fig. 20.1**).
   b. PET has no role in screening for HCC in patients with cirrhosis.[3]
2. ***Extrahepatic disease***
   a. The primary tumor must have fluorodeoxyglucose (FDG) uptake for PET results to be valid.
   b. PET can detect distant disease for staging and recurrence, altering management in up to 30% of patients.[4]
   c. PET may be valuable in patients with treated HCC and a rising serum α-fetoprotein and normal conventional imaging. In these cases, the accuracy of PET for detecting recurrence is 74%.[5]
3. ***Monitoring therapy.*** PET is more accurate than computed tomography (CT) (after iodized oil injection) for evaluating tumor viability postchemoembolization (**Fig. 20.2**).[6] PET may also detect recurrence after radiofrequency ablation earlier than CT.[7]
4. ***Prognosis***
   a. A standardized uptake value (SUV) ratio (tumor to nontumor SUV) > 2 predicts poor prognosis after resection.[8]
   b. Tumor recurrence is more likely after liver transplantation in patients with PET-positive HCC.[9]

Accuracy and Comparison with Other Modalities

1. ***Primary lesion detection***
   a. *PET.* Sensitivity 50 to 70%[10,11]
      - Low sensitivity is due to low uptake in well-differentiated HCC.
      - Tumors that are visualized by PET (**Fig. 20.1**) usually are higher grade and larger in size, with elevated circulating α-fetoprotein.
   b. PET is less sensitive than CT, magnetic resonance imaging (MRI), or ultrasound.
2. ***Extrahepatic disease.***[12] PET has a relatively high detection rate (83%) for extrahepatic metastases > 1 cm in size but a low detection rate for metastases < 1 cm.
   a. PET can detect lesions that are negative or equivocal on conventional imaging.
   b. Patients with rising tumor markers and negative PET exams usually do not have extrahepatic metastases; however, HCCs are often detected in the liver within

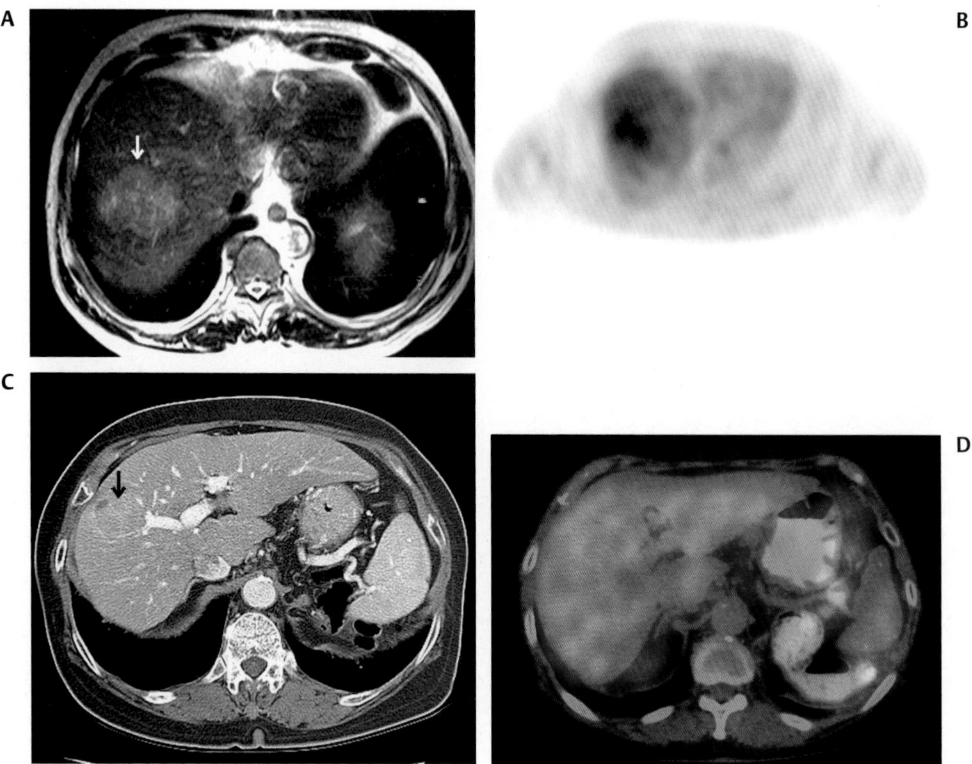

Fig. 20.1 Hepatocellular carcinoma: high-grade versus low grade. (**A**) Axial T2-weighted magnetic resonance imaging scan demonstrates a focal area of hyperintensity corresponding to a hepatoma (*arrow*) in the right dome of the liver. (**B**) Axial positron emission tomography (PET) scan demonstrates increased uptake in this high-grade hepatoma. (**C**) Axial computed tomography (CT) in a different patient demonstrates a mostly isodense right lobe lesion with an enhancing capsule and a peripheral area of low density (*arrow*). (**D**) Axial PET/CT at the same level demonstrates that this low-grade hepatoma has uptake equal to normal liver.

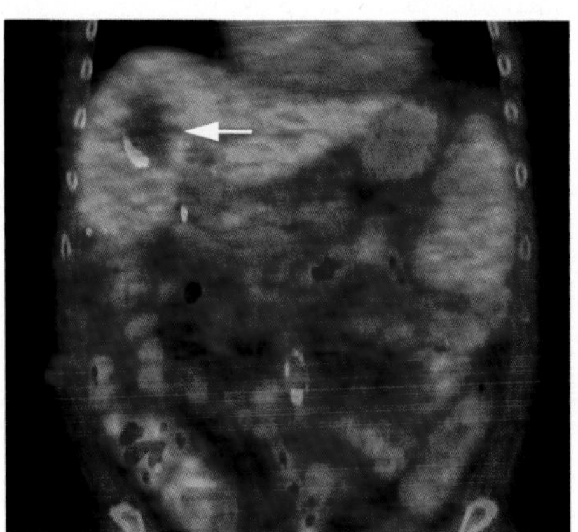

Fig. 20.2 Hepatic chemoembolization. Coronal positron emission tomography/computed tomography scan demonstrates lack of fluorodeoxyglucose uptake in hepatoma (*arrow*) after chemoembolization.

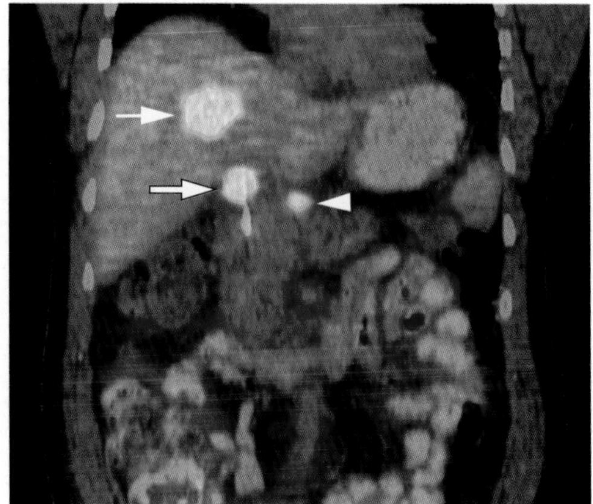

Fig. 20.3 Metastatic cholangiocarcinoma. Coronal positron emission tomography/computed tomography scan demonstrates both intrahepatic (*arrow*) and extrahepatic (*open arrow*) cholangiocarcinoma and a local nodal metastasis (*arrowhead*).

months. Thus, these patients should be closely followed with liver imaging.

Pearls

1. ***SUV.*** HCCs usually have lower SUVs than metastases or cholangiocarcinoma.[13]
2. ***Fibrolamellar HCC.*** Fibrolamellar HCCs, which are pathologically low grade, can have increased FDG uptake (these tumors have intratumoral fibrous stromata, which are associated with increased FDG uptake).[4]
3. ***Delayed imaging.*** Delayed imaging at 2 or 3 hours may detect more lesions.[14]

Pitfalls

- ***Cirrhosis/hepatitis.*** Patients with cirrhosis and chronic hepatitis can have slightly increased FDG activity in the liver, which could limit detection of HCC.

◆ Cholangiocarcinoma[1]

Clinical Indication: C

PET can detect the primary tumor, regional lymph nodes (**Fig. 20.3**), and distant disease (**Fig. 20.4**). The primary value is in detecting distant disease. In patients with cholangiocarcinoma and gallbladder carcinoma, PET/CT findings change management in 17% of patients deemed resectable after initial work-up.[15]

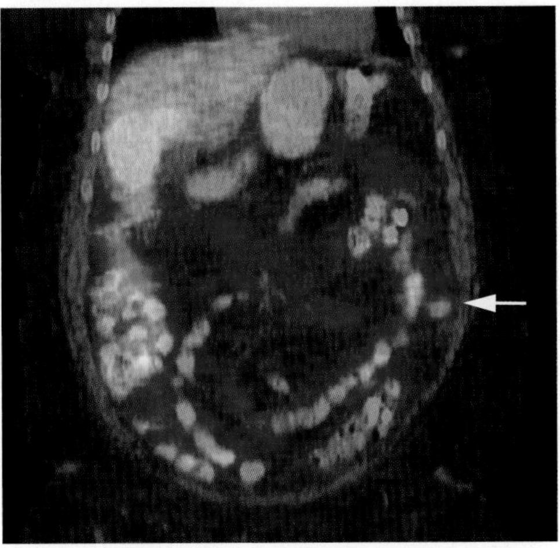

Fig. 20.4 Metastatic cholangiocarcinoma. Coronal positron emission tomography/computed tomography scan demonstrates a large right intrahepatic cholangiocarcinoma with peritoneal metastases (*arrow*) in the left paracolic gutter.

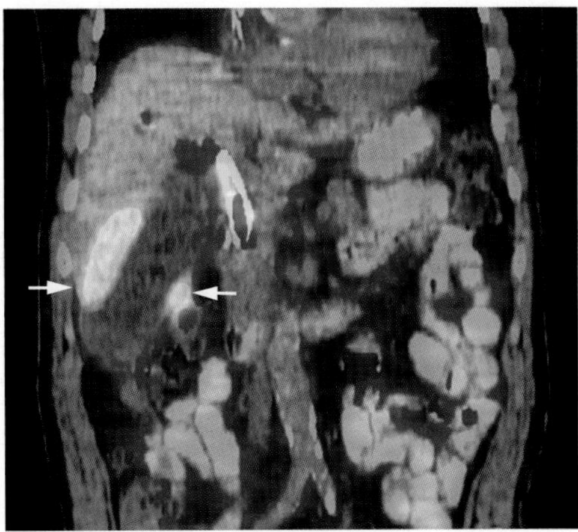

Fig. 20.5 Gallbladder cancer. Coronal positron emission tomography/computed tomography scan demonstrates intense uptake in the gallbladder wall (*arrows*) secondary to gallbladder carcinoma. Inflammatory uptake is also noted around a common bile duct stent.

1. ***Primary tumor***
   a. PET is highly sensitive for the detection of cholangiocarcinoma.
   b. *Gallbladder carcinoma.* PET is highly sensitive for the detection of gallbladder carcinoma (**Fig. 20.5**).[15]
      - However, benign gallbladder polyps can have FDG uptake.
   c. PET is particularly useful when other imaging techniques are equivocal.
   d. *Primary sclerosing cholangitis.* Limited data suggest PET may be valuable for the detection of cholangiocarcinoma in patients with biliary strictures and/or

Table 20.1 Sensitivity and Specificity of Positron Emission Tomography (PET) versus Computed Tomography (CT) in the Detection of Regional Lymph Node Metastases

	Sensitivity %	Specificity %
PET	38	100
CT	59	54

primary sclerosing cholangitis.[16–18] However, in the setting of primary sclerosing cholangitis, false-positives secondary to inflammation have been reported.[18] Dynamic scanning with determination of the metabolic clearance of FDG may be helpful in avoiding false-positives.[16]

- An SUV cutoff of 3.6 is helpful in differentiating benign from malignant strictures in the liver hilum.[17]

2. *Metastatic disease*

a. PET is more sensitive for distant metastases than for regional nodal spread.[19]

b. In particular, distant metastases are often detected in peripheral intrahepatic cholangiocarcinoma.[20]

Accuracy and Comparison with Other Modalities

1. *Primary tumor*

a. *PET.* Sensitivity 92%, specificity 93%[19]

b. *Anatomical region.* The sensitivity for perihilar cholangiocarcinoma is lower than for intrahepatic and common bile duct cancers.[21]

c. Overall, PET is more accurate than CT; however, the sensitivity for perihilar cancer is lower than that of CT.[21]

2. *Regional lymph nodes*[22]

a. **Table 20.1**

b. PET is less sensitive but more specific than CT for regional lymph node metastases.

3. *Distant disease.* PET/CT is much more sensitive than CT for the detection of distant disease.[15]

Pitfalls

1. Mucinous adenocarcinoma can be false-negative.

2. False-positive biliary tract uptake can be seen with recent stent placement (as seen in **Fig. 6.33**, p. 60).

3. Inflammatory disorders such as primary sclerosing cholangitis, cholangitis from any etiology, and cholecystitis can cause false-positives.

4. Sensitivity for carcinomatosis is limited.[23]

5. Sensitivity for infiltrative cholangiocarcinoma is much lower than for nodular cholangiocarcinoma.[23]

References

1. Hustinx R. PET imaging in assessing gastrointestinal tumors. Radiol Clin North Am 2004;42(6):1123–1139
2. Lin EC, Kuni CC. Radionuclide imaging of hepatic and biliary disease. Semin Liver Dis 2001;21(2):179–194
3. Teefey SA, Hildeboldt CC, Dehdashti F, et al. Detection of primary hepatic malignancy in liver transplant candidates: prospective comparison of CT, MR imaging, US, and PET. Radiology 2003;226(2):533–542
4. Wudel LJ Jr, Delbeke D, Morris D, et al. The role of [^{18}F]fluorodeoxyglucose positron emission tomography imaging in the evaluation of hepatocellular carcinoma. Am Surg 2003;69(2):117–124
5. Chen YK, Hsieh DS, Liao CS, et al. Utility of FDG-PET for investigating unexplained serum AFP elevation in patients with suspected hepatocellular carcinoma recurrence. Anticancer Res 2005;25(6C):4719–4725
6. Torizuka T, Tamaki N, Inokuma T, et al. Value of fluorine-18-FDG-PET to monitor hepatocellular carcinoma after interventional therapy. J Nucl Med 1994;35(12):1965–1969
7. Paudyal B, Oriuchi N, Paudyal P, et al. Early diagnosis of recurrent hepatocellular carcinoma with ^{18}F-FDG PET after radiofrequency ablation therapy. Oncol Rep 2007;18(6):1469–1473
8. Hatano E, Ikai I, Higashi T, et al. Preoperative positron emission tomography with fluorine-18-fluorodeoxyglucose is predictive of prognosis in patients with hepatocellular carcinoma after resection. World J Surg 2006;30(9):1736–1741
9. Yang SH, Suh KS, Lee HW, et al. The role of (18)F-FDG-PET imaging for the selection of liver transplantation candidates among hepatocellular carcinoma patients. Liver Transpl 2006;12(11):1655–1660
10. Khan MA, Combs CS, Brunt EM, et al. Positron emission tomography scanning in the evaluation of hepatocellular carcinoma. J Hepatol 2000;32(5):792–797
11. Trojan J, Schroeder O, Raedle J, et al. Fluorine-18 FDG positron emission tomography for imaging of hepatocellular carcinoma. Am J Gastroenterol 1999;94(11):3314–3319
12. Sugiyama M, Sakahara H, Torizuka T, et al. ^{18}F-FDG PET in the detection of extrahepatic metastases from hepatocellular carcinoma. J Gastroenterol 2004;39(10):961–968
13. Shiomi S, Nishiguchi S, Ishizu H, et al. Usefulness of positron emission tomography with fluorine-18-fluorodeoxyglucose for predicting outcome in patients with hepatocellular carcinoma. Am J Gastroenterol 2001;96(6):1877–1880
14. Lin WY, Tsai SC, Hung GU. Value of delayed ^{18}F-FDG-PET imaging in the detection of hepatocellular carcinoma. Nucl Med Commun 2005;26(4):315–321
15. Petrowsky H, Wildbrett P, Husarik DB, et al. Impact of integrated positron emission tomography and computed tomography on staging and management of gallbladder cancer and cholangiocarcinoma. J Hepatol 2006;45(1):43–50

16. Prytz H, Keiding S, Bjornsson E, et al. Dynamic FDG-PET is useful for detection of cholangiocarcinoma in patients with PSC listed for liver transplantation. Hepatology 2006;44(6):1572–1580
17. Reinhardt MJ, Strunk H, Gerhardt T, et al. Detection of Klatskin's tumor in extrahepatic bile duct strictures using delayed ^{18}F-FDG PET/CT: preliminary results for 22 patient studies. J Nucl Med 2005;46(7):1158–1163
18. Wakabayashi H, Akamoto S, Yachida S, et al. Significance of fluorodeoxyglucose PET imaging in the diagnosis of malignancies in patients with biliary stricture. Eur J Surg Oncol 2005;31(10):1175–1179
19. Kluge R, Schmidt F, Caca K, et al. Positron emission tomography with [(18)F]fluoro-2-deoxy-D-glucose for diagnosis and staging of bile duct cancer. Hepatology 2001;33(5):1029–1035
20. Kim YJ, Yun M, Lee WJ, et al. Usefulness of ^{18}F-FDG PET in intrahepatic cholangiocarcinoma. Eur J Nucl Med Mol Imaging 2003;30(11):1467–1472
21. Moon CM, Bang S, Chung JB, et al. Usefulness of (18)F-fluorodeoxyglucose positron emission tomography in differential diagnosis and staging of cholangiocarcinomas. J Gastroenterol Hepatol 2008;23:759–765
22. Kato T, Tsukamoto E, Kuge Y, et al. Clinical role of (18)F-FDG PET for initial staging of patients with extrahepatic bile duct cancer. Eur J Nucl Med Mol Imaging 2002;29(8):1047–1054
23. Anderson CD, Rice MH, Pinson CW, et al. Fluorodeoxyglucose PET imaging in the evaluation of gallbladder carcinoma and cholangiocarcinoma. J Gastrointest Surg 2004;8(1):90–97

21

Pancreatic Cancer

Eugene C. Lin and Abass Alavi

◆ Pancreatic Masses and Adenocarcinoma

Clinical Indication: B

Positron emission tomography (PET) can be useful in differentiating benign pancreatic masses from adenocarcinoma.

Accuracy and Comparison with Other Modalities

1. ***PET*** **(Table 21.1)**
2. ***Location.*** The sensitivity for periampullary neoplasms is less than for neoplasm elsewhere in the pancreas.[1]
3. ***Tumor size.*** The sensitivity of PET is not substantially affected by tumor size if lesions are > 1 cm.
4. ***Comparison with computed tomography (CT)***
   - ***a.*** PET is most helpful compared with CT for lesions < 2 cm.[2]
   - ***b.*** For lesions > 4 cm, CT is superior, as large pancreatic tumors often contain areas of low metabolism.
   - ***c.*** If CT shows no discrete mass, a positive PET is highly predictive of malignancy.[3]
   - ***d.*** If CT is indeterminate, a positive PET is less specific for malignancy but is very sensitive.[3]

Table 21.1 Sensitivity and Specificity of Positron Emission Tomography (PET) versus Computed Tomography (CT) in the Detection of Pancreatic Cancer

	Sensitivity %	Specificity %
PET	92	85
CT	65	62

Pearls

1. ***Clinical history***[4]
   - ***a.*** The absence of clinical and laboratory findings of acute pancreatitis does not rule out an inflammatory etiology for a pancreatic mass.
   - ***b.*** Obtaining a C-reactive protein may be helpful, as false-positive results due to inflammation are more likely to occur when C-reactive protein is elevated.
2. ***Characteristics of malignant versus inflammatory masses***
   - ***a.*** Inflammatory lesions are often more diffuse than focal.
   - ***b.*** However, acute or chronic pancreatitis secondary to duct obstruction can be seen in conjunction with pancreatic malignancy. In these cases, it is difficult to distinguish tumor from pancreatitis on PET (**Fig. 21.1**).
   - ***c.*** Although chronic pancreatitis can cause false-positive results, the majority (87%) of

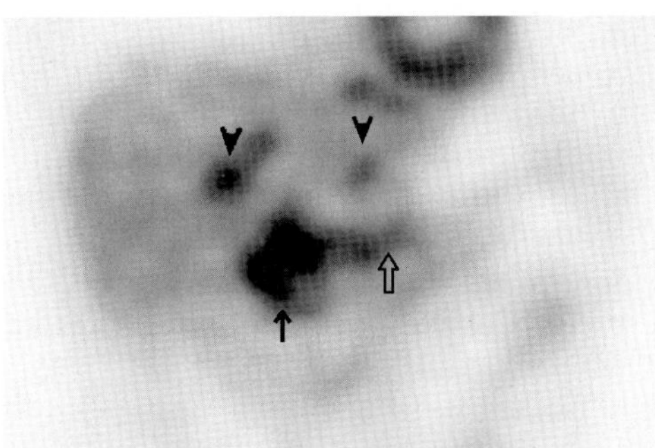

Fig. 21.1 Metastatic pancreatic cancer with chronic pancreatitis. Coronal positron emission tomography scan demonstrates focal uptake in a pancreatic head adenocarcinoma (*solid arrow*). Increased uptake in the pancreatic body (*open arrow*) is not tumor, but secondary to chronic pancreatitis from the obstructing pancreatic head mass. Liver metastases are present in both the right and left lobes (*arrowheads*).

patients with chronic pancreatitis have negative PET exams. The possibility of malignancy should still be pursued in patients with chronic pancreatitis and positive PET.[5]

3. ***Standardized uptake values (SUV)***
   a. There is no generally agreed upon SUV cutoff for differentiating benign from malignant lesions: published values range from 2.0 to 4.0.[6,7]
   b. If the patient has a history of pancreatitis, using SUV cutoff in the higher range helps to avoid false-positive results because pancreatic inflammatory lesions can have substantial uptake.
   c. SUV values should be corrected for glucose level if possible.
4. ***Delayed imaging***[8]
   a. Delayed imaging at 2 hours can help differentiate between malignant lesions and benign inflammatory lesions.
   b. Malignant lesions will have increasing uptake over time, whereas inflammatory lesions will have a decline in uptake.
   c. However, 19% of malignant pancreatic tumors show a decline in uptake from 1 to 2 hours.[9]

Table 21.2 Sensitivity and Specificity of Positron Emission Tomography/Computed Tomography (PET/CT) versus Computed Tomography in the Detection of Malignant Cystic Pancreatic Tumors

	Sensitivity %	Specificity %
PET/CT	86	91
CT	67 to 71	87 to 90

Pitfalls

1. ***Hyperglycemia.*** Hyperglycemia is a confounding factor for all oncologic PET but is the most problematic in pancreatic PET, where it causes a high false-negative rate. PET must be interpreted with caution in hyperglycemic patients with a pancreatic mass.

A

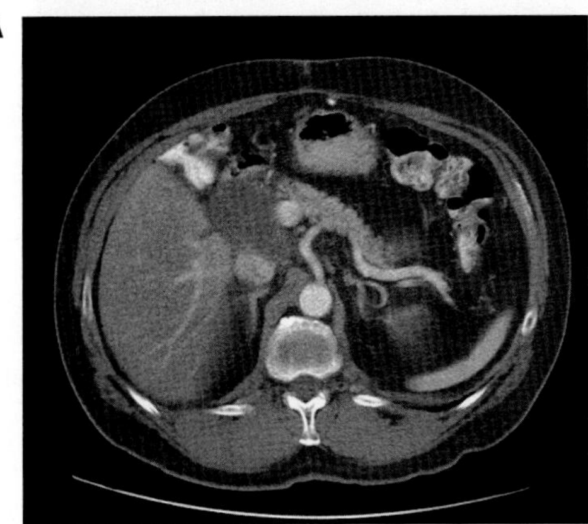

B

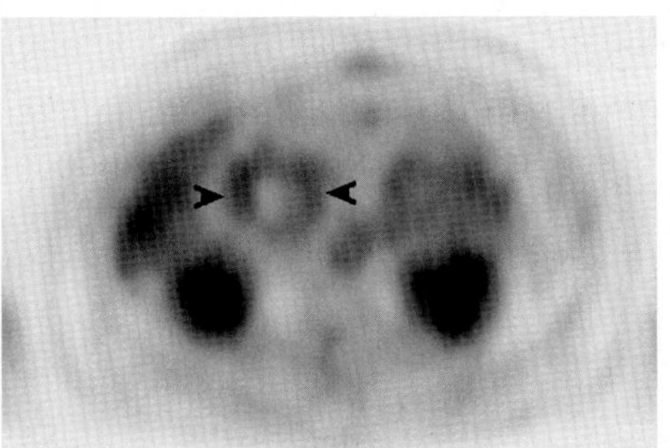

Fig. 21.2 Pancreatic pseudocyst. **(A)** Computed tomography scan demonstrates a cystic lesion in the pancreatic head region. **(B)** Axial positron emission tomography scan at a slightly more inferior level demonstrates uptake around the cyst (*arrowheads*) but no uptake within the cyst. This appearance is consistent with a pseudocyst.

- If the plasma glucose is > 130 mg/dL, the detection rate of pancreatic malignancies is only 42%.[10]

2. ***False-positives.*** Pancreatitis (chronic, acute, autoimmune), benign lesions (serous cystadenoma, hemorrhagic pseudocyst)
3. ***False-negatives.*** Early-stage tumors, elevated glucose

◆ Cystic Tumors

Clinical Indication: C

1. ***Accuracy.*** PET or PET/CT can differentiate benign from malignant cystic tumors (**Fig. 21.2**) with greater accuracy than CT, using an SUV cutoff of 2.5 (**Table 21.2**).[11,12]
2. ***Intraductal papillary mucinous tumor (IPMT).*** IPMT usually has increased fluorodeoxyglucose (FDG) uptake.[13,14]
   - *a.* Malignant IPMT has more uptake than benign IPMT.
   - *b.* Solid components have more uptake than the cystic components.
   - *c.* The cystic component usually has diffuse uptake greater than normal pancreas.
3. ***Solid pseudopapillary tumors.*** Benign solid pseudo-papillary tumors with increased uptake have been reported.[15]

◆ Islet Cell Tumors

Clinical Indication: C

1. Sensitivity of PET is low (53%) (**Fig. 21.3**) but comparable to CT, magnetic resonance imaging (MRI), and ultrasound.[14]
2. Small tumors not identified by other imaging methods are also usually not identified by PET.

A

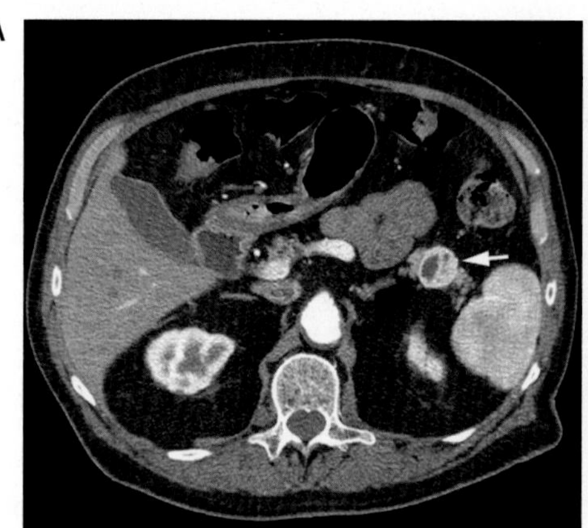

B

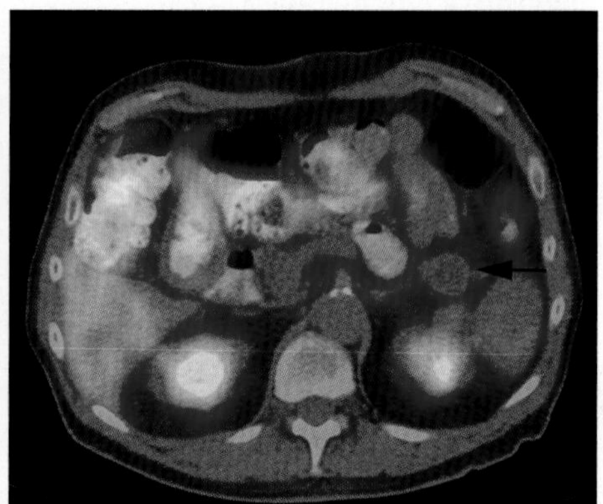

C

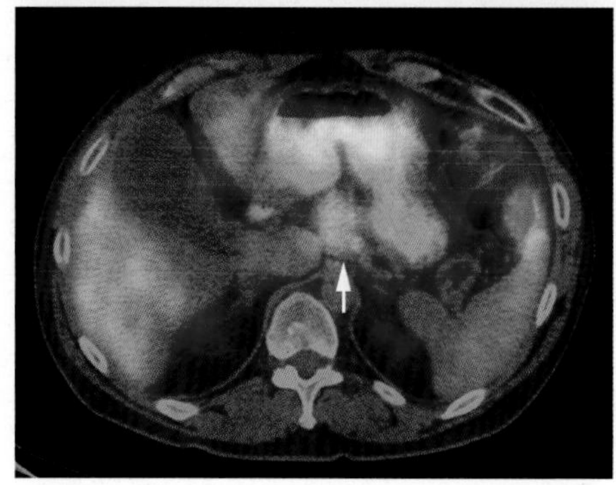

Fig. 21.3 Pancreatic islet cell tumors with variable fluorodeoxyglucose (FDG) uptake. **(A)** Axial computed tomography (CT) scan demonstrates a hypervascular islet cell tumor in the tail of the pancreas (*arrow*). **(B)** Axial positron emission tomography (PET)/CT scan demonstrates lack of FDG uptake in the islet cell tumor (*arrow*). **(C)** Axial PET/CT scan in another patient demonstrates moderate FDG uptake in an islet cell tumor (*arrow*) arising from the body of the pancreas.

◆ Staging

Clinical Indication: B

1. PET cannot replace CT, as it cannot assess local resectability. However, it can identify local and distant disease (**Fig. 21.4**) not seen on CT and help avoid unnecessary surgery.
   - The use of PET or PET/CT avoids unnecessary surgery by upstaging disease in ~17% of patients originally considered resectable by CT and angiography.[16,17]
2. PET is more useful for staging of distant metastases rather than local nodal disease.
3. PET is helpful for evaluating indeterminate liver lesions seen on CT.[18,19]

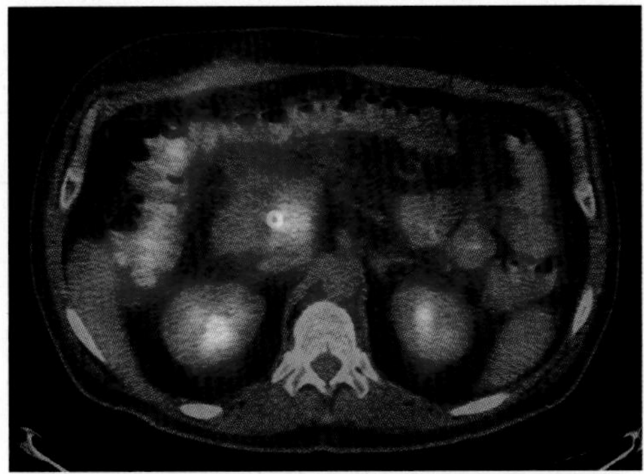

Fig. 21.5 Pancreatic cancer. Uptake is noted in a small pancreatic head cancer. This can be differentiated from inflammatory uptake around the stent by its eccentric location relative to the stent.

Accuracy and Comparison with Other Modalities

1. ***PET.*** Sensitivity 70%, specificity 93%[20]
2. ***Accuracy by site***
   a. *Liver*[21]
      - Very sensitive for metastases > 1 cm (97%)
      - Low sensitivity for metastases < 1 cm (43%)
      - High specificity (95%)

   b. *Lymph nodes.* Sensitivity 49%, specificity 63%[22]
   c. *Peritoneal metastasis.* Sensitivity 25% (does not detect microscopic spread)[22]
3. PET and CT are complementary in the detection of distant metastases in patients with pancreatic cancer. PET can miss liver and lung metastases, but it can detect nodal, peritoneal, and osseous metastases missed by CT.[23]

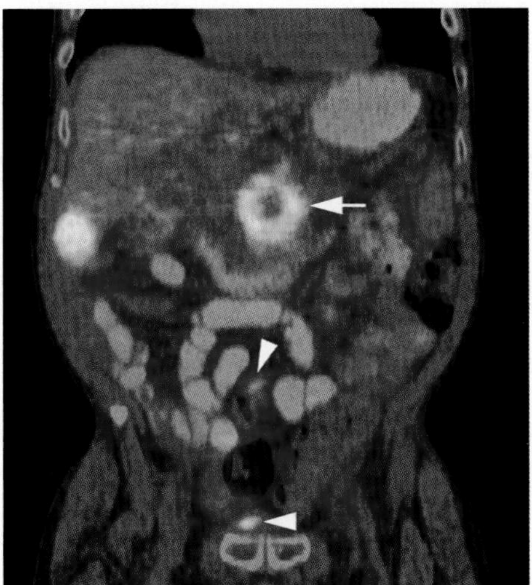

Fig. 21.4 Metastastic pancreatic cancer. Coronal positron emission tomography/computed tomography demonstrates ringlike uptake in a necrotic pancreatic carcinoma (*arrow*). A liver metastasis is present, as are multiple peritoneal metastases (*arrowheads*).

Pitfalls

1. ***Cholestasis.*** Cholestasis secondary to intrahepatic biliary dilatation can cause false-positive liver lesions.
2. ***Biliary stents.*** Recent biliary stent insertion can cause increased uptake along the stent tract. This can mimic nodal or liver metastases, particularly on axial images (as seen in **Fig. 6.33**, p. 60). It may be difficult to distinguish uptake along a stent from a pancreatic lesion (**Fig. 21.5**).

◆ Therapy Response and Prognosis

Clinical Indication: C

1. ***Therapy response.*** PET can assess response to neoadjuvant chemoradiation and intraoperative radiotherapy.[2,17] PET can predict tumor response before CT.

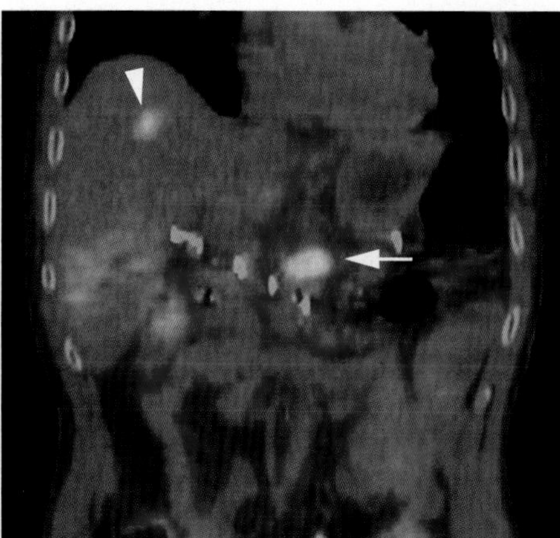

Fig. 21.6 Recurrent pancreatic cancer. Coronal positron emission tomography/computed tomography demonstrates a recurrence in the pancreatic bed (*arrow*) status post Whipple procedure. A liver metastasis (*arrowhead*) is present.

2. ***Postoperative recurrence.*** PET can detect disease recurrence after resection (**Fig. 21.6**).[24]
   a. PET is valuable in this setting, as it is may be difficult to evaluate the pancreatic region on CT after surgery and radiation secondary to scarring and inflammation.
   b. CT should be the first-line imaging modality for follow-up, with PET performed if CT is equivocal or if CT is negative and tumor markers are rising.
   c. PET is superior to CT for detecting local, nonlocoregional, and extra-abdominal recurrences. CT or MRI is superior for the detection of liver metastases.[25]
3. ***Prognosis***
   a. The degree of initial FDG uptake correlates with survival.[26–28]
   b. The degree of FDG uptake 1 month after chemotherapy correlates with survival.[29]

References

1. Kalady MF, Clary BM, Clark LA, et al. Clinical utility of positron emission tomography in the diagnosis and management of periampullary neoplasms. Ann Surg Oncol 2002;9(8):799–806
2. Rose DM, Delbeke D, Beauchamp RD, et al. 18Fluorodeoxyglucose-positron emission tomography in the management of patients with suspected pancreatic cancer. Ann Surg 1999;229(5):729–737
3. Orlando LA, Kulasingam SL, Matchar DB. Meta-analysis: the detection of pancreatic malignancy with positron emission tomography. Aliment Pharmacol Ther 2004;20(10):1063–1070
4. Shreve PD. Focal fluorine-18 fluorodeoxyglucose accumulation in inflammatory pancreatic disease. Eur J Nucl Med 1998;25(3):259–264
5. van Kouwen MC, Jansen JB, van Goor H, et al. FDG-PET is able to detect pancreatic carcinoma in chronic pancreatitis. Eur J Nucl Med Mol Imaging 2004; 32(4):399–404
6. Delbeke D, Rose DM, Chapman WC, et al. Optimal interpretation of FDG PET in the diagnosis, staging and management of pancreatic carcinoma. J Nucl Med 1999;40(11):1784–1791
7. Imdahl A, Nitzsche E, Krautmann F, et al. Evaluation of positron emission tomography with 2-[^{18}F]fluoro-2-deoxy-D-glucose for the differentiation of chronic pancreatitis and pancreatic cancer. Br J Surg 1999; 86(2):194–199
8. Nakamoto Y, Higashi T, Sakahara H, et al. Delayed (18)F-fluoro-2-deoxy-D-glucose positron emission tomography scan for differentiation between malignant and benign lesions in the pancreas. Cancer 2000; 89(12):2547–2554
9. Higashi T, Saga T, Nakamoto Y, et al. Diagnosis of pancreatic cancer using fluorine-18 fluorodeoxyglucose positron emission tomography (FDG PET)—usefulness and limitations in "clinical reality." Ann Nucl Med 2003;17(4):261–279
10. Diederichs CG, Staib L, Glatting G, et al. FDG PET: elevated plasma glucose reduces both uptake and detection rate of pancreatic malignancies. J Nucl Med 1998;39(6):1030–1033
11. Sperti C, Pasquali C, Decet G, et al. F-18-fluorodeoxyglucose positron emission tomography in differentiating malignant from benign pancreatic cysts: a prospective study. J Gastrointest Surg 2005;9(1): 22–29
12. Tann M, Sandrasegaran K, Jennings SG, Skandarajah A, McHenry L, Schmidt CM. Positron-emission tomography and computed tomography of cystic pancreatic masses. Clin Radiol 2007;62(8):745–751
13. Yoshioka M, Sato T, Furuya T, et al. Positron emission tomography with 2-deoxy-2-[(18)F] fluoro-D-glucose for diagnosis of intraductal papillary mucinous tumor of the pancreas with parenchymal invasion. J Gastroenterol 2003;38(12):1189–1193
14. Nakamoto Y, Higashi T, Sakahara H, et al. Evaluation of pancreatic islet cell tumors by fluorine-18 fluorodeoxyglucose positron emission tomography: comparison with other modalities. Clin Nucl Med 2000;25(2):115–119
15. Sato M, Takasaka I, Okumura T, et al. High F-18 fluorodeoxyglucose accumulation in solid pseudopapillary tumors of the pancreas. Ann Nucl Med 2006;20(6):431–436
16. Heinrich S, Goerres GW, Schafer M, et al. Positron emission tomography/computed tomography influences on the management of resectable pancreatic cancer and its cost-effectiveness. Ann Surg 2005;242(2):235–243
17. Kalra MK, Maher MM, Boland GW, et al. Correlation of positron emission tomography and CT in evaluating pancreatic tumors: technical and clinical implications. AJR Am J Roentgenol 2003;181(2):387–393
18. Hustinx R. PET imaging in assessing gastrointestinal tumors. Radiol Clin North Am 2004;42(6):1123–1139

19. Mertz HR, Sechopoulos P, Delbeke D, Leach SD. EUS, PET, and CT scanning for evaluation of pancreatic adenocarcinoma. Gastrointest Endosc 2000;52(3): 367–371
20. Gambhir SS, Czernin J, Schwimmer J, et al. A tabulated summary of the FDG PET literature. J Nucl Med 2001; 42(5, Suppl)1S–93S
21. Frohlich A, Diederichs CG, Staib L, et al. Detection of liver metastases from pancreatic cancer using FDG PET. J Nucl Med 1999;40(2):250–255
22. Diederichs CG, Staib L, Vogel J, et al. Values and limitations of 18F-fluorodeoxyglucose-positron-emission tomography with preoperative evaluation of patients with pancreatic masses. Pancreas 2000;20(2): 109–116
23. Nishiyama Y, Yamamoto Y, Yokoe K, et al. Contribution of whole body FDG-PET to the detection of distant metastasis in pancreatic cancer. Ann Nucl Med 2005;19(6):491–497
24. Franke C, Klapdor R, Meyerhoff K, Schauman M. 18-FDG positron emission tomography of the pancreas: diagnostic benefit in the follow-up of pancreatic carcinoma. Anticancer Res 1999;19(4A):2437–2442
25. Ruf J, Lopez HE, Oettle H, et al. Detection of recurrent pancreatic cancer: comparison of FDG-PET with CT/ MRI. Pancreatology 2005;5(2–3):266–272
26. Nakata B, Chung YS, Nishimura S, et al. ^{18}F-fluorodeoxyglucose positron emission tomography and the prognosis of patients with pancreatic adenocarcinoma. Cancer 1997;79(4):695–699
27. Sperti C, Pasquali C, Chierichetti F, et al. 18-Fluorodeoxyglucose positron emission tomography in predicting survival of patients with pancreatic carcinoma. J Gastrointest Surg 2003;7(8):953–959
28. Zimny M, Fass J, Bares R, et al. Fluorodeoxyglucose positron emission tomography and the prognosis of pancreatic carcinoma. Scand J Gastroenterol 2000;35(8):883–888
29. Maisey NR, Webb A, Flux GD, et al. FDG-PET in the prediction of survival of patients with cancer of the pancreas: a pilot study. Br J Cancer 2000;83(3): 287–293

22

Gynecologic Tumors

Eugene C. Lin and Abass Alavi

◆ Cervical Cancer[1,2]

The primary value of positron emission tomography (PET) in cervical cancer is in diagnosis of extrapelvic disease in initial staging and in detection of recurrence.

Primary Tumor

Clinical Indication: D

PET will detect the majority of primary tumors (**Figs. 22.1** and **22.2**), but is not as accurate as magnetic resonance imaging (MRI) for assessing locoregional involvement.[3] The degree of uptake in the primary tumor at diagnosis negatively correlates with treatment response and prognosis.[4]

Staging

Clinical Indication: B

PET is useful in staging locally advanced untreated cervical carcinoma. There are conflicting data on the value of PET in early-stage resectable cervical cancer.[5]

1. PET is more accurate than conventional imaging for evaluating lymph node metastases (**Figs. 22.1** and **22.2**).[6]
2. PET is particularly useful for evaluating disease in paraaortic nodes when computed tomography (CT) and MRI do not demonstrate adenopathy.[7]
3. ***Prognosis.*** Standardized uptake value (SUV) ≥ 3.3 in para-aortic lymph nodes is a negative prognostic factor.[8]
4. ***Radiation planning.*** When nodal radiotherapy is planned, the radiation field can be determined based on PET results.[9] There

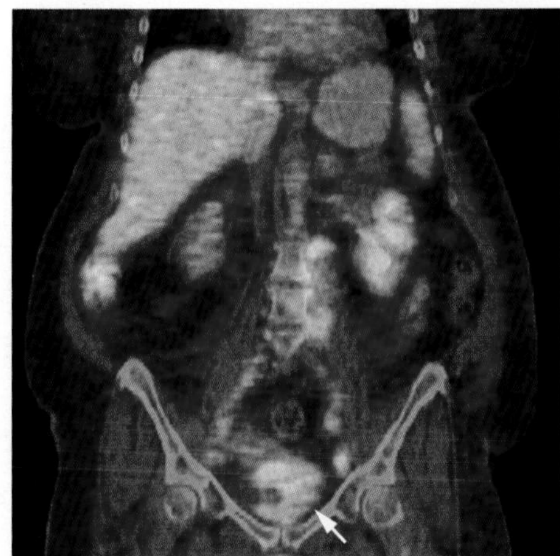

Fig. 22.1 Metastatic cervical cancer. Coronal positron emission tomography/computed tomography scan demonstrates uptake in a primary cervical carcinoma (*arrow*) with multiple pelvic and retroperitoneal nodal metastases.

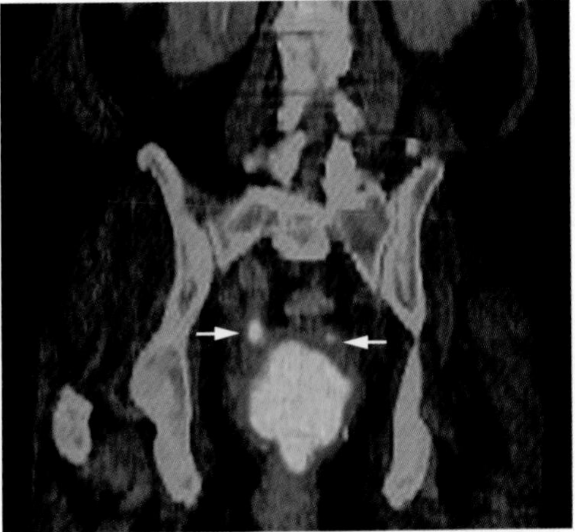

Fig. 22.2 Primary cervical cancer with pelvic nodal metastases. Coronal positron emission tomography/computed tomography scan demonstrates intense uptake in a primary cervical cancer with pelvic nodal metastases (*arrows*). Given the location of these nodal metastases, ureteral activity if present could potentially decrease sensitivity. (Courtesy of Bruce Higginbotham, Little Rock, AR.)

are also potential applications of PET in planning intracavitary brachytherapy.
- PET is particularly useful for detecting para-aortic nodal disease when only pelvic nodal enlargement is seen on CT and MRI. This results in changing the appropriate treatment field accordingly.

5. ***Positive PET.*** The positive predictive value of PET for pelvic and para-aortic nodes is high (90%+), and a positive PET study is sufficient to justify treatment by radiation or surgery.[10]
6. ***Negative PET.*** However, a negative PET does not preclude histologic lymph node sampling, as microscopic disease cannot be not excluded.

Accuracy and Comparison with Other Modalities

1. ***Body region (PET).*** **Table 22.1**[11]
2. ***MRI.*** PET is more accurate than MRI for pelvic nodal metastases.[11] PET/CT is more sensitive than MRI for pelvic nodal metastases, but there is no difference in specificity (**Table 22.2**).[12]
3. ***CT.*** PET detects more abnormal pelvic lymph nodes than CT (79% vs 47%).[11] Increased uptake in lymph nodes on PET even when CT is negative is associated with poor prognosis.[13]
4. ***Early-stage cervical cancer.*** PET and PET/CT have low to moderate sensitivity but high specificity for the lymph nodes metastases in early-stage cervical cancer. PET has a sensitivity of 53% and specificity of 90% for pelvic lymph node metastases in early-stage (IA to IIA) cervical cancer. The sensitivity for para-aortic nodes is even lower (25%).[14] Therefore, PET may have limited value in early-stage cervical cancer if MRI is negative.[15] PET/CT performs considerably better in early cervical cancer staging, with a sensitivity of 73% and specificity of 97%.[16]

Table 22.1 Sensitivity and Specificity of Positron Emission Tomography in the Detection of Nodal Metastases

Body Region	Sensitivity %	Specificity %
Aortic nodes	84	95
Pelvic nodes	79	99

Pearls

1. ***Urinary activity.*** Minimizing the effects of radioactive urine in the bladder and ureters is important in cervical cancer, as the specific areas of concern are the pelvic and para-aortic nodes (**Fig. 22.2**).
2. ***Dual time point imaging.*** Dual time point imaging (an additional delayed 3-hour scan) increases accuracy in para-aortic lymph nodes, particularly inferior para-aortic nodes.[17]

Pitfalls

1. In patients with early-stage disease, most of the false-negative results will be seen in the pelvis.

Table 22.2 Sensitivity and Specificity of Positron Emission Tomography (PET) versus Magnetic Resonance Imaging (MRI) in the Detection of Pelvic Nodal Metastases

	Sensitivity %	Specificity %
PET	79	99
MRI	72	96

2. In patients' advanced stages of disease, more false-negative results will be noted in para-aortic nodes.
3. Lymphangiography can cause false-positive nodal uptake.[18]
4. A short axis diameter > 0.5 cm is the size threshold for accurate identification of metastatic lymph nodes from cervical cancer by PET/CT.[16]

Recurrence

Clinical Indication: C

Limited data suggest that PET is more sensitive than conventional imaging for recurrent cervical cancer. PET might be best employed in patients with better prognoses (e.g., determined by squamous cell carcinoma antigen levels and symptoms) and possibility of salvage therapies. In these patients, accurate determination of recurrence location can help decide between salvage therapy and chemoradiation.[19,20]

Accuracy and Comparison with Other Modalities

1. ***PET.*** Sensitivity 96%, specificity 81%[11]
2. ***Body region.*** The sensitivity for recurrence is poor in the lung, retrovesical, and para-aortic lymph nodes.[21]
3. ***CT/MRI.*** PET is more sensitive than CT/MRI, but there is no difference in specificity.
   - PET is more sensitive than CT/MRI for metastases (89% vs 39%), but there is no difference in local lesion detection.[20]

Pearls

1. ***Symptoms.*** PET is useful in both symptomatic and asymptomatic women.[22]
2. ***Squamous carcinoma antigen.*** PET is useful in detecting recurrence if serum squamous carcinoma antigen is elevated.[23]

Pitfalls

Focal rectal activity on PET is a possible cause of false-positive results for recurrent local disease.

Therapy Response and Prognosis

Clinical Indication: C

1. ***Therapy response.*** There are limited data on the utility of PET for evaluation of therapy response in cervical carcinoma.
   a. *Radiotherapy effect.*[24] Following irradiation, increased fluorodeoxyglucose (FDG) activity is common from inflammation; therefore, increased FDG activity is sensitive but nonspecific for active tumor.
   b. *Neoadjuvant chemotherapy.*[25] Decrease in SUV correlates better with histological response than MRI in patients undergoing neoadjuvant therapy prior to radical hysterectomy.
2. ***Prognosis***
   a. *Pretherapy.* A visual grading system, which incorporates the primary tumor size, its shape, the degree of nonuniformity of FDG uptake, and the level of pelvic or para-aortic nodal involvement by PET, can estimate prognosis.[26]
   b. *Posttherapy.* Persistent FDG uptake following therapy, particularly in para-aortic nodes, is a strong predictor of poor prognosis.[27]

◆ Ovarian Cancer: Ovarian Masses[1,2]

Clinical Indication: C

PET has little role as a primary modality in the evaluation of primary ovarian masses.

1. PET employed alone results in a substantial number of false-positive and -negative results.
2. However, PET can complement the results of ultrasound and/or MRI findings and improve the overall accuracy of diagnostic imaging in patients with ovarian masses (as seen in **Fig. 6.38**).[28]

Accuracy and Comparison with Other Modalities

1. ***PET.*** Sensitivity 58 to 86%, specificity 54 to 86%[28]
2. ***Comparison:*** **Table 22.3**[28]

Table 22.3 Sensitivity and Specificity of Positron Emission Tomography versus Other Imaging Modalities in the Evaluation of Primary Ovarian Masses

	Sensitivity %	Specificity %
PET	58	76
US	92	60
MRI	83	84
Combined	92	85

Abbreviations: MRI, magnetic resonance imaging; PET, positron emission tomography; US, ultrasound.

Pearls

1. ***Standardized uptake value.*** There is no established SUV threshold for distinguishing malignant from benign ovarian lesions: published values range from 3.25 to 7.9.[29,30]
2. ***Visual threshold.*** One arbitrary visual threshold for malignancy includes any uptake equal to or greater than that of the liver.[28]
3. ***Postmenopausal uptake.*** Ovarian uptake in the postmenopausal woman is much more worrisome than in a premenopausal woman, and malignancy should be strongly suspected.[30]

Pitfalls

1. ***False-negatives.*** Low-grade tumors, early-stage ovarian carcinomas
2. ***False-positives***
   a. Inflammatory processes, endometriomas, benign cystic lesions (e.g., corpus luteum cyst, dermoid cyst, serous cyst), thecoma, physiologic uptake
   b. In premenopausal women, physiologic ovarian uptake is most common around ovulation and during the early luteal phase of the menstrual cycle.[31] Physiologic ovarian uptake can be minimized by scheduling PET just after menstruation.
   c. Bowel or iliac node activity on PET can be difficult to differentiate from ovarian activity (as seen in **Fig. 10.13**, p. 111).

Recurrence

Clinical Indication: B

1. PET is most useful when conventional imaging is inconclusive and cancer antigen (CA-) 125 is elevated.
2. ***Second look laparotomy.*** Although PET is accurate in the diagnosis of ovarian cancer recurrence (particularly if used in conjunction with conventional imaging techniques), it is still limited because a second-look laparotomy is still necessary if recurrence is strongly suspected. The sensitivity of PET for small volume disease (< 1 cm) is low compared with second-look laparotomy.[32] Despite this, PET can change management due to its high positive predictive value.[33,34]
   a. A positive PET scan can preclude the need for invasive surgical assessment.
   b. Tumor deposits large enough to be identified by PET may be considered for sur-

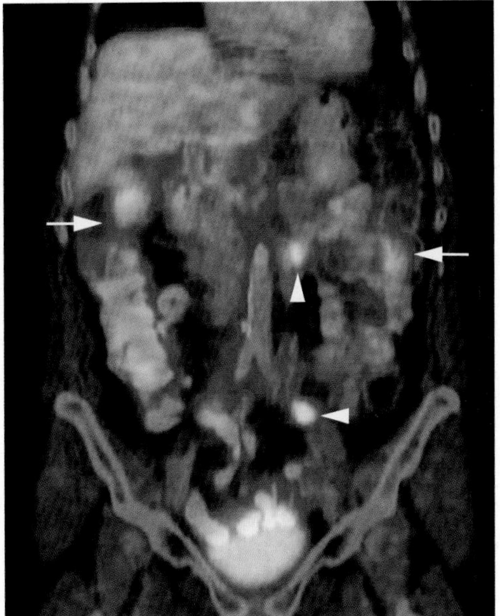

Fig. 22.3 Metastatic ovarian cancer. Coronal positron emission tomography/computed tomography (PET/CT) scan demonstrates both nodal (*arrowheads*) and peritoneal (*arrows*) metastases from ovarian cancer. PET has better sensitivity for nodal metastases than peritoneal metastases in ovarian cancer. (Courtesy of Carolyn Meltzer, MD, Atlanta, GA).

gical resection because these lesions may not respond to chemotherapy.

c. The small lesions that are missed by PET may be responsive to chemotherapy.

3. *Clinical suspicion.* The sensitivity of PET depends upon the level of clinical suspicion.

a. PET sensitivity is high if there is clinical suspicion of recurrence, particularly if this suspicion is based upon rising CA-125 levels.

- PET has the highest yield if used when CA-125 is 30 U/mL or greater.[35]

b. Sensitivity is lower if PET is used in patients who are judged to be disease-free based on clinical assessment. However, in a minority of patients with a normal CA-125, recurrence will be identified only with PET.[36]

c. The sensitivity of combined PET and CA-125 is high (98%).[36]

4. *Prognosis.* There is limited evidence as to the prognostic value of PET in suspected recurrent ovarian cancer. Patients with localized or no disease identified by PET may have improved survival,[37,38] but CA-125 may be more useful for prognosis than PET.[37]

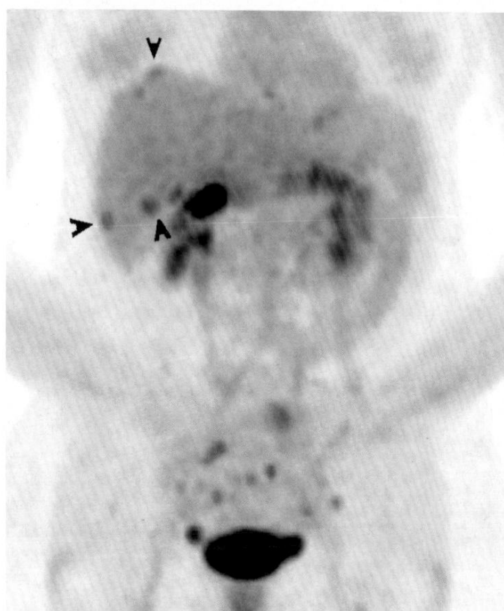

Fig. 22.4 Metastatic ovarian cancer. Coronal positron emission tomography scan in a patient with ovarian cancer demonstrates multiple serosal metastases around the liver (*arrowheads*) as well as multiple pelvic peritoneal metastases. (Courtesy of Ronald Korn, MD, PhD, Scottsdale, AZ.)

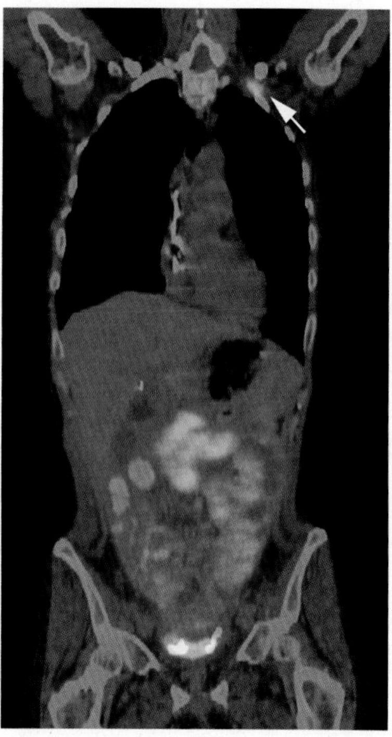

Fig. 22.5 Metastatic ovarian cancer. Coronal positron emission tomography/computed tomography scan demonstrates extensive peritoneal carcinomatosis secondary to ovarian cancer. This carcinomatosis has both a focal soft tissue component in the central omentum and a diffuse fluid component (note the poor visualization of the inferior border of the liver). There is also a left supraclavicular node metastasis (*arrow*).

Accuracy and Comparison with Other Modalities

1. *Clinical situation.* The accuracy of PET depends upon the clinical situation.[11]

a. Clinical suspicion of recurrence. Sensitivity 90%, specificity 86%

b. Rising CA-125, negative conventional imaging. Sensitivity 96%, specificity 80%

c. Negative conventional imaging and CA-125. Sensitivity 54%, specificity 73%

2. PET is most useful when interpreted in conjunction with conventional imaging modalities (CT, MRI).[33]

a. The accuracy increases from 79 to 94% when PET is interpreted in conjunction with conventional imaging modalities.[33]

b. PET is more specific than CT (94% vs 77%).[39]

3. ***PET/CT.*** Sensitivity 93%, specificity 97%[40]
   - PET/CT detects more lesions than PET or CT alone[41]
4. ***Body region***
   a. *Retroperitoneal nodes.* In ovarian cancer patients, PET is more sensitive in the retroperitoneum than the peritoneum.[42] However, the sensitivity of PET/CT for isolated retroperitoneal nodal disease is only 41%, with a specificity of 94%.[43] Thus, regional lymphadenectomy may still be necessary with a negative PET study, but PET has a high positive predictive value for retroperitoneal nodal disease with negative or equivocal CT findings.
   b. PET is more sensitive for lymph node metastases than peritoneal metastases (**Figs. 22.3, 22.4,** and **22.5**). With PET/CT, lesions as small as 0.5 cm can be detected,[34] but even with PET/CT imaging, sensitivity for peritoneal metastases < 1 cm is low.[39]
   c. The sensitivity is lowest in the pelvis.[34]

Pearls

It is important to understand the classic patterns of peritoneal spread when evaluating patients with ovarian cancer (see Chapter 10).

Pitfalls

Diffuse peritoneal carcinomatosis (**Fig. 22.5**) may not cause focal lesions and could be interpreted as a falsely negative study if windowed incorrectly.

Therapy Response

Clinical Indication: C

Limited data suggest that PET is useful for early prediction of response to neoadjuvant chemotherapy. Sequential PET studies after the first cycle of neoadjuvant chemotherapy may be more accurate than clinical or histopathological response criteria, including CA-125, in predicting response and survival.[44]

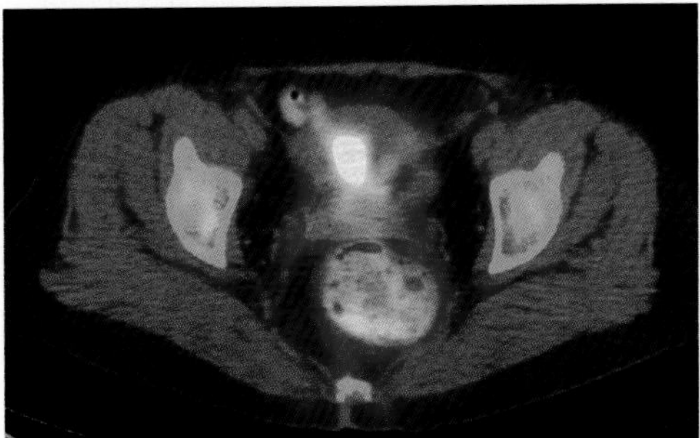

Fig. 22.6 Endometrial carcinoma. Axial positron emission tomography/computed tomography scan demonstrates intense endometrial uptake secondary to endometrial carcinoma. In a postmenopausal woman, this would be very suspicious for neoplasm; however, premenopausal women can have physiologic endometrial uptake, which varies during the menstrual cycle (see Chapter 6).

◆ Endometrial Cancer

Clinical Indication: C

There are limited data on the role of PET in endometrial cancer. The primary tumor is visible on PET in the majority of cases (**Fig. 22.6**).[45] PET has moderate sensitivity for predicting lymph node metastases preoperatively;[46] however, sensitivity is poor for lymph node metastases < 1 cm.[45] PET may be helpful for further evaluating equivocal extrauterine lesions seen on CT or MRI. PET may be more useful in primary advanced (stage III or IV) cancer.[47] In posttherapy surveillance, PET may be more accurate than CT or MRI[47,48] and is helpful in both suspected recurrence and detection of asymptomatic recurrent disease.[49]

References

1. Dehdashti F, Siegel BA. Evaluation of breast and gynecologic cancers by positron emission tomography. Semin Roentgenol 2002;37(2):151–168
2. Zimny M, Siggelkow W. Positron emission tomography scanning in gynecologic and breast cancers. Curr Opin Obstet Gynecol 2003;15(1):69–75
3. Belhocine T, Thille A, Fridman V, et al. Contribution of whole-body ^{18}FDG PET imaging in the management of cervical cancer. Gynecol Oncol 2002;87(1):90–97
4. Kidd EA, Siegel BA, Dehdashti F, Grigsby PW. The standardized uptake value for F-18 fluorodeoxyglucose is a sensitive predictive biomarker for cervical cancer treatment response and survival. Cancer 2007;110(8):1738–1744

5. Lai CH, Yen TC, Chang TC. Positron emission tomography imaging for gynecologic malignancy. Curr Opin Obstet Gynecol 2007;19(1):37–41
6. Rose PG, Adler LP, Rodriguez M, et al. Positron emission tomography for evaluating para-aortic nodal metastasis in locally advanced cervical cancer before surgical staging: a surgicopathologic study. J Clin Oncol 1999;17(1):41–45
7. Lin WC, Hung YC, Yeh LS, et al. Usefulness of (18)F-fluorodeoxyglucose positron emission tomography to detect para-aortic lymph nodal metastasis in advanced cervical cancer with negative computed tomography findings. Gynecol Oncol 2003;89(1):73–76
8. Yen TC, See LC, Lai CH, et al. Standardized uptake value in para-aortic lymph nodes is a significant prognostic factor in patients with primary advanced squamous cervical cancer. Eur J Nucl Med Mol Imaging 2008;25(3):493–501
9. Tsai CS, Chang TC, Lai CH, et al. Preliminary report of using FDG-PET to detect extrapelvic lesions in cervical cancer patients with enlarged pelvic lymph nodes on MRI/CT. Int J Radiat Oncol Biol Phys 2004;58(5):1506–1512
10. Narayan K, Hicks RJ, Jobling T, et al. A comparison of MRI and PET scanning in surgically staged loco-regionally advanced cervical cancer: potential impact on treatment. Int J Gynecol Cancer 2001;11(4):263–271
11. Havrilesky LJ, Kulasingam SL, Matchar DB, Myers ER. FDG-PET for management of cervical and ovarian cancer. Gynecol Oncol 2005;97(1):183–191
12. Choi HJ, Roh JW, Seo SS, et al. Comparison of the accuracy of magnetic resonance imaging and positron emission tomography/computed tomography in the presurgical detection of lymph node metastases in patients with uterine cervical carcinoma: a prospective study. Cancer 2006;106(4):914–922
13. Grigsby PW, Siegel BA, Dehdashti F. Lymph node staging by positron emission tomography in patients with carcinoma of the cervix. J Clin Oncol 2001;19(17):3745–3749
14. Wright JD, Dehdashti F, Herzog TJ, et al. Preoperative lymph node staging of early-stage cervical carcinoma by [^{18}F]-fluoro-2-deoxy-D-glucose-positron emission tomography. Cancer 2005;104(11):2484–2491
15. Chou HH, Chang TC, Yen TC, et al. Low value of [^{18}F]-fluoro-2-deoxy-D-glucose positron emission tomography in primary staging of early-stage cervical cancer before radical hysterectomy. J Clin Oncol 2006;24(1):123–128
16. Sironi S, Buda A, Picchio M, et al. Lymph node metastasis in patients with clinical early-stage cervical cancer: detection with integrated FDG PET/CT. Radiology 2006;238(1):272–279
17. Ma SY, See LC, Lai CH, et al. Delayed (18)F-FDG PET for detection of paraaortic lymph node metastases in cervical cancer patients. J Nucl Med 2003;44(11):1775–1783
18. Reinhardt MJ, Ehritt-Braun C, Vogelgesang D, et al. Metastatic lymph nodes in patients with cervical cancer: detection with MR imaging and FDG PET. Radiology 2001;218(3):776–782
19. Belhocine TZ. ^{18}F-FDG PET imaging in posttherapy monitoring of cervical cancers: from diagnosis to prognosis. J Nucl Med 2004;45(10):1602–1604
20. Yen TC, See LC, Chang TC, et al. Defining the priority of using ^{18}F-FDG PET for recurrent cervical cancer. J Nucl Med 2004;45(10):1632–1639
21. Ryu SY, Kim MH, Choi SC, et al. Detection of early recurrence with ^{18}F-FDG PET in patients with cervical cancer. J Nucl Med 2003;44(3):347–352
22. Chung HH, Kim SK, Kim TH, et al. Clinical impact of FDG-PET imaging in post-therapy surveillance of uterine cervical cancer: from diagnosis to prognosis. Gynecol Oncol 2006;103(1):165–170
23. Chang TC, Law KS, Hong JH, et al. Positron emission tomography for unexplained elevation of serum squamous cell carcinoma antigen levels during follow-up for patients with cervical malignancies: a phase II study. Cancer 2004;101(1):164–171
24. Nakamoto Y, Eisbruch A, Achtyes ED, et al. Prognostic value of positron emission tomography using F-18-fluorodeoxyglucose in patients with cervical cancer undergoing radiotherapy. Gynecol Oncol 2002;84(2):289–295
25. Yoshida Y, Kurokawa T, Kawahara K, et al. Metabolic monitoring of advanced uterine cervical cancer neoadjuvant chemotherapy by using [F-18]-fluorodeoxyglucose positron emission tomography: preliminary results in three patients. Gynecol Oncol 2004;95(3):597–602
26. Miller TR, Pinkus E, Dehdashti F, Grigsby PW. Improved prognostic value of ^{18}F-FDG PET using a simple visual analysis of tumor characteristics in patients with cervical cancer. J Nucl Med 2003;44(2):192–197
27. Grigsby PW, Siegel BA, Dehdashti F, Mutch DG. Posttherapy surveillance monitoring of cervical cancer by FDG-PET. Int J Radiat Oncol Biol Phys 2003;55(4):907–913
28. Fenchel S, Grab D, Nuessle K, et al. Asymptomatic adnexal masses: correlation of FDG PET and histopathologic findings. Radiology 2002;223(3):780–788
29. Hubner KF, McDonald TW, Niethammer JG, et al. Assessment of primary and metastatic ovarian cancer by positron emission tomography (PET) using 2-[^{18}F]deoxyglucose (2-[18F]FDG). Gynecol Oncol 1993;51(2):197–204
30. Lerman H, Metser U, Grisaru D, et al. Normal and abnormal ^{18}F-FDG endometrial and ovarian uptake in pre- and postmenopausal patients: assessment by PET/CT. J Nucl Med 2004;45(2):266–271
31. Kim SK, Kang KW, Roh JW, et al. Incidental ovarian ^{18}F-FDG accumulation on PET: correlation with the menstrual cycle. Eur J Nucl Med Mol Imaging 2005;32(7):757–763
32. Rose PG, Faulhaber P, Miraldi F, Abdul-Karim FW. Positive emission tomography for evaluating a complete clinical response in patients with ovarian or peritoneal carcinoma: correlation with second-look laparotomy. Gynecol Oncol 2001;82(1):17–21
33. Nakamoto Y, Saga T, Ishimori T, et al. Clinical value of positron emission tomography with FDG for recurrent ovarian cancer. AJR Am J Roentgenol 2001;176(6):1449–1454
34. Sironi S, Messa C, Mangili G, et al. Integrated FDG PET/CT in patients with persistent ovarian cancer: correlation with histologic findings. Radiology 2004;233(2):433–440
35. Menzel C, Dobert N, Hamscho N, et al. The influence of CA 125 and CEA levels on the results of (18)F-deoxyglucose positron emission tomography in suspected recurrence of epithelial ovarian cancer. Strahlenther Onkol 2004;180(8):497–501
36. Murakami M, Miyamoto T, Iida T, et al. Whole-body positron emission tomography and tumor marker CA125 for detection of recurrence in epithelial ovarian cancer. Int J Gynecol Cancer 2006;16(Suppl 1):99–107

37. Kurosaki H, Oriuchi N, Okazaki A, et al. Prognostic value of FDG-PET in patients with ovarian carcinoma following surgical treatment. Ann Nucl Med 2006;20(3):171–174
38. Simcock B, Neesham D, Quinn M, et al. The impact of PET/CT in the management of recurrent ovarian cancer. Gynecol Oncol 2006;103(1):271–276
39. Pannu HK, Cohade C, Bristow RE, et al. PET-CT detection of abdominal recurrence of ovarian cancer: radiologic-surgical correlation. Abdom Imaging 2004;29(3):398–403
40. Chung HH, Kang WJ, Kim JW, et al. Role of [(18)F]FDG PET/CT in the assessment of suspected recurrent ovarian cancer: correlation with clinical or histological findings. Eur J Nucl Med Mol Imaging 2007;34(4):480–486
41. Hauth EA, Antoch G, Stattaus J, et al. Evaluation of integrated whole-body PET/CT in the detection of recurrent ovarian cancer. Eur J Radiol 2005;56(2):263–268
42. Drieskens O, Stroobants S, Gysen M, et al. Positron emission tomography with FDG in the detection of peritoneal and retroperitoneal metastases of ovarian cancer. Gynecol Obstet Invest 2003;55(3):130–134
43. Bristow RE, Giuntoli RL, Pannu HK, et al. Combined PET/CT for detecting recurrent ovarian cancer limited to retroperitoneal lymph nodes. Gynecol Oncol 2005; 99(2):294–300
44. Avril N, Sassen S, Schmalfeldt B, et al. Prediction of response to neoadjuvant chemotherapy by sequential F-18-fluorodeoxyglucose positron emission tomography in patients with advanced-stage ovarian cancer. J Clin Oncol 2005;23(30):7445–7453
45. Suzuki R, Miyagi E, Takahashi N, et al. Validity of positron emission tomography using fluoro-2-deoxyglucose for the preoperative evaluation of endometrial cancer. Int J Gynecol Cancer 2007;17(4):890–896
46. Horowitz NS, Dehdashti F, Herzog TJ, et al. Prospective evaluation of FDG-PET for detecting pelvic and para-aortic lymph node metastasis in uterine corpus cancer. Gynecol Oncol 2004;95(3):546–551
47. Chao A, Chang TC, Ng KK, et al. ^{18}F-FDG PET in the management of endometrial cancer. Eur J Nucl Med Mol Imaging 2006;33(1):36–44
48. Saga T, Higashi T, Ishimori T, et al. Clinical value of FDG-PET in the follow up of post-operative patients with endometrial cancer. Ann Nucl Med 2003;17(3):197–203
49. Belhocine T, De BC, Hustinx R, Willems-Foidart J. Usefulness of (18)F-FDG PET in the post-therapy surveillance of endometrial carcinoma. Eur J Nucl Med Mol Imaging 2002;29(9):1132–1139

23

Urologic Tumors

Eugene C. Lin and Abass Alavi

◆ Renal Cell Carcinoma:[1] Renal Masses

Clinical Indication: C

The role of positron emission tomography (PET) in the evaluation of renal masses is somewhat limited. Both solid and cystic renal masses can be evaluated. Renal masses are sometimes detected incidentally on PET images.

1. ***Solid lesions.*** PET imaging is of limited value in solid lesions demonstrated by conventional imaging techniques because resection is usually necessary.
2. ***Indeterminate renal cysts***
   a. A positive PET scan in an indeterminate renal cyst (**Fig. 23.1**) is very specific for malignancy, and further diagnostic tests such as cyst aspiration can be avoided before resection.[2]
   b. However, a negative PET scan does not completely rule out malignancy.
3. ***Renal metastases.*** Limited data suggest that PET can detect renal metastases.[3] Primary and metastatic renal tumors have a similar degree of fluorodeoxyglucose (FDG) uptake.[4]

Accuracy and Comparison with Other Modalities[5]

FDG PET is specific for the diagnosis of malignancy in renal masses, but sensitivity will vary depending upon lesion size and location (**Table 23.1**).

Pearls and Pitfalls

1. ***Necessity of diuresis.*** Diuresis is extremely important if PET is performed to evaluate a renal mass.

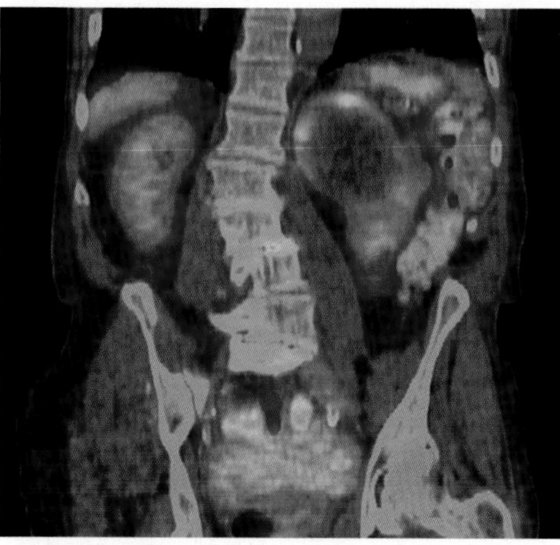

Fig. 23.1 Cystic renal cell carcinoma. Coronal positron emission tomography/computed tomography demonstrates focal areas of peripheral uptake in a large left upper pole renal cyst, consistent with cystic renal cell carcinoma. However, the lack of fluorodeoxyglucose in a complex renal cyst would not exclude renal cell carcinoma.

Table 23.1 Sensitivity and Specificity of Positron Emission Tomography (PET) versus Computed Tomography (CT) in the Detection of Renal Tumors

	Sensitivity %	Specificity %
PET	60	100
CT	92	100

a. False-negative results can result from the presence of urinary activity adjacent to and obscuring the lesion (**Fig. 23.2**).
b. False-positive results can occur from focal collections of urine that mimic a lesion.

2. ***Adjacent lesions.*** Lesions outside but adjacent to the kidney can sometimes appear to be exophytic renal masses on PET (see **Fig. 7.5**, p. 82).
   - Correlation with anatomical imaging is necessary before a diagnosis of an exophytic renal mass is made.
3. ***Degree of uptake.*** FDG uptake greater than that of renal parenchyma is noted in the majority of renal cell carcinomas, but the degree of uptake is sometimes only minimally more than the surrounding tissues and may be difficult to differentiate from normal parenchyma (**Fig. 23.3**).

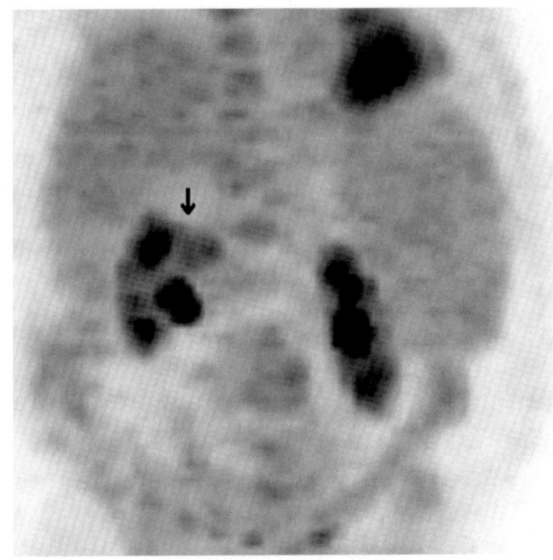

Fig. 23.3 Subtle renal cell carcinoma. Coronal positron emission tomography scan demonstrates a subtle medial right upper pole renal mass (*arrow*). Note that this is only slightly more intense than normal renal parenchyma and can only be diagnosed by the contour deformity. Most renal cell carcinomas are more intense than this.

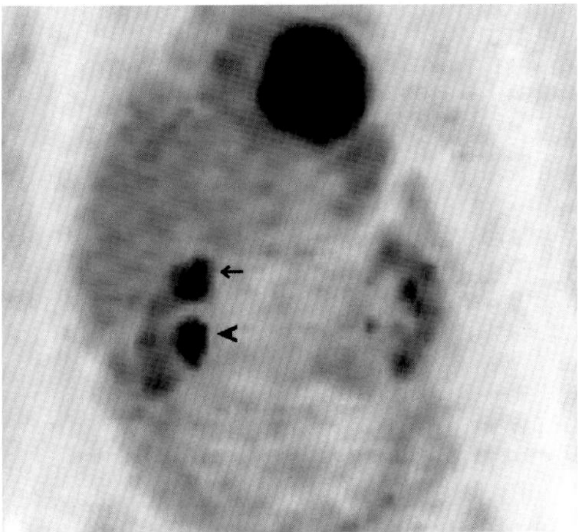

Fig. 23.2 Renal mass or collecting system? Coronal positron emission tomography scan demonstrates focal activity in the upper pole of the right kidney (*arrow*). Note the similarity of appearance to renal collecting system activity (*arrowhead*). In this case, it is difficult to determine whether this is uptake in a renal mass or stasis in the upper pole collecting system. The uptake was secondary to a renal cell carcinoma.

4. ***Oncocytomas.*** Oncocytomas are usually isointense with the adjacent renal parenchyma, although uptake can occasionally be in the range of carcinoma.[6,7]
5. ***Angiomyolipomas.*** The spectrum of uptake in angiomyolipomas has not been reported, but there has been one reported case of false-positive uptake in an angiomyolipoma.[8]
6. ***Inflammatory lesions.*** Inflammatory lesions such as xanthogranulomatous pyelonephritis can have false-positive increased uptake.[9]

Staging and Restaging

Clinical Indication: C

1. PET is primarily useful in
   a. Identifying distant metastases (**Fig. 23.4**)
   b. Evaluating indeterminate lesions seen on anatomical imaging techniques
   c. Solitary metastasis being considered for resection

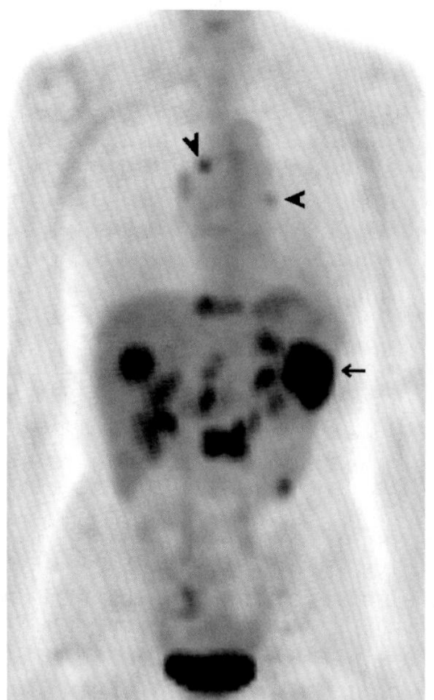

Fig. 23.4 Metastatic renal cell carcinoma. Coronal positron emission tomography scan demonstrates a left renal cell carcinoma (*arrow*) metastatic to the bone, liver, abdominal nodes, and mediastinum (*arrowheads*).

2. PET is unlikely to be helpful in tumors with a low histological grade and limited local stage (≤ T2).[6]
3. ***Restaging.*** PET is most helpful in further evaluating patients with indeterminate lesions seen on anatomical imaging modalities.

Accuracy and Comparison with Other Modalities

1. ***Staging and PET.*** Sensitivity 64%, specificity 100%[10]
   a. PET is insensitive but specific.
   b. PET is less sensitive than computed tomography (CT) in all anatomical sites but is more specific in the lungs and bone marrow.[5]
   c. PET can sometimes detect bone marrow metastases from renal cell carcinoma, which are not detected on a bone scan.
2. ***Restaging and PET.*** Sensitivity 71%, specificity 75%[11]

Pitfalls

Given the relatively low sensitivity, a negative PET scan does not exclude the presence of disease for either staging or restaging purposes.

◆ Testicular Cancer

Staging

Clinical Indication: C

The accuracy of PET in detected testicular neoplasms is unknown, but PET can sometimes detect unsuspected testicular neoplasms (**Fig. 23.5**). PET is valuable in staging stage II testicular germ cell tumors (**Fig. 23.6**), but may not be of additional value in patients with stage I tumors.[12]

Accuracy and Comparison with Other Modalities

1. ***PET.*** Sensitivity 82%, specificity 94%[13]
2. The primary value of PET compared with CT is in reducing false-positive results.

Pitfalls

1. Both PET and CT will miss disease in small retroperitoneal nodes (≤ 1 cm).
2. PET cannot detect mature teratoma.

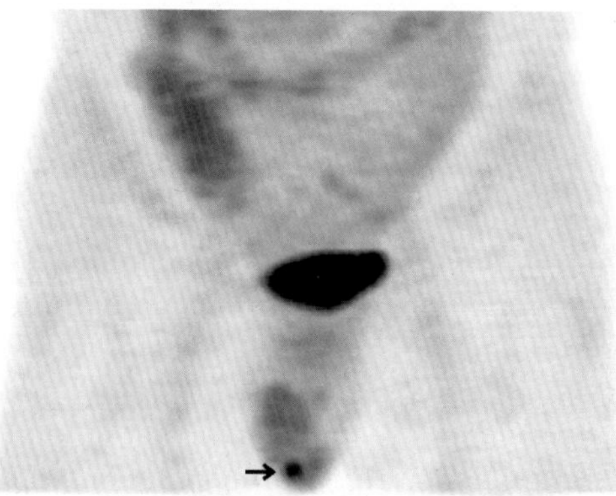

Fig. 23.5 Testicular tumor. Focal testicular uptake is noted (*arrow*) on a coronal positron emission tomography scan. This was an incidentally detected right testicular seminoma.

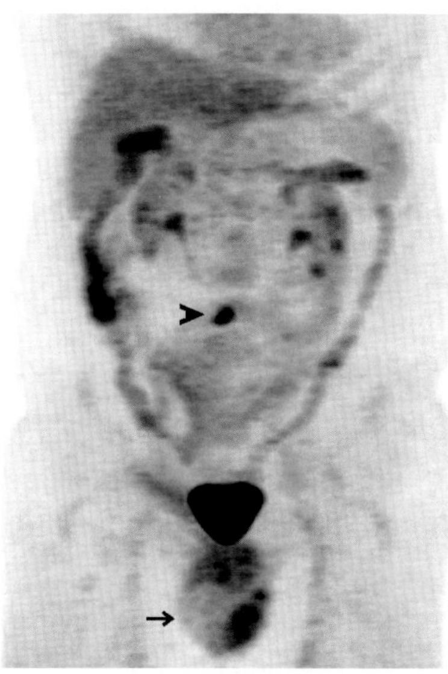

Fig. 23.6 Metastatic testicular cancer. Coronal positron emission tomography scan demonstrates uptake in a metastatic retroperitoneal node (*arrowhead*). The patient is status post right orchiectomy (*arrow*) for testicular cancer.

Recurrence

Clinical Indication: B

PET is useful in evaluating tumor recurrence in both seminomas and nonseminomatous germ cell tumors (NSGCT), although it is more useful in seminomas.

1. ***Histology.*** It is important to know whether the primary tumor was a seminoma or NSGCT. Mature teratoma does not have increased uptake. Because mature teratoma is present in more than 40% of resected masses in NSGCT, it is a major source of false-negative results (mature teratoma is benign but is removed due to risk of malignant transformation). In seminomas only 4% of residual lesions are mature teratoma. Thus, FDG PET has a greater role in evaluating tumor recurrence in seminoma than in NSGCT (**Table 23.2**).[14,15]
2. ***Lesion size.*** The management of postchemotherapy masses in patients with seminoma is controversial. Lesions < 3 cm are usually followed by imaging. Lesions > 3 cm are more likely to contain residual tumor, and management ranges from observation to resection.
   - PET is very effective in differentiating residual tumor from fibrosis in lesions ≥ 3 cm (**Fig. 23.7**).[14–16]
3. ***Elevated tumor markers***
   - ***a.*** PET is helpful in patients with elevated tumor markers regardless of whether a residual mass is seen on CT.
   - ***b.*** In patients with elevated markers and a residual mass, the negative predictive value is low (50%), but PET is often the first modality to identify the recurrence on follow-up studies.[17]

Table 23.2 Sensitivity and Specificity of Positron Emission Tomography (PET) versus Computed Tomography (CT) in the Detection of Recurrent Seminomas

	Sensitivity %	Specificity %
PET	80	100
CT	70	74

Accuracy and Comparison with Other Modalities

1. ***Seminomas***[15]
   - ***a.*** PET is more accurate than CT, primarily due to the higher specificity of PET.
   - ***b.*** However, there have been reported cases of residual masses, some > 3 cm, with

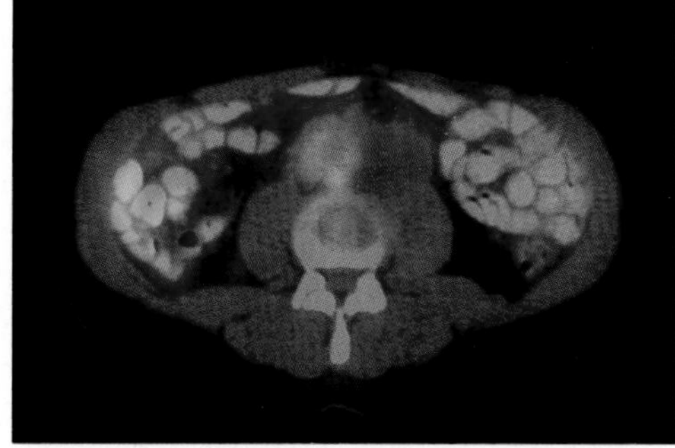

Fig. 23.7 Seminoma with retroperitoneal mass. Axial positron emission tomography/computed tomography in a patient with seminoma demonstrates a large retroperitoneal mass. The right aspect has fluorodeoxyglucose (FDG) uptake consistent with tumor; the left aspect is cystic-appearing without FDG uptake.

false-positive uptake secondary to necrosis or inflammation.[18]

2. ***NSGST (stage I).*** Sensitivity 70%, specificity 100%[19]
   - However, in one study high-risk (lymphovascular invasion–positive) patients with clinical stage I NSGSTs and a negative PET had a high risk of relapse.[20] Thus, PET may not be sufficiently sensitive in this setting.

Pearls

1. ***Standardized uptake value (SUV)***
   a. Seminomas usually have higher SUVs than nonseminomatous lesions.[21]
   b. If SUV is > 5 in a lesion, it is much more likely to be viable tumor than mature teratoma or necrosis/fibrosis.[22]
2. ***Timing.*** PET should be performed between 4 and 12 weeks after chemotherapy.[14,15]
   - Earlier imaging may result in false-positive results from inflammation following therapy.

Pitfalls

1. PET does not detect mature teratomas.
2. False-positives secondary to necrosis or inflammation are possible in residual masses, some > 3 cm in size.[23]

◆ Bladder Cancer

Clinical Indication: C

PET can detect both regional lymph node disease (**Fig. 23.8**) and distant metastases from bladder cancer. A major obstacle to detecting regional lymph node disease is bladder activity; therefore, bladder catheterization is often necessary. There are very limited data evaluating PET in bladder cancer. Potential uses are preoperative staging, detection of pelvic recurrence, differentiation of fibrosis from tumor, and detection of distant metastases.[8] PET may have prognostic value, as patients with PET-positive disease during preoperative staging have lower median survival time.[23]

Accuracy

1. ***Preoperative staging***
   a. *PET.* Sensitivity 60%, specificity 88%[23]
   b. Correlation of PET and CT improves accuracy.

◆ Prostate Cancer

Clinical Indication: D

FDG PET is of limited value in prostate cancer due to the low FDG avidity of most prostate cancer cells. In addition, urinary activity limits pelvic evaluation unless bladder catheterization and diuresis are used. The C-11 labeled tracers (acetate, choline, and methionine) have shown more promise than FDG. The primary use of FDG PET is in recurrent disease with a rising prostate-specific antigen (PSA).

1. ***Primary tumor***
   a. Most (81%) primary prostate tumors (**Fig. 23.9**) have low FDG uptake.[24]

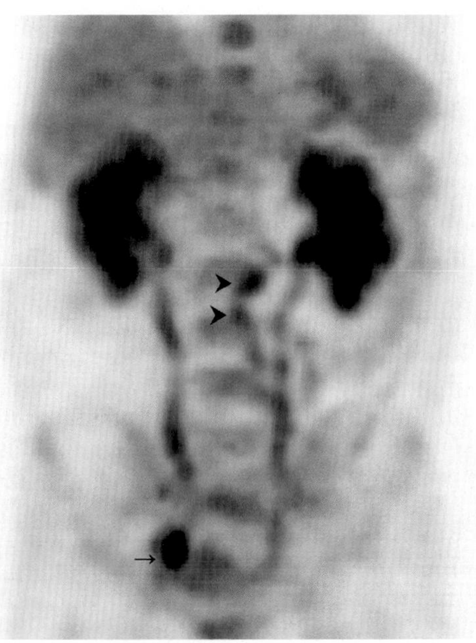

Fig. 23.8 Metastatic bladder cancer. Coronal positron emission tomography scan demonstrates a right bladder cancer (*arrow*) metastatic to retroperitoneal nodes (*arrowheads*). The bladder cancer is visualized only because the bladder is empty from Foley catheter placement.

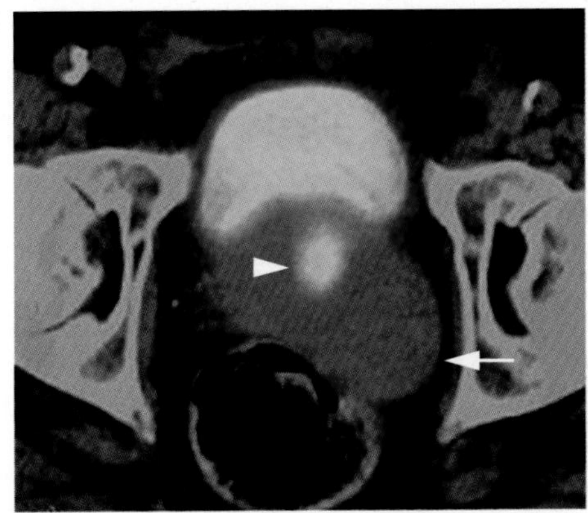
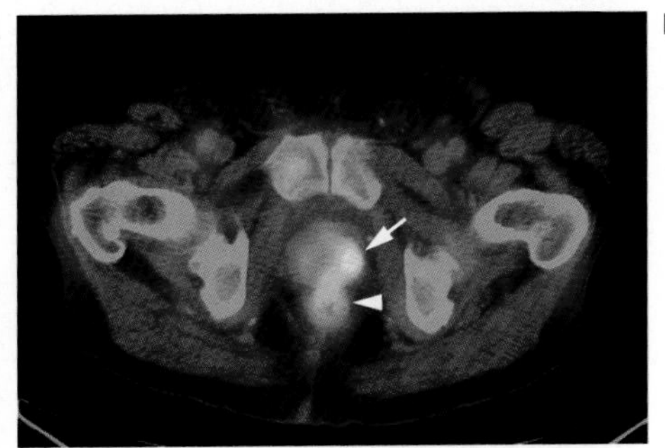

Fig. 23.9 Variable uptake in prostate cancer. **(A)** Axial positron emission tomography/computed tomography (PET/CT) scan demonstrates a large exophytic left prostate carcinoma (*arrow*) with no fluorodeoxyglucose uptake. Central prostatic activity (*arrowhead*) is in the urethra. **(B)** Axial PET/CT demonstrates focal uptake is present in a left prostate cancer (*arrow*). Many prostate carcinomas do not demonstrate this degree of uptake. Note the proximity of the prostate to rectal activity (*arrowhead*), which is a common cause of false-positive results when evaluating for local recurrence. (**[A]** Courtesy of Bruce Higginbotham, MD, Seattle, WA.)

b. The amount of uptake overlaps with benign prostate hyperplasia and does not correlate with stage or grade.

2. Preoperative staging

a. PET is insensitive for staging pelvic lymph nodes prior to surgery.

b. PET is not useful for evaluating organ-confined prostate cancer defined by conventional work-up.

3. Recurrence

a. *Clinical/imaging factors*. PET has potential value where the following are applicable:[25–27]

- PSA > 4 ng/mL or increases > 0.2 ng/mL per month
- Advanced cancer
- Untreated patient
- Incomplete or lack of response to treatment
- Negative bone scan
- Equivocal pelvic CT findings

b. *Local recurrence*

- PET has poor accuracy for differentiating local recurrence and scar.[28]

c. *Metastatic disease*

- PET has limited sensitivity for metastatic disease.
- However, PET is more likely to detect distant metastases than local recurrence.[8]

4. Therapy response

a. PET may have some role as a surrogate marker of response to chemotherapy in hormone-resistant disease.[29]

b. *Antiandrogenic treatment*. PET may have some value in monitoring antiandrogenic treatment.[8]

- Patients with a flare phenomenon seen on bone scan may be more accurately assessed with PET.

Accuracy and Comparison with Other Modalities

1. Recurrence

a. *PET*. Sensitivity 79%, specificity 66%[8]

b. These values were obtained at PSA levels > 2.4 ng/mL.

c. Overall FDG PET detects local or systemic disease in 31% of patients with a PSA relapse.[30]

d. PET is superior to CT but inferior to MRI for detection of recurrence in the prostate bed.

e. PET may be able to replace CT in the setting of suspected recurrence, but other modalities such as endorectal MRI for local recurrence and bone scan for bone metastases would still be necessary.

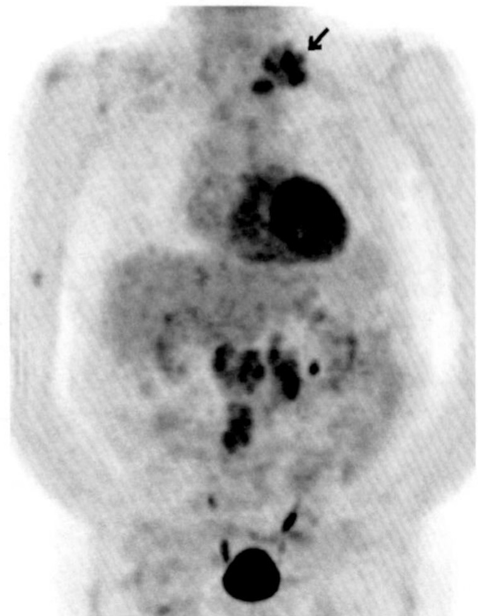

Fig. 23.10 Metastatic prostate cancer. Coronal positron emission tomography (PET) scan demonstrates metastatic disease from prostate cancer to retroperitoneal and left supraclavicular nodes (*arrow*). The left supraclavicular nodes are a common area of nonregional nodal spread (via the thoracic duct) from prostate cancer. (Courtesy of Ronald Korn, MD, PhD, Scottsdale, AZ.)

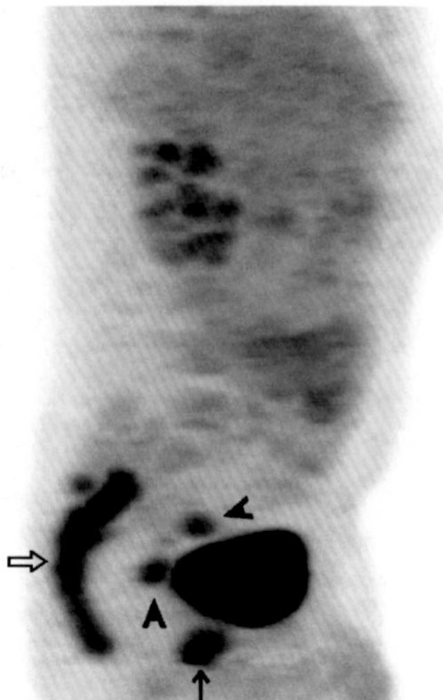

Fig. 23.11 Metastatic prostate cancer. Sagittal positron emission tomography (PET) scan demonstrates uptake in a primary prostate carcinoma (*arrow*) with sacral (*open arrow*) and pelvic nodal (*arrowheads*) metastases.

2. ***Body region.*** PET is more useful for soft tissue and nodal metastases (**Figs. 23.10** and **23.11**) than for bone metastases.
3. ***Bone metastasis***
   a. PET is significantly less sensitive but more specific than bone scan for sclerotic prostate cancer metastasis.
   b. The reported sensitivity of PET is as low as 18% (androgen-independent disease) relative to bone scan.[31]
   c. Lesions seen on bone scan only are usually quiescent (stable compared with prior scans).[5]
   d. Lesions seen on PET scan only are usually active (and become positive on subsequent bone scans).
4. ***Comparison to CT.*** PET is as sensitive as or more sensitive than CT for overall detection of metastatic disease (however, CT has poor sensitivity in prostate cancer).

Pitfalls

1. ***Antiandrogenic treatment.*** Androgen ablation decreases tumor glucose utilization.[32] PET is less sensitive in patients who are being treated with antiandrogenic hormones. However, PET may have value in predicting response to antiandrogenic treatment.

References

1. Mathews D, Oz OK. Positron emission tomography in prostate and renal cell carcinoma. Curr Opin Urol 2002;12(5):381–385
2. Goldberg MA, Mayo-Smith WW, Papanicolaou N, et al. FDG PET characterization of renal masses: preliminary experience. Clin Radiol 1997;52(7):510–515
3. Kaneta T, Hakamatsuka T, Yamada T, et al. FDG PET in solitary metastatic/secondary tumor of the kidney: a report of three cases and a review of the relevant literature. Ann Nucl Med 2006;20(1):79–82
4. Kumar R, Chauhan A, Lakhani P, et al. 2-deoxy-2-[F-18]fluoro-D-glucose-positron emission tomography in characterization of solid renal masses. Mol Imaging Biol 2005;7(6):431–439
5. Kang DE, White RL Jr, Zuger JH, et al. Clinical use of fluorodeoxyglucose F 18 positron emission tomography for detection of renal cell carcinoma. J Urol 2004;171(5):1806–1809
6. Aide N, Cappele O, Bottet P, et al. Efficiency of [(18)F]FDG PET in characterising renal cancer and detecting distant metastases: a comparison with CT. Eur J Nucl Med Mol Imaging 2003;30(9):1236–1245
7. Ramdave S, Thomas GW, Berlangieri SU, et al. Clinical role of F-18 fluorodeoxyglucose positron emission tomography for detection and management of renal cell carcinoma. J Urol 2001;166(3):825–830
8. Schoder H, Larson SM. Positron emission tomography for prostate, bladder, and renal cancer. Semin Nucl Med 2004;34(4):274–292

9. Ak I, Can C. F-18 FDG PET in detecting renal cell carcinoma. Acta Radiol 2005;46(8):895–899
10. Majhail NS, Urbain JL, Albani JM, et al. F-18 fluorodeoxyglucose positron emission tomography in the evaluation of distant metastases from renal cell carcinoma. J Clin Oncol 2003;21(21):3995–4000
11. Jadvar H, Kherbache HM, Pinski JK, Conti PS. Diagnostic role of [F-18]-FDG positron emission tomography in restaging renal cell carcinoma. Clin Nephrol 2003;60(6):395–400
12. Albers P, Bender H, Yilmaz H, et al. Positron emission tomography in the clinical staging of patients with stage I and II testicular germ cell tumors. Urology 1999;53(4):808–811
13. Gambhir SS, Czernin J, Schwimmer J, et al. A tabulated summary of the FDG PET literature. J Nucl Med 2001;42(5, Suppl):1S–93S
14. De Santis M, Bokemeyer C, Becherer A, et al. Predictive impact of 2-18fluoro-2-deoxy-D-glucose positron emission tomography for residual postchemotherapy masses in patients with bulky seminoma. J Clin Oncol 2001;19(17):3740–3744
15. De Santis M, Becherer A, Bokemeyer C, et al. 2-18fluoro-deoxy-D-glucose positron emission tomography is a reliable predictor for viable tumor in postchemotherapy seminoma: an update of the prospective multicentric SEMPET trial. J Clin Oncol 2004;22(6):1034–1039
16. Becherer A, De Santis M, Karanikas G, et al. FDG PET is superior to CT in the prediction of viable tumour in post-chemotherapy seminoma residuals. Eur J Radiol 2005;54(2):284–288
17. Hain SF, O'Doherty MJ, Timothy AR, et al. Fluorodeoxyglucose positron emission tomography in the evaluation of germ cell tumours at relapse. Br J Cancer 2000;83(7):863–869
18. Lewis DA, Tann M, Kesler K, et al. Positron emission tomography scans in postchemotherapy seminoma patients with residual masses: a retrospective review from Indiana University Hospital. J Clin Oncol 2006;24(34):e54–e55
19. Lassen U, Daugaard G, Eigtved A, et al. Whole-body FDG-PET in patients with stage I non-seminomatous germ cell tumours. Eur J Nucl Med Mol Imaging 2003; 30(3):396–402
20. Huddart RA, O'Doherty MJ, Padhani A, et al. 18fluorodeoxyglucose positron emission tomography in the prediction of relapse in patients with high-risk, clinical stage I nonseminomatous germ cell tumors: preliminary report of MRC Trial TE22—the NCRI Testis Tumour Clinical Study Group. J Clin Oncol 2007; 25(21):3090–3095
21. Cremerius U, Effert PJ, Adam G, et al. FDG PET for detection and therapy control of metastatic germ cell tumor. J Nucl Med 1998;39(5):815–822
22. Stephens AW, Gonin R, Hutchins GD, Einhorn LH. Positron emission tomography evaluation of residual radiographic abnormalities in postchemotherapy germ cell tumor patients. J Clin Oncol 1996;14(5):1637–1641
23. Drieskens O, Oyen R, Van Poppel H, et al. FDG-PET for preoperative staging of bladder cancer. Eur J Nucl Med Mol Imaging 2005;32(12):1412–1417
24. Effert PJ, Bares R, Handt S, et al. Metabolic imaging of untreated prostate cancer by positron emission tomography with 18fluorine-labeled deoxyglucose. J Urol 1996;155(3):994–998
25. Sung J, Espiritu JI, Segall GM, Terris MK. Fluorodeoxyglucose positron emission tomography studies in the diagnosis and staging of clinically advanced prostate cancer. BJU Int 2003;92(1):24–27
26. Seltzer MA, Barbaric Z, Belldegrun A, et al. Comparison of helical computerized tomography, positron emission tomography and monoclonal antibody scans for evaluation of lymph node metastases in patients with prostate specific antigen relapse after treatment for localized prostate cancer. J Urol 1999;162(4):1322–1328
27. Chang CH, Wu HC, Tsai JJ, et al. Detecting metastatic pelvic lymph nodes by ^{18}F-2-deoxyglucose positron emission tomography in patients with prostate-specific antigen relapse after treatment for localized prostate cancer. Urol Int 2003;70(4):311–315
28. Hofer C, Laubenbacher C, Block T, et al. Fluorine-18-fluorodeoxyglucose positron emission tomography is useless for the detection of local recurrence after radical prostatectomy. Eur Urol 1999;36(1):31–35
29. Powles T, Murray I, Brock C, Oliver T, Avril N. Molecular positron emission tomography and PET/CT imaging in urological malignancies. Eur Urol 2007;51(6):1511–1520
30. Schoder H, Herrmann K, Gonen M, et al. 2-[^{18}F]fluoro-2-deoxyglucose positron emission tomography for the detection of disease in patients with prostate-specific antigen relapse after radical prostatectomy. Clin Cancer Res 2005;11(13):4761–4769
31. Morris MJ, Akhurst T, Osman I, et al. Fluorinated deoxyglucose positron emission tomography imaging in progressive metastatic prostate cancer. Urology 2002;59(6):913–918
32. Oyama N, Akino H, Suzuki Y, et al. FDG PET for evaluating the change of glucose metabolism in prostate cancer after androgen ablation. Nucl Med Commun 2001;22(9):963–969

24

Colorectal Cancer

Eugene C. Lin and Abass Alavi

◆ Primary Colonic Neoplasms

Clinical Indication: C

Positron emission tomography (PET) has no role in screening for colonic neoplasm, but colonic lesions may be detected incidentally on PET scans performed for other indications (**Fig. 24.1**).

Accuracy and Comparison with Other Modalities

1. ***PET.*** Sensitivity 74%, specificity 84% for colonic neoplasm (adenomas or carcinoma) compared with colonoscopy.[1]
   - If there is a known colon cancer, it will usually be detectable by PET. Tumor size and depth of invasion are associated with higher standardized uptake values (SUVs).[2] One study suggests that PET is unlikely to miss a colon cancer,[3] but another suggests that the sensitivity of PET for colon cancers < 2 cm is limited.[4]
2. ***Lesion size.*** The detectability of colonic adenomas depends on lesion size. Other factors influencing detectability are shape (decreased sensitivity for flat morphology) and grade of dysplasia.[3,4]
   - Seventy-two percent of adenomas > 11 mm in size are detected by PET.[3]

Pearls and Pitfalls

1. Both adenomas (**Fig. 24.1**) and carcinomas (**Fig. 24.2**) may appear with increased uptake on PET. One study suggests that carcinomas generally have greater uptake than adenomas,[5] but other studies suggest there is no difference in uptake.[3,6]

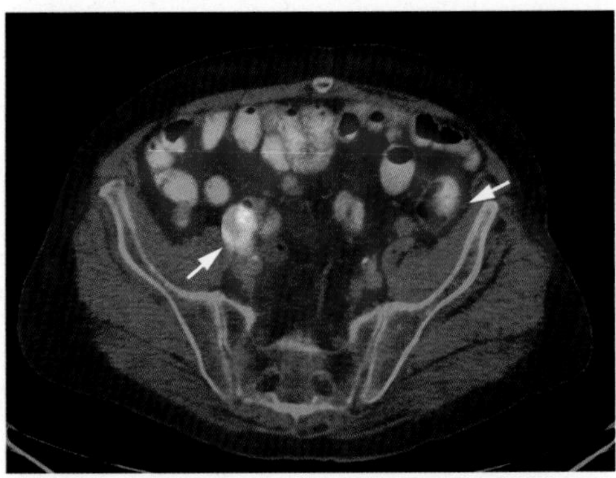

Fig. 24.1 Colon polyps. Axial positron emission tomography/computed tomography (PET/CT) scan demonstrates uptake in two colonic polyps (*arrows*). Focal colonic uptake should usually be further evaluated. However, focal colonic uptake on PET/CT will be false-positive in ~30% of cases. Standardized uptake value is not helpful in distinguishing pathologic from physiologic uptake. Focal uptake in the ascending colon or cecum is more likely to be physiologic than elsewhere in the colon.

2. ***Nonmalignant causes of uptake***[7]
   a. Focal physiologic uptake can cause false-positive findings.
      - With PET/CT, focal bowel uptake is false-positive approximately one third of the time.[6,8] The false-positive rate is higher with PET alone.
      - SUV values cannot distinguish between focal physiologic uptake and neoplasm.[6,8]
   b. Uptake in hyperplastic polyps has been described, although this is unusual.
   c. Hemorrhoids can have increased uptake likely secondary to inflammation.
3. ***Uptake pattern.*** The pattern of uptake is helpful in differential diagnosis.
   a. Nodular colonic uptake is often due to a focal lesion.
   b. Segmental uptake is often secondary to inflammation.
   c. Diffuse uptake is usually normal. There is usually more uptake in the right colon, particularly in the cecum.[9]

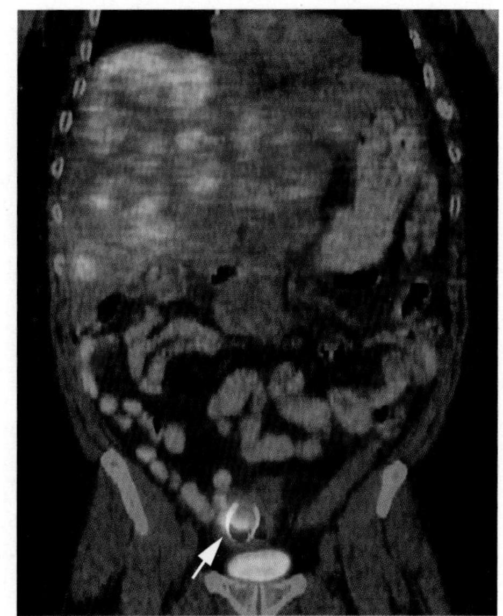

Fig. 24.2 Metastatic primary colon cancer. Coronal positron emission tomography/computed tomography demonstrates a primary sigmoid colon cancer (*arrow*) with extensive hepatic metastases. A stent has been placed in the region of the tumor to relieve obstruction.

◆ Initial Staging

Clinical Indication: B

1. Preoperative staging in colorectal cancer with PET is not commonly performed because patients will often undergo colectomy to relieve obstruction, and intraoperative staging can be done during surgery. PET is helpful in patients with a normal computed tomography (CT) scan and high carcinoembryonic antigen (CEA), where demonstration of metastatic disease may preclude surgery. In patients with advanced disease (**Fig. 24.2**), PET may allow optimal staging compared with findings during surgery.
   - PET/CT colonography is more accurate in defining TNM (tumor-nodes-metastasis) stage than CT alone, primarily because of its more accurate definition of the T stage. The bowel distention during PET/CT colonography is helpful for evaluating the bowel wall and surrounding soft tissue. However, T stage is often of minor clinical relevance in colon cancer (accurate assessment of T stage preoperatively is more important in rectal cancer). Thus, the change in patient management from PET/CT in colorectal cancer staging is often due to detection of synchronous tumors.[10]
2. ***Rectal cancer.*** PET may have value in advanced primary rectal cancer, particularly if neoadjuvant chemoradiation is being considered. In these patients it can detect distant metastatic or synchronous disease and upstage disease in 8 to 24% of patients.[11–13]
   - Discordant findings (usually lymph node metastases) between PET/CT and CT are more common in low rectal cancers than in mid or high rectal cancers; therefore, PET/CT will more frequently add staging information in low rectal cancers.[14]

◆ Recurrence and Restaging[15,16]

Clinical Indication: A

PET is a standard modality for evaluating colon cancer recurrence. The primary uses are

1. Searching for suspected recurrent disease (rising CEA), when anatomical imaging is equivocal or negative (**Figs. 24.3, 24.4,** and **24.5**)

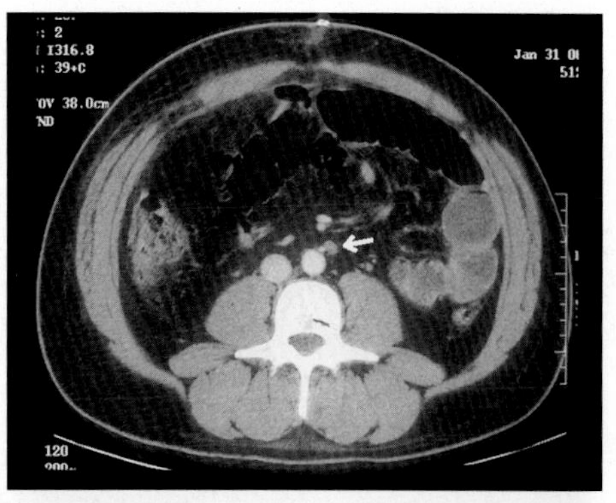

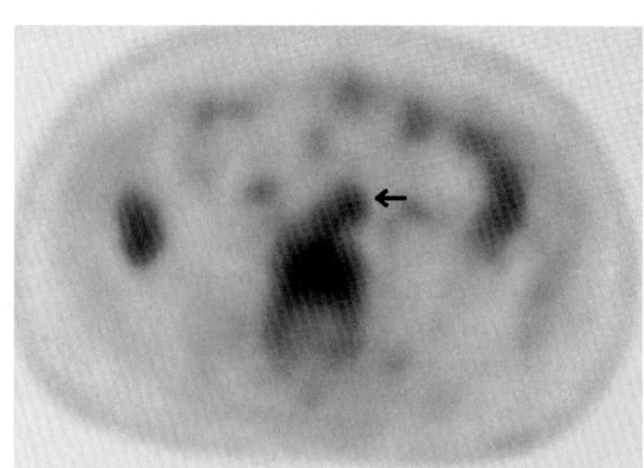

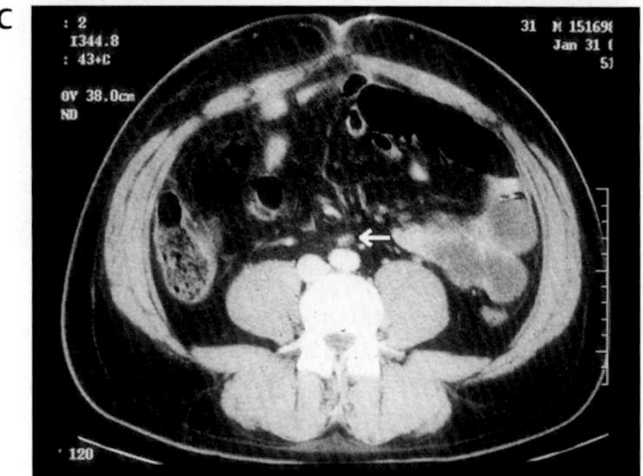

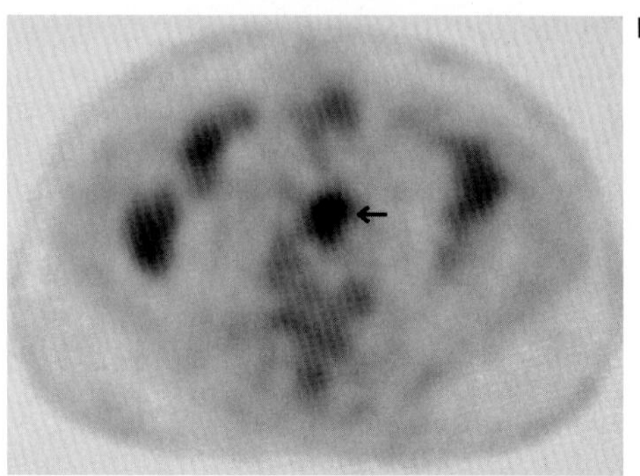

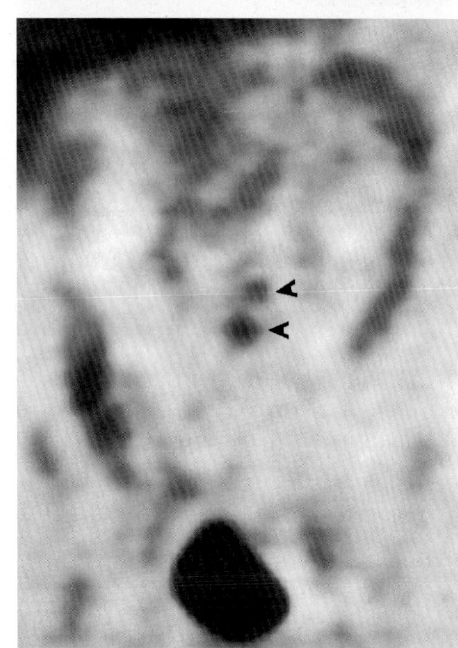

Fig. 24.3 Small metastatic nodes from colon cancer. **(A,C)** Axial computed tomography (CT) scans in a patient with colon cancer demonstrate small retroperitoneal nodes (*arrows*). These measure ~5 mm in short axis dimension and would be considered normal by CT. **(B,D)** Axial positron emission tomography (PET) scans demonstrate focal increased uptake (*arrows*) corresponding to these nodes. This degree of uptake in nodes of this small size is highly suggestive for malignancy. A low standardized uptake value (SUV) value would not change the diagnosis of malignancy, as partial volume effects could lower SUV substantially. **(E)** Coronal PET scan demonstrates uptake in the two nodes (*arrowheads*). Note that even though the nodes are < 1 cm on CT, the contrast-to-noise ratio is greater on PET, and the nodes are very clearly seen. Lesion detection on PET is improved in regions with little motion and surrounding physiologic activity (e.g., the retroperitoneum). Although the superior node to the left of midline is comparable in size to the midline inferior node on the CT, the inferior node is more intense and appears "larger" on PET. PET is not accurate for size determination.

- The exact utility of PET depends upon the level of CEA elevation. If CEA < 25 ng/mL, PET is helpful for triaging patients for appropriate management. If CEA > 25 ng/mL, PET is mainly helpful in confirming the presence of advanced disease and occasionally in identifying potentially resectable disease.[17] A cost-effective cutoff

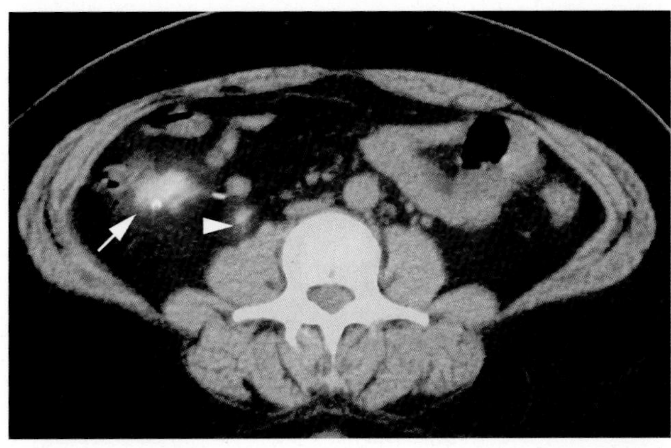

Fig. 24.4 Recurrent colon cancer. Axial positron emission tomography/computed tomography scan in a patient with colon cancer demonstrates recurrent disease (*arrow*) near an anastomosis. A small medial focus of activity (*arrowhead*) is in the ureter.

for utilizing PET to evaluate unexplained CEA elevation may be 10 ng/mL.

2. Restaging of a known recurrence if surgery is planned
    - In patients screened with preoperative PET before hepatic resection, PET detects unsuspected tumor in 25% and reduces the number of unnecessary laparotomies.[18] The overall 5-year survival rate after hepatic resection is 58% in colon cancer patients who have been examined with PET (compared with 30% in patients who have been assessed by conventional techniques).[19]
3. Differentiation of posttreatment changes from recurrence
    - This is a common problem in rectal cancer, as both recurrence and postradiation scars can result in abnormal soft tissue masses in the presacral space (**Fig. 24.6**).

Accuracy

1. ***PET, hepatic.*** Sensitivity 80%, specificity 92%[21]

    PET, extrahepatic. Sensitivity 91%, specificity 98%
    1. *Lesion size.* Sensitivity of PET is much lower for liver lesions < 1 cm in size.

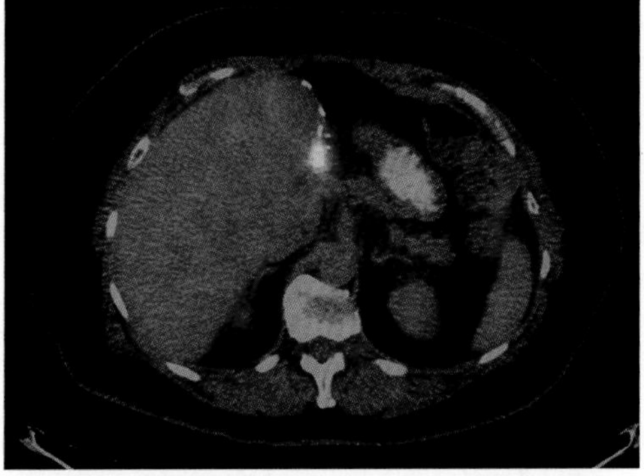

Fig. 24.5 Recurrent colon cancer. Axial positron emission tomography/computed tomography in a patient with colon cancer demonstrates recurrence at the margin of a prior hepatic resection.

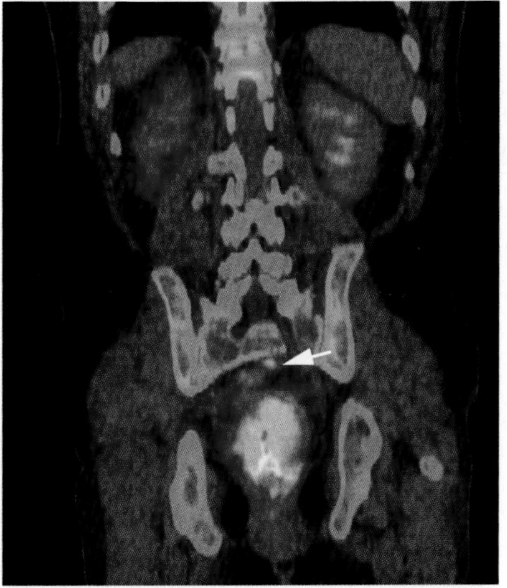

Fig. 24.6 Recurrent rectal cancer. Coronal positron emission tomography/computed tomography (PET/CT) demonstrates a large presacral recurrence of rectal cancer. A small local nodal metastasis (arrow) is present.

b. *Mucinous tumors*. Sensitivity is low for mucinous tumors (58%), possibly due to hypocellularity of the malignant mass.[22]
c. *Body region*. The specificity is very high in the liver and in local pelvic recurrence and lower elsewhere in the body.

2. ***PET/CT***
    a. PET/CT increases the accuracy to 90% from 75% for PET alone.[23]
    b. The primary advantage of PET/CT over PET is in increasing specificity for extra-abdominal and hepatic recurrences.

Local Recurrence

1. ***PET.*** Sensitivity 84%, specificity 88%[24]
    a. The best results are obtained when PET is performed more than 12 months after radiation.
    b. PET is more accurate than immunoscintigraphy, with equal or greater sensitivity than MRI.
2. ***PET/CT.*** PET/CT increases accuracy in differentiating benign from malignant uptake in the pelvis and in presacral masses compared with PET alone (**Fig. 24.6**).[25]
    a. Pelvic uptake: Sensitivity 96%, specificity 90%
    b. Presacral mass: Sensitivity 100%, specificity 96%

Comparison to Other Modalities

Liver Metastases

1. ***PET.*** Sensitivity 80%, specificity 92%[21]
    CT. Sensitivity 83%, specificity 84%
    a. PET is the most sensitive modality for detecting liver metastases with equivalent degree of specificity.[27]
    b. CT portography has a higher degree of sensitivity, but a much lower degree of specificity for identifying liver metastases than PET.[27]
2. **PET/CT.** PET/CT and CT have comparable sensitivity for detection of liver metastases, but PET/CT has superior sensitivity for detecting intrahepatic recurrence after hepatectomy (100% vs 50%).[28]
3. **MRI.** PET is more sensitive than magnetic resonance imaging (MRI) for detecting liver metastases on a per patient basis but not a per lesion basis.[29] However, MRI with liver-specific contrast agents such as mangafodipir trisodium and superparamagnetic iron oxide particles can detect more liver lesions than PET.[30,31]

Extrahepatic Metastases

1. ***PET***. Sensitivity 91%, specificity 98%[21]
2. ***CT.*** Sensitivity 61%, specificity 91%
    a. *Peritoneal recurrence*. PET sensitivity 88%, CT 38%[32]
    b. *Body region*. PET is more sensitive than CT in the abdomen, pelvis, and retroperitoneum, and is comparable to CT in the lungs.[33]
    c. *Immunoscintigraphy*. Compared with immunoscintigraphy (technetium 99m anti-CEA antibody), PET is significantly superior for the detection of distant metastases.[34]
3. ***PET/CT.***[28] PET/CT is superior to CT for both detecting both extrahepatic metastases and local recurrence.
    a. *Extrahepatic metastases (sensitivity)*. PET/CT 89%, CT 64%
    b. *Local recurrence at primary colorectal resection site (sensitivity)*. PET/CT 93%, CT 53%
    c. PET/CT changes management in 21% of patients.

Pearls

1. In patients with known liver metastases by anatomical imaging, PET can detect additional liver metastases, but it is most useful in detecting extrahepatic metastases and therefore precluding liver resection.
2. If hepatic resection is planned, it is difficult to localize liver lesions to specific segments on PET, as anatomical landmarks such as the hepatic veins are not visualized. Thus, correlation with anatomical imaging is necessary before surgery. PET/CT is ideally suited for this purpose.
3. ***Prognosis.*** Primary tumor grade and SUV of liver metastases are prognostic variables in patients undergoing liver resection after PET imaging

a. Standard prognostic variables for outcome after liver metastases resection such as number of lesions, size, and synchronicity may be less important if PET is performed. These prognostic variables are a surrogate for extrahepatic disease, but PET can often detect this extrahepatic disease. However, primary tumor grade may be more valuable as a prognostic variable if PET is performed because poor differentiation could suggest a greater likelihood of small-volume disease not detectable by PET. Therefore, patients who have poorly differentiated primary tumors may still have a high chance of recurrence and poor outcome even if PET is negative for extrahepatic disease.[19]

b. Survival is significantly longer in patients with a low SUV in liver metastases than for patients with a high SUV.[20]

Pitfalls

1. ***Normal CEA.*** Positive PET findings in patients with normal CEA, even if symptoms suggest recurrence, should be interpreted with caution because most often no disease is found on follow-up examinations.
2. ***Postsurgical.*** A common cause of false-positive results in evaluating pelvic recurrence of rectal cancer is posterior displacement of pelvic contents following surgery. PET/CT is very helpful in reducing false-positive findings as a result of this type of intervention.[25] Minimizing bladder activity by voiding/catheterization is also helpful.
3. ***Neoadjuvant chemotherapy.*** The sensitivity of PET in detecting colorectal hepatic metastases decreases following neoadjuvant chemotherapy.[26] This is true even if PET imaging is performed with a minimal interval of 2 weeks following chemotherapy and may be related to decreased size of the metastases.

◆ Therapy Response[35]

Clinical Indication: C

PET has multiple uses in assessing therapy response in colorectal carcinomas.[36]

1. ***Chemotherapy response in advanced colorectal cancer.*** PET is useful for predicting response to chemotherapy in patients with unresectable colorectal cancer liver metastases.
   a. *Early prediction.* PET can differentiate responders from nonresponders early in the course of chemotherapy for hepatic metastases. PET should be performed at least 4 weeks after initiating therapy, as false-positive results from inflammation can be seen in the first 2 weeks of treatment.[37]
   b. *Late prediction.* After completion of therapy, PET findings correlate better with pathological response than the findings on CT. However, one study suggests that liver metastases that have a complete metabolic response on PET and disappear on CT or MRI can still contain viable tumor.[38] Thus, if patients with unresectable liver metastases are treated to render them resectable, negative PET findings should not preclude curative resection.
   c. *Prognosis.* There is a significant survival benefit in patients with low FDG uptake in colorectal cancer metastases.[39] This is true for both patients who undergo resection and those who are treated with chemotherapy.
2. ***Monitoring response to local ablative therapy for liver metastases.*** PET can be used to monitor the results of minimally invasive therapies, such as radiofrequency (RF) ablation and interarterial yttrium-90 (90Y) microsphere radioembolization.
   a. *RF ablation.* PET/CT is more sensitive (65%) than CT (44%) for detection of residual tumor after RF ablation.[40]
      - On CT and MRI, a nonpathologic rim of increased contrast enhancement is found immediately after RF ablation, which often cannot be differentiated from residual tumor.[41] PET may be helpful in this scenario, as the area of increased contrast enhancement has been reported to not demonstrate increased uptake.[41] However, there is conflicting evidence as a peripheral rim of FDG activity in surrounding normal tissue was noted after RF ablation in another study of liver metastases[42] and also in lung tumors.[43] Macroscopic residual tumor usually appears as focal uptake[42] rather than a peripheral

rim of uptake; however, inflammatory uptake could obscure residual tumor. Possible ways to avoid potential inflammatory uptake are to image early (within 2 days of ablation) or late (after 4 weeks).[42]
   - PET-negative lesions after ablation are very unlikely to develop local recurrence.
   - ***b.*** *90Y radioembolization.* PET/CT provides a more accurate and earlier assessment of therapy response to 90Y radioembolization than does CT.[44]
3. ***Response evaluation in preoperative chemoradiotherapy for primary rectal cancer***
   - ***a.*** *Early prediction.* PET performed as early as 12 days after preoperative chemoradiotherapy predicts pathologic response.[45]
   - ***b.*** *Late prediction.* PET performed after preoperative chemoradiotherapy predicts response[46] and prognosis.[47]

References

1. Drenth JP, Nagengast FM, Oyen WJ. Evaluation of (pre-)malignant colonic abnormalities: endoscopic validation of FDG-PET findings. Eur J Nucl Med 2001;28(12):1766–1769
2. Gu J, Yamamoto H, Fukunaga H, et al. Correlation of GLUT-1 overexpression, tumor size, and depth of invasion with ^{18}F–2-fluoro-2-deoxy-D-glucose uptake by positron emission tomography in colorectal cancer. Dig Dis Sci 2006;51(12):2198–2205
3. van Kouwen MC, Nagengast FM, Jansen JB, et al. 2-(^{18}F)-fluoro-2-deoxy-D-glucose positron emission tomography detects clinical relevant adenomas of the colon: a prospective study. J Clin Oncol 2005;23(16): 3713–3717
4. Friedland S, Soetikno R, Carlisle M, et al. 18-fluorodeoxyglucose positron emission tomography has limited sensitivity for colonic adenoma and early stage colon cancer. Gastrointest Endosc 2005;61(3):395–400
5. Chen YK, Kao CH, Liao AC, et al. Colorectal cancer screening in asymptomatic adults: the role of FDG PET scan. Anticancer Res 2003;23(5b):4357–4361
6. Israel O, Yefremov N, Bar-Shalom R, et al. PET/CT detection of unexpected gastrointestinal foci of ^{18}F-FDG uptake: incidence, localization patterns, and clinical significance. J Nucl Med 2005;46(5):758–762
7. Kamel EM, Thumshirn M, Truninger K, et al. Significance of incidental ^{18}F-FDG accumulations in the gastrointestinal tract in PET/CT: correlation with endoscopic and histopathologic results. J Nucl Med 2004;45(11):1804–1810
8. Gutman F, Alberini JL, Wartski M, et al. Incidental colonic focal lesions detected by FDG PET/CT. AJR Am J Roentgenol 2005;185(2):495–500
9. Tatlidil R, Jadvar H, Bading JR, Conti PS. Incidental colonic fluorodeoxyglucose uptake: correlation with colonoscopic and histopathologic findings. Radiology 2002;224(3):783–787
10. Veit-Haibach P, Kuehle CA, Beyer T, et al. Diagnostic accuracy of colorectal cancer staging with whole-body PET/CT colonography. JAMA 2006;296(21):2590–2600
11. Heriot AG, Hicks RJ, Drummond EG, et al. Does positron emission tomography change management in primary rectal cancer? A prospective assessment. Dis Colon Rectum 2004;47(4):451–458
12. Nahas CS, Akhurst T, Yeung H, et al. Positron emission tomography detection of distant metastatic or synchronous disease in patients with locally advanced rectal cancer receiving preoperative chemoradiation. Ann Surg Oncol 2008;15(3):704–711
13. Muthusamy VR, Chang KJ. Optimal methods for staging rectal cancer. Clin Cancer Res 2007;13(22 Pt 2):6877s–6884s
14. Gearhart SL, Frassica D, Rosen R, et al. Improved staging with pretreatment positron emission tomography/computed tomography in low rectal cancer. Ann Surg Oncol 2006;13(3):397–404
15. Vitola J, Delbeke D. Positron emission tomography for evaluation of colorectal carcinoma. Semin Roentgenol 2002;37(2):118–128
16. Chin BB, Wahl RL. ^{18}F-fluoro-2-deoxyglucose positron emission tomography in the evaluation of gastrointestinal malignancies. Gut 2003;52(Suppl 4):iv23–iv29
17. Liu FY, Chen JS, Changchien CR, et al. Utility of 2-fluoro-2-deoxy-D-glucose positron emission tomography in managing patients of colorectal cancer with unexplained carcinoembryonic antigen elevation at different levels. Dis Colon Rectum 2005;48(10):1900–1912
18. Wiering B, Krabbe PF, Dekker HM, et al. The role of FDG-PET in the selection of patients with colorectal liver metastases. Ann Surg Oncol 2007;14(2):771–779
19. Fernandez FG, Drebin JA, Linehan DC, et al. Five-year survival after resection of hepatic metastases from colorectal cancer in patients screened by positron emission tomography with F-18 fluorodeoxyglucose (FDG-PET). Ann Surg 2004;240(3):438–447
20. Riedl CC, Akhurst T, Larson S, et al. ^{18}F-FDG PET scanning correlates with tissue markers of poor prognosis and predicts mortality for patients after liver resection for colorectal metastases. J Nucl Med 2007;48(5):771–775
21. Wiering B, Krabbe PF, Jager GJ, et al. The impact of fluor-18-deoxyglucose-positron emission tomography in the management of colorectal liver metastases. Cancer 2005;104(12):2658–2670
22. Whiteford MH, Whiteford HM, Yee LF, et al. Usefulness of FDG-PET scan in the assessment of suspected metastatic or recurrent adenocarcinoma of the colon and rectum. Dis Colon Rectum 2000;43(6):759–767
23. Votrubova J, Belohlavek O, Jaruskova M, et al. The role of FDG-PET/CT in the detection of recurrent colorectal cancer. Eur J Nucl Med Mol Imaging 2006;33(7):779–784
24. Moore HG, Akhurst T, Larson SM, et al. A case-controlled study of 18-fluorodeoxyglucose positron emission tomography in the detection of pelvic recurrence in previously irradiated rectal cancer patients. J Am Coll Surg 2003;197(1):22–28
25. Even-Sapir E, Parag Y, Lerman H, et al. Detection of recurrence in patients with rectal cancer: PET/CT after abdominoperineal or anterior resection. Radiology 2004;232(3):815–822

26. Lubezky N, Metser U, Geva R, et al. The role and limitations of 18-fluoro-2-deoxy-D-glucose positron emission tomography (FDG-PET) scan and computerized tomography (CT) in restaging patients with hepatic colorectal metastases following neoadjuvant chemotherapy: comparison with operative and pathological findings. J Gastrointest Surg 2007;11(4):472–478
27. Delbeke D, Vitola JV, Sandler MP, et al. Staging recurrent metastatic colorectal carcinoma with PET. J Nucl Med 1997;38(8):1196–1201
28. Selzner M, Hany TF, Wildbrett P, et al. Does the novel PET/CT imaging modality impact on the treatment of patients with metastatic colorectal cancer of the liver? Ann Surg 2004;240(6):1027–1034
29. Bipat S, van Leeuwen MS, Comans EF, et al. Colorectal liver metastases: CT, MR imaging, and PET for diagnosis—meta-analysis. Radiology 2005;237(1):123–131
30. Sahani DV, Kalva SP, Fischman AJ, et al. Detection of liver metastases from adenocarcinoma of the colon and pancreas: comparison of mangafodipir trisodium-enhanced liver MRI and whole-body FDG PET. AJR Am J Roentgenol 2005;185(1):239–246
31. Rappeport ED, Loft A, Berthelsen AK, et al. Contrast-enhanced FDG-PET/CT vs. SPIO-enhanced MRI vs. FDG-PET vs. CT in patients with liver metastases from colorectal cancer: a prospective study with intraoperative confirmation. Acta Radiol 2007;48(4):369–378
32. Tanaka T, Kawai Y, Kanai M, et al. Usefulness of FDG-positron emission tomography in diagnosing peritoneal recurrence of colorectal cancer. Am J Surg 2002;184(5):433–436
33. Valk PE, Abella-Columna E, Haseman MK, et al. Whole-body PET imaging with [^{18}F]fluorodeoxyglucose in management of recurrent colorectal cancer. Arch Surg 1999;134(5):503–511
34. Willkomm P, Bender H, Bangard M, et al. FDG PET and immunoscintigraphy with 99mTc-labeled antibody fragments for detection of the recurrence of colorectal carcinoma. J Nucl Med 2000;41(10):1657–1663
35. Kostakoglu L, Goldsmith SJ. ^{18}F-FDG PET evaluation of the response to therapy for lymphoma and for breast, lung, and colorectal carcinoma. J Nucl Med 2003;44(2):224–239
36. de Geus-Oei LF, Ruers TJ, Punt CJ, et al. FDG-PET in colorectal cancer. Cancer Imaging 2006;6:S71–S81
37. Findlay M, Young H, Cunningham D, et al. Noninvasive monitoring of tumor metabolism using fluorodeoxyglucose and positron emission tomography in colorectal cancer liver metastases: correlation with tumor response to fluorouracil. J Clin Oncol 1996;14(3):700–708
38. Tan MC, Linehan DC, Hawkins WG, Siegel BA, Strasberg SM. Chemotherapy-induced normalization of FDG uptake by colorectal liver metastases does not usually indicate complete pathologic response. J Gastrointest Surg 2007;11(9):1112–1119
39. de Geus-Oei LF, Wiering B, Krabbe PF, et al. FDG-PET for prediction of survival of patients with metastatic colorectal carcinoma. Ann Oncol 2006;17(11):1650–1655
40. Veit P, Antoch G, Stergar H, et al. Detection of residual tumor after radiofrequency ablation of liver metastasis with dual-modality PET/CT: initial results. Eur Radiol 2006;16(1):80–87
41. Antoch G, Vogt FM, Veit P, et al. Assessment of liver tissue after radiofrequency ablation: findings with different imaging procedures. J Nucl Med 2005;46(3):520–525
42. Khandani AH, Calvo BF, O'Neil BH, Jorgenson J, Mauro MA. A pilot study of early ^{18}F-FDG PET to evaluate the effectiveness of radiofrequency ablation of liver metastases. AJR Am J Roentgenol 2007;189(5):1199–1202
43. Okuma T, Matsuoka T, Okamura T, et al. ^{18}F-FDG small-animal PET for monitoring the therapeutic effect of CT-guided radiofrequency ablation on implanted VX2 lung tumors in rabbits. J Nucl Med 2006;47(8):1351–1358
44. Bienert M, McCook B, Carr BI, et al. 90Y microsphere treatment of unresectable liver metastases: changes in ^{18}F-FDG uptake and tumour size on PET/CT. Eur J Nucl Med Mol Imaging 2005;32(7):778–787
45. Cascini GL, Avallone A, Delrio P, et al. ^{18}F-FDG PET is an early predictor of pathologic tumor response to preoperative radiochemotherapy in locally advanced rectal cancer. J Nucl Med 2006;47(8):1241–1248
46. Denecke T, Rau B, Hoffmann KT, et al. Comparison of CT, MRI and FDG-PET in response prediction of patients with locally advanced rectal cancer after multimodal preoperative therapy: is there a benefit in using functional imaging? Eur Radiol 2005;15(8):1658–1666
47. Capirci C, Rubello D, Chierichetti F, et al. Long-term prognostic value of ^{18}F-FDG PET in patients with locally advanced rectal cancer previously treated with neoadjuvant radiochemotherapy. AJR Am J Roentgenol 2006;187(2):W202–W208

25

Musculoskeletal Tumors

Eugene C. Lin and Abass Alavi

◆ Distinguishing Benign from Malignant Musculoskeletal Tumors

In a known bone or soft tissue lesion, positron emission tomography (PET) is of some value in determining whether the lesion is benign or malignant and in grading malignant lesions. In addition, bone or soft tissue lesions are detected incidentally on PET performed for other indications. The degree of fluorodeoxyglucose (FDG) uptake in the lesion can aid in differential diagnosis when correlated with conventional imaging modalities.

Benign versus Malignant Bone Tumors

Clinical Indication: C

1. ***Low uptake.*** A low level of uptake suggests that a bone lesion is likely benign (although there are false-negative results in plasmacytoma and low-grade chondrosarcoma).
2. ***High uptake.*** A high level of uptake is less specific. Although lesions with high uptake are more likely to represent malignancy (primary or metastatic), high uptake can be seen in a large number of benign lesions (see Pitfalls section).
3. ***Chondrosarcoma versus enchondroma***[1]
   a. Chondrosarcomas (**Fig. 25.1**) usually have less uptake than other sarcomas but more uptake than enchondromas.
   b. PET cannot distinguish between benign tumors and grade I chondrosarcomas.
   c. Grade II and III chondrosarcomas have higher glucose metabolism than low-grade cartilage tumors.
      - A standardized uptake value (SUV) cutoff of 2.3 is helpful in differentiating grade II and III chondrosarcomas from low-grade tumors.
4. ***Chondrosarcoma versus osteochondroma.*** Limited data suggest an SUV cutoff of 2.0 may differentiate benign from malignant osteochondromas.[2]

Accuracy

1. ***PET.*** Sensitivity 93%, specificity 67%[3]
   - These results were obtained using tumor-to-background ratio of 3.0 as a positive result.

Pearls

1. In general, malignant bone lesions have higher FDG uptake than benign lesions.
2. Metastases have the highest uptake, usually more than primary malignant bone lesions.[4]

A

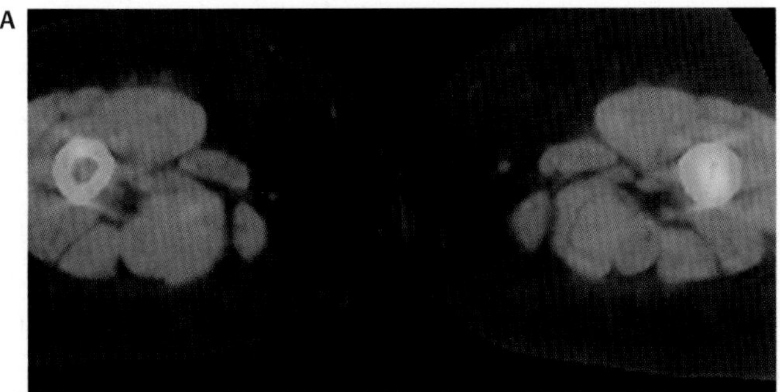

B

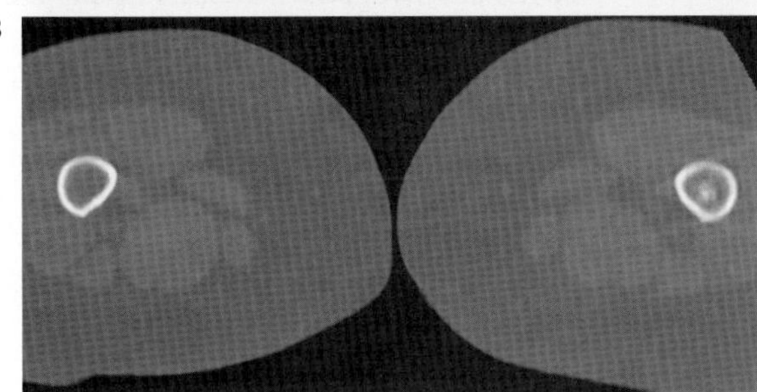

C

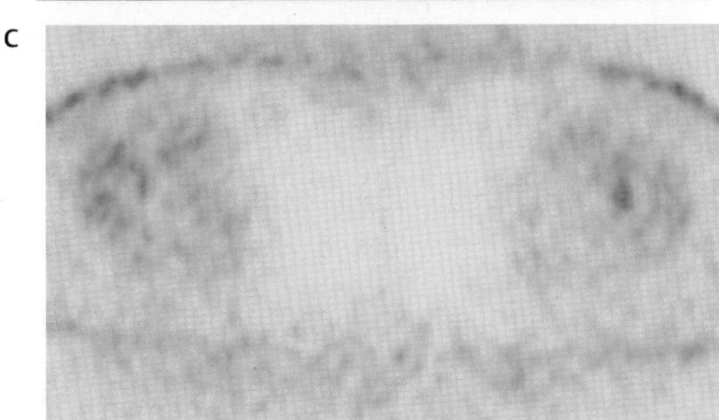

Fig. 25.1 Chondrosarcoma. **(A)** Axial positron emission tomography/computed tomography (PET/CT) demonstrates uptake in a low-grade chondrosarcoma of the left femur. **(B)** As the CT demonstrates there is a dense chondroid matrix in this region. **(C)** The nonattenuation-corrected image should be reviewed to determine that the visualized activity is not artifactual. However, it is unlikely that the degree of increased attenuation from a chondroid matrix would be enough to result in artifactually increased activity.

3. However, benign bone tumors can have substantial FDG accumulation (> 2.0 SUV).
   - Particularly true for histiocytic or giant cell-containing lesions (**Fig. 25.2**)

Pitfalls

1. ***False-negatives.***[3,5] Low-grade chondrosarcoma, plasmacytoma, myxoid tumors
2. ***False-positives.***[6,7] Giant cell tumor, chondroblastoma, fibrous dysplasia, sarcoidosis, Langerhans cell histiocytosis, nonossifying fibroma, osteoblastoma, aneurysmal bone cyst, Paget disease (active), enchondroma, chondromyxoid fibroma, desmoplastic fibroma, brown tumor, fibro-osseous defects, osteomyelitis, bone infarct, acute or subacute fracture

Benign versus Malignant Soft Tissue Tumors

Clinical Indication: C

1. ***Low uptake.*** Low FDG uptake is of limited value in differentiating benign from malignant soft tissue tumors, as it could be represent either a nonmalignant lesion or a low-grade sarcoma.
2. ***High uptake.*** High uptake is more useful, as it usually indicates intermediate or high-grade malignancy. Although some benign

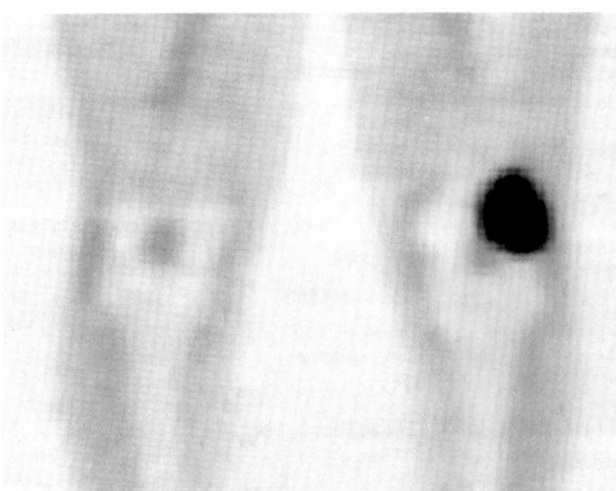

Fig. 25.2 Giant cell tumor. Coronal positron emission tomography (PET) scan demonstrates intense uptake (standardized uptake value [SUV] = 10.8) in a giant cell tumor of the left knee. This is a classic location for giant cell tumor involving the metaphysis with subarticular extension. Many benign bone tumors can have high levels of fluorodeoxyglucose (FDG) uptake. (Courtesy of Janet Eary, MD, Seattle, WA.)

lesions can have high uptake, radiographic correlation can often differentiate these lesions from sarcomas.

3. ***Liposarcoma versus lipoma.*** Limited data suggest that an SUV cutoff of 0.81 may differentiate liposarcomas (**Fig. 25.3**) from lipomas.[8]

Accuracy

1. ***PET.*** Sensitivity 92%, specificity 73%[9]
   - These results were obtained using qualitative interpretation.

Pearls and Pitfalls

1. ***Tumor grade.*** FDG uptake correlates with tumor grade.[10]
   a. Lesions with SUV ≥ 1.6 are usually high grade.
   b. Lesions with SUV < 1.6 are usually low grade or benign.
2. ***Benign lesions.*** Benign soft tissue lesions usually do not have substantial FDG uptake.[11]
   a. Lipomas and hemangiomas have the lowest uptake.
   b. *False-positives.* High uptake can be seen in giant cell tumor of the tendon sheath, sarcoid, desmoid, and schwannomas. Uptake in a hibernoma can mimic a liposarcoma.[12]
3. ***Delayed imaging.*** Delayed imaging can help differentiate benign from malignant tumors, as malignant lesions show an increase in uptake on delayed images.

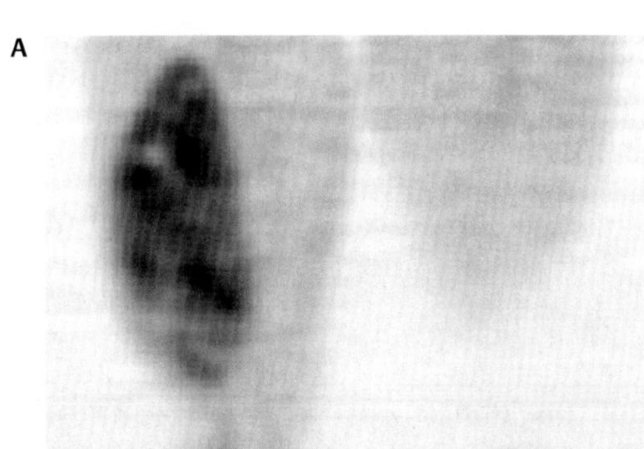

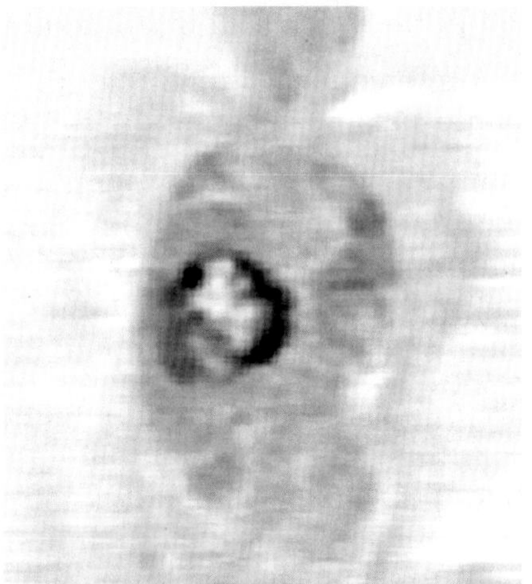

Fig. 25.3 Liposarcomas. Coronal positron emission tomography (PET) scans demonstrate fluorodeoxyglucose uptake in liposarcomas in the **(A)** thigh and **(B)** abdomen. The abdominal liposarcoma is heterogeneous with a standardized uptake value (SUV) of 11.7, consistent with a poor prognosis tumor. Given the heterogeneity of uptake, the PET scan would be helpful in guiding biopsy. The thigh liposarcoma has a much lower SUV of 2.7, consistent with a better prognosis tumor. However, there is some degree of heterogeneity, suggesting myxoid degeneration and a poorer prognosis than might be predicted by the SUV alone. (Courtesy of Janet Eary, MD, Seattle, WA.)

- Benign lesions reach maximum uptake early (30 minutes), whereas high-grade malignant lesions reach maximum uptake late (4 hours).[13]

◆ Evaluation of Known Musculoskeletal Tumors

PET is valuable in both osseous and soft tissue malignancies. The primary uses are staging, guiding biopsy, detecting recurrence, therapy response, and tumor grading.

Osteosarcoma and Soft Tissue Sarcomas[14,15]

Clinical Indication: B

The primary applications of PET are in guiding biopsy, therapy monitoring, and diagnosing local recurrence.

1. ***Staging.*** PET is of limited value in staging osteosarcoma (**Fig. 25.4**).
   a. PET is less sensitive than bone scan for the detection of bone metastases from osteosarcoma.[16]
   b. PET cannot substitute for CT in detecting lung metastases from osteosarcoma.[17]
2. ***Tumor grading***
   a. In known sarcomas, high SUV correlates with high histologic tumor grade (**Fig. 25.3**). Within the subset of high-grade sarcomas, the degree of FDG uptake at the time of diagnosis provides additional prognostic information.[18]
   b. Benign lesions can occasionally have uptake levels comparable to those of sarcomas.
3. ***Guiding biopsy in heterogeneous tumors*** **(Fig. 25.3)**. Fusion with computed tomography (CT) or magnetic resonance imaging (MRI) is helpful.
4. ***Therapy monitoring***
   a. PET predicts tumor response to preoperative neoadjuvant chemotherapy and eventual outcome (**Fig. 25.5**).[14]
   b. PET may be superior to bone scintigraphy in monitoring osteosarcoma therapy.[19]
5. ***Diagnosis of local recurrence*** **(Fig. 25.6)**
6. ***Prognosis.*** FDG uptake in sarcomas correlates negatively with survival and positively with disease progression.[20]

A

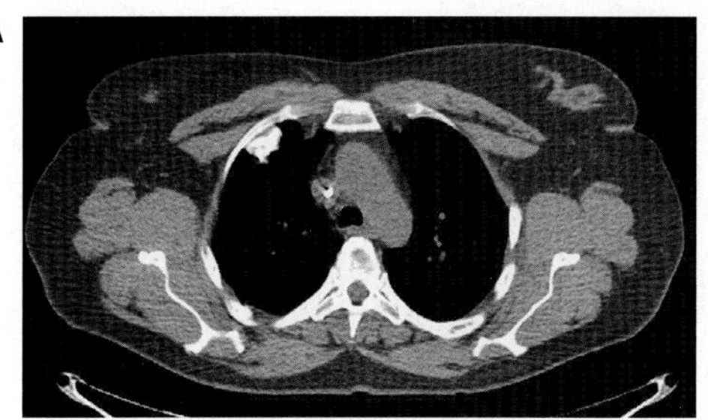

B

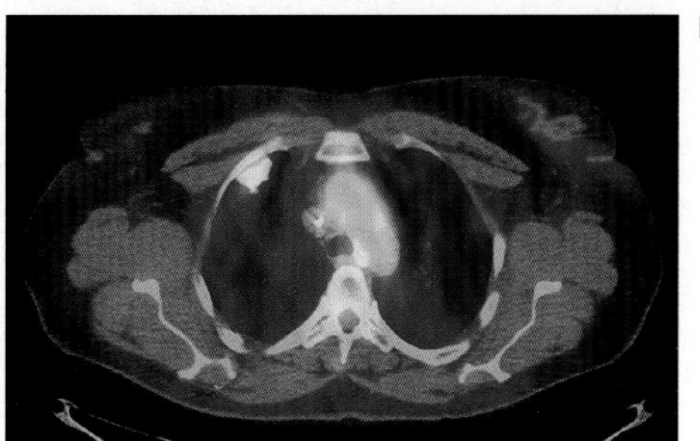

C

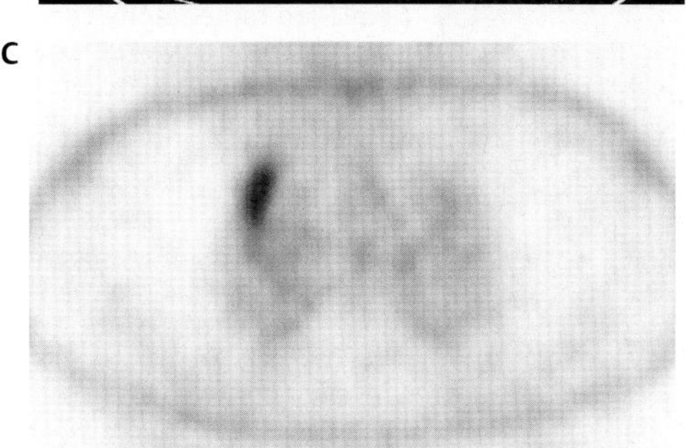

Fig. 25.4 Osteosarcoma lung metastasis. **(A)** Computed tomography (CT) scan in a patient with osteosarcoma demonstrates a calcified right upper lobe lesion. **(B)** Axial positron emission tomography (PET)/CT scan demonstrates uptake in this lesion consistent with metastasis. **(C)** In this case, it is important to review the nonattenuation-corrected image to determine that the uptake is not artifactual secondary to the increased density of the lesion. Although PET can detect lung metastases from osteosarcoma, CT is more sensitive for this purpose.

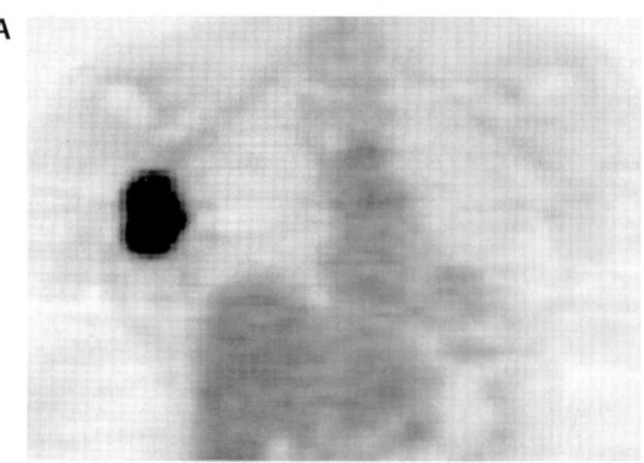

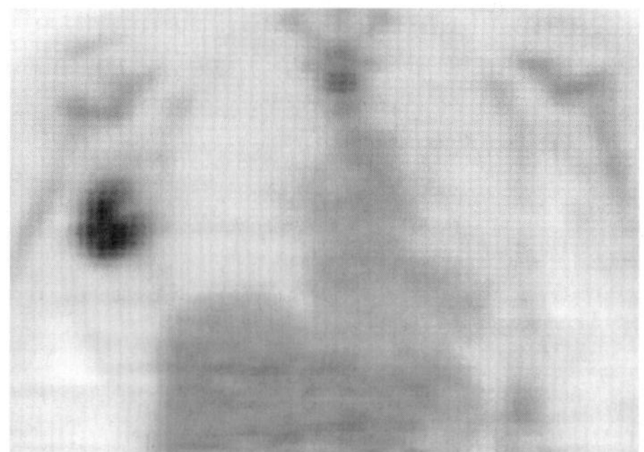

Fig. 25.5 Sarcoma response to therapy. Coronal positron emission tomography scans demonstrate therapy response in a right axillary soft tissue sarcoma **(A)** pretherapy and **(B)** posttherapy. (Courtesy of Janet Eary, MD, Seattle, WA.)

Accuracy and Comparison with Other Modalities

1. ***Staging.*** Combined PET/CT and conventional imaging results in correct N staging in 97% and correct M staging in 93% of patients.[21] The accuracy is significantly higher than PET alone.
2. ***Tumor recurrence***
   a. *Conventional imaging.* PET has a small advantage compared with conventional imaging for detection of soft tissue and bone metastases (**Table 25.1**).[22]
   b. *MRI.* PET is useful for the evaluation of potential recurrence when MRI is equivocal.[23]
      i. One specific situation where PET is valuable is when metallic prosthesis artifact will limit MRI.
      ii. PET has the additional advantage over MRI for evaluating the whole body for distant metastatic sites.
   c. *Sestamibi.* PET is more accurate than sestamibi (**Table 25.2**).[24]

Pitfalls

1. ***Staging***
   - *Lung.* A negative PET scan in the presence of suspicious CT findings does not exclude

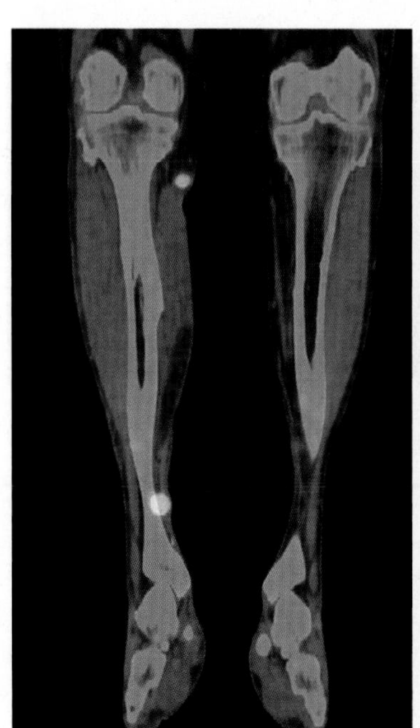

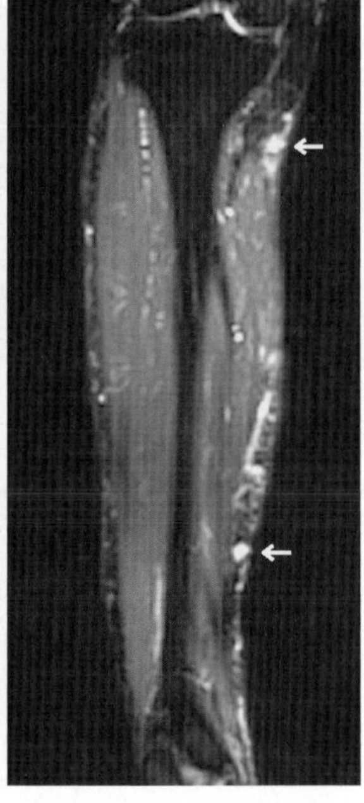

Fig. 25.6 Recurrent sarcoma. **(A)** Coronal positron emission tomography/computed tomography (PET/CT) demonstrates two foci of uptake in the soft tissue of the medial right calf secondary to recurrent sarcoma. **(B)** Coronal short TI inversion recovery magnetic resonance imaging (STIR MRI) in the same patient demonstrates two hyperintense foci (*arrows*) corresponding to the fluorodeoxyglucose (FDG) uptake.

Table 25.1 Sensitivity and Specificity of Positron Emission Tomography (PET) versus Conventional Imaging (CI) in the Detection of Soft Tissue and Bone Metastases in Recurrent Sarcomas

Modality	Sensitivity %	Specificity %
PET	96	81
CT	100	56

metastases, as a significant percentage of pulmonary metastases < 1 cm are negative on PET.[25]

2. ***Postamputation evaluation***[26]
   a. *Diffuse uptake.* Diffuse increased uptake can be seen in the stump up to 18 months postamputation.
   b. *Focal uptake.* Focal areas of uptake can been seen in areas of skin breakdown from pressure. Clinical correlation is necessary, as focal areas of uptake without correlative skin breakdown usually represent recurrence.
3. ***Therapy response***[11]
   - Lesions that respond completely sometimes have a peripheral rim of FDG uptake, which corresponds to a fibrous pseudocapsule containing inflammatory tissue.

Ewing Sarcoma

Clinical Indication: C

PET is more accurate than a bone scan in detecting bone metastases (**Table 25.3**).[16]

Multiple Myeloma

Clinical Indication: C

PET is useful in evaluating initial extent of disease and treatment response. PET may be most useful in nonsecretory disease, solitary osseous plasmacytoma, and extramedullary plasmacytoma. PET is also useful in the posttransplant setting where patients are nonsecretors, but the lesions still have FDG uptake.[27]

Table 25.2 Sensitivity and Specificity of Positron Emission Tomography (PET) versus Sestamibi in Recurrent Sarcomas

Modality	Sensitivity %	Specificity %
PET	98	90
Sestamibi	82	80

Table 25.3 Sensitivity and Specificity of Positron Emission Tomography (PET) versus Bone Scan in the Detection of Bone Metastases in Ewing Sarcoma

Modality	Sensitivity %	Specificity %
PET	100	96
Bone scan	68	87

Accuracy and Comparison with Other Modalities

1. ***PET.*** Sensitivity 84 to 92%, specificity 83 to 100%[28]
2. ***Plain radiographs.*** PET reveals more disease than plain radiographs in over 60% of patients (**Fig. 25.7**).[28]
   - In addition, PET can identify extramedullary disease.
3. ***Sestamibi.*** There are conflicting data as to whether sestamibi or PET identifies more lesions.[29,30]
   - Sestamibi uptake correlates with extent of marrow infiltration better than PET.
   - FDG uptake correlates with active disease progression.
4. ***Therapy follow-up.*** PET may be more accurate than a bone scan or plain radiographs for treatment follow-up.[31]
   a. PET is useful in identifying focal recurrence for radiation therapy in nonsecretory disease.
   b. Residual disease, particularly extramedullary, after therapy is a poor prognostic factor.[31]

Pitfalls

1. If PET/CT is used as the sole imaging modality in myeloma, it will miss some small lytic bone lesions and could miss diffuse spine involvement.[32] MRI may be superior to PET/CT in diagnosing infiltrative disease in the spine.[33]
2. PET is limited when there is diffuse bone marrow activity, as widespread disease is

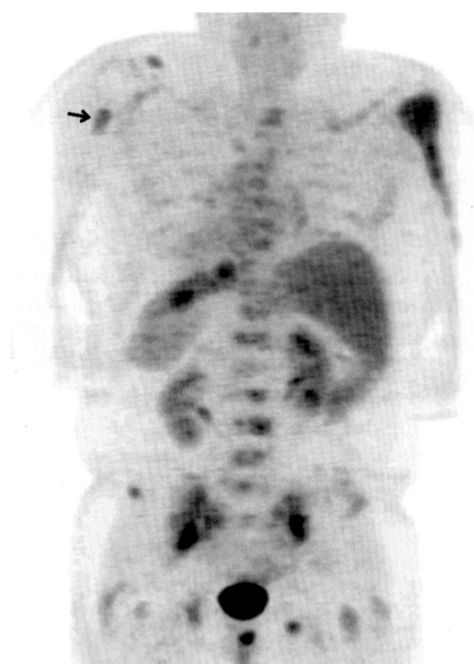
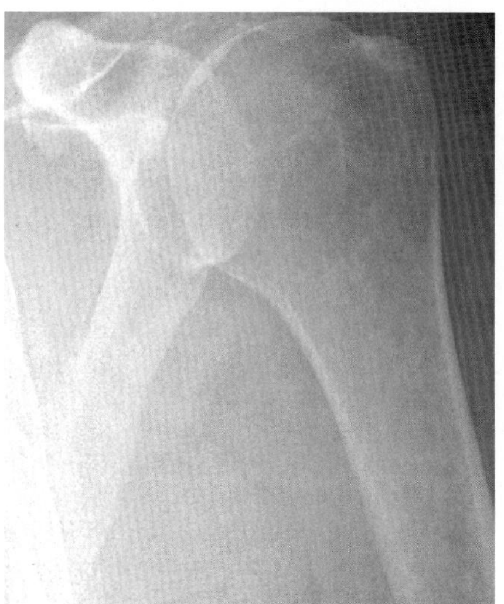

Fig. 25.7 Multiple myeloma: positron emission tomography (PET) versus plain film. **(A)** Coronal PET scan (posterior projection) in a patient with multiple myeloma demonstrates multiple osseous lesions. Although there is a lesion of the proximal left humeral shaft seen on PET (*arrow*), the corresponding radiograph **(B)** is negative.

difficult to differentiate from activated normal marrow.

References

1. Lee FY, Yu J, Chang SS, et al. Diagnostic value and limitations of fluorine-18 fluorodeoxyglucose positron emission tomography for cartilaginous tumors of bone. J Bone Joint Surg Am 2004;86-A(12):2677–2685
2. Feldman F, Vanheertum R, Saxena C. 18fluorodeoxyglucose positron emission tomography evaluation of benign versus malignant osteochondromas: preliminary observations. J Comput Assist Tomogr 2006;30(5):858–864
3. Schulte M, Brecht-Krauss D, Heymer B, et al. Grading of tumors and tumorlike lesions of bone: evaluation by FDG PET. J Nucl Med 2000;41(10):1695–1701
4. Watanabe H, Shinozaki T, Yanagawa T, et al. Glucose metabolic analysis of musculoskeletal tumours using 18fluorine-FDG PET as an aid to preoperative planning. J Bone Joint Surg Br 2000;82(5):760–767
5. Hicks RJ, Toner GC, Choong PF. Clinical applications of molecular imaging in sarcoma evaluation. Cancer Imaging 2005;5(1):66–72
6. Aoki J, Watanabe H, Shinozaki T, et al. FDG PET of primary benign and malignant bone tumors: standardized uptake value in 52 lesions. Radiology 2001; 219(3):774–777
7. Goodin GS, Shulkin BL, Kaufman RA, McCarville MB. PET/CT characterization of fibroosseous defects in children: ^{18}F-FDG uptake can mimic metastatic disease. AJR Am J Roentgenol 2006;187(4):1124–1128
8. Suzuki R, Watanabe H, Yanagawa T, et al. PET evaluation of fatty tumors in the extremity: possibility of using the standardized uptake value (SUV) to differentiate benign tumors from liposarcoma. Ann Nucl Med 2005;19(8):661–670
9. Ioannidis JP, Lau J. ^{18}F-FDG PET for the diagnosis and grading of soft-tissue sarcoma: a meta-analysis. J Nucl Med 2003;44(5):717–724
10. Adler LP, Blair HF, Makley JT, et al. Noninvasive grading of musculoskeletal tumors using PET. J Nucl Med 1991;32(8):1508–1512
11. Aoki J, Endo K, Watanabe H, et al. FDG-PET for evaluating musculoskeletal tumors: a review. J Orthop Sci 2003;8(3):435–441
12. Lin D, Jacobs M, Percy T, et al. High 2-deoxy-2[F-18]fluoro-D-glucose uptake on positron emission tomography in hibernoma originally thought to be myxoid liposarcoma. Mol Imaging Biol 2005;7(3):201–212
13. Lodge MA, Lucas JD, Marsden PK, et al. A PET study of 18FDG uptake in soft tissue masses. Eur J Nucl Med 1999;26(1):22–30
14. Brenner W, Bohuslavizki KH, Eary JF. PET imaging of osteosarcoma. J Nucl Med 2003;44(6):930–942
15. Jadvar H, Gamie S, Ramanna L, Conti PS. Musculoskeletal system. Semin Nucl Med 2004;34(4):254–261
16. Franzius C, Sciuk J, Daldrup-Link HE, et al. FDG-PET for detection of osseous metastases from malignant

primary bone tumours: comparison with bone scintigraphy. Eur J Nucl Med 2000;27(9):1305–1311

17. Franzius C, Daldrup-Link HE, Sciuk J, et al. FDG-PET for detection of pulmonary metastases from malignant primary bone tumors: comparison with spiral CT. Ann Oncol 2001;12(4):479–486

18. Schuetze SM. Utility of positron emission tomography in sarcomas. Curr Opin Oncol 2006;18(4):369–373

19. Franzius C, Sciuk J, Brinkschmidt C, et al. Evaluation of chemotherapy response in primary bone tumors with F-18 FDG positron emission tomography compared with histologically assessed tumor necrosis. Clin Nucl Med 2000;25(11):874–881

20. Eary JF, O'Sullivan F, Powitan Y, et al. Sarcoma tumor FDG uptake measured by PET and patient outcome: a retrospective analysis. Eur J Nucl Med Mol Imaging 2002;29(9):1149–1154

21. Tateishi U, Yamaguchi U, Seki K, Terauchi T, Arai Y, Kim EE. Bone and soft-tissue sarcoma: preoperative staging with fluorine 18 fluorodeoxyglucose PET/CT and conventional imaging. Radiology 2007;245(3): 839–847

22. Franzius C, Daldrup-Link HE, Wagner-Bohn A, et al. FDG-PET for detection of recurrences from malignant primary bone tumors: comparison with conventional imaging. Ann Oncol 2002;13(1):157–160

23. Bredella MA, Caputo GR, Steinbach LS. Value of FDG positron emission tomography in conjunction with MR imaging for evaluating therapy response in patients with musculoskeletal sarcomas. AJR Am J Roentgenol 2002;179(5):1145–1150

24. Garcia R, Kim EE, Wong FC, et al. Comparison of fluorine-18-FDG PET and technetium-99m-MIBI SPECT in evaluation of musculoskeletal sarcomas. J Nucl Med 1996;37(9):1476–1479

25. Iagaru A, Chawla S, Menendez L, Conti PS. 18F-FDG PET and PET/CT for detection of pulmonary metastases from musculoskeletal sarcomas. Nucl Med Commun 2006;27(10):795–802

26. Mulligan ME, Badros AZ. PET/CT and MR imaging in myeloma. Skeletal Radiol 2007;36(1):5–16

27. Hain SF, O'Doherty MJ, Lucas JD, Smith MA. Fluorodeoxyglucose PET in the evaluation of amputations for soft tissue sarcoma. Nucl Med Commun 1999;20(9):845–848

28. Schirrmeister H, Bommer M, Buck AK, et al. Initial results in the assessment of multiple myeloma using 18F-FDG PET. Eur J Nucl Med Mol Imaging 2002; 29(3):361–366

29. Hung GU, Tsai CC, Tsai SC, Lin WY. Comparison of Tc-99m sestamibi and F-18 FDG-PET in the assessment of multiple myeloma. Anticancer Res 2005; 25(6C):4737–4741

30. Mileshkin L, Blum R, Seymour JF, et al. A comparison of fluorine-18 fluoro-deoxyglucose PET and technetium-99m sestamibi in assessing patients with multiple myeloma. Eur J Haematol 2004;72(1): 32–37

31. Durie BG, Waxman AD, D'Agnolo A, Williams CM. Whole-body (18)F-FDG PET identifies high-risk myeloma. J Nucl Med 2002;43(11):1457–1463

32. Breyer RJ III, Mulligan ME, Smith SE, et al. Comparison of imaging with FDG PET/CT with other imaging modalities in myeloma. Skeletal Radiol 2006;35(9): 632–640

33. Nanni C, Zamagni E, Farsad M, et al. Role of ^{18}F-FDG PET/CT in the assessment of bone involvement in newly diagnosed multiple myeloma: preliminary results. Eur J Nucl Med Mol Imaging 2006;33(5): 525–531

IV

Nononcologic Applications

26

Pediatric PET/CT

M. Beth McCarville

The use of positron emission tomography/computed tomography (PET/CT) in children requires consideration of several unique technical and logistic issues. Young children often require sedation for PET/CT, and personnel trained in the management of children are vital to patient safety. Pregnant guardians of young patients should not be allowed in the fluorodeoxyglucose (FDG) uptake room, and arrangements must be made for the supervision of such patients. Before administration of the radioisotope, young female patients themselves must be questioned regarding their childbearing potential. This delicate subject is best handled by a technologist with experience working with young girls. Additionally, interpretation of pediatric PET/CT imaging requires familiarity with pediatric anatomy and physiology because, compared with adults, children have more metabolically active brown fat and less retroperitoneal fat (**Fig. 26.1**).[1] PET/CT is becoming an increasingly important adjunct to the care of the pediatric oncology patient. Several indications for its use in children are discussed herein.

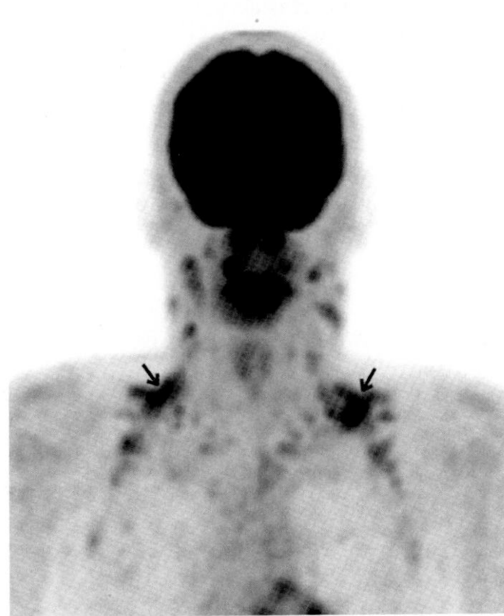

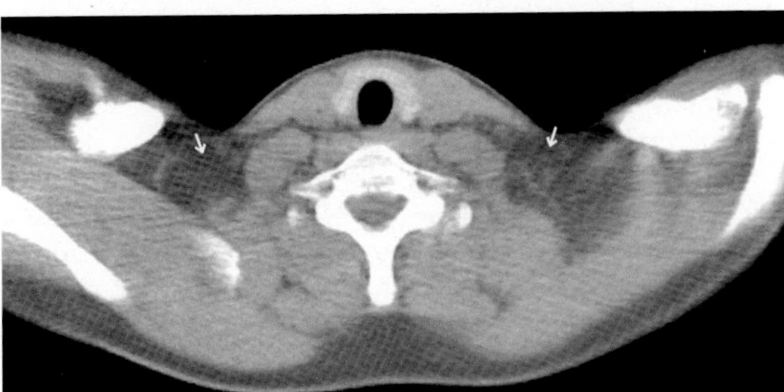

Fig. 26.1 A 16-year-old boy previously treated for Hodgkin lymphoma. **(A)** Maximum intensity projection positron emission tomography (MIP PET) image showing intense fluorodeoxyglucose (FDG) activity in the supraclavicular areas (*arrows*) that is difficult to accurately localize by positron emission tomography (PET) alone. **(B)** This is coregistered axial computed tomography (CT).

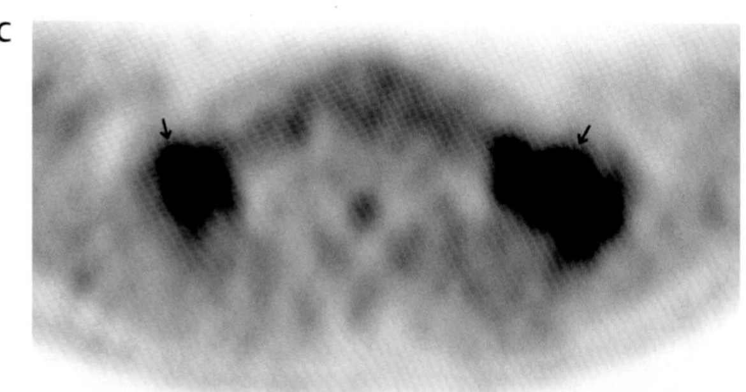

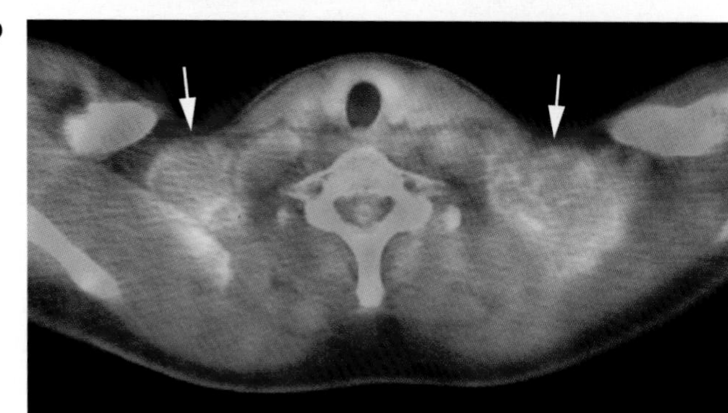

Fig. 26.1 (*Continued*) Coregistered axial **(B)** computed tomography (CT), **(C)** PET, and **(D)** fused PET/CT images allow confident localization of FDG activity to brown fat (*arrows*). Children often have abundant metabolically active brown fat, such as shown here.

◆ Bone Tumors

Clinical Indication

PET/CT has shown value in detecting bone metastases from primary Ewing sarcoma of bone and in the response evaluation of primary Ewing sarcoma and osteosarcoma.

Accuracy

1. In one study, on an examination-based analysis, the sensitivity, specificity, and accuracy of PET for detecting bone metastases from Ewing sarcoma of bone were 1.00, 0.96, and 0.97, respectively.[2]
2. A study evaluating the maximum standardized uptake value (SUV) of primary tumors before initiation of neoadjuvant chemotherapy (SUV1) and after neoadjuvant chemotherapy (SUV2) in patients with either osteosarcoma (n = 18) or Ewing sarcoma of bone (n = 15) found that the positive predictive value (PPV) for a favorable response (≥ 90% tumor necrosis) of an SUV2 < 2 was 93%, and the negative predictive value (NPV) for unfavorable response (< 90% necrosis) was 75%. The PPV and NPV for favorable and unfavorable response using an SUV2:SUV1 cutpoint of 0.5 were 78% and 63%, respectively.[3]

Pearls

1. It is postulated that bone marrow metastases, such as commonly seen in Ewing sarcoma, are FDG avid but often lack avidity for the bone-seeking agent, technetium 99m methylene diphosphonate (^{99m}Tc MDP). PET has the additional potential advantage of demonstrating extraosseous metastases.[2]

Pitfalls

1. On PET alone, skull metastases may be obscured by intense brain FDG activity. Evaluation of the skull in the bone window setting on correlative CT imaging, obtained during PET/CT, may increase the sensitivity for detection of skull metastases.[2,4]
2. In children, benign fibro-osseous lesions can mimic bone metastases on PET imaging. Furthermore, maximum SUVs of these

benign lesions overlap those of malignant lesions. Information gained from correlative CT or MR images is useful in determining the benign nature of such lesions (**Fig. 26.2**).[5,6]

3. Maximum SUVs of primary Ewing sarcoma and osteosarcoma may not accurately reflect overall tumor necrosis because small metabolically active foci may be present within tumor that is > 90% necrotic.[3,7]
4. After chemotherapy or radiation therapy, SUVs may remain high within primary bone tumors due to inflammation or reactive fibrosis rather than viable tumor.[3,7]

◆ Soft Tissue Tumors

Clinical Indication

In children with soft tissue malignancies, PET/CT has shown value in identifying the site of an unknown primary tumor, staging, monitoring response to therapy, and detecting recurrence.

Accuracy

1. Because soft tissue malignancies in children are rare, there have been no formal studies

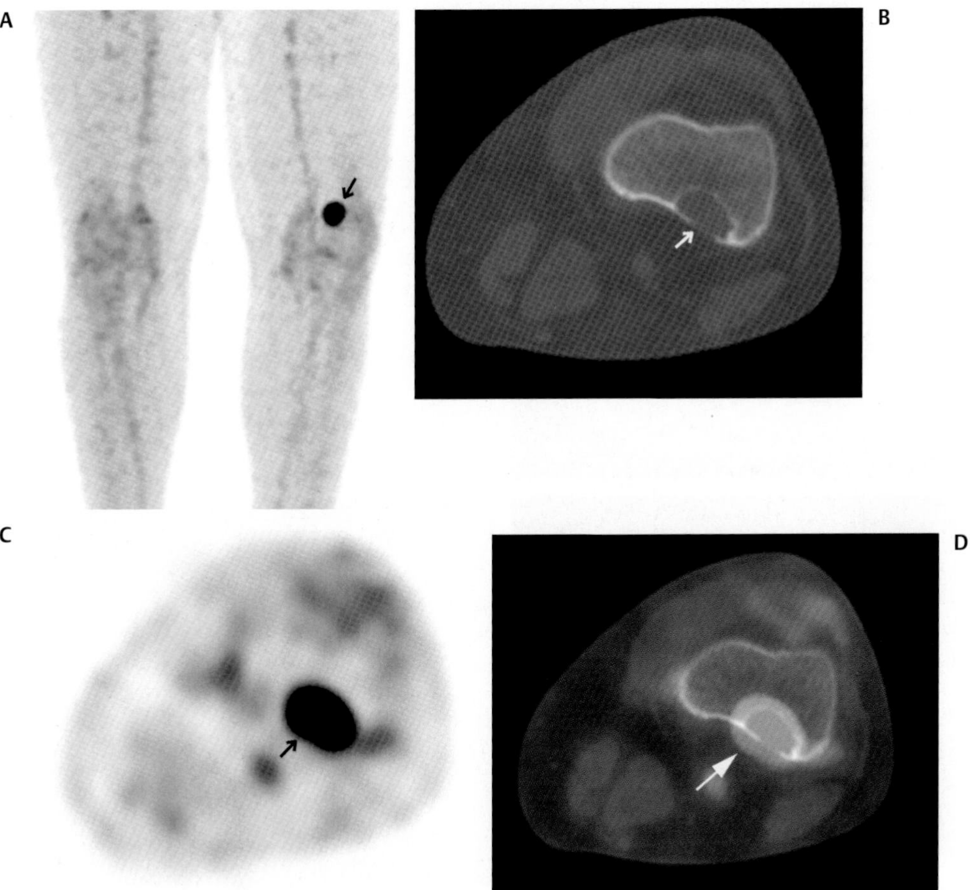

Fig. 26.2 A 19-year-old boy under treatment for metastatic paraganglioma. **(A)** Maximum intensity projection positron emission tomography (MIP PET) image of the knees shows intense fluorodeoxyglucose (FDG) activity in the distal left femur (*arrow*), worrisome for metastatic deposit. Coregistered axial **(B)** computed tomography (CT), **(C)** PET, and **(D)** fused PET/CT images, viewed in a bone window setting, allow identification of a benign nonossifying fibroma (*arrows*). Benign fibro-osseous lesions, such as this, are relatively common in children and can demonstrate minimal to intense FDG avidity.

of the accuracy of PET or PET/CT in the diagnosis or follow-up of these tumors.

Pearls

1. About 4% of rhabdomyosarcoma (RMS) will present with widely metastatic disease and unknown primary site.[8] PET/CT allows examination of the entire body in one sitting and can reveal the primary RMS as well as metastatic foci.[9]
2. One retrospective review showed that, in children with a variety of soft tissue malignancies, PET/CT detected sites of metastatic disease missed by physical examination and conventional imaging, including ^{99m}Tc MDP bone scintigraphy and CT. PET/CT appears to be especially valuable in the assessment of children with alveolar RMS, which has a propensity to metastasize to unusual soft tissue sites (**Fig. 26.3**).[9]
3. After chemotherapy, FDG avidity of primary and metastatic foci, from childhood soft tissue malignancies, appears to reflect tumor viability (**Fig. 26.4**).[9]
4. About 25 to 35% of children with sarcomas experience recurrence after therapy.[10] PET/CT is sensitive to recurrent disease in children with a variety of soft tissue sarcomas, particularly those with alveolar RMS.[9]

Pitfalls

1. In children with soft tissue malignancies, PET/CT cannot reliably distinguish benign

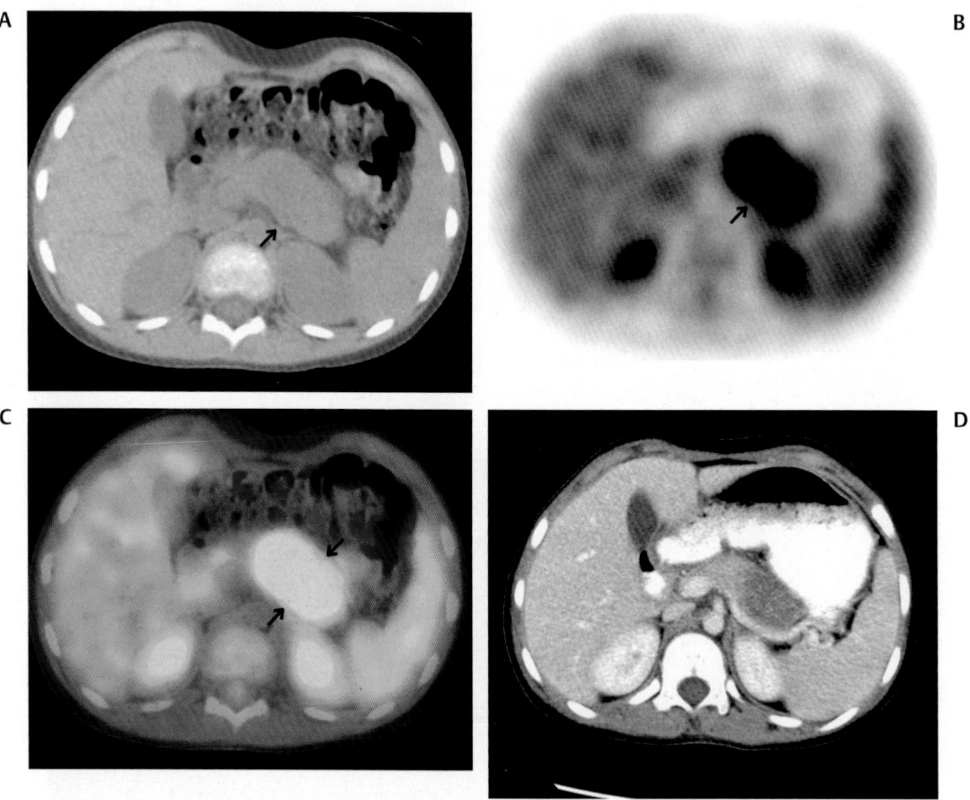

Fig. 26.3 A 10-year-old girl with metastatic alveolar rhabdomyosarcoma. Coregistered axial **(A)** computed tomography (CT), **(B)** positron emission tomography (PET), and **(C)** fused PET/CT images demonstrate an intensely fluorodeoxyglucose-avid pancreas metastasis (*arrows*) that was not clinically suspected. **(D)** This diagnostic CT, with oral and intravenous contrast, confirms the pancreatic location of the mass (*arrows*). PET/CT is useful in detecting clinically occult sites of metastatic disease in children with a variety of soft tissue and bone sarcomas.

from malignant lymph nodes. Enlarged nodes due to follicular hyperplasia and sinus histiocytosis can appear intensely FDG avid (**Fig. 26.5**).[9] Conversely, enlarged, malignant lymph nodes may show only minimal FDG avidity.[11]

◆ Langerhans Cell Histiocytosis

Clinical Indications

PET/CT may be useful in the baseline evaluation, response to therapy, and detection of reactivation of Langerhans cell histiocytosis (LCH).[12]

Accuracy

1. Because of the rarity of LCH, there has been no systematic investigation of the accuracy of PET/CT in its diagnosis and management.

Pearls

1. At baseline, PET/CT may detect sites of disease not evident on physical examination or conventional imaging examinations (**Fig. 26.6**).[12]
2. During therapy, FDG PET/CT may be more sensitive to LCH disease activity than plain film radiography and ^{99m}Tc MDP bone scintigraphy.[12]

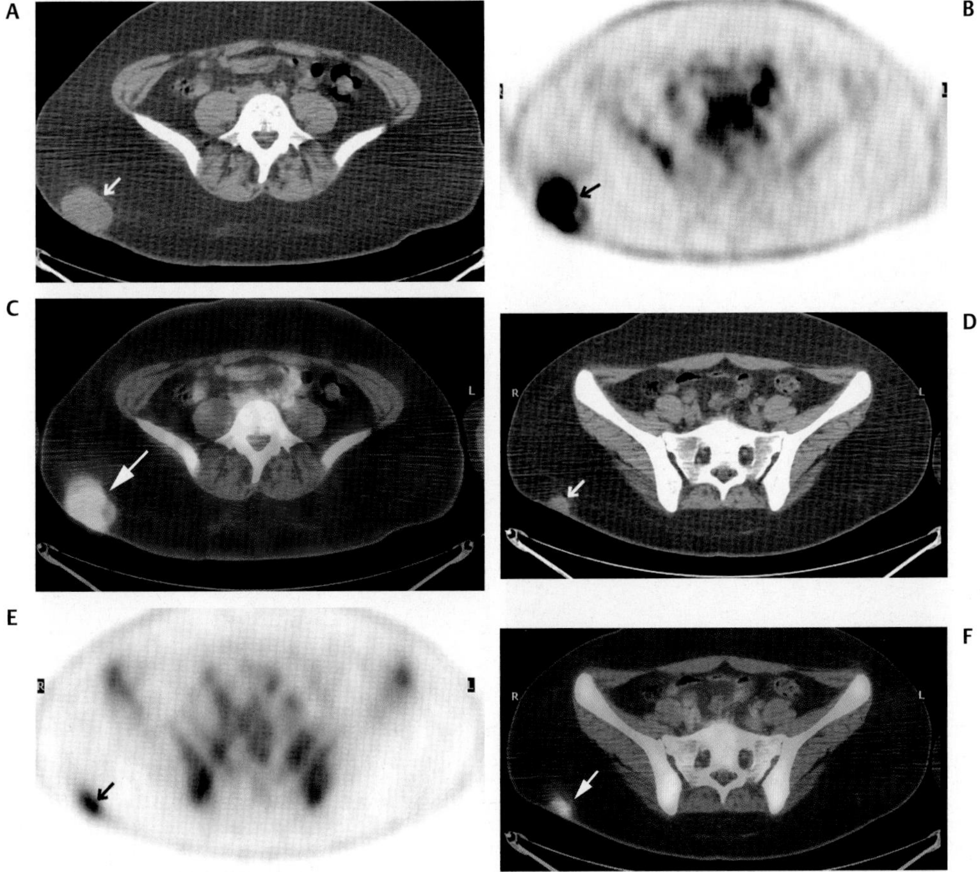

Fig. 26.4 An 18-year-old girl with extraosseous Ewing sarcoma family of tumor. Baseline coregistered, axial **(A)** computed tomography (CT), **(B)** positron emission tomography (PET), and **(C)** fused PET/CT images show the intensely fluorodeoxyglucose (FDG)-avid primary tumor in the right buttock. **(D–F)** At completion of chemotherapy, the tumor had become smaller but remained intensely FDG avid (*arrows*). Histology confirmed the majority of this residual tumor was viable.

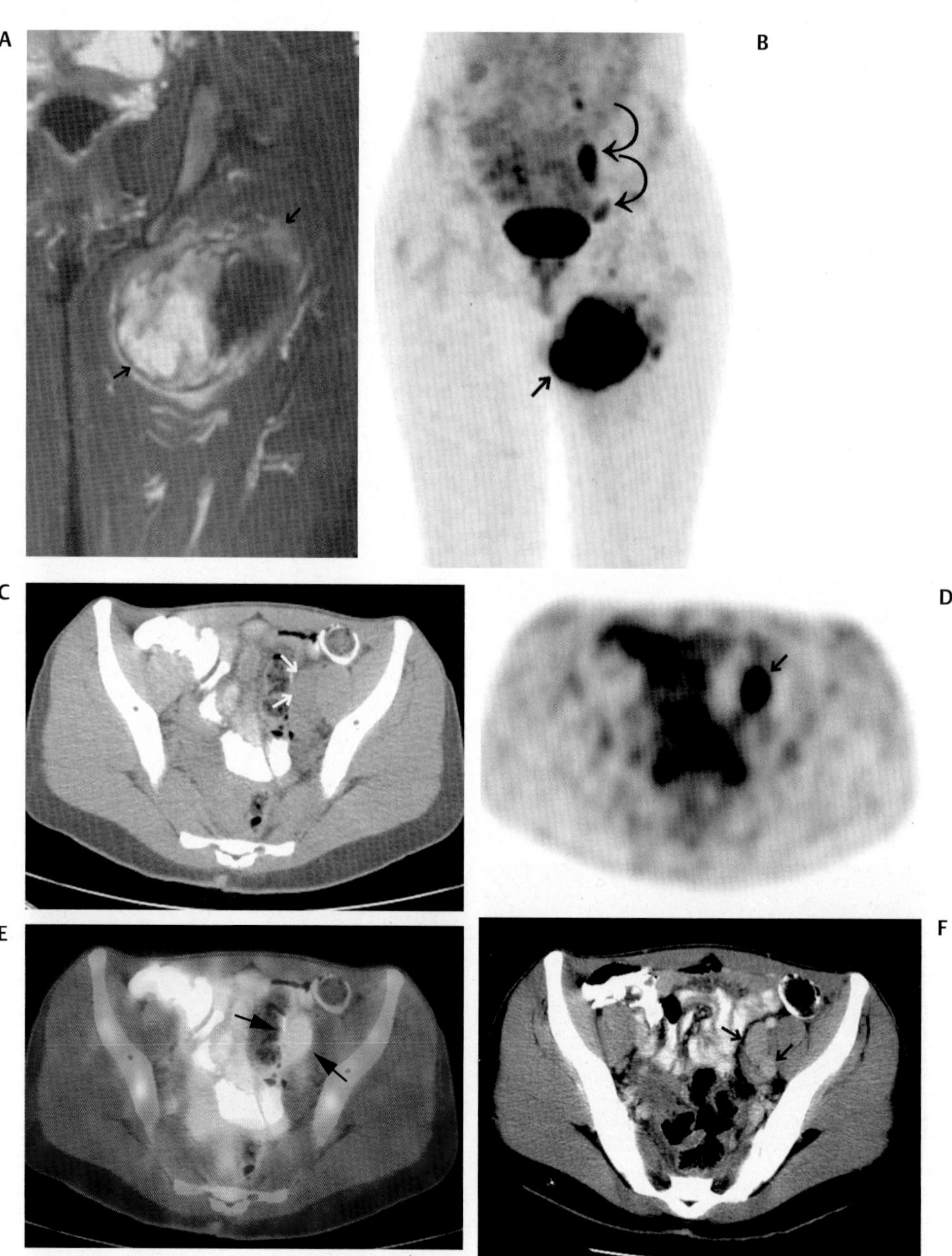

Fig. 26.5 A 19-year-old girl with malignant peripheral nerve sheath tumor. **(A)** Coronal short tau inversion recovery magnetic resonance image (STIR MRI) shows the primary left thigh tumor (*arrows*) at diagnosis. **(B)** This baseline maximum intensity projection positron emission tomography (MIP PET) image demonstrates intense fluorodeoxyglucose (FDG) activity in the primary tumor (*straight arrow*) and several foci of intense FDG activity in the left pelvis (*curved arrows*). Coregistered axial **(C)** computed tomography (CT), **(D)** PET, and **(E)** fused PET/CT images localize the left pelvic activity to enlarged iliac nodes (*arrows*). **(F)** This diagnostic CT with oral and intravenous contrast confirms the presence of enlarged left iliac nodes (*arrows*). These were worrisome for nodal spread from the left thigh malignancy, but on pathologic inspection they contained only follicular hyperplasia and sinus histiocytosis.

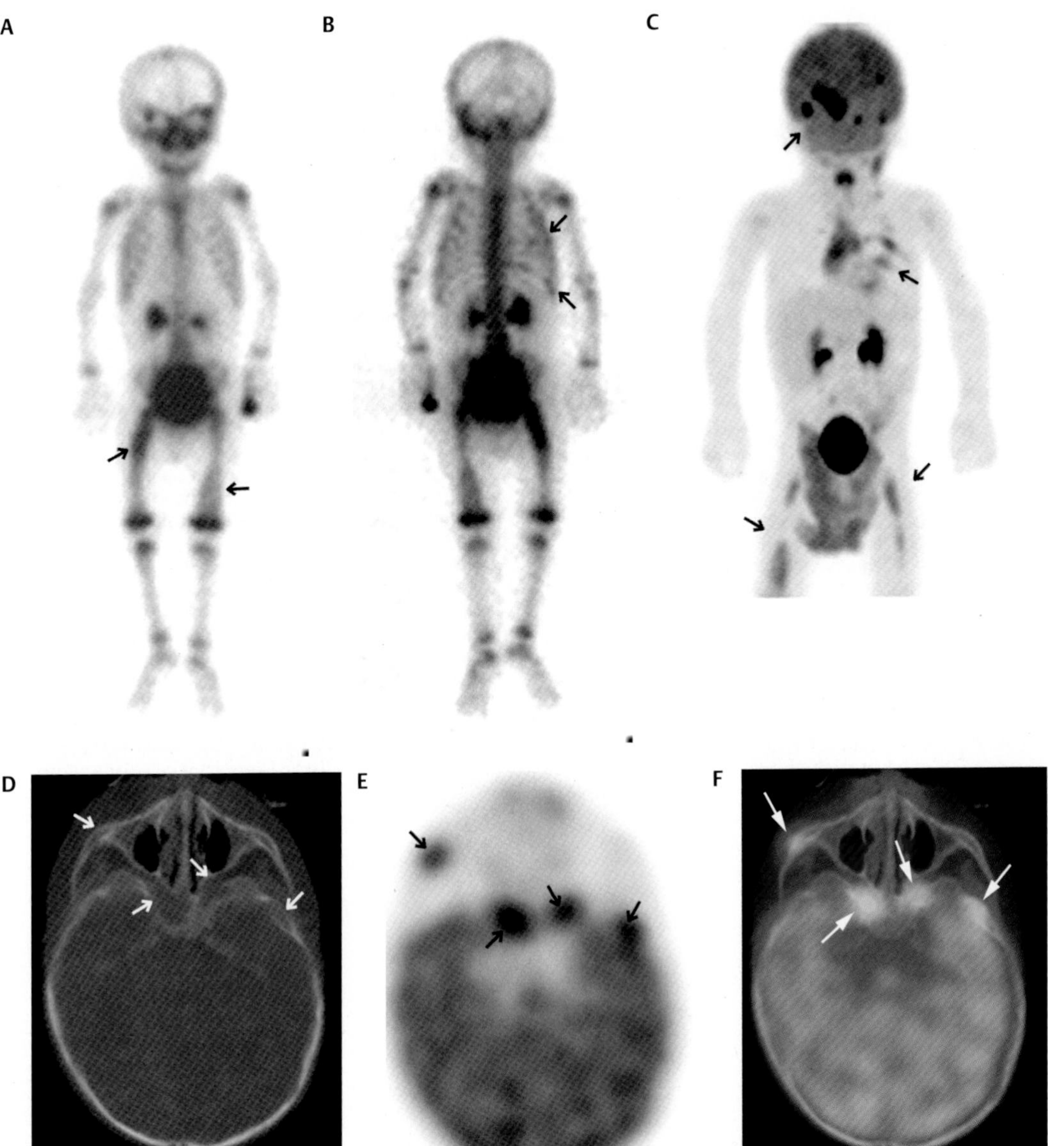

Fig. 26.6 A 17-month-old boy presented with right proptosis and was suspected to have neuroblastoma. **(A)** This baseline anterior technetium 99m (^{99m}Tc) bone scan image shows abnormal activity in both femora (*arrows*). **(B)** This posterior ^{99m}Tc bone scan image shows subtle activity in several posterior right ribs (*arrows*). **(C)** This baseline maximum intensity projection positron emission tomography (MIP PET) image shows abnormal fluorodeoxyglucose (FDG) activity in both femora, in several left ribs, and in the head (*arrows*). The foci of abnormal activity in the head were localized to the skull by these coregistered axial **(D)** computed tomography (CT), **(E)** PET, and **(F)** fused PET/CT images (*arrows*). The skull lesions and left rib abnormalities were not well seen on the ^{99m}Tc bone scan.

3. After therapy, patients with solitary bone lesions have a 10% risk of disease reactivation, whereas those with multiple bone lesions are 7 times more likely to recur. Risk of reactivation also depends on site of bone lesions; 39% of patients with multiple lesions that include the skull will have disease reactivation compared with 18% of those without skull lesions.[12] PET/CT may be more sensitive to disease reactivation than plain radiography.

References

1. Kaste SC. Issues specific to implementing PET-CT for pediatric oncology: what we have learned along the way. Pediatr Radiol 2004;34(3):205–213
2. Franzius C, Sciuk J. drup-Link HE, Jurgens H, Schober O. FDG-PET for detection of osseous metastases from malignant primary bone tumours: comparison with bone scintigraphy. Eur J Nucl Med 2000;27(9):1305–1311
3. Hawkins DS, Rajendran JG, Conrad EU III, Bruckner JD, Eary JF. Evaluation of chemotherapy response in pediatric bone sarcomas by [F-18]-fluorodeoxy-D-glucose positron emission tomography. Cancer 2002;94(12):3277–3284
4. Kushner BH, Yeung HW, Larson SM, Kramer K, Cheung NK. Extending positron emission tomography scan utility to high-risk neuroblastoma: fluorine-18 fluorodeoxyglucose positron emission tomography as sole imaging modality in follow-up of patients. J Clin Oncol 2001;19(14):3397–3405
5. Aoki J, Watanabe H, Shinozaki T, et al. FDG PET of primary benign and malignant bone tumors: standardized uptake value in 52 lesions. Radiology 2001;219(3):774–777
6. Goodin GS, Shulkin BL, Kaufman RA, McCarville MB. PET/CT characterization of fibroosseous defects in children: 18F-FDG uptake can mimic metastatic disease. AJR Am J Roentgenol 2006;187(4):1124–1128
7. Hawkins DS, Schuetze SM, Butrynski JE, et al. [^{18}F]Fluorodeoxyglucose positron emission tomography predicts outcome for Ewing sarcoma family of tumors. J Clin Oncol 2005;23(34):8828–8834
8. Etcubanas E, Peiper S, Stass S, Green A. Rhabdomyosarcoma, presenting as disseminated malignancy from an unknown primary site: a retrospective study of ten pediatric cases. Med Pediatr Oncol 1989; 17(1):39–44
9. McCarville MB, Christie R, Daw NC, Spunt SL, Kaste SC. PET/CT in the evaluation of childhood sarcomas. AJR Am J Roentgenol 2005;184(4):1293–1304
10. Pizzo PA, Poplack DG. Section IV: Management of common cancers of childhood. In: Principles and Practice of Pediatric Oncology. Philadelphia, PA: Lippincott, Williams and Wilkins; 2002:489–1176
11. Ben Arush MW, Bar SR, Postovsky S, et al. Assessing the use of FDG-PET in the detection of regional and metastatic nodes in alveolar rhabdomyosarcoma of extremities. J Pediatr Hematol Oncol 2006;28(7):440–445
12. Kaste SC, Rodriguez-Galindo C, McCarville ME, Shulkin BL. PET-CT in pediatric Langerhans cell histiocytosis. Pediatr Radiol 2007;37(7):615–622

27

PET and PET/CT in Radiation Therapy Planning

Sandip Basu, Guobin Song, Abass Alavi, and Eugene C. Lin

The introduction of metabolic imaging into the radiation therapy planning (RTP) process is a major advance in the management of cancer patients. The impact can be seen in

- More accurate staging
- Delineating the accurate volume and the extent of the disease
- Dose painting and theragnostic imaging

◆ More Accurate Staging

Conventional imaging techniques may up- or downstage patients with a variety of cancers. When radiation therapy is employed for optimal management of the diseased sites, understaging may result in partial treatment, and overstaging may lead to unnecessary radiation toxicity to the site(s) without disease. Positron emission tomography (PET) allows accurate staging not only at the primary site, but also at the locoregional level and distant regions. Staging with fluorodeoxyglucose (FDG) PET may change the intent of treatment from curative to palliative in 10 to 26% of cases when a new distant metastasis is detected. Several studies have documented that the improved staging with FDG PET can be used to improve patient management and significantly impact RTP (**Table 27.1**) and therefore improve outcome and minimize toxicity.[1–4]

◆ Tumor Volume Delineation

1. The functional information from PET images can be fused to the anatomical data from computed tomography (CT) and/or magnetic resonance imaging (MRI) within the RTP system to aid in detecting tumor and delineating the target volume for RTP. There is a considerable interest on the impact of such combined information on treatment planning, as the interobserver variability is substantially reduced compared with when these modalities are individually used.
2. Thresholding is the most commonly adopted method to determine volumes automatically from PET images. Most algorithms have been derived from the study of spheres of various sizes with differing levels of background signal. Some investigators have chosen to use a threshold based upon a percentage of the maximum standardized uptake value (SUVmax); others have relied on a threshold based on an absolute SUVmax value.[6] Contours are based upon the maximum in the lesion of interest, with values

Table 27.1 Impact of (Staging-) PET Scan on Radiotherapy Treatment

	Changes in Staging	Effect on Radiotherapy
T-stage	Larger extension of primary tumor (upstaging)	Enlargement of radiotherapy fields to avoid geographic miss Change of radiotherapy indication from curative to palliative
	Less extension of primary tumor (downstaging)	Decrease in radiotherapy fields and hence decrease in radiation exposure of normal tissues, thus allowing dose escalation Change of radiotherapy indication from palliative to curative
N-stage	Detection of new site of lymph node involvement (upstaging)	Enlargement of radiotherapy fields to avoid geographic miss Change of radiotherapy indication from curative to palliative
	Omission of enlarged lymph nodes, diagnosed as malignant on CT or MRI (downstaging)	Change of radiotherapy indication from palliative to curative Decrease in radiotherapy fields and hence decrease in radiation exposure of normal tissues, thus allowing dose escalation
M-stage	Detection of distant metastases	Change of radiotherapy indication from curative to palliative

Source: From van Baardwijk A, et al. The current status of FDG-PET in tumor volume definition in radiotherapy treatment planning. Cancer Treat Rev 2006;32(4):245–260. Reprinted with permission.
Abbreviations: CT, computed tomography; MRI, magnetic resonance imaging; PET, positron emission tomography.

ranging from 30 to 50% of the SUVmax used by various investigators.

3. In lung cancer, incorporation of PET data improves tumor volume and dose coverage and spares normal tissues, leading to less toxicity with the potential option of escalating dose to tumor tissue. In esophageal cancer and in lymphoma, a PET scan can be used to include PET-positive lymph nodes in the target volume.
4. In most other tumor sites, not enough data are currently available to draw definitive conclusions, though a few studies demonstrate its promise.
5. Daisne et al[7] compared CT, MRI, and PET with pathologic findings in head and neck patients. Smaller gross tumor volume (GTV) was observed with FDG PET for oropharyngeal, laryngeal, and hypopharyngeal tumors.
6. Three major issues to be addressed (the majority of studies are presently focused on this issues as well) are (a) whether it allows accurate tumor delineation; (b) whether its incorporation influences GTV, clinical target volume (CTV), and planning target volume (PTV); and (c) whether there is an improvement in treatment outcome.[7–9]

Target Volumes in Radiation Therapy Planning

1. ***Gross tumor volume (GTV).*** Derived from the gross demonstrable extent and location of tumor identified with the CT or simulator images
2. ***Clinical target volume (CTV).*** Expanded GTV to include subclinical disease based on additional clinical information
3. ***Planning target volume (PTV).*** Expanded CTV by the addition of a variable margin to take into account internal organ movement as well as patient motion and setup uncertainties[10,11]

4. ***Biological target volumes (BTV).*** Derived from the biological information about tumors and surrounding normal tissue obtained from the PET component of PET/CT.[12] BTV can have different implications based upon the PET radiotracer used for scanning; for example, BTV determined from FDG might be considered to represent the viable tumor cells and can be used to determine a minimum dose for the entire tumor. However, a BTV resulting from fluoromisonidazol (FMISO; a PET tracer for hypoxia) would represent a smaller tumor subvolume, where the maximum tumor dose requires delivery to the hypoxic cells associated with radioresistance.

Clinical Applications

Integration of PET images in radiotherapy planning has been primarily studied in non–small cell lung cancer (NSCLC),[13–15] with some studies published on esophageal carcinoma,[16] head and neck cancer (HNC),[17] and rectal carcinoma.[18]

Study Results for Lung Cancer

1. A survey of the published findings shows that treatment volumes are significantly altered in 30 to 60% patients with NSCLC with the addition of biologic targeting with FDG PET.[19]
2. In a series of 44 patients of NSCLC, FDG PET altered the stage of the disease in 25% of the cases by downstaging the disease in a majority of them.[20] GTV based on FDG PET was on average smaller than the GTV defined by CT. Also, in a different study it was found that for the same radiotoxicity to the lungs, spinal cord, and esophagus, the dose to the tumor can be enhanced by 25%; this resulted in a potentially higher tumor control probability (24% for PET/CT planning compared with 6.3% for CT-only planning).[21]
3. FDG PET also alters the delineation of the GTV by discriminating tumor tissue from atelectasis or necrosis.[19,22,23] Modifications in target volume delineation allows delivering a tumoricidal dose to the target while minimizing the radiation dose to the uninvolved tissue.

Study Results for Head and Neck Carcinoma

Studies have shown excellent treatment outcomes in HNC patients treated with intensity-modulated radiation therapy (IMRT),[24,25] in which many small pencil beams are used to conform the volume irradiated to any irregular shape. IMRT has the ability to deliver high doses of radiation to the tumor target with very high precision; thus, accurate tumor targeting and delineation are required more than ever.

Studies in patients with locally advanced head neck squamous cell carcinoma have demonstrated that PET/CT-based radiation treatment would significantly change the dose distribution.[26,27]

PET/CT has also been found helpful in the management of occult primary head and neck tumors by determining a site of origin of the primary tumor in 60%.[28] This translates into reduced dose distribution to uninvolved mucosal sites compared with the results of CT scan only–based plans.

◆ Dose Painting and Theragnostic Imaging

These novel concepts are primarily based upon the results of scanning with novel imaging markers of tumor hypoxia or proliferation and variations in tumor volume as well as viability during radiotherapy that could modify the delineation of target volumes.

Dose Painting

Information obtained from other novel tracers like those of hypoxia, proliferation, apoptosis, and receptor expression can be integrated with that of FDG PET imaging, which provides greater insight into the biologic pathways involved in radiation responses.[29–34] Taken together, these can be utilized by the new sophisticated software planning algorithms to deliver IMRT treatments,[35–39] where the intensity through the treatment beam is varied. Combining several IMRT treatment portals can result in complex cross-sectional dose distributions being achieved and even the delivery of high-dose areas within the target, a technique that has been referred to as "dose painting."[12]

This concept depends on the ability to visualize tumor subvolumes, which are potentially radioresistant, and then paint some additional dose restricted to those subvolumes.

PET/CT for Adaptive Radiotherapy during Course of Treatment: Theragnostic Imaging

This is based upon calculation of the mean dose delivery during the early part of the treatment and the tumor response during this initial period of therapy and revision of the subsequent treatment plan.[40–43] This replanning of the radiotherapy during the course of treatment can help in substantial sparing of the surrounding nontarget tissues and is the major advantage of "theragnostic" imaging, a term coined by Bentzen.[43]

◆ Respiratory Gating of PET

1. The aim is to accurately target the dose of radiation to the "diseased" tissue volume with relative sparing of the surrounding normal tissue.
2. Gating systems that can be coupled with the development of treatment plans and target volumes in equivalent physiologic state are under active research. These will allow the radiation to be delivered in synchrony with physiologic motion such as respiration.[44–47]
3. These are especially relevant to the treatment of the thoracic neoplasms.

◆ Future Developments for Incorporating PET into Routine Radiotherapy Planning

1. Interpretation of PET images for contouring target volumes
2. Proper coregistration of PET and CT images
3. Computer software for easy image transfer to and acceptance by treatment planning systems from the PET systems
4. Mechanisms to account for tumor motion

◆ Promising Approaches

1. Use of four-dimensional PET/CT can correct for respiratory motion artifacts seen in conventional PET/CT imaging. It has the potential to reduce smearing and improve the accuracy in PET/CT coregistration.
2. Employing PET/CT for radiosurgery treatment planning for the purpose of improved local control rates following radiosurgery and to reduce subsequent tumor recurrence rates.

◆ Summary

The literature with regard to the clinical impact and patient outcome of using PET/CT to modify dose in metabolically active tumor cells is evolving at this time, and further clinical studies are needed. The detailed structural and functional imaging information potentially improves RTP by minimizing unnecessary irradiation of normal tissues and by reducing the risk of geographic miss. The potential of PET to quantify metabolism and identify new imaging targets within tumor tissue such as cellular proliferation, hypoxia, tumor receptors, and gene expression, thereby helping in the biological optimization of dose delivery, is an exciting area of research.[45–49] However, the impact of PET/CT-based IMRT dose painting RTP on tumor control and clinical outcome can only be determined with prospective research studies of patients.

References

1. Mah K, Caldwell CB, Ung YC, et al. The impact of (18)FDG-PET on target and critical organs in CT-based treatment planning of patients with poorly defined non-small-cell lung carcinoma: a prospective study. Int J Radiat Oncol Biol Phys 2002;52:339–350
2. Ciernik IF, Dizendorf E, Baumert BG, et al. Radiation treatment planning with an integrated positron emission and computer tomography (PET/CT): a feasibility study. Int J Radiat Oncol Biol Phys 2003;57:853–863
3. Dizendorf EV, Baumert BG, von Schulthess GK, et al. Impact of whole-body ^{18}F-FDG PET on staging and managing patients for radiation therapy. J Nucl Med 2003;44:24–29
4. Kalff V, Hicks RJ, MacManus MP, et al. Clinical impact of (18)F fluorodeoxyglucose positron emission tomography in patients with non-small-cell lung cancer: a prospective study. J Clin Oncol 2001;19:111–118
5. van Baardwijk A, Baumert BG, Bosmans G, et al. The current status of FDG-PET in tumour volume

definition in radiotherapy treatment planning. Cancer Treat Rev 2006;32(4):245–260

6. Black QC, Grills IS, Kestin LL, et al. Defining a radiotherapy target with positron emission tomography. Int J Radiat Oncol Biol Phys 2004;60:1272–1282
7. Daisne J-F, Sibomana M, Bol A, Doumont T, Lonneux M, Gregoire V. Tri-dimensional automatic segmentation of PET volumes based on measured source-to-background ratios: influence of reconstruction algorithms. Radiother Oncol 2003;69:247–250
8. Erdi YE, Mawlawi O, Larson SM, et al. Segmentation of lung lesion volume by adaptive positron emission tomography image thresholding. Cancer 1997; 80(12, Suppl)2505–2509
9. Yaremko B, Riauka T, Robinson D, Murray B, Mc Ewan A, Roa W. Threshold modification for tumour imaging in non-small cell lung cancer using positron emission tomography. Nucl Med Commun 2005;26: 433–440
10. International Commission on Radiation Units and Measurements. Prescribing, recording and reporting photon beam therapy, ICRU Report 50. Bethesda, MD: International Commission on Radiation Units and Measurements; 1993
11. International Commission on Radiation Units and Measurements. Prescribing, recording and reporting photon beam therapy (Supplement to ICRU Report 50), ICRU Report 62. Bethesda, MD: International Commission on Radiation Units and Measurements; 1999
12. Ling CC, Humm J, Larson S, et al. Towards multidimensional radiotherapy (MD-CRT): biological imaging and biological conformality. Int J Radiat Oncol Biol Phys 2000;47:551–560
13. Caldwell CB, Mah K, Ung YC, et al. Observer variation in contouring gross tumour volume in patients with poorly defined non-small-cell lung tumours on CT: the impact of 18FDG-hybrid PET fusion. Int J Radiat Oncol Biol Phys 2001;51:923–931
14. Erdi YE, Rosenzweig K, Erdi AK, et al. Radiotherapy treatment planning for patients with non-small cell lung cancer using positron emission tomography (PET). Radiother Oncol 2002;62:51–60
15. Fox JL, Ramesh R, O'Meara W, et al. Does registration of PET and planning CT images decrease interobserver and intraobserver variation in delineating tumour volumes for non-small cell lung cancer? Int J Radiat Oncol Biol Phys 2005;62:70–75
16. Moureau-Zabotto L, Touboul E, Lerouge D, et al. Impact of CT and ^{18}F-deoxyglucose positron emission tomography image fusion for conformal radiotherapy in esophageal carcinoma. Int J Radiat Oncol Biol Phys 2005;63:340–345
17. Scarfone C, Lavely WC, Cmelak AJ, et al. Prospective feasibility trial of radiotherapy target definition for head and neck cancer using 3 dimensional PET and CT imaging. J Nucl Med 2004;45:543–552
18. Roels S, Duthoy W, Haustermans K, et al. Definition and delineation of the clinical target volume for rectal cancer. Int J Radiat Oncol Biol Phys 2006;65:1129–1142
19. Bradley JD, Perez CA, Dehdashti F, et al. Implementing biologic target volumes in radiation treatment planning for non-small cell lung cancer. J Nucl Med 2004;45(suppl II):S96–S101
20. De Ruysscher D, Wanders S, van Haren E, et al. Selective mediastinal node irradiation based on FDG-PET scan data in patients with non-small-cell lung cancer: a prospective clinical study. Int J Radiat Oncol Biol Phys 2005;62:988–994
21. De Ruysscher D, Wanders S, Minken A, et al. Effects of radiotherapy planning with a dedicated combined PET-CT-simulator of patients with non-small cell lung cancer on dose limiting normal tissues and radiation dose-escalation: a planning study. Radiother Oncol 2005;77:5–10
22. Nestle U, Walter K, Schmidt S, et al. ^{18}F-deoxyglucose positron emission tomography (FDG-PET) for the planning of radiotherapy in lung cancer: high impact in patients with atelectasis. Int J Radiat Oncol Biol Phys 1999;44:593–597
23. Bradley J, Thorstad WL, Mutic S, et al. Impact of FDG-PET on radiation therapy volume delineation in non-small-cell lung cancer. Int J Radiat Oncol Biol Phys 2004;59:78–86
24. Chao KS, Deasy JO, Markman J, et al. A prospective study of salivary function sparing in patients with head-and-neck cancers receiving intensity-modulated or three-dimensional radiation therapy: Initial results. Int J Radiat Oncol Biol Phys 2001;49:907–916
25. Lee N, Xia P, Quivey JM, et al. Intensity-modulated radiotherapy in the treatment of nasopharyngeal carcinoma: an update of the UCSF experience. Int J Radiat Oncol Biol Phys 2002;53:12–22
26. Schwartz DL, Ford E, Rajendran J, et al. FDG-PET/CT imaging for preradiotherapy staging of head-and-neck squamous cell carcinoma. Int J Radiat Oncol Biol Phys 2005;61:129–136 [Medline]
27. Schwartz DL, Ford EC, Rajendran J, et al. FDG-PET/CT-guided intensity modulated head and neck radiotherapy: a pilot investigation. Head Neck 2005;27: 478–487
28. Wong WL, Saunders M. The impact of FDG PET on the management of occult primary head and neck tumors. Clin Oncol (R Coll Radiol) 2003;15:461–466
29. Fujibayashi Y, Taniuchi H, Yonekura Y, Ohtani H, Konishi J, Yokoyama A. Copper-62-ATSM: a new hypoxia imaging agent with high membrane permeability and low redox potential. J Nucl Med 1997;38:1155–1160
30. Shields AF, Grierson JR, Dohmen BM, et al. Imaging proliferation in vivo with [F-18]FLT and positron emission tomography. Nat Med 1998;4:1334–1336
31. Borbath I, Gregoire V, Bergstrom M, Laryea D, Langstrom B, Pauwels S. Use of 5-[(76)Br]bromo-2'-fluoro-2'-deoxyuridine as a ligand for tumour proliferation: validation in an animal tumour model. Eur J Nucl Med Mol Imaging 2002;29:19–27
32. Gronroos T, Bentzen L, Marjamaki P, et al. Comparison of the biodistribution of two hypoxia markers [^{18}F]FETNIM and [^{18}F]FMISO in an experimental mammary carcinoma. Eur J Nucl Med Mol Imaging 2004;31:513–520
33. Mahy P, De Bast M, Leveque PH, et al. Preclinical validation of the hypoxia tracer 2-(2-nitroimidazol-1-yl)-N-(3,3,3-[(18)F]trifluoropropyl)acetamide, [(18)F]EF3. Eur J Nucl Med Mol Imaging 2004;31:1263–1272
34. Mishani E, Abourbeh G, Jacobson O, et al. High-affinity epidermal growth factor receptor (EGFR) irreversible inhibitors with diminished chemical reactivities as positron emission tomography (PET)-imaging agent candidates of EGFR overexpressing tumors. J Med Chem 2005;48:5337–5348
35. Chao KS, Bosch WR, Mutic S, et al. A novel approach to overcome hypoxic tumor resistance: Cu-ATSM-guided intensity-modulated radiation therapy. Int J Radiat Oncol Biol Phys 2001;49:1171–1182
36. Douglas JG, Stelzer KJ, Mankoff DA, et al. [F-18]-fluorodeoxyglucose positron emission tomography

for targeting radiation dose escalation for patients with glioblastoma multiforme: clinical outcomes and patterns of failure. Int J Radiat Oncol Biol Phys 2006;64:886–891

37. Mutic S, Malyapa RS, Grigsby PW, et al. PET-guided IMRT for cervical carcinoma with positive para-aortic lymph nodes: a dose-escalation treatment planning study. Int J Radiat Oncol Biol Phys 2003;55:28–35

38. Vanuytsel LJ, Vansteenkiste JF, Stroobants SG, et al. The impact of (18)F-fluoro-2-deoxy-D-glucose positron emission tomography (FDG-PET) lymph node staging on the radiation treatment volumes in patients with non-small cell lung cancer. Radiother Oncol 2000;55:317–324

39. Lee NY, Mechalakos JG, Nehmeh S, et al. Fluorine-18-labeled fluoromisonidazole positron emission and computed tomography-guided intensity-modulated radiotherapy for head and neck cancer: a feasibility study. Int J Radiat Oncol Biol Phys 2008;70:2–13

40. Geets X, Lee L, Lonneux M, Coche E, Cosnard G, Grégoire V. Re-assessment of HNSCC tumor volume during radiotherapy with anatomic and functional imaging. [abstract] Radiother Oncol 2006;78(Suppl 1):S59

41. Humm JL, Lee J, O'Donoghue JA, et al. Changes in FDG tumor uptake during and after fractionated radiation therapy in a rodent tumor xenograft. Clin Positron Imaging 1999;2:289–296

42. Brahme A. Biologically optimized 3-dimensional in vivo predictive assay-based radiation tberapy using positron emission tomography-computerized tomography imaging. Acta Oncol 2003;42:123–136

43. Bentzen SM. Theragnostic imaging for radiation oncology: dose-painting by numbers. Lancet Oncol 2005;6:112–117

44. Livieratos L, Stegger L, Bloomfield PM, et al. Rigid body transformation of list mode projection data for respiratory motion correction in cardiac PET. IEEE Medical Imaging Conference records. Piscataway, NJ: IEEE; 2003

45. Wang Y, Baghaei H, Li H, et al. A simple respiration gating technique and its application in high resolution PET. IEEE Medical Imaging Conference records. Piscataway, NJ: IEEE; 2003

46. Guivarc'h O, Turzo A, Visvikis D, et al. Synchronisation of pulmonary scintigraphy by respiratory flow and by impedance plethysmography. Proc SPIE Medical Imaging #5370. Bellingham, WA: SPIE;2004:1166–1175

47. Erdi YE, Nehmeh SA, Pan T, et al. The CT motion quantitation of lung lesions and its impact on PET measured SUV's. J Nucl Med 2004;45:1287–1292

48. Grégoire V, Haustermans K, Geets X, Roels S, Lonneux M. PET-based treatment planning in radiotherapy: a new standard? J Nucl Med 2007;48(Suppl 1): 68S–77S

49. Senan S, De Ruysscher D. Critical review of PET-CT for radiotherapy planning in lung cancer. Crit Rev Oncol Hematol 2005;56(3):345–351

28

FDG PET in the Evaluation of Infection and Inflammation

Sandip Basu, Abass Alavi, and Eugene C. Lin

Although several molecular mechanisms have been proposed as the basis for fluorodeoxyglucose (FDG) uptake in cells, overexpression of glucose transport protein 1 (GLUT1) subtype in the stimulated macrophages, neutrophils, and lymphocytes is considered the most likely underlying biological phenomenon responsible for this observation. The data on the role of combined positron emission tomography/computed tomography (PET/CT) in the assessment of infection and inflammation are sparse at this time, but undoubtedly this modality may prove to be even more effective than PET alone for evaluating certain clinical scenarios where surgical interventions are being considered.

◆ Comparison of FDG PET with Other Imaging Modalities for Evaluating Infection and Inflammation

Conventional Nuclear Medicine Techniques

1. ***Advantages of FDG PET***
   - Securing results within a short period of time (1.5 to 2 hours)
   - High-resolution tomographic images
   - High target-to-background contrast ratio
   - Sensitive for chronic infections
   - Technically not demanding or less labor-intensive
   - High interobserver agreement
   - Radiation dose 2 to 3 times lower than that of conventional nuclear medicine techniques
   - Useful in detecting infection in the axial skeleton, where white blood cell (WBC) scanning is of limited value
2. ***Disadvantages of FDG PET***
   - Not widely available in most of the world
   - Relatively high cost
   - Differentiation between tumor and infection or inflammation is not possible, but delayed imaging and dual-time-point PET is of help.

Anatomical Imaging Modalities (Computed Tomography/Magnetic Resonance Imaging [CT/MRI])

1. ***Advantages of FDG PET***
   - Whole-body technique
   - Not affected by metallic implants
   - Assessment of metabolic activity of inflammatory process is more specific in the right setting than hyperperfusion or edema (CT/MRI).

2. ***Disadvantages of FDG PET***
   - Not widely available in most of the world
   - Relatively low spatial resolution compared with structural techniques

◆ Potential Clinical Applications

Chronic Osteomyelitis

Overview

1. Limited added value in the diagnosis of uncomplicated cases of acute osteomyelitis compared with the combination of physical examination, biochemical alterations in combination with three-phase bone scanning or MRI
2. Several studies have documented the important role of FDG PET in diagnosing patients with chronic osteomyelitis (**Figs. 28.1, 28.2,** and **28.3**).
3. In contrast to other nuclear medicine modalities, such as gallium scintigraphy and labeled leukocyte imaging, FDG has high resolution and can distinguish soft tissue infection from osteomyelitis.
4. It is expected that FDG PET imaging will be used routinely in the near future to determine the presence or the absence of an infectious focus, to monitor response to antimicrobial treatment, and to develop criteria for deciding when the treatment can be safely stopped.

Accuracy

1. Guhlmann et al[1,2] reported a higher accuracy for FDG PET than antigranulocyte antibody scintigraphy in imaging the central skeleton for infection in patients with suspected chronic osteomyelitis.
2. De Winter et al[3] reported a sensitivity of 100%, a specificity of 86%, and an accuracy of 93% in 60 patients with suspected chronic musculoskeletal infections.
3. Another prospective study by Meller et al[4] on 30 patients with suspected active chronic osteomyelitis concluded that FDG PET is superior to indium 111–labeled leukocyte imaging in the diagnosis of chronic osteomyelitis in the central skeleton.
4. FDG PET accurately detects spinal osteomyelitis (**Fig. 28.2**) and could potentially replace gallium 67 (^{67}Ga) for this purpose.[5–7]
5. A recent meta-analysis showed that FDG PET is not only the most sensitive imaging modality for detecting chronic osteomyelitis,

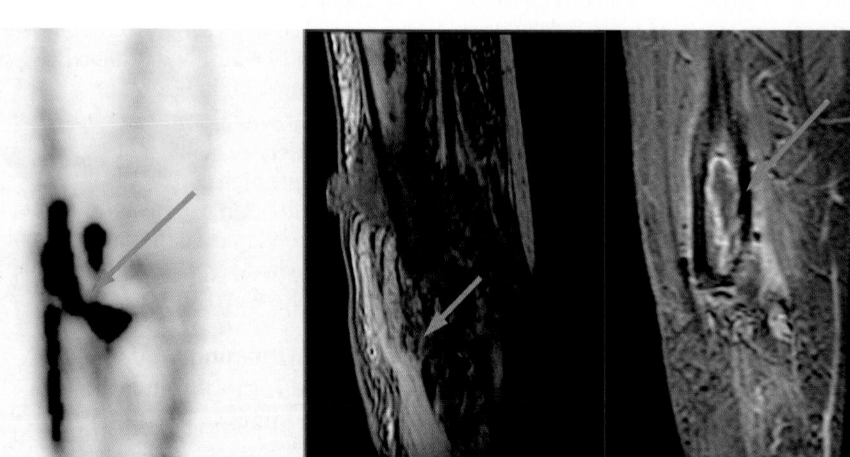

Fig. 28.1 **(A)** Sagittal fluorodeoxyglucose positron emission tomography (FDG PET). **(B)** Precontrast spoiled gradient (SPGR). **(C)** Postcontrast SPGR. Avid FDG uptake in the sinus tract (*arrow*) connecting soft tissue abscess with the medullary track of the femur in a patient of proven chronic osteomyelitis. Corresponding magnetic resonance imaging abnormalities are also shown in this figure. (From Kumar R, Basu S, Torigian D, Anand V, Zhuang H, Alavi A. Role of modern imaging techniques for diagnosis of infection in the era of ^{18}F-fluorodeoxyglucose positron emission tomography. Clin Microbiol Rev 2008;21(1):209–224. Reprinted with permission.)

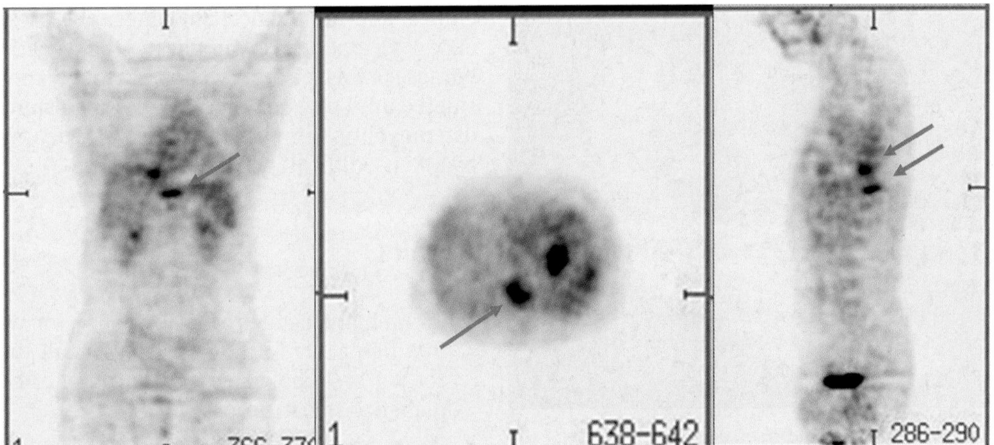

Fig. 28.2 Foci of fluorodeoxyglucose uptake in chronic osteomyelitis of the thoracic spine in two adjacent vertebral bodies. Radiolabeled white blood cell imaging in general has a low yield in this setting. (From Zhuang H, Alavi A. 18-fluorodeoxyglucose positron emission tomographic imaging in the detection and monitoring of infection and inflammation. Semin Nucl Med 2002;32:47–59. Reprinted with permission.)

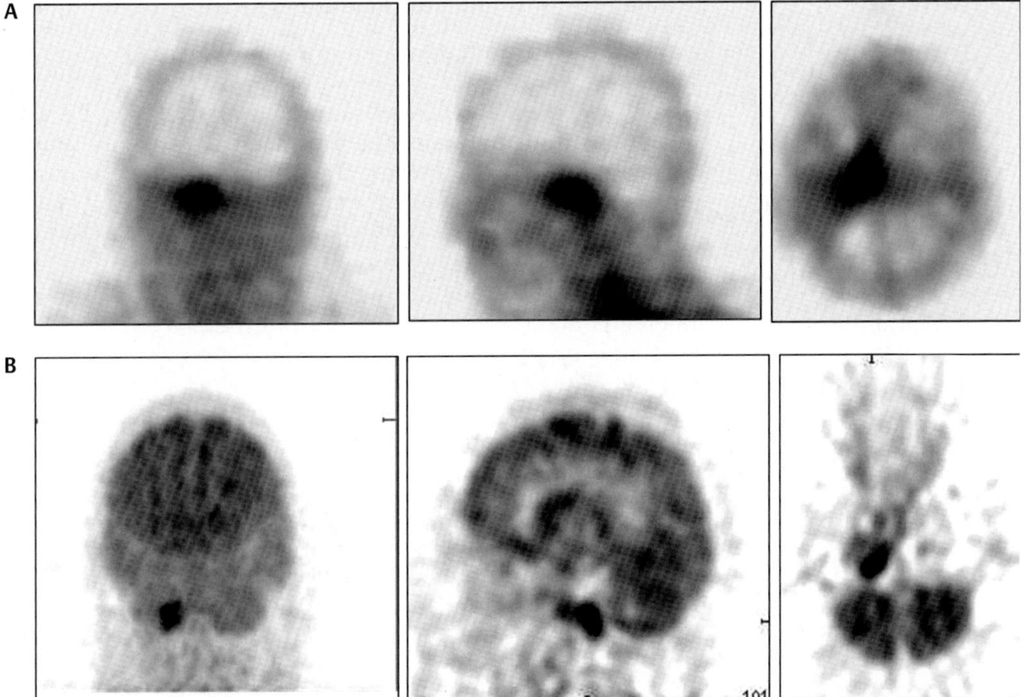

Fig. 28.3 **(A)** Gallium single-photon emission tomography (SPECT). **(B)** Fluorodeoxyglucose positron emission tomography (FDG PET). Avid FDG uptake in the focus of infection in a patient of proven malignant otitis with corresponding gallium 67 citrate–SPECT images. Note that PET images reveal the site of the disease more precisely than those of SPECT. (From Zhuang H, Alavi A. 18-fluorodeoxyglucose positron emission tomographic imaging in the detection and monitoring of infection and inflammation. Semin Nucl Med 2002;32:47–59. Reprinted with permission.)

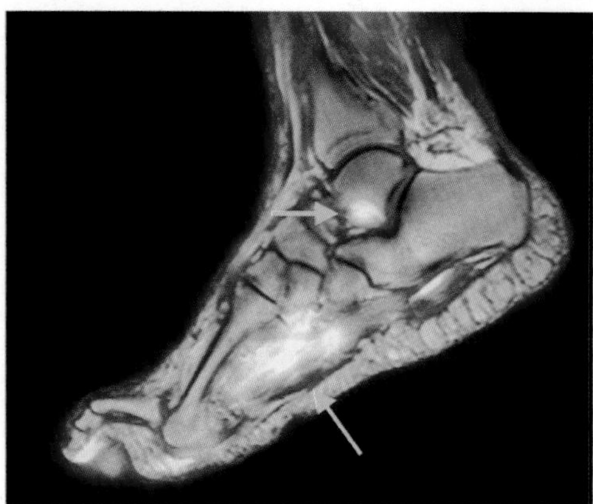

Fig. 28.4 Fused fluorodeoxyglucose positron emission tomography (FDG PET) and magnetic resonance (MR) images of a patient with a diabetic foot and a suspected bone infection. FDG PET image shows significant uptake in the soft tissue in the plantar aspect of the foot (suggestive of cellulitis); in addition, it reveals a focus of abnormal activity in the talus (consistent with talar bone osteomyelitis). (From Basu S, Alavi A. FDG-PET takes lead role in suspected or proven infection. Diagnostic Imaging San Francisco 2007; 29(11):59–64. Reproduced with permission.)

but also has a greater specificity than radiolabeled WBC scintigraphy, bone scintigraphy, or MRI.[8–10]

Complicated Diabetic Foot

Overview

Detection of infection and differentiating it from acute neuropathic osteoarthropathy in the setting of a complicated diabetic foot is a clinical and radiological challenge. The presence of ulceration also complicates the scenario because in this setting infection is strongly considered until proven otherwise. Distinguishing osteomyelitis from Charcot osteoarthropathy by MRI is a difficult task.

Accuracy

1. Preliminary data provide evidence for an important role for FDG PET imaging in the setting of complicated and uncomplicated diabetic osteoarthropathy.[10,11]
2. It can differentiate between Charcot neuroarthropathy and osteomyelitis and also soft tissue infection.[12,13]
3. FDG PET/CT was found to be highly accurate in detection of osteomyelitis (**Fig. 28.4**) by Keidar et al.[11]

Infected Prosthesis

Overview

1. One particular challenge for orthopedic surgeons has been differentiating mechanical loosening of prosthesis from superimposed infection and has been the subject of multiple research studies during the past several years.
2. FDG PET has a great potential for detecting infection in hip prostheses (**Figs. 28.5, 28.6,** and **28.7**), and to a lesser extent in knee prostheses.

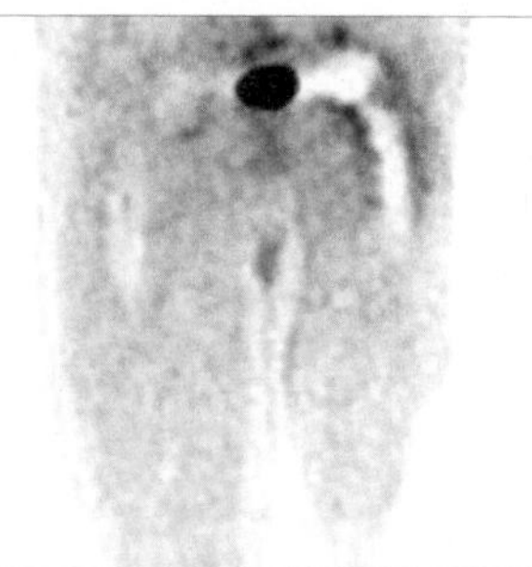
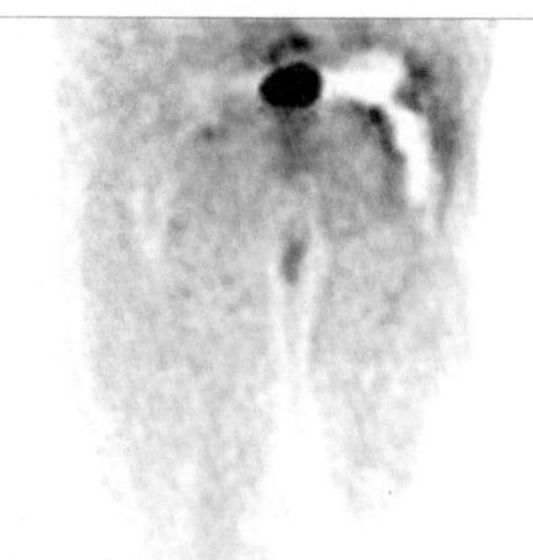
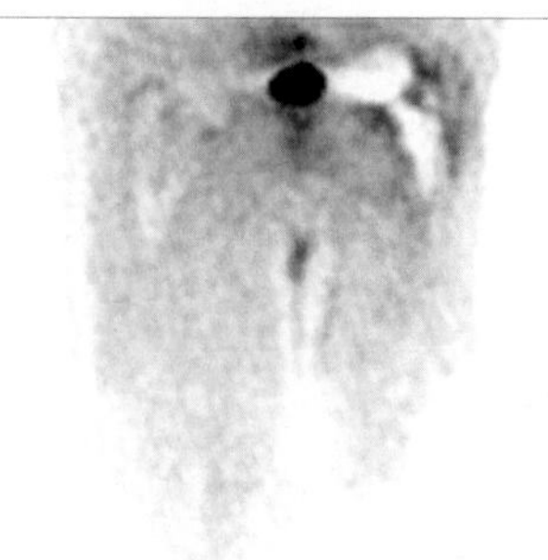

Fig. 28.5 The coronal images shown above belong to a patient with a painful left hip following arthroplasty. Although there is some inflammation seen around the neck of the prosthesis and the proximal femur, this is a common reaction in patients after insertion of hip prostheses. The images show no clear evidence of infection due to lack of fluorodeoxyglucose uptake at the bone–prosthesis interface; this aseptic diagnosis was confirmed by surgical intervention in this patient.

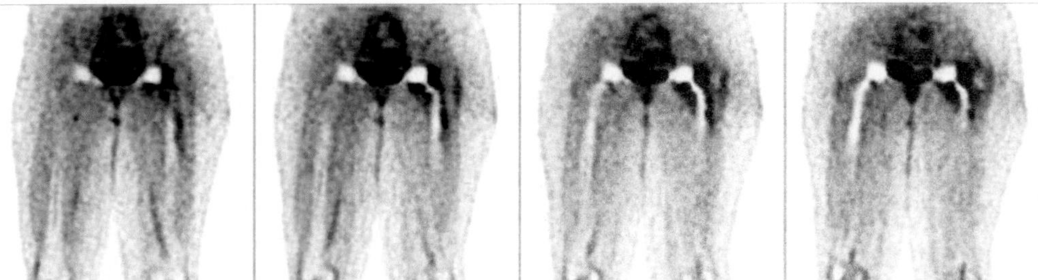

Fig. 28.6 Coronal images of the pelvis and thigh regions show no evidence of infection in the right hip prosthesis. On the left side, however, there is significant uptake of fluorodeoxyglucose at the bone–prosthesis interface surrounding the acetabular component and in the proximal half of the femoral stem. There is also evidence of extension of infection into the proximal soft tissue structures. The right prosthesis appears aseptic, and the left prosthesis appears infected. This was confirmed by surgical exploration.

3. FDG PET is advantageous over anatomical imaging modalities because it is not affected by the metal implants and provides better resolution images than those of the conventional nuclear medicine techniques, and it is exquisitely sensitive.
4. Noninfectious reactions are common months and even years after surgery, and the recognition of such reactions is important in managing these patients. Increased FDG uptake around the neck and/or head of the prosthesis is very common and should not be interpreted as a finding suggestive of infection. Most infection is found at the bone–prosthesis interface, and most noninfectious inflammatory reactions are found outside the bone–prosthesis junction.
5. Presently, the potential of FDG PET in the evaluation of prostheses is relatively well defined. More research may further enhance the role of FDG PET in the evaluation of prostheses.

Accuracy

1. In a prospective study involving 89 patients with 92 painful hip prostheses, our group[14] reported that the respective sensitivity, specificity, positive predictive value (PPV), and negative predictive value (NPV) of FDG PET for detecting infection was 95.2, 93, 80, and 98.5%, respectively. Similar figures of technetium 99m sulfur colloid indium 111-labeled white blood cell scintigraphy (TcSC-Ind BM/WBC) in the diagnosis of periprosthetic infection for hip prostheses was 50, 95.1, 41, and 88.6%, respectively.

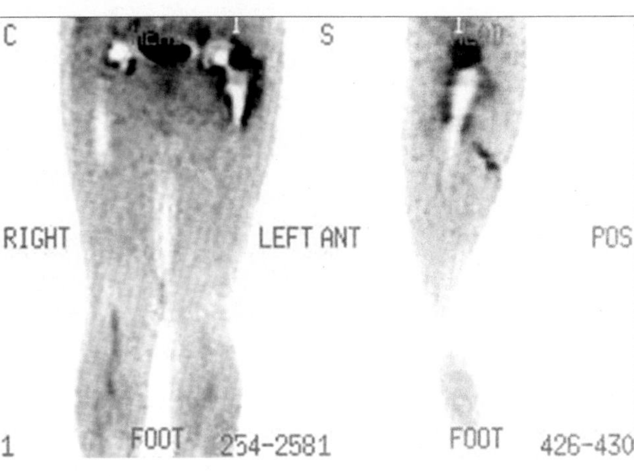

Fig. 28.7 The images shown above represent fluorodeoxyglucose positron emission tomography images of the pelvis and thighs taken in a patient with bilateral hip prostheses complaining of pain in the left hip. A fistula tract leading to the posterior thigh can be clearly seen in the sagittal image. The right prosthesis, meanwhile, appears uncomplicated and free of infection. The infection of the left hip was confirmed by surgical intervention.

Fever of Unknown Origin

Overview

Fever of unknown origin (FUO) is a clinical challenge, especially in the elderly, and appears to be an accepted indication for FDG PET in clinical practice. The nonspecificity of FDG is of great value in evaluating patients with FUO because it accumulates in infections, malignancies, and inflammatory diseases, which are the three major causes of FUO. Being a "catch-all" tracer, it has the potential to replace ^{67}Ga and labeled leukocyte imaging in this setting. However, overall, FDG PET has had an added value to conventional techniques in 40 to 70% of the patients.

Accuracy

1. In a subgroup of 40 patients who had both PET and a ^{67}Ga study, Blockmans et al[15] found that FDG PET revealed more abnormalities than the gallium scintigraphy (77 vs 67%, respectively).
2. Stumpe et al[16] reported 98% sensitivity, 75% specificity, and 91% accuracy for FDG PET in 39 patients with suspected infections.
3. Meller et al[17] compared FDG and gallium scanning in patients referred for assessment for FUO and reported a sensitivity of 81% and a specificity of 86% for FDG PET in detecting the cause of the fever and a sensitivity and specificity of 67 and 78%, respectively, for gallium scanning.
4. Bleeker-Rovers et al[18] evaluated 35 patients with FUO and reported that FDG PET was clinically helpful in 37% of cases, with a sensitivity and specificity of 93 and 90%, respectively, a PPV 87%, and an NPV of 95%.
5. A pilot study suggests that, in spite of the normal myocardial FDG uptake, FDG PET accurately helps identify sites of infective endocarditis and is a promising supplement to conventional echocardiography.[19]

AIDS Patients

Overview

PET has a major role to play in the management of human immunodeficiency virus (HIV)–infected patients and is especially valuable in the assessment of diseases affecting the central nervous system (CNS). Quantitative assessment has shown that the standardized uptake values

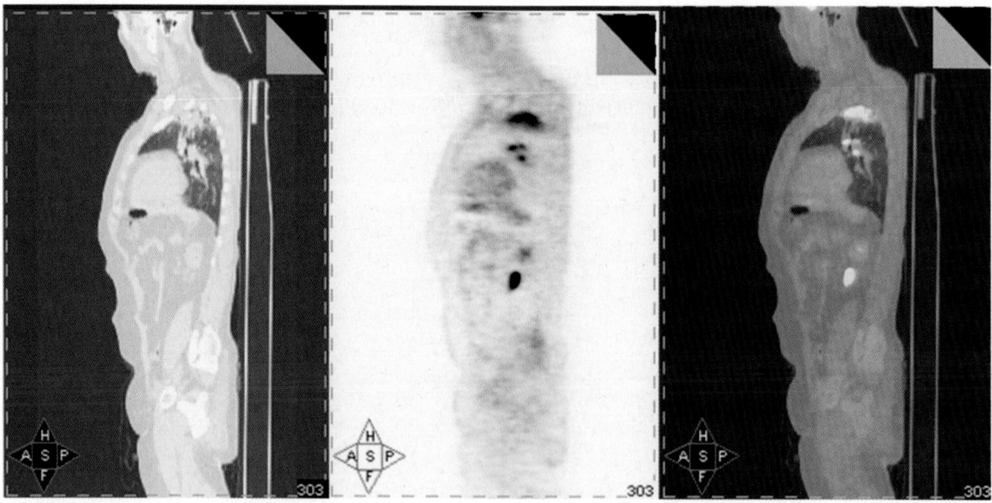

Fig. 28.8 Tubercular inflammatory lesion in the apex of the left lung, which shows intense fluorodeoxyglucose uptake fused with the corresponding computed tomography scan. (From Kumar R, Basu S, Torigian D, Anand V, Zhuang H, Alavi A. Role of modern imaging techniques for diagnosis of infection in the era of ^{18}F-fluorodeoxyglucose positron emission tomography. Clin Microbiol Rev 2008;21(1):209–224. Reprinted with permission.)

(SUVs) of toxoplasmosis are significantly lower than those of lymphoma, with virtually no overlap between the uptake values of the two conditions.

Accuracy

1. Hoffman et al[20] studied 11 individuals with acquired immunodeficiency syndrome (AIDS) and CNS lesions and found FDG PET imaging to be more accurate than CT or MRI in differentiating between malignant and nonmalignant etiologies for the CNS lesions.
2. O'Doherty et al[21] showed that PET had an overall sensitivity and specificity of 92 and 94%, respectively, in the detection of infections (**Fig. 28.8**) or malignancies in patients with AIDS.
3. Using FDG PET in 47 AIDS patients, Santiago et al[22] found a lesion sensitivity of 82.5% for FDG imaging.

Sarcoidosis

Overview

Assessment of disease activity in sarcoidosis largely determines the type of therapy to be instituted. FDG PET can help in the correct assessment of disease activity in sarcoidosis, which is critical for initiating an optimal management plan because most patients will have a self-limited course, whereas a small percentage may die without treatment soon after diagnosis. FDG uptake patterns in sarcoidosis (**Fig. 28.9**) can be misinterpreted as malignancy; thus, this test is not useful for initial diagnosis.

Accuracy

1. Several groups have reported FDG uptake by sarcoid granulomas,[23–25] which appear as typically active lymph nodes in the mediastinum and hilar regions.
2. By quantifying glucose metabolism in sarcoidosis, Brudin et al[23] have suggested that FDG uptake reflects likely disease activity and its extent at different stages of this unpredictable systemic disorder.

Atherosclerosis

Overview

FDG PET imaging has the potential to assess atherosclerosis as an inflammatory process at the early stages of the disease, during its natural course, and following therapeutic intervention. The mechanism of this uptake is unclear, and possibilities include high glucose metabolism by macrophages in the atherosclerotic plaque, by smooth muscle in the media, or by proliferating subendothelial muscles.

Accuracy

1. Our group has investigated the frequency of FDG uptake in the large arteries in relation to the atherogenic risk factors.[26] The positive correlation of arterial FDG uptake with the atherogenic risk factors suggested a promising role for FDG PET imaging in the diagnosis of atherosclerosis and follow-up after treatment intervention.[27,28] In a population of 149 subjects, the mean SUVs of the ascending aorta, aortic arch, descending thoracic aorta, iliac arteries, and femoral arteries increased with age ($p < .01$).[29]
2. High correlation is reported between the FDG uptake in the aorta and macrophage content of atherosclerotic lesions.[30]
3. Locally increased concentration of FDG is readily demonstrable in experimental lesions by ex vivo autoradiography. The feasibility of detection of vulnerable atheroma by intravascular catheter and positron-sensitive probe has been explored by various investigators.[31,32]
4. In animal studies, a promising application of FDG PET for monitoring the therapeutic effect of anti-inflammatory drugs on stabilization of vulnerable atherosclerotic plaques has been demonstrated. FDG PET was able to image the reduction of inflammation by probucol.[33] FDG PET, by its ability to image reduction of macrophage infiltration, may

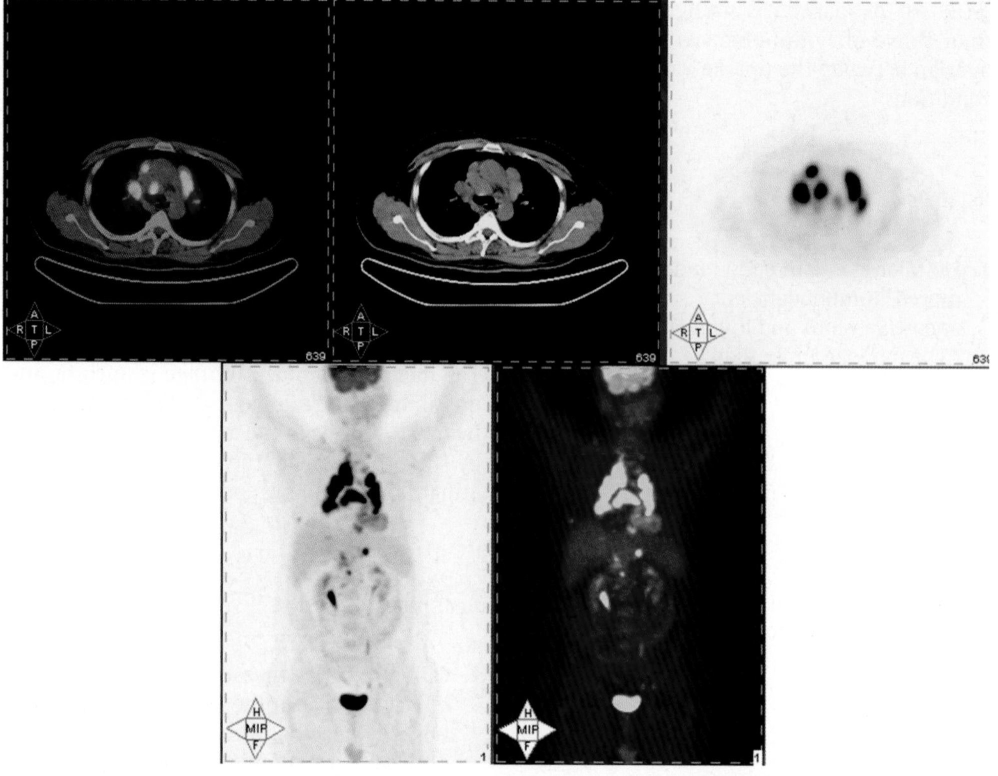

Fig. 28.9 Fluorodeoxyglucose positron emission tomography images of a case of sarcoidosis where typical uptake is seen in the chest. In patients with active sarcoidosis, significant uptake is seen at the disease sites and can be mistaken for lymphoma or other lymphoproliferative disorders. (From Kumar R, Basu S, Torigian D, Anand V, Zhuang H, Alavi A. Role of modern imaging techniques for diagnosis of infection in the era of ^{18}F-fluorodeoxyglucose positron emission tomography. Clin Microbiol Rev 2008;21(1):209–224. Reprinted with permission.)

be useful for evaluating the therapeutic effect of new drugs clinically that can stabilize vulnerable plaques.

Vasculitis

Overview

Histology is considered the gold standard for the diagnosis of vasculitis, but histopathological confirmation of the diagnosis of vasculitis is not always possible. FDG PET has the potential to be added to the imaging armamentarium as a functional technique for scanning and detection of metabolically active processes along large- and medium-sized arteries. It has been reported to be useful in the diagnosis and treatment of patients with vasculitis by several investigators. It appears to have great potential in the diagnosis and treatment of patients with aortitis.

Accuracy

1. In a series of 15 patients with early aortitis, Meller et al[34] compared FDG PET and MRI for the initial diagnosis and following immunosuppressive therapy. The results of FDG PET and MRI for the initial diagnosis were comparable, but FDG PET detected more inflammatory vascular regions and was more reliable in assessing disease activity following therapy than the latter modality.

2. Webb et al[35] found that FDG PET had a sensitivity of 92%, a specificity of 100%, and NPVs and PPVs of 85 and 100%, respectively, in the initial assessment of active vasculitis in Takayasu arteritis. Their conclusion was that FDG PET could be used to evaluate the activity of the disease and to monitor the effectiveness of treatment.
3. In the initial studies of FDG PET examining CNS involvement in patients with systemic lupus erythematosus (SLE), cerebral blood flow and glucose uptake were found to be reduced during active focal and diffuse CNS lupus.[36] In these and the subsequent studies, FDG PET was considered to be the most sensitive method for demonstrating reversible deficits and for correlating the functional imaging results with neurologic findings.[37–39]

Inflammatory Bowel Disease

FDG PET has been reported to be useful in detecting disease activity in patients with inflammatory bowel disease (IBD). Normal FDG uptake in the bowel varies in distribution and intensity due to several factors[40–42] and can affect the sensitivity and specificity of this technique in this disorder. FDG PET can play a major role in the evaluation of IBD in the pediatric age group because this population has low FDG activity in the bowel.

Follow-up with FDG PET

A potential future use of FDG PET includes following disease activity after therapeutic interventions.[43] Further well-designed studies are

A

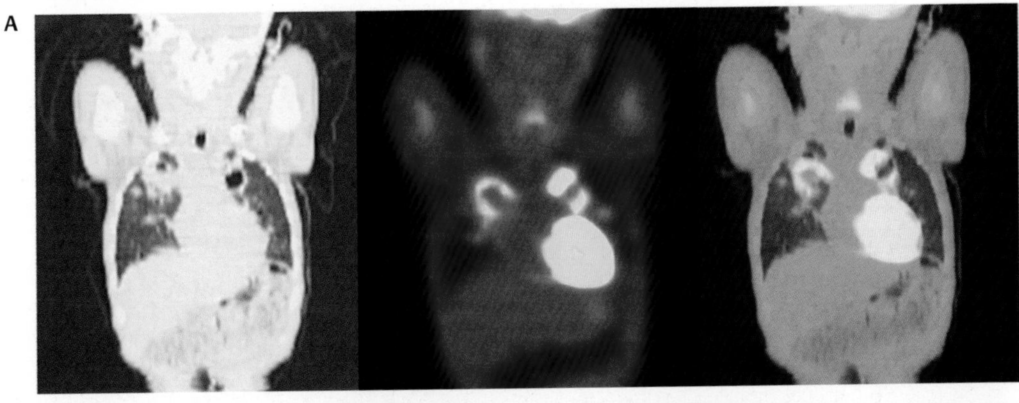

B

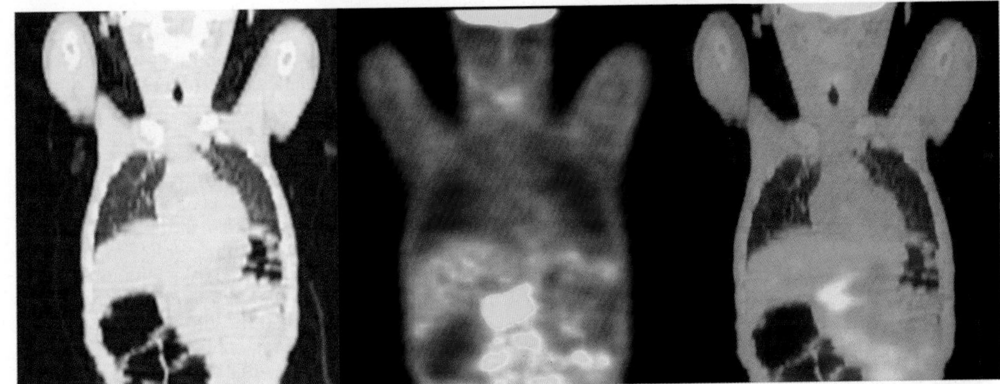

Fig. 28.10 **(A)** Pre- and **(B)** posttreatment fluorodeoxyglucose positron emission tomography in a proven case of pneumonia showing therapeutic response. Corresponding computed tomography and fused images are shown in this figure. (From Kumar R, Basu S, Torigian D, Anand V, Zhuang H, Alavi A. Role of modern imaging techniques for diagnosis of infection in the era of ^{18}F-fluorodeoxyglucose positron emission tomography. Clin Microbiol Rev 2008;21(1):209–224. Reprinted with permission.)

warranted to investigate whether FDG PET has an incremental value in this setting when compared with other techniques. Theoretically, it can be argued that imaging activated inflammatory cells (**Fig. 28.10**) with FDG is likely to be more sensitive and specific than changes in perfusion or edema detected by CT/MRI or scintigraphic techniques (**Fig. 28.11**).

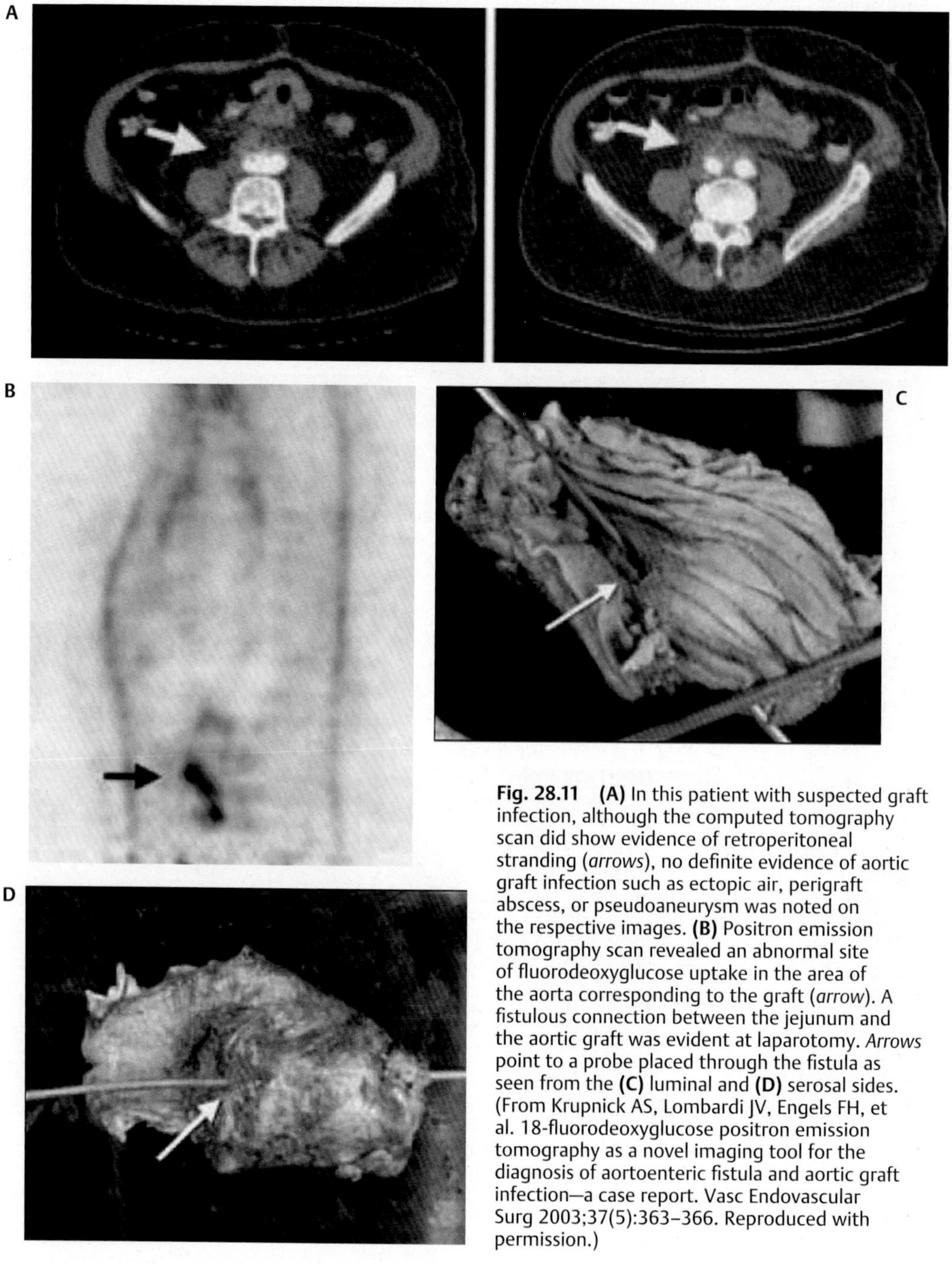

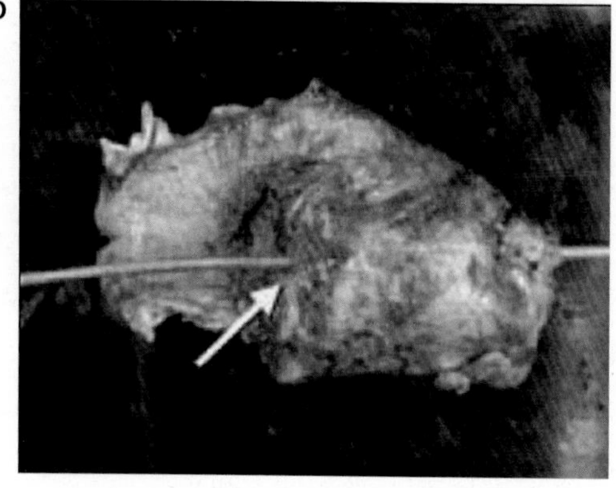

Fig. 28.11 **(A)** In this patient with suspected graft infection, although the computed tomography scan did show evidence of retroperitoneal stranding (*arrows*), no definite evidence of aortic graft infection such as ectopic air, perigraft abscess, or pseudoaneurysm was noted on the respective images. **(B)** Positron emission tomography scan revealed an abnormal site of fluorodeoxyglucose uptake in the area of the aorta corresponding to the graft (*arrow*). A fistulous connection between the jejunum and the aortic graft was evident at laparotomy. *Arrows* point to a probe placed through the fistula as seen from the **(C)** luminal and **(D)** serosal sides. (From Krupnick AS, Lombardi JV, Engels FH, et al. 18-fluorodeoxyglucose positron emission tomography as a novel imaging tool for the diagnosis of aortoenteric fistula and aortic graft infection—a case report. Vasc Endovascular Surg 2003;37(5):363–366. Reproduced with permission.)

Nonspecific Uptake in the Joints: Potential for Assessing Arthritis

1. FDG accumulation is frequently observed in various joints (particularly inferior glenohumeral joints at the shoulder); this is likely to represent inflammatory reactions.[44,45]
2. The exact location of FDG accumulation at these sites is unclear, but it is likely in the synovial tissue surrounding the joint. These are usually chronic in nature and represent a long-standing process that is detected as an incidental finding on FDG PET scan.
3. The degree of FDG uptake as an indication of the severity of the inflammatory process may become an important source of information in rheumatologic conditions like osteoarthritis and rheumatoid arthritis.[46]

References

1. Guhlmann A, Brecht-Krauss D, Suger G, et al. Chronic osteomyelitis Detection with FDG PET and correlation with histopathologic findings. Radiology 1998; 206:749–754
2. Guhlmann A, Brecht-Krauss D, Suger G, et al. Fluorine-18-FDG PET and technetium-99m antigranulocyte antibody scintigraphy in chronic osteomyelitis. J Nucl Med 1998;39:2145–2152
3. De Winter F, Van de Wiele C, Vogelaers D, et al. Fluorine-18 fluorodeoxyglucose-positron emission tomography: a highly accurate imaging modality for the diagnosis of chronic musculoskeletal infections. J Bone Joint Surg Am 2001;83-A:651–666
4. Meller J, Koster G, Liersch T, et al. Chronic bacterial osteomyelitis prospective comparison of F-18-FDG imaging with a dual-head coincidence camera and In-111-labelled autologous leucocyte scintigraphy. Eur J Nucl Med 2002;29:53–60
5. Gratz S, Dorner J, Fischer U, et al. ^{18}F-FDG hybrid PET in patients with suspected spondylitis. Eur J Nucl Med Mol Imaging 2002;29:516–524
6. Stumpe KD, Zanetti M, Weishaupt D, Hodler J, Boos N, Von Schulthess GK. FDG positron emission tomography for differentiation of degenerative and infectious endplate abnormalities in the lumbar spine detected on MR imaging. AJR Am J Roentgenol 2002;179: 1151–1157
7. Love C, Palestro CJ. ^{18}F-FDG and ^{67}Ga-SPECT imaging in suspected vertebral osteomyelitis: an intraindividual comparison. [abstract] J Nucl Med 2003; 45(suppl):148P
8. Crymes WB Jr, Demos H, Gordon L. Detection of musculoskeletal infection with ^{18}F-FDG PET: review of the current literature. J Nucl Med Technol 2004;32(1): 12–15
9. Zhuang H, Alavi A. 18-fluorodeoxyglucose positron emission tomographic imaging in the detection and monitoring of infection and inflammation. Semin Nucl Med 2002;32(1):47–59
10. Alnafisi N, Yun M, Alavi A. F-18 FDG positron emission tomography to differentiate diabetic osteoarthropathy from septic arthritis. Clin Nucl Med 2001;26(7):638–639
11. Keidar Z, Militianu D, Melamed E, Bar-Shalom R, Israel O. The diabetic foot: initial experience with ^{18}F-FDG PET/CT. J Nucl Med 2005;46(3):444–449
12. Basu S, Chryssikos T, Houseni M, et al. Potential role of FDG PET in the setting of diabetic neuro-osteoarthropathy: can it differentiate uncomplicated Charcot's neuroarthropathy from osteomyelitis and soft-tissue infection? Nucl Med Commun 2007; 28(6):465–472
13. Höpfner S, Krolak C, Kessler S, Tiling R. Preoperative imaging of Charcot neuroarthropathy: does the additional application of (18)F-FDG-PET make sense? Nucl Med (Stuttg) 2006;45(1):15–20
14. Pill SG, Parvizi J, Tang PH, et al. Comparison of fluorodeoxyglucose positron emission tomography and (111)indium-white blood cell imaging in the diagnosis of periprosthetic infection of the hip. J Arthroplasty 2006; 21(6, Suppl 2)91–97
15. Blockmans D, Knockaert D, Maes A, et al. Clinical value of [F-18]fluoro-deoxyglucose positron emission tomography for patients with fever of unknown origin. Clin Infect Dis 2001;32:191–196
16. Stumpe KDM, Dazzi H, Schaffner A, et al. Infection imaging using whole-body FDG-PET. Eur J Nucl Med 2000;27:822–832
17. Meller J, Altenvoerde G, Munzel U, et al. Fever of unknown origin Prospective comparison of [F-18]FDG imaging with a double-head coincidence camera and gallium-67 citrate SPECT. Eur J Nucl Med 2000; 27:1617–1625
18. Bleeker-Rovers CP, de Kleijn EM, Corstens FH, van der Meer JW, Oyen WJ. Clinical value of FDG PET in patients with fever of unknown origin and patients suspected of focal infection or inflammation. Eur J Nucl Med Mol Imaging 2004;31:29–37
19. Yen RF, Chen YC, Wu YW, Pan MH, Chang SC. Using 18-fluoro-2-deoxyglucose positron emission tomography in detecting infectious endocarditis/endoarteritis: a preliminary report. Acad Radiol 2004;11: 316–321
20. Hoffman JM. A. WH and T. Schifter, FDG-PET in differentiating lymphoma from nonmalignant central nervous system lesions in patients with AIDS. J Nucl Med 1993;34:567–575
21. O'Doherty MJ, Barrington SF, Campbell M, et al. PET scanning and the human immunodeficiency virus-positive patient. J Nucl Med 1997;38:1575–1583
22. Santiago JF, Jana S, Gilbert HM, Salem S, Bellman PC, Hsu RKS. Naddaf Sleiman, Abdel-Dayem H: Role of fluorine-18-fluorodeoxyglucose in the work-up of febrile AIDS patients: experience with dual head coincidence imaging. Clin Positron Imaging 1999;2:301–309
23. Brudin LH, Valind SO, Rhodes CG, et al. Fluorine-18 deoxyglucose uptake in sarcoidosis measured with positron emission tomography. Eur J Nucl Med 1994;21:297–305
24. Lewis PJ, Salama A. Uptake of fluorine-18-fluorodeoxyglucose in sarcoidosis. J Nucl Med 1994;35:1647–1649
25. Yasuda S, Shohtsu A, Ide M, et al. High fluorine-18 labeled deoxyglucose uptake in sarcoidosis. Clin Nucl Med 1996;21:983–984
26. Yun M, Jang S, Cucchiara A, et al. F-18 FDG uptake in the large arteries: a correlation study with the atherogenic risk factors. Semin Nucl Med 2002;32:70–76

27. Zhang Z, Machac J, Helft G, et al. Noninvasive serial monitoring of atherosclerotic progression and regression with FDG-PET in a rabbit model. J Nucl Med 2000;41:7P

28. Lin EC, Quaife R. FDG uptake in chronic superior vena cava thrombus on positron emission tomographic imaging. Clin Nucl Med 2001;26:241–242

29. Bural GG, Torigian DA, Chamroonrat W, et al. FDG-PET is an effective imaging modality to detect and quantify age-related atherosclerosis in large arteries. Eur J Nucl Med Mol Imaging 2008 35(3):562–569

30. Vallabhajosula S, Machac J, Knesaurek KK, et al. Imaging atherosclerotic macrophage density by positron emission tomography using F-18-fluorodeoxyglucose (FDG) (abstr). J Nucl Med 1996;37:144

31. Lederman RJ, Raylman R, Fisher S, et al. Detection of atherosclerosis using a novel positron-sensitive probe and 18-fluorodeoxyglucose (FDG). Nucl Med Commun 2001;22:747–753

32. Strauss HW, Mari C, Patt BE, Ghazarossian V. Intravascular radiation detectors for the detection of vulnerable atheroma. J Am Coll Cardiol 2006; 47(8, Suppl)C97–C100

33. Ogawa M, Magata Y, Kato T, et al. Application of 18F-FDG PET for monitoring the therapeutic effect of antiinflammatory drugs on stabilization of vulnerable atherosclerotic plaques. J Nucl Med 2006;47(11):1845–1850

34. Meller J, Strutz F, Siefker J, et al. Early diagnosis and follow-up of aortitis with F-18 FDG PET and MRI. Eur J Nucl Med Mol Imaging 2003;30:730–736

35. Webb M, Chambers A, Al-Nahhas A, et al. The role of F-18-FDG PET in characterising disease activity in Takayasu arteritis. Eur J Nucl Med Mol Imaging 2004;31:627–634

36. van Dam AP. Diagnosis and pathogenesis of CNS lupus. Rheumatol Int 1991;11(1):1–11

37. Stoppe G, Wildhagen K, Seidel JW, et al. Positron emission tomography in neuropsychiatric lupus erythematosus. Neurology 1990;40(2):304–308

38. Sailer M, Burchert W, Ehrenheim C, et al. Positron emission tomography and magnetic resonance imaging for cerebral involvement in patients with systemic lupus erythematosus. J Neurol 1997;244(3):186–193

39. Weiner SM, Otte A, Schumacher M, et al. Diagnosis and monitoring of central nervous system involvement in systemic lupus erythematosus: value of F-18 fluorodeoxyglucose PET. Ann Rheum Dis 2000;59(5):377–385

40. Shreve PD, Anzai Y, Wahl RL. Pitfalls in oncologic diagnosis with FDG PET imaging physiologic and benign variants. Radiographics 1999;19:61–77

41. Miraldi F, Vesselle H, Faulhaber PF, et al. Elimination of artifactual accumulation of FDG in PET imaging of colorectal cancer. Clin Nucl Med 1998;23:3–7

42. Pio BS, Byrne F, Aranda R, et al. Noninvasive quantification of bowel inflammation through positron emission tomography imaging of 2-deoxy-2-[^{18}F]fluoro-D-glucose-labeled white blood cells. Mol Imaging Biol 2003;5:271–277

43. Zhuang H, Alavi A. 18-fluorodeoxyglucose positron emission tomographic imaging in the detection and monitoring of infection and inflammation. Semin Nucl Med 2002;32:47–59

44. von Schulthess G, Meier N, Stumpe K. Joint accumulations of FDG in whole body PET scans. Nucl Med (Stuttg) 2001;40:193–197

45. Wandler E, Kramer EL, Sherman O, Babb J, Scarola J, Rafii M. Diffuse FDG shoulder uptake on PET is associated with clinical findings of osteoarthritis. AJR Am J Roentgenol 2005;185(3):797–803

46. Polisson RP, Schoenberg OI, Fischman A, et al. Use of magnetic resonance imaging and positron emission tomography in the assessment of synovial volume and glucose metabolism in patients with rheumatoid arthritis. Arthritis Rheum 1995;38:819–825

47. Kumar R, Basu S, Torigian D, Anand V, Zhuang H, Alavi A. Role of modern imaging techniques for diagnosis of infection in the era of ^{18}F-fluorodeoxyglucose positron emission tomography. Clin Microbiol Rev 2008;21(1):209–224

48. Basu S, Alavi A. FDG-PET takes lead role in suspected or proven infection. Diagnostic Imaging San Francisco 2007; 29(11):59–64

49. Krupnick AS, Lombardi JV, Engels FH, et al. 18-fluorodeoxyglucose positron emission tomography as a novel imaging tool for the diagnosis of aortoenteric fistula and aortic graft infection–a case report. Vasc Endovascular Surg 2003;37(5):363–366

29

Neurologic Applications

Eugene C. Lin and Abass Alavi

◆ Seizure Localization[1]

Clinical Indication: B

Positron emission tomography (PET) is useful in lateralizing epileptogenic foci in patients with equivocal clinical, electroencephalographic (EEG), and magnetic resonance imaging (MRI) examinations. PET does not add value in patients localized by ictal scalp EEG and MRI.[2]

Accuracy[3,4]

1. Ipsilateral PET hypometabolism is an indicator for good postoperative outcome in the presurgical evaluation of drug-resistant temporal lobe epilepsy. Ipsilateral PET hypometabolism has a predictive value of 86% for good outcome (80% in patients with a normal MRI and 72% in patients with a nonlocalized scalp EEG).[2]
2. PET is more accurate for temporal epilepsy.
3. ***Interictal PET***
   a. *Temporal lobe epilepsy*. Sensitivity 84%, specificity 86%
   b. *Extratemporal lobe epilepsy*. Sensitivity 33%, specificity 95%

Comparison with Other Modalities

1. Interictal PET is more sensitive than interictal single-photon emission computed tomography (SPECT) but less sensitive than ictal SPECT.
2. ***SPECT.*** Temporal epilepsy:
   a. *Ictal SPECT.* Sensitivity 90%, specificity 73%
   b. *Interictal SPECT.* Sensitivity 66%, specificity 68%

Pearls[5,6]

1. In the interictal state, the involved region will be hypometabolic (**Fig. 29.1**). The extent of hypometabolism may be a dynamic process related to the frequency of seizures.[7] During ictus, the involved region is hypermetabolic.
2. Temporal lobe hypometabolism usually involves the entire temporal lobe.
   a. Lateral hypometabolism may be more pronounced.
   b. Even if a focal lesion is present on anatomical images, the temporal lobe hypometabolism is usually diffuse.
3. ***MRI negative.*** PET is accurate even when there is no MRI evidence of mesial temporal sclerosis.[8] In patients with a negative MRI, the hypometabolism tends to involve the inferolateral temporal lobe rather than the mesial temporal lobe.[9]
4. ***Contralateral temporal lobe.*** Rarely, the temporal lobe contralateral to the seizure focus may appear mildly hypermetabolic.

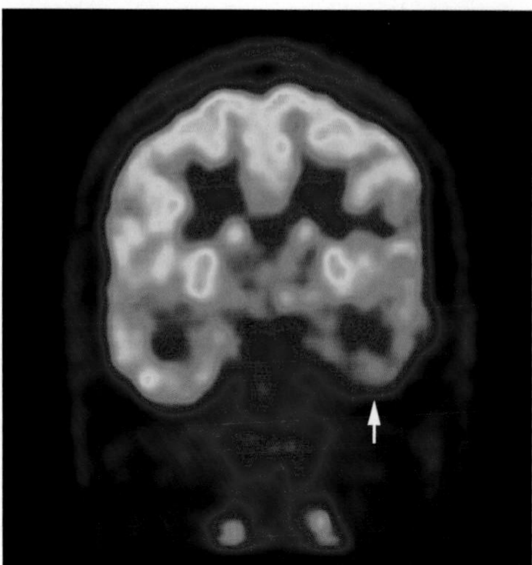

Fig. 29.1 Seizure focus. Coronal positron emission tomography scan demonstrates decreased left temporal lobe activity (*arrow*) consistent with an interictal seizure focus.

5. ***Interpretation criteria.*** In patients with suspected temporal lobe epilepsy, any degree of hypometabolism on visual inspection should be considered significant. A quantitative difference of 15% or more between the temporal lobes is usually significant.[10]
6. ***Extratemporal hypometabolism.*** Ipsilateral extratemporal hypometabolism is relatively common.
   a. The hypometabolism is most common in the thalamus and very uncommon in the occipital lobes and basal ganglia. The greatest degree of hypometabolism is seen in the ipsilateral frontal lobe.[11]
   b. Bilateral cerebellar hypometabolism is common, which is likely related to chronic use of antiepilepsy drugs. Crossed cerebellar diaschisis contralateral to the seizure focus can also be seen.[12]
   c. Extratemporal areas of cortical hypometabolism are usually contiguous with each other and the main site in the temporal lobe.
   d. Extratemporal hypometabolism is less severe than the temporal hypometabolism.
7. ***Thalamic hypometabolism***[1]
   a. Ipsilateral thalamic hypometabolism is associated with long-standing epilepsy and secondary generalization of seizures.
   b. Contralateral thalamic hypometabolism is a predictor of a higher risk of postoperative seizures.
8. ***Prognosis.*** Unilateral focal temporal hypometabolism is associated with a good surgical outcome. Symmetric bilateral temporal, extratemporal, or thalamic hypometabolism is associated with a higher incidence of postoperative seizures.[13]

Pitfalls[6]

1. ***Localization.*** PET is primarily useful in lateralizing the epileptogenic focus rather than in exact localization. As hypometabolism often diffusely involves the temporal lobe and extends into extratemporal regions, hypometabolism on PET should not guide the extent of surgical resection without further supportive evidence.[8]
2. ***Intracranial electrodes.*** Intracranial electrode insertion can cause areas of hypometabolism.
   - PET should be performed before intracranial electroencephalogram.
3. ***Subclinical seizures.*** Unrecognized subclinical seizure activity during the administration of FDG can result in false-positive apparent hypometabolism in the contralateral temporal lobe (relative to the ictal hypermetabolism in the involved temporal lobe). Therefore, patients should be monitored if possible before the dose is injected.
4. ***Children.*** Interictal hypermetabolism in the seizure focus can occur in children, but rarely in adults.
5. ***Focal cortical malformations.*** Focal cortical malformations can be associated with decreased, normal, or increased uptake. Focal subcortical heterotopia and lobar dysplasia can be associated with increased uptake on interictal PET.[14]

◆ Dementia: Alzheimer Disease[15,16]

Clinical Indication: B

PET is the most valuable imaging study for patients with suspected Alzheimer disease

(AD) with mild to moderate cognitive impairment, who (1) meet standard criteria for dementia without identifiable cause after full work-up or (2) exhibit progressive cognitive dysfunction during a period of observation.

PET can be helpful in

1. ***Differentiation.*** Differentiating AD from other dementias
2. ***Diagnosis.*** Aiding in the diagnosis of early AD
3. ***Prognosis.*** The degree of hypometabolism seen on PET correlates with rate the degree of cognitive decline after the study.

Accuracy and Comparison with Other Modalities

1. ***PET.*** Sensitivity 86%, specificity 86%[17]
   - PET is sensitive for differentiating both AD versus normal and AD versus non-AD disorders.
2. ***Early AD.*** Decreased metabolism in the parietotemporal areas predicts decline, with an overall accuracy of 86% and sensitivity and specificity ranging from 75 to 100%.[15,18]
3. ***SPECT.*** PET is ~15 to 20% more accurate than SPECT.[15]
   - PET is superior to SPECT in differentiating AD from vascular and other dementias.

Pearls

1. ***Interpretation criteria for a positive study***[19]
   - ***a.*** Bilateral symmetric temporoparietal hypometabolism (**Fig. 29.2**)
     - Parietal activity is usually decreased more than temporal activity.
   - ***b.*** Posterior cingulate cortex hypometabolism
   - ***c.*** Hypometabolism may be asymmetric or unilateral early during the disease (**Fig. 29.3**).
   - ***d.*** Hypometabolism can involve frontal lobes in advanced disease (**Fig. 29.4**).
     - Frontal lobe abnormalities are not seen without temporoparietal disease.
   - ***e.*** Preserved metabolism in the sensorimotor and visual cortices (**Fig. 29.2**), cerebellum, basal ganglia, and thalamus
   - ***f.*** Cerebellar activity remains constant throughout the stages of the disease; therefore, it can be used as a reference point for generating semiquantitative indices for affected sites.
   - ***g.*** Glucose metabolism is lower throughout the cortex in patients with AD compared with normal individuals.[20]
2. ***Differentiation from other dementias.*** AD can usually be differentiated from
   - ***a.*** *Frontotemporal dementia (Pick disease).*[15] Frontal and temporal hypometabolism is the dominant pattern (**Fig. 29.5**).
     - Reduced activity in the posterior cingulate cortex seen in AD is not noted in frontotemporal dementia.[21] Anterior cingulate hypometabolism is often seen in frontotemporal dementia.[22]
     - Frontotemporal dementia affects the anterior and medial temporal more than lateral temporal cortices.
     - The greatest decrease is often in the medial frontal cortices.
     - There is relative sparing of parietal lobes in frontotemporal dementia.
   - ***b.*** *Vascular dementia (multi-infarct dementia).* Multiple focal cortical and subcortical defects are seen in this type of dementia.
     - Areas of decreased metabolism differentiating vascular dementia from AD are the deep gray nuclei, cerebellum, primary cortices, middle temporal gyrus, and anterior cingulate gyrus.[23]
     - Note that these defects should be accounted for by areas of abnormal signal on MRI. If these defects have no MRI correlate, this pattern could suggest a primary neurodegenerative disorder rather than vascular dementia.[15]
     - However, frontal lobe metabolism is usually decreased in patients with white matter signal abnormalities on MRI secondary to subcortical ischemic vascular disease, regardless of the location of the signal abnormalities.[24]
3. ***Early versus late-onset AD.*** Glucose metabolism is most severely affected in the

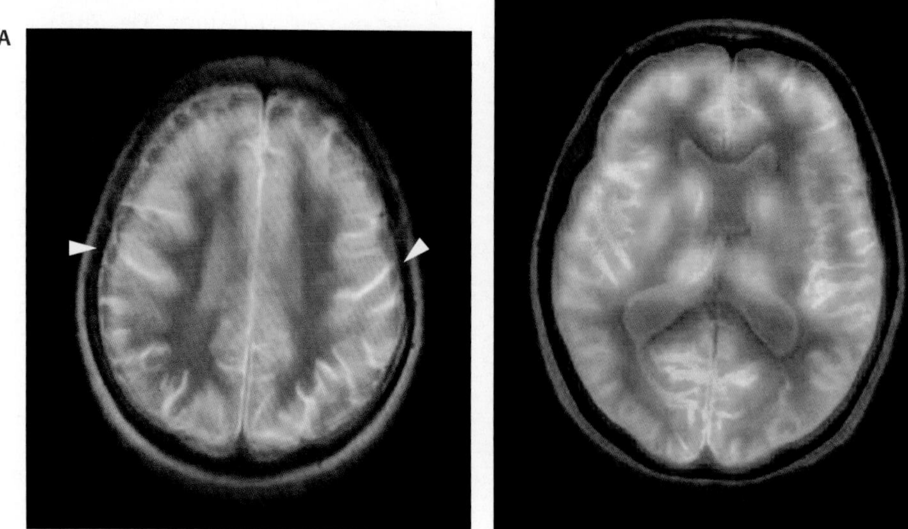

Fig. 29.2 Alzheimer disease. **(A)** Fused axial positron emission tomography/magnetic resonance imaging (PET/MRI) demonstrates bilateral parietal hypometabolism consistent with Alzheimer disease. Preserved activity in the motor-sensory cortex (*arrowheads*) around the central sulcus is characteristic in Alzheimer disease. **(B)** Fused axial PET/MRI in the same patient demonstrates preservation of activity in the visual cortex.

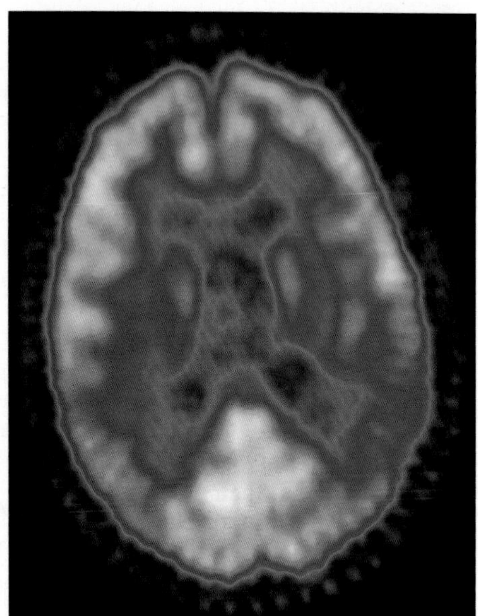

Fig. 29.3 Alzheimer disease. Axial positron emission tomography scan demonstrates bilateral parietal hypometabolism in a patient with Alzheimer disease. The hypometabolism is greater in the left parietal region.

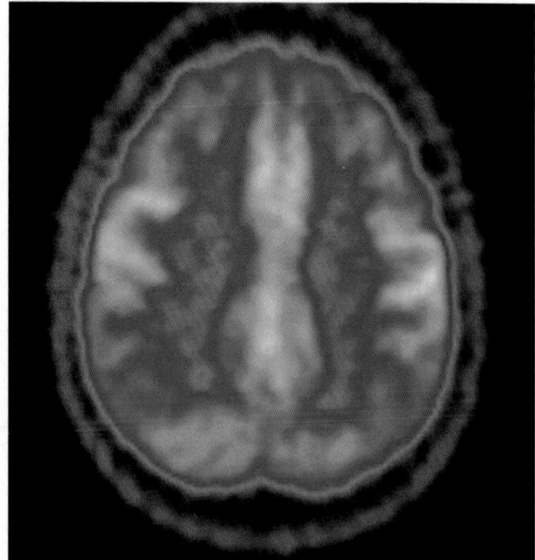

Fig. 29.4 Late-stage Alzheimer disease. Axial positron emission tomography scan demonstrates bilateral frontal and parietal hypometabolism. The frontal lobe hypometabolism is seen in the later stages of Alzheimer disease.

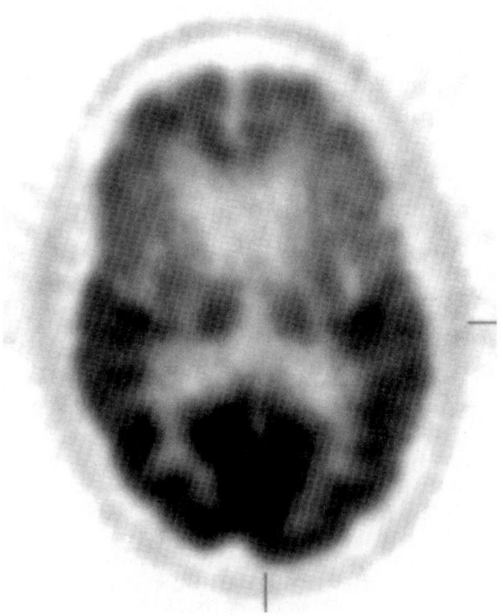

Fig. 29.5 Pick disease. Axial positron emission tomography scan demonstrates frontal hypometabolism characteristic for Pick disease.

parietal, frontal, posterior cingulate cortices, and subcortical area in early-onset AD and in the limbic system and medial frontal lobe in late-onset AD.[25,26] The overall hypometabolism in early-onset AD is greater in magnitude and extent.[26]

Pitfalls

1. ***False-positives.*** Dementia with Lewy bodies (DLB) and Parkinson dementia can mimic AD on PET.
   a. ***Dementia with Lewy bodies***
      - DLB has bilateral temporoparietal hypometabolism like AD, but it also involves the occipital lobes (**Fig. 29.6**).
      - The most prominent difference between DLB and AD is reduction in visual cortex activity in DLB.[27]
      - In mild DLB, hypometabolism usually involves substantially larger portions of the cortex than in mild AD. In mild AD, there is often hypometabolism in the medial temporal lobe (hippocampus), which is not present in mild DLB.[28]
      - In practice, DLB may be difficult to distinguish from AD with PET; the accuracy is around 70% for this purpose.[29]

   b. ***Parkinson dementia***
      - Parkinson disease with dementia can have the same pattern of hypometabolism as AD and DLB.
      - However, compared with AD, Parkinson dementia tends to have greater reduction in the visual cortex and less reduction in the medial temporal lobe.[30]

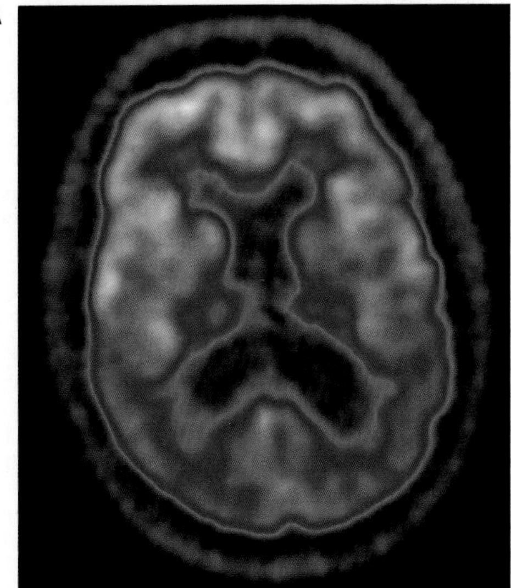

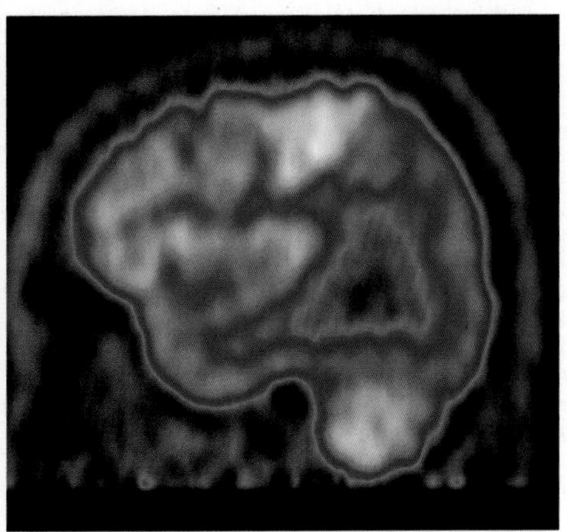

Fig. 29.6 Lewy body dementia. **(A)** Axial and **(B)** sagittal positron emission tomography scans demonstrate hypometabolism involving the bilateral parietal, temporal, and occipital lobes. The occipital and visual cortex involvement distinguishes Lewy body dementia from Alzheimer disease.

- Compared with DLB, there is less reduction in the anterior cingulate cortex in Parkinson dementia.[31]

2. ***False-negatives.*** Decreased activity due to depression or hypometabolism from thyroid disease may be a confounding factor. In particular, coexisting depression or thyroid disease may be problematic if the degree of decreased uptake on an initial PET scan is used as a prognostic factor.

References

1. Newberg AB, Alavi A. PET in seizure disorders. Radiol Clin North Am 2005;43(1):79–92
2. Willmann O, Wennberg R, May T, Woermann FG, Pohlmann-Eden B. The contribution of ^{18}F-FDG PET in preoperative epilepsy surgery evaluation for patients with temporal lobe epilepsy: A meta-analysis. Seizure 2007;16(6):509–520
3. Bernal B, Altman NR. Evidence-based medicine: neuroimaging of seizures. Neuroimaging Clin N Am 2003;13(2):211–224
4. Spencer SS. The relative contributions of MRI, SPECT, and PET imaging in epilepsy. Epilepsia 1994;35(Suppl 6):S72–S89
5. Bohnen N. Neurological applications. In: Wahl R, ed. Principles and Practice of Positron Emission Tomography. Philadelphia, PA: Lippincott Williams & Wilkins; 2002: 276–297
6. Henry TR, Van Heertum RL. Positron emission tomography and single photon emission computed tomography in epilepsy care. Semin Nucl Med 2003;33(2):88–104
7. Van Paesschen W, Dupont P, Sunaert S, Goffin K, Van Laere K. The use of SPECT and PET in routine clinical practice in epilepsy. Curr Opin Neurol 2007;20(2):194–202
8. Knowlton RC. The role of FDG-PET, ictal SPECT, and MEG in the epilepsy surgery evaluation. Epilepsy Behav 2006;8(1):91–101
9. Carne RP, Cook MJ, MacGregor LR, et al. "Magnetic resonance imaging negative positron emission tomography positive" temporal lobe epilepsy: FDG-PET pattern differs from mesial temporal lobe epilepsy. Mol Imaging Biol 2007;9(1):32–42
10. Delbeke D, Lawrence SK, Abou-Khalil BW, et al. Postsurgical outcome of patients with uncontrolled complex partial seizures and temporal lobe hypometabolism on 18FDG-positron emission tomography. Invest Radiol 1996;31(5):261–266
11. Nelissen N, Van Paesschen W, Baete K, et al. Correlations of interictal FDG-PET metabolism and ictal SPECT perfusion changes in human temporal lobe epilepsy with hippocampal sclerosis. Neuroimage 2006;32(2):684–695
12. Kawai N, Kawanishi M, Tamiya T, Nagao S. Crossed cerebellar glucose hypermetabolism demonstrated using PET in symptomatic epilepsy–case report. Ann Nucl Med 2005;19(3):231–234
13. Salmenpera TM, Duncan JS. Imaging in epilepsy. J Neurol Neurosurg Psychiatry 2005;76(Suppl 3):iii2–iii10
14. Poduri A, Golja A, Takeoka M, Bourgeois BF, Connolly L, Riviello JJ Jr. Focal cortical malformations can show asymmetrically higher uptake on interictal fluorine-18 fluorodeoxyglucose positron emission tomography (PET). J Child Neurol 2007;22(2):232–237
15. Silverman DH. Brain 18F-FDG PET in the diagnosis of neurodegenerative dementias: comparison with perfusion SPECT and with clinical evaluations lacking nuclear imaging. J Nucl Med 2004;45(4):594–607
16. Van Heertum RL, Greenstein EA, Tikofsky RS. 2-deoxy-fluoroglucose-positron emission tomography imaging of the brain: current clinical applications with emphasis on the dementias. Semin Nucl Med 2004;34(4):300–312
17. Patwardhan MB, McCrory DC, Matchar DB, et al. Alzheimer disease: operating characteristics of PET–a meta-analysis. Radiology 2004;231(1):73–80
18. Mosconi L. Brain glucose metabolism in the early and specific diagnosis of Alzheimer's disease: FDG-PET studies in MCI and AD. Eur J Nucl Med Mol Imaging 2005;32(4):486–510
19. Van Heertum RL, Tikofsky RS. Positron emission tomography and single-photon emission computed tomography brain imaging in the evaluation of dementia. Semin Nucl Med 2003;33(1):77–85
20. Coleman RE. Positron emission tomography diagnosis of Alzheimer's disease. Neuroimaging Clin N Am 2005;15(4):837–846 x
21. Bonte FJ, Harris TS, Roney CA, Hynan LS. Differential diagnosis between Alzheimer's and frontotemporal disease by the posterior cingulate sign. J Nucl Med 2004;45(5):771–774
22. Foster NL, Heidebrink JL, Clark CM, et al. FDG-PET improves accuracy in distinguishing frontotemporal dementia and Alzheimer's disease. Brain 2007;130(Pt 10):2616–2635
23. Kerrouche N, Herholz K, Mielke R, et al. 18FDG PET in vascular dementia: differentiation from Alzheimer's disease using voxel-based multivariate analysis. J Cereb Blood Flow Metab 2006;26(9):1213–1221
24. Tullberg M, Fletcher E, DeCarli C, et al. White matter lesions impair frontal lobe function regardless of their location. Neurology 2004;63(2):246–253
25. Ishii K, Minoshima S. PET is better than perfusion SPECT for early diagnosis of Alzheimer's disease. Eur J Nucl Med Mol Imaging 2005;32(12):1463–1465
26. Kim EJ, Cho SS, Jeong Y, et al. Glucose metabolism in early onset versus late onset Alzheimer's disease: an SPM analysis of 120 patients. Brain 2005;128(Pt 8):1790–1801
27. Gilman S, Koeppe RA, Little R, et al. Differentiation of Alzheimer's disease from dementia with Lewy bodies utilizing positron emission tomography with [(18)F] fluorodeoxyglucose and neuropsychological testing. Exp Neurol 2005;191(Suppl 1):S95–S103
28. Ishii K, Soma T, Kono AK, et al. Comparison of regional brain volume and glucose metabolism between patients with mild dementia with Lewy bodies and those with mild Alzheimer's disease. J Nucl Med 2007;48(5):704–711
29. Koeppe RA, Gilman S, Joshi A, et al. 11C-DTBZ and 18F-FDG PET measures in differentiating dementias. J Nucl Med 2005;46(6):936–944
30. Vander Borght T, Minoshima S, Giordani B, et al. Cerebral metabolic differences in Parkinson's and Alzheimer's diseases matched for dementia severity. J Nucl Med 1997;38(5):797–802
31. Yong SW, Yoon JK, An YS, Lee PH. A comparison of cerebral glucose metabolism in Parkinson's disease, Parkinson's disease dementia and dementia with Lewy bodies. Eur J Neurol 2007;14(12):1357–1362

30

Cardiac PET and PET/CT

Amol Takalkar, Eugene C. Lin, Elias Botvinick, Adam M. Alessio, and Luis Araujo

◆ Myocardial Perfusion Assessment

Clinical Indication: A

Myocardial perfusion assessment at rest and with stress (exercise or pharmacologic) is important in patients with known or suspected coronary artery disease (CAD). Single-photon emission tomography (SPECT) myocardial perfusion imaging with thallium or technetium 99m labeled agents is routinely practiced. However, SPECT imaging has several limitations and myocardial perfusion imaging with positron emission tomography (PET) is superior to SPECT. In practice, PET myocardial perfusion imaging is constrained by the need for an on-site cyclotron to perform nitrogen 13 ammonia imaging. Rubidium 82 imaging can be performed with a generator. Given the cost of the generator and current reimbursements, 2 to 3 studies a day may need to be performed for PET to be cost-effective.

Tracers

Nitrogen 13 (^{13}N) ammonia (cyclotron-produced) and rubidium 82 (^{82}Rb) chloride (generator produced) are Food and Drug Administration (FDA)–approved PET radiopharmaceuticals for assessing myocardial blood flow. Oxygen 15 (^{15}O) labeled water and ^{62}Cu-pyruvaldehyde bis (N4-methylthiosemicarbazone) (Cu-PTSM) can also be used but are mostly restricted to the research setting.

^{82}Rb can be eluted from a strontium 82 generator, which needs to be replaced approximately every 4 weeks. The half-life of ^{82}Rb is 75 seconds.

^{13}N ammonia has a half-life of ~10 minutes.

The advantages of ^{82}Rb are that a cyclotron is not needed, and it is ideal for peak dipyridamole or regadenosan stress gated imaging. Rb-82 as imaging typically starts 90 to 120 seconds after injection compared with 3 to 5 minutes with ^{13}N ammonia. The disadvantages are poorer resolution (due to a positron range of 2.6 mm), lower extraction, and more difficulty with quantitation compared with ^{13}N ammonia. It is also very difficult to perform exercise stress testing with ^{82}Rb, given the short half-life of the tracer.

Protocols

Generally, similar protocols (except for dose of radiotracer and imaging time and duration) to those used for SPECT are followed; however,

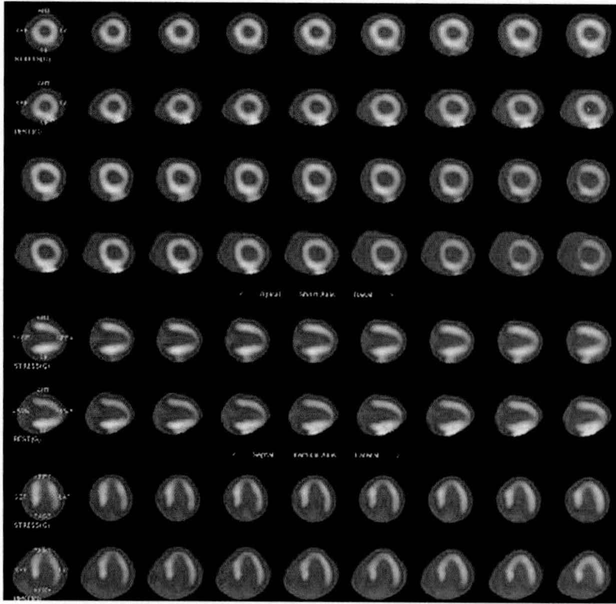

Fig. 30.1 Rest and dipyridamole stress myocardial perfusion positron emission tomography rubidium 82 images displayed conventionally in the short, vertical, and horizontal long axes, showing normal myocardial perfusion at rest and stress. (Courtesy of Elias Botvinick, MD, San Francisco, CA.)

usually pharmacologic stress testing is performed. Exercise stress testing is difficult due to the short half-life of the tracers. With ^{13}N ammonia, exercise stress testing can be done, but it requires meticulous coordination and setup. The images are displayed and reviewed similar to the cardiac SPECT images (**Fig. 30.1** and **Fig. 30.2**).

Accuracy and Comparison with Other Modalities

PET imaging provides better spatial and temporal resolution and hence is better suited in patients with thick/muscular chest wall, large breast tissue, or overall body habitus that frequently leads to indeterminate SPECT myocardial perfusion studies (**Fig. 30.3**). Due to the short half-life of the PET tracers, pure stress-related images uncontaminated by the prior rest injection can be obtained. Unlike gated SPECT, left ventricular ejection fraction can be assessed at peak stress, as imaging is performed soon after injection. PET imaging, with absolute quantification of regional radiotracer uptake, is better suited when serial studies are required to assess perfusion in a particular myocardial segment. It also allows better evaluation of endothelial dysfunction and coronary flow reserve as a measure of coronary stenosis. Moreover, PET allows for more efficient imaging protocols, leading to faster studies (around 45 minutes compared with 3 to 4 hours for SPECT studies) and lower radiation exposure.

Numerous studies have shown that myocardial perfusion PET has higher accuracy,[2] sensitivity,[3] and specificity[4] compared with SPECT.

Pitfalls

1. If ^{13}N ammonia is used for perfusion imaging, there is decreased lateral wall activity in ~10% of normal patients. The etiology of this is unknown.
2. Misregistration artifact during a cardiac PET/ computed tomography (CT) scan can result in artifactual defects (see Pitfalls in Myocardial Viability section).

◆ Myocardial Viability

Clinical Indication: A

1. PET imaging with fluorodeoxyglucose (FDG) with myocardial perfusion imaging is the

A

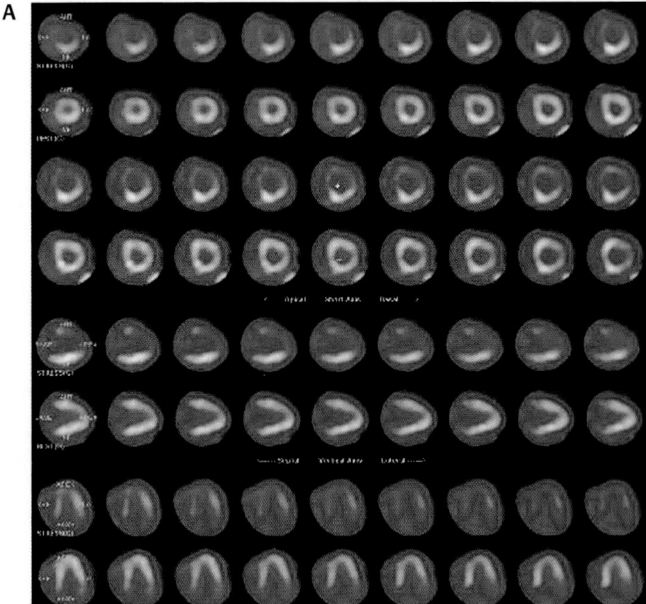

B

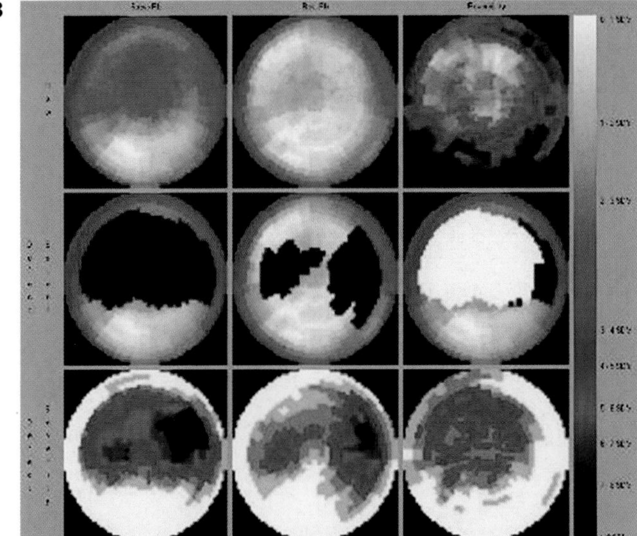

C

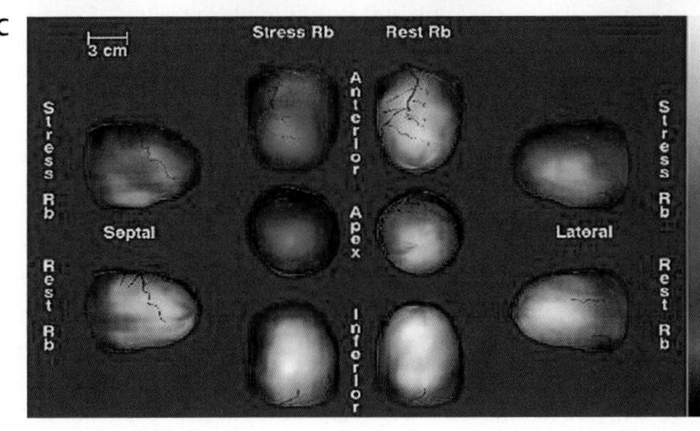

Fig. 30.2 **(A)** Rest and dipyridamole stress myocardial perfusion positron emission tomography (PET) rubidium 82 images showing a large region of ischemia in the anterior wall, anterior septum, and anterior and midlateral walls and gross stress-induced cavitary dilation by conventional display. **(B)** The polar map shows the defect distribution and magnitude. **(C)** A model three-dimensional ventricle fused with a model coronary tree (can be patient's own coronary tree if the patient had undergone a PET study with computed tomography coronary angiography) showing the extent and density of the abnormality. (Courtesy of Elias Botvinick, MD, San Francisco, CA.)

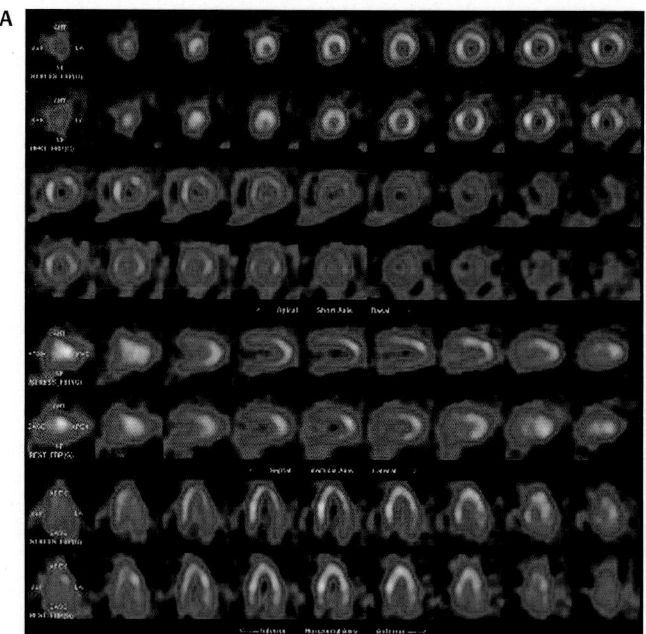

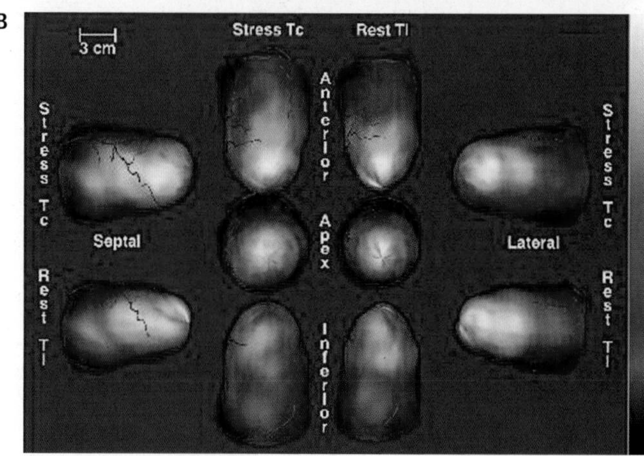

current gold standard for the assessment of myocardial viability.

2. Demonstration of significant viable myocardium in a patient with chronic ischemic heart disease with left ventricular (LV) dysfunction indicates a need for prompt revascularization and predicts low perioperative mortality and morbidity, significant improvement in left ventricular ejection fraction (LVEF) and congestive heart failure (CHF) symptoms, and improved survival.
3. Absence of viable myocardium in a patient with chronic ischemic heart disease with LV dysfunction supports the decision for medical management and/or cardiac transplantation.

Clinical Scenario

Patients with severe LV dysfunction and CAD continue to pose a significant management dilemma to clinicians who frequently need to choose between aggressive medical treatment and revascularization therapy.[5] Revascularization therapy results in better long-term survival rates, and several investigators have

C

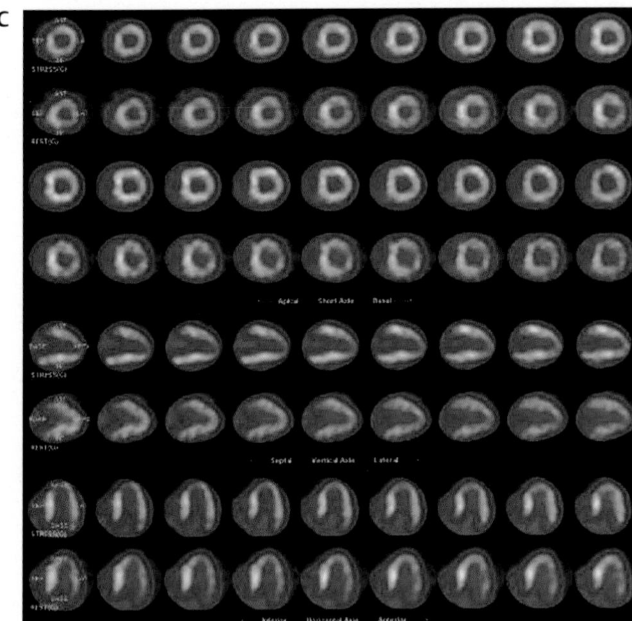

D

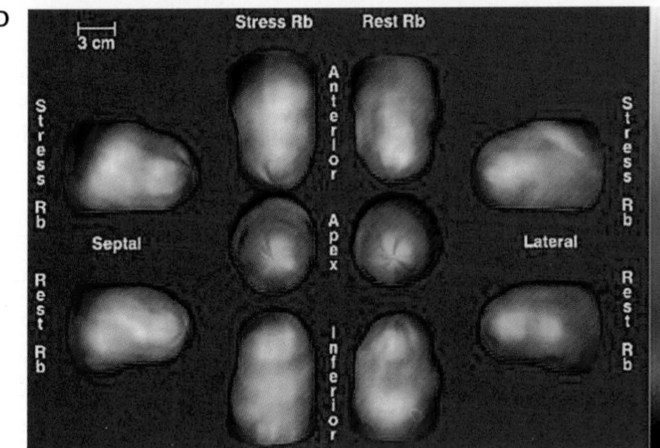

Fig. 30.3 (*Continued*) **(A)** Rest thallium 201 and dipyridamole pharmacologic stress technetium 99m sestamibi single-photon emission tomography myocardial perfusion images of an obese 63-year-old woman with atypical chest pain showing irregular uptake with an apparent fixed inferior wall defect with possible stress induced abnormality in the lateral wall, **(B)** also well seen on the model left ventricular display. **(C)** A repeat pharmacologic stress imaging study performed with positron emission tomography shows normal rest and stress perfusion **(D)** with normal ventricular model of myocardial uptake. (Courtesy of Elias Botvinick, MD, San Francisco, CA.)

demonstrated the benefit of revascularization in CAD patients with poor LV function.[6–14] However, it is associated with significant periprocedure morbidity and mortality, making identification and selection of only those patients who will benefit maximally from revascularization extremely crucial. Improvement in the LV function after revascularization is mainly dependent on the reversibility of contractile dysfunction. Dysfunctional but “viable” myocardium is said to be reversibly dysfunctional, whereas scar tissue usually results in nonreversibly dysfunctional myocardium. Thus, accurate identification of myocardial viability is a critical component in the diagnostic work-up of these patients.

Mechanism of Myocardial Ischemia

Myocardial ischemia may result from acute coronary artery occlusion or from chronic hypoperfusion or repetitive ischemic processes. The severity and duration of myocardial ischemia will determine the myocardial response to the ischemic process. Although the myocardium has several immediate as well as sustained mechanisms of adaptations (e.g., hibernation, stunning

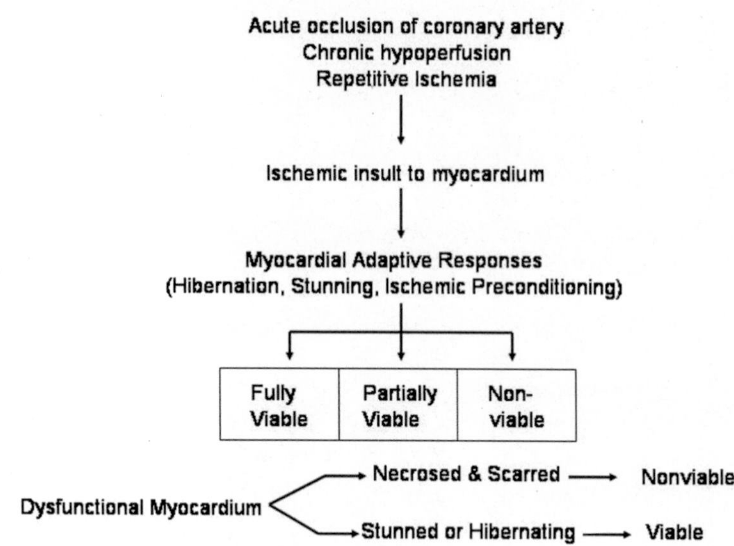

Fig. 30.4 Myocardial response to ischemia.

and ischemic preconditioning[15–17]) to withstand acute and chronic ischemia, the end result of ischemic injury is a mechanically dysfunctional myocardium. The dysfunctional myocardium may be related to ischemic but viable myocardium, such as stunned or hibernating myocardium or necrosed and scarred myocardium that may be completely nonviable (**Fig. 30.4**).

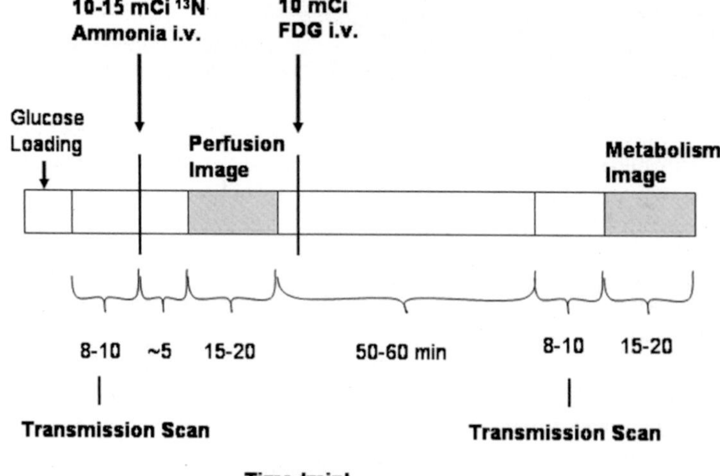

Fig. 30.5 Protocol to assess myocardial viability with positron emission tomography. FDG, fluorodeoxyglucose.

A

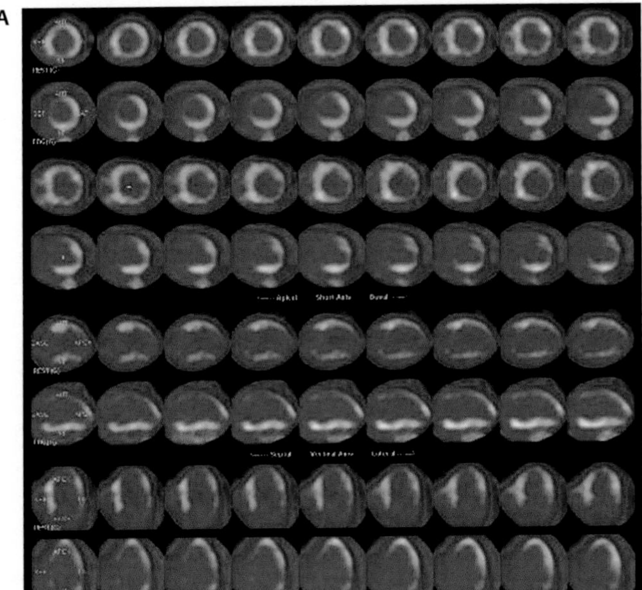

B

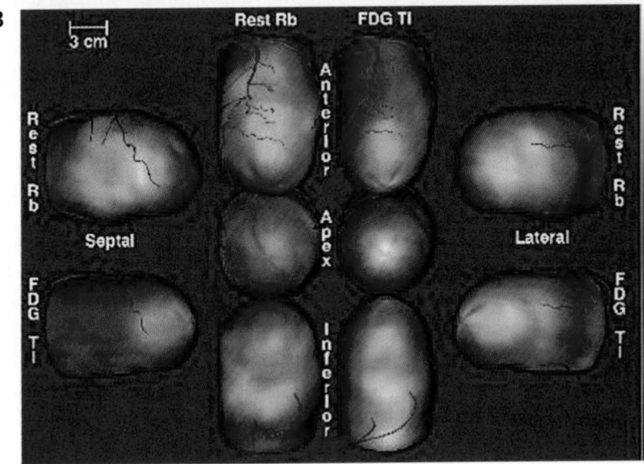

Fig. 30.6 (A) A rest rubidium 82 perfusion image with a rest fluorine 18 fluorodeoxyglucose (FDG) scan in a patient with known coronary artery disease and recent myocardial infarction for viability evaluation showing perfusion in all regions except the left ventricular apex, related anterior wall, and inferior-lateral wall, which show positive FDG uptake (mismatch), indicating regional viability and a high likelihood of functional improvement after bypass graft surgery. **(B)** The findings are superimposed on a model left ventricle, where defects are shown in blue. (Courtesy of Elias Botvinick, MD, San Francisco, CA.)

Identification of Myocardial Viability by PET

The normal myocardium preferentially uses free fatty acids (FFAs) as energy substrates during normal fasting conditions. During hypoxia and ischemia, FFA oxidation is markedly decreased, and the rate of anaerobic glycolysis is enhanced. Thus, the ischemic myocardium uses glucose in preference to FFAs as the energy substrate.[18–27] FDG PET can reliably and accurately assess the initial steps of glucose metabolism in the ischemic myocardium by evaluating myocardial glucose uptake. The protocol for assessing myocardial viability using PET and

Table 30.1 Sensitivity and Specificity of Various Methods to Assess Myocardial Viability

Imaging Method	Sensitivity %	Specificity %
PET	93	58
Thallium rest-redistribution	86	59
Thallium reinjection	88	50
Technetium tracers	81	66
Dobutamine echo	81	80

Abbreviations: echo, echocardiogram; PET, positron emission tomography.

A

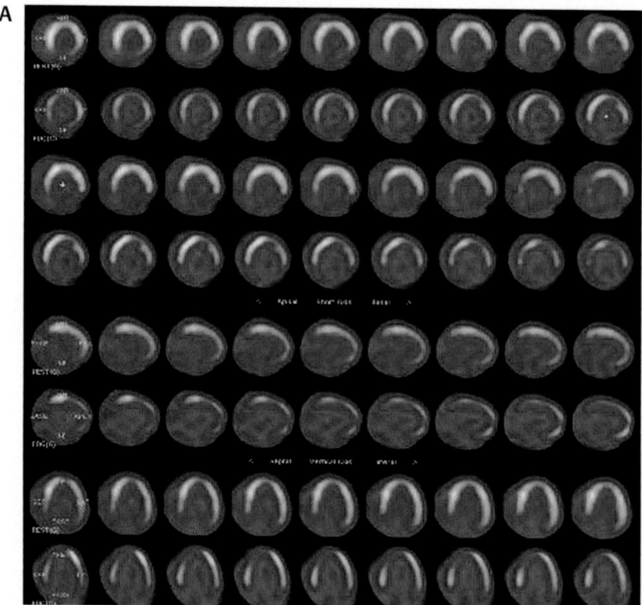

B

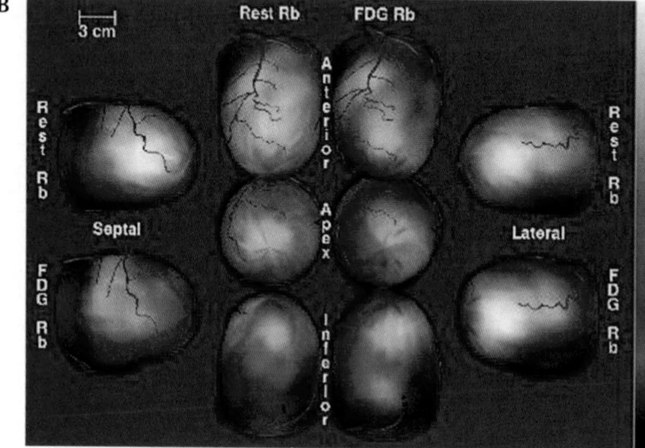

Fig. 30.7 **(A)** Rest rubidium 82 (^{82}Rb) myocardial perfusion images above fluorodeoxyglucose positron emission tomography (FDG PET) myocardial metabolic images showing a large, dense, matched defect in the inferior wall, extending into posteroseptal and basal posterolateral regions, that suggests a scar in the right coronary and the basal region of the left circumflex coronary artery territories. There is apparent paradox of ^{82}Rb uptake (indicating viability) with reduced FDG uptake in the distal left ventricular septum (likely a metabolic variation without implications of nonviability). **(B)** A color-coded model of the left ventricle also shows the defects well. (Courtesy of Elias Botvinick, MD, San Francisco, CA.)

^{13}N ammonia for myocardial perfusion imaging and FDG for myocardial metabolism imaging is depicted in **Fig. 30.5**.

Using the combination of myocardial blood flow and myocardial metabolism, three possible patterns have been described in the dysfunctional myocardium: (1) normal myocardial blood flow and FDG activity, (2) decreased myocardial blood flow with normal or increased FDG activity—"flow-metabolism mismatch" (**Fig. 30.6**), and (3) decreased myocardial blood flow and FDG activity—"matched defect" (**Fig. 30.7**).[28,29] The first two patterns represent viable myocardium; the third pattern represents nonviable myocardium. The flow–metabolism mismatch pattern is considered to be the scintigraphic hallmark of dysfunctional, ischemic, but viable myocardium.

Accuracy and Comparison with Other Modalities

Methods to Assess Myocardial Viability

Myocardial viability can be assessed by several imaging modalities that assess different biological characteristics of the myocardium.

1. ***Assessment of contractile reserve.*** Stress echocardiography or magnetic resonance

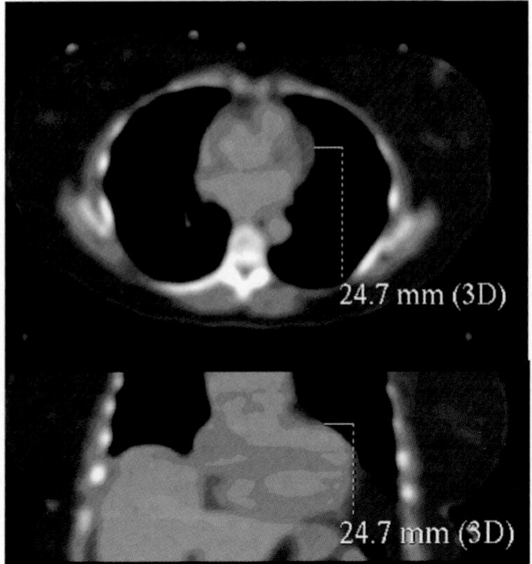

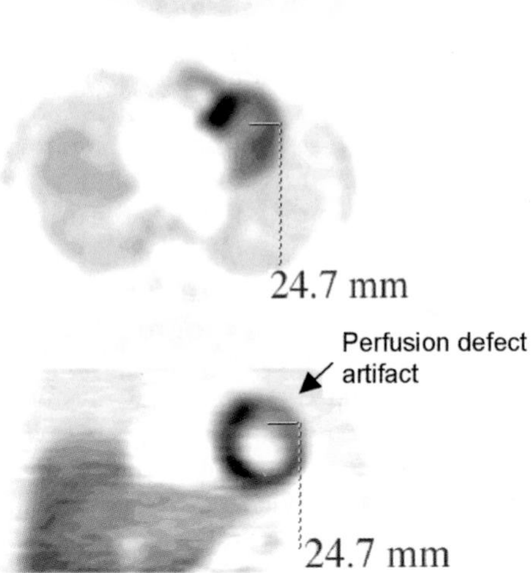

Fig. 30.8 Axial and coronal slices from a $^{13}NH_3$ stress study performed on a positron emission tomography/computed tomography (PET/CT) scanner. This is an example of attenuation and emission scan mismatch in cardiac PET/CT, which often occurs along the lateral free wall or right diaphragm. The left column shows images from a helical CT scan used for attenuation correction of the PET images in the second column. The same line in three-dimensional space is drawn from the edge of the cardiac lateral wall in the CT to the edge of the wall on the PET, marking the 2.5 cm mismatch at the lateral wall between the attenuation and emission images. This mismatch leads to the artifactual defect highlighted on the same PET slices. (Courtesy of Adam Alessio, PhD, Seattle, WA.)

imaging (MRI) with low- or high-dose dobutamine.

2. ***Assessment of sarcolemma integrity.*** Thallium 201 rest–redistribution studies
3. ***Assessment of myocardial perfusion and mitochondrial membrane integrity.*** SPECT with technetium 99m agents such as sestamibi and tetrofosmin, with or without nitrate enhancement
4. ***Assessment of myocardial metabolism.*** PET with myocardial perfusion and fluorine 18 [^{18}F]FDG[30]
5. ***Assessment of cell membrane integrity.*** Contrast-enhanced MRI[31,32]

Accuracy of Methods to Assess Myocardial Viability33

All techniques have a higher sensitivity than specificity (**Table 30.1**). However, PET may be the most sensitive technique, and dobutamine stress echo may be the most specific technique. PET has the greatest value relative to other techniques in patients with severe LV dysfunction. Contrast-enhanced MRI is a newer technique for evaluation of hibernating myocardium. Initial data suggest that the MRI findings correlate well with PET and has a high sensitivity as well as specificity.

Pearls

Clinical Implications of Myocardial Viability

1. ***Prediction of postrevascularization functional recovery.*** The ability of PET to predict functional recovery in the form of improved global and regional LV function after revascularization by assessing myocardial viability prior to treatment has been well documented by several investigators.[34–38] Studies have demonstrated a linear correlation between the number of viable segments and the changes in LVEF, and a significantly higher functional improvement occurs in patients with large flow–metabolism mismatches compared with those with minimal or no mismatch on PET.

2. ***Prediction of improvement in CHF symptoms, exercise capacity, and quality of life.*** The preoperative size of myocardial viability as determined by PET correlates directly to the degree of improvement in heart failure symptoms after coronary artery bypass grafting; thus, myocardial viability evaluation also predicts the level of improvement in CHF symptoms after revascularization.
3. ***Prediction of cardiac events, remodeling, and long-term survival.*** Chronic ischemic heart disease patients with LV dysfunction are at increased risk for future cardiac events, and the presence of dysfunctional but viable myocardium appears to be a risk indicator for recurrent ischemic events. The natural history of disease progression in heart failure patients is significantly affected by LV remodeling, and measures that halt or reverse ventricular remodeling result in more favorable outcomes in such patients. In chronic ischemic heart disease patients with LV dysfunction, viable myocardium is independently associated with improved long-term survival after revascularization.
4. ***Prediction of perioperative complications and short-term survival.*** Establishing the presence of a viable myocardium before revascularization in addition to the clinical and angiographic assessment in the decision-making process results in a low perioperative morbidity and mortality (fewer perioperative complications, less need for inotropic drugs, low early mortality, and promising short-term survival).[39,40]

Interpretation[41]

1. ***Partial mismatch.*** A partial mismatch is seen when FDG uptake is reduced, but not as much as the perfusion deficit. This may be secondary to a combination of scar and hibernating myocardium.
2. ***Stunning.*** Normal FDG uptake with a focal wall motion abnormality suggests stunning.
   - If the wall motion abnormality is global with normal FDG uptake, this could be secondary to a cardiomyopathy or three-vessel disease.
3. ***Reverse mismatch***
   - ***a.*** Reverse mismatch (normal perfusion with decreased FDG uptake) is often artifactual secondary to normalization errors (see Pitfalls).
   - ***b.*** Also associated with recent myocardial infarction, multivessel disease, diabetes, and left bundle branch block (septal reverse mismatch)

Pitfalls[41]

1. ***Reverse mismatch.*** As areas of hibernating myocardium can have increased FDG uptake relative to normal myocardium, it is important to normalize the FDG uptake to the area of maximum perfusion. Failure to do so can result in artifactual reverse mismatched defects (normal perfusion and decreased FDG uptake) in the normal myocardium.
2. ***Recent myocardial infarction.*** FDG uptake can be seen in recently infarcted myocardium, secondary to leukocytes in the infarct region.
3. ***Perfusion imaging***
   - ***a.*** If PET tracers are not available to assess perfusion, SPECT imaging with standard tracers such as technetium sestamibi can be substituted. However, correlation between PET and SPECT images will be inexact due to attenuation on the SPECT images. Transmission-based attenuation-corrected SPECT imaging may be more accurate for correlation with PET.
   - ***b.*** *^{13}N ammonia.* If ^{13}N ammonia is used as the perfusion tracer, there is decreased lateral wall activity in ~10% of normal patients. The etiology of this is unknown.
4. ***Artifacts.***[42–47] One limitation of cardiac PET imaging on a PET/CT system is that misalignment between emission and attenuation image can lead to global and regional perfusion errors. The PET attenuation correction is often formed from a helical CT acquisition, representing a snapshot of the respiratory cycle, whereas the PET image is acquired over multiple respirations. Misalignment of these temporally different scans is common and often occurs in the diagnostic region of interest (along the lateral wall of the myocardium), leading to moderate to severe perfusion artifacts in 40% of cardiac PET–helical CT acquisitions. These misalignment artifacts are well ap-

preciated in cardiac PET/CT (**Fig. 30.8**) and have been shown to cause errors up to ± 35% over conventional cardiac PET imaging in which attenuation maps are formed over multiple respirations with a transmission rod source.

Several approaches have been proposed to minimize these artifacts. Groups have explored the option of performing the CT scan at an optimal time during respiration, such as at mid-expiration, to minimize potential mismatches. Our clinical experience has found that asking a patient to hold his or her breath at a certain point in the respiratory cycle causes highly variable results. Another approach is to acquire the attenuation map with a cine CT acquisition, which acquires multiple low-dose CT scans over a period of time at each slice in the patient. The average or intensity maximum of these cine images can be used to reduce the potential of artifact-forming mismatches. If a mismatch is evident, most vendors offer a realignment tool to manually fix major errors.

References

1. Di Carli MF, Dorbala S, Meserve J, et al. Clinical myocardial perfusion PET/CT. J Nucl Med 2007;48(5): 783–793
2. Bateman TM, Heller GV, McGhie AI, et al. Diagnostic accuracy of rest/stress ECG-gated Rb-82 myocardial perfusion PET: comparison with ECG-gated Tc-99m sestamibi SPECT. J Nucl Cardiol 2006;13(1):24–33
3. Go RT, Marwick TH, MacIntyre WJ, et al. A prospective comparison of rubidium-82 PET and thallium-201 SPECT myocardial perfusion imaging utilizing a single dipyridamole stress in the diagnosis of coronary artery disease. J Nucl Med 1990;31(12):1899–1905
4. Stewart RE, Schwaiger M, Molina E, et al. Comparison of rubidium-82 positron emission tomography and thallium-201 SPECT imaging for detection of coronary artery disease. Am J Cardiol 1991;67(16):1303–1310
5. Schelbert HR. ^{18}F-deoxyglucose and the assessment of myocardial viability. Semin Nucl Med 2002;32(1): 60–69
6. Alderman EL, Fisher LD, Litwin P, et al. Results of coronary artery surgery in patients with poor left ventricular function (CASS). Circulation 1983;68(4):785–795
7. Emond M, Mock MB, Davis KB, et al. Long-term survival of medically treated patients in the Coronary Artery Surgery Study (CASS) Registry. Circulation 1994;90(6):2645–2657
8. Passamani E, Davis KB, Gillespie MJ, Killip T. A randomized trial of coronary artery bypass surgery: survival of patients with a low ejection fraction. N Engl J Med 1985;312(26):1665–1671
9. Alderman EL, Corley SD, Fisher LD, et al. Five-year angiographic follow-up of factors associated with progression of coronary artery disease in the Coronary Artery Surgery Study (CASS). CASS Participating Investigators and Staff. J Am Coll Cardiol 1993;22(4):1141–1154
10. Mickleborough LL, Maruyama H, Takagi Y, Mohamed S, Sun Z, Ebisuzaki L. Results of revascularization in patients with severe left ventricular dysfunction. Circulation 1995; 92(9, Suppl)II73–II79
11. Kaul TK, Agnihotri AK, Fields BL, Riggins LS, Wyatt DA, Jones CR. Coronary artery bypass grafting in patients with an ejection fraction of twenty percent or less. J Thorac Cardiovasc Surg 1996;111(5):1001–1012
12. Miller DC, Stinson EB, Alderman EL. Surgical treatment of ischemic cardiomyopathy; is it ever too late? Am J Surg 1981;141(6):688–693
13. Luciani GB, Faggian G, Razzolini R, Livi U, Bortolotti U, Mazzucco A. Severe ischemic left ventricular failure: coronary operation or heart transplantation? Ann Thorac Surg 1993;55(3):719–723
14. Ellis SG, Fisher L, Dushman-Ellis S, et al. Comparison of coronary angioplasty with medical treatment for single- and double-vessel coronary disease with left anterior descending coronary involvement: long-term outcome based on an Emory-CASS registry study. Am Heart J 1989;118(2):208–220
15. Wijns W, Vatner SF, Camici PG. Hibernating myocardium. N Engl J Med 1998;339(3):173–181
16. Bengel FM, Schwaiger M. Assessment of myocardial viability by PET. In: Valk P, ed. Positron Emission Tomography: Principles and Clinical Practice. Heidelberg, Germany: Springer Verlag;2003:447-463
17. Kloner RA, Bolli R, Marban E, Reinlib L, Braunwald E. Medical and cellular implications of stunning, hibernation and preconditioning: an NHLBI workshop. Circulation 1998;97:1848–1867
18. Liedtke AJ. Alterations of carbohydrate and lipid metabolism in the acutely ischemic heart. Prog Cardiovasc Dis 1981;23(5):321–336
19. Liedtke AJ. The origins of myocardial substrate utilization from an evolutionary perspective: the enduring role of glucose in energy metabolism. J Mol Cell Cardiol 1997;29(4):1073–1086
20. Liedtke AJ, Renstrom B, Hacker TA, Nellis SH. Effects of moderate repetitive ischemia on myocardial substrate utilization. Am J Physiol 1995;269(1 Pt 2): H246–H253
21. Liedtke AJ, Renstrom B, Nellis SH, Hall JL, Stanley WC. Mechanical and metabolic functions in pig hearts after 4 days of chronic coronary stenosis. J Am Coll Cardiol 1995;26(3):815–825
22. Vanoverschelde JL, Wijns W, Depre C, et al. Mechanisms of chronic regional postischemic dysfunction in humans: new insights from the study of noninfarcted collateral-dependent myocardium. Circulation 1993;87(5):1513–1523
23. Schelbert HR, Henze E, Phelps ME, Kuhl DE. Assessment of regional myocardial ischemia by positron-emission computed tomography. Am Heart J 1982;103(4 Pt 2):588–597
24. Schwaiger M, Fishbein MC, Block M, et al. Metabolic and ultrastructural abnormalities during ischemia in canine myocardium: noninvasive assessment by positron emission tomography. J Mol Cell Cardiol 1987;19(3):259–269
25. Kalff V, Schwaiger M, Nguyen N, McClanahan TB, Gallagher KP. The relationship between myocardial blood flow and glucose uptake in ischemic canine myocardium determined with fluorine-18-deoxyglucose. J Nucl Med 1992;33(7):1346–1353

26. Marwick TH, Nemec JJ, Lafont A, Salcedo EE, MacIntyre WJ. Prediction by postexercise fluoro-18 deoxyglucose positron emission tomography of improvement in exercise capacity after revascularization. Am J Cardiol 1992;69(9):854–859

27. Taegtmeyer H. Myocardial Metabolism. In: Phelps M, Mazziotta J, Schelbert H, eds. Positron Emission Tomography and Autoradiography: Principles and Applications for the Brain and Heart. New York: Raven Press; 1986:149-195

28. Keng FY. Clinical applications of positron emission tomography in cardiology: a review. Ann Acad Med Singapore 2004;33(2):175–182

29. Schelbert HR. ^{18}F-deoxyglucose and the assessment of myocardial viability. Semin Nucl Med 2002;32(1): 60–69

30. Bax JJ, Wijns W, Cornel JH, Visser FC, Boersma E, Fioretti PM. Accuracy of currently available techniques for prediction of functional recovery after revascularization in patients with left ventricular dysfunction due to chronic coronary artery disease: comparison of pooled data. J Am Coll Cardiol 1997;30(6):1451–1460

31. Shan K, Constantine G, Sivananthan M, Flamm SD. Role of cardiac magnetic resonance imaging in the assessment of myocardial viability. Circulation 2004;109(11):1328–1334

32. Lekx KS, Pereira RS, Prato FS, Sykes J, Wisenberg G. Determining myocardial viability in a chronic occlusion canine model using MRI with a constant infusion of Gd-DTPA. Proceedings of the 8th Meeting of International Society for Magnetic Resonance in Medicine (ISMRM). Berkeley, CA: ISMRM; 2000:311

33. Bax JJ, Poldermans D, Elhendy A, Boersma E, Rahimtoola SH. Sensitivity, specificity, and predictive accuracies of various noninvasive techniques for detecting hibernating myocardium. Curr Probl Cardiol 2001;26(2):147–186

34. Baer FM, Voth E, Deutsch HJ, et al. Predictive value of low dose dobutamine transesophageal echocardiography and fluorine-18 fluorodeoxyglucose positron emission tomography for recovery of regional left ventricular function after successful revascularization. J Am Coll Cardiol 1996;28(1):60–69

35. Bax JJ, Cornel JH, Visser FC, et al. F18-fluorodeoxyglucose single-photon emission computed tomography predicts functional outcome of dyssynergic myocardium after surgical revascularization. J Nucl Cardiol 1997;4(4):302–308

36. Knuuti MJ, Saraste M, Nuutila P, et al. Myocardial viability: fluorine-18-deoxyglucose positron emission tomography in prediction of wall motion recovery after revascularization. Am Heart J 1994;127(4 Pt 1): 785–796

37. Schoder H, Campisi R, Ohtake T, et al. Blood flow-metabolism imaging with positron emission tomography in patients with diabetes mellitus for the assessment of reversible left ventricular contractile dysfunction. J Am Coll Cardiol 1999;33(5):1328–1337

38. Tillisch J, Brunken R, Marshall R, et al. Reversibility of cardiac wall-motion abnormalities predicted by positron tomography. N Engl J Med 1986;314(14):884–888

39. Haas F, Haehnel CJ, Picker W, et al. Preoperative positron emission tomographic viability assessment and perioperative and postoperative risk in patients with advanced ischemic heart disease. J Am Coll Cardiol 1997;30(7):1693–1700

40. Landoni C, Lucignani G, Paolini G, et al. Assessment of CABG-related risk in patients with CAD and LVD. Contribution of PET with [^{18}F]FDG to the assessment of myocardial viability. J Cardiovasc Surg (Torino) 1999;40(3):363–372

41. Beanlands RSB, Ruddy TD, Mahhadi J. Myocardial viability. In: RL Wahl, ed. Principles and Practice of Positron Emission Tomography. Philadelphia, PA: Lippincott Williams & Wilkins; 2002:334-350

42. Gould KL, Pan T, Loghin C, et al. Frequent diagnostic errors in cardiac PET/CT due to misregistration of CT attenuation and emission PET images: a definitive analysis of causes, consequences, and corrections. J Nucl Med 2007;48(7):1112–1121

43. Goerres GW, Burger C, Kamel E, et al. Respiration-induced attenuation artifact at PET/CT: technical considerations. Radiology 2003;226(3):906–910

44. Goerres GW, Kamel E, Heidelberg T-NH, Schwitter MR, Burger C. Schulthess GKv. PET-CT image co-registration in the thorax: influence of respiration. Eur J Nucl Med Mol Imaging 2002;29(3):351–360

45. Nakamoto Y, Osman M, Cohade C, et al. PET/CT: comparison of quantitative tracer uptake between germanium and CT transmission attenuation-corrected images. J Nucl Med 2002;43(9):1137–1143

46. Pan T, Mawlawi O, Nehmeh SA, et al. Attenuation correction of PET images with respiration-averaged CT images in PET/CT. J Nucl Med 2005;46(9):1481–1487

47. Alessio AM, Kohlmyer S, Branch K, et al. Cine CT for attenuation correction in cardiac PET/CT. J Nucl Med 2007;48(5):794–801

Index

Note: Page numbers followed by *f* and *t* indicate figures and tables, respectively.

A

Abdomen, lesions in
  mislocalization, PET/CT and, 92
Abscess
  breast, 156
  hepatic, 105
  mimicking gastric cancer, 90*f*
AC. *See* Attenuation correction
AC images. *See* Attenuation-corrected (AC) images
Acipimox, and myocardial glucose uptake, 37
Acute respiratory distress syndrome, and pulmonary FDG uptake, 53
Adenocarcinoma, differentiated, in lung, 144
Adenoids, FDG uptake, 49
Adenoma(s)
  adrenal, 114
  of breast, ductal, 156
  colonic
    detection of, 212
  hepatic, 105
  parathyroid, 51–54, 137
  pituitary, 121, 122*f*
Adenomyomatosis, in gallbladder, and FDG uptake, 59
Adrenal cancer, and FDG uptake, 59
Adrenal gland(s)
  adenomas, 114–115
  FDG uptake
    bilateral, 60*f*, 62
    focal, 60
    in metastatic disease, 114–115, 115*f*
    nonmetastatic causes of, 115
    normal pattern, 60
  giant myelolipoma, and FDG uptake, 60
  hemorrhage, 115
    and FDG uptake, 60
  histoplasmosis of, 115
    and FDG uptake, 60
  masses, PET of, 115
  metastases to, 115, 115*f*
  oncological PET imaging of, 115, 115*f*
    false negatives, 115
Adrenal hyperplasia, and FDG uptake, 60*f*, 62, 115, 119*f*, 148
Aerobic glycolysis, 28
  cancer therapy directed at, 28
Age, and thymic uptake, 52
AIDS patients, management of, FDG PET in, 250–251, 250*f*
AKT, 28
Alcohol, and FDG uptake, 34
Alzheimer disease
  diagnosis of, 258–262, 260*f*
  differential diagnosis of, 258–262
  early- *versus* late-onset, 259–261
  prognosis for, 259
Amyloidosis, and pulmonary FDG uptake, 53
Aneurysmal bone cyst, 220
Angiomyolipoma, renal, and FDG uptake, 62, 205

Annihilation photons, 3*f*, 4, 6, 7*f*
Antiandrogen treatment, for prostate cancer, 209, 210
Anticonvulsants, and brain FDG uptake, 121
Anxiety, and FDG uptake, in skeletal muscle, 68
Aorta, artifacts in, intravenous contrast and, 96
Aortic graft, suspected infection of, evaluation for, FDG PET for, 254*f*
Arterial phase imaging, artifacts in, intravenous contrast and, 96
Arthritis
  evaluation, FDG PET for, 254*f*, 255
  and FDG uptake, 66–67, 67*f*
Artifact(s)
  in cardiac PET and PET/CT, 96, 271*f*, 272–273
  dense material and, 95
  increased FDG uptake around metallic prostheses as, 75, 96
  intravenous contrast and, 95, 96*f*
  metallic materials and, 75, 96
  misregistration, 88–93, 103
    correction for, 92
    at heart–lung interface, 91*f*, 92
    at liver–lung interface, 144
    at lung–diaphragm interface, 91*f*, 92
    peridiaphragmatic, 165
  motion, 241
  noise, 59, 106*f*
  oral contrast and, 94*f*, 95
  in PET/CT, 88–96
  truncation, 90, 96
    and standardized uptake value (SUV), 39
Ascites, malignant, 107, 107*f*
ASCT. *See* Autologous stem cell transplantation (ASCT)
Astrocytoma, pilocytic, 121
Atelectasis. *See also* Round atelectasis
  and pulmonary FDG uptake, 53, 55*f*
  secondary to obstructing tumor, and pulmonary FDG uptake, 53, 55*f*
Atherosclerosis
  evaluation, FDG PET in, 251
  FDG uptake in, in vascular wall, 70, 71*f*
ATP citrate lyase, and cancer therapy, 28
Atrial fibrillation, FDG uptake in, 44, 47*f*
Atrium, cardiac, FDG uptake, 44, 46*f*, 47*f*
Attenuation artifacts, dense material and, 95
Attenuation correction, 8, 9*f*
  CT-based, 8, 13–14, 14*f*, 39, 88
    and artifactual FDG uptake around metallic prostheses, 75
    and standardized uptake value (SUV), 39
  and standardized uptake value (SUV), 39
Autologous stem cell transplantation (ASCT), for lymphoma, and pretreatment PET, 179
Axilla, FDG uptake, 52
Axillary staging
  of breast cancer, 108, 158

B

Baastrup disease, lumbar FDG uptake in, 68, 68*f*
Barium, oral, and attenuation artifacts, 95, 95*f*
Barrett esophagus, and FDG uptake, 55
Becquerel (unit), 4
Biliary tract
  FDG uptake, 60, 60*f*
  stent, and FDG uptake, 60, 60*f*, 187, 192*f*, 193
Bilinear scaling method, 14, 14*f*
Biological target volumes (BTV), 240
Biopsy, and oncological PET imaging, 36
Bismuth germinate (BGO) scintillator, 5, 5*t*
Bladder activity, reduction of, and minimization of physiologic FDG uptake, for oncological PET, 35
Bladder cancer
  metastatic, 208, 208*f*
  oncological PET imaging of, 208, 208*f*
  staging, 208
Bladder irrigation, and minimization of physiologic FDG uptake, for oncological PET, 36
Block detector, 6, 6*f*
Blood flow, and FDG uptake, 25
Body surface area, and standardized uptake value (SUV), 38
Body weight, and standardized uptake value (SUV), 38
Bone
  benign fractures, and FDG uptake, 64–65, 64*f*, 65*f*
  breast cancer metastases to, 157
  FDG uptake
    focal, 68
    G-CSF therapy and, 58*f*, 64, 66*f*
    normal pattern, 64
  lymphoma of, treated, flip-flop phenomenon of, 66*f*
Bone infarct, 222
Bone lesion(s), FDG uptake, 68
Bone marrow
  breast cancer metastases to, 157
  FDG uptake
    diffuse, 64, 176
    focal, 176
    normal pattern, 64

lymphoma and, 176
metastases to, 111–114, 112*f*, 113*f*
on bone scan, 111, 112*f*
FDG uptake, 111, 112*f*
lytic *versus* sclerotic, 111–112, 112*f*, 113*f*
PET *versus* bone scan of, 113–114
treated, 113, 113*f*, 114
oncological PET imaging of, 111–114, 112*f*, 113*f*
correlation with CT, 113*f*, 114
Bone scan
bone marrow metastases on, 111, 112*f*
of Ewing sarcoma, 225, 226*t*
and flare phenomenon, 119–120
in lymphoma, 178
Bone tumor(s)
benign and malignant, differentiation of, 220–223, 221*f*, 222*f*
grade, and FDG uptake, 222
histiocytic, 220
in pediatric patients, 232–233, 233*f*
Bowel activity, 90*f*
and FDG uptake, 58
and peritoneal metastases, differentiation of, 104*f*, 108
PET/CT and, 92, 94*f*
PET/CT and SUV for, 94*f*
reduction of, and minimization of physiologic FDG uptake, for oncological PET, 35
Brain
edema, and FDG uptake, 121
FDG uptake, 25
age-related changes in, 41
asymmetry in, 41
blood glucose and, 121
comparison with SPECT, 41
crossed cerebellar diaschisis and, 41, 43*f*
factors affecting, 121
normal pattern of, 41
renal function and, 41
and standardized uptake value (SUV), 121
symmetry of, 41
focal cortical malformations, 258
glucose metabolism, factors affecting, 121
hypometabolism in, 257–258, 258*f*
lymphoma in, PET imaging for, 125–126
metastases to, 114*f*, 115
oncological PET imaging of, 114*f*, 115, 122–126
seizure focus in, localization, 257–258, 258*f*
toxoplasmosis in, PET imaging for, 125–126
Brain tumor(s), 115
biopsy site for, 121
FDG uptake
delayed imaging and, 121
factors affecting, 121
grade, and detectability on PET, 121, 124
metabolic grading of, 121
positron emission tomography of, 122–126
false negatives, 122
false positives, 122, 122*f*, 124*f*
primary, 122–126
radiation effects on, and PET imaging, 123–126
versus radiation necrosis, 123–126
recurrence, 123, 124*f*, 125*f*
FDG uptake levels in, 124, 125*f*
magnetic resonance imaging of, 124, 124*f*, 125*f*
PET imaging for
correlation with anatomical imaging, 123
interpretation, 124
postsurgical changes and, 123
Breast(s)
abscess, 156
benign neoplasms of, 156
dense, and FDG uptake, 156
ductal adenoma, 156
FDG uptake
focal, 52, 155
incidental, 156
fibroadenomas, 156
fibrous dysplasia, 156
hematoma in, 156
inflammatory disorders, 156
lesions of, misregistration, PET/CT and, 92, 93*f*
masses in, detection of, 155–156
postbiopsy, 156
postmenopausal, FDG uptake, 52
premenopausal, FDG uptake, 52, 52*f*
seroma in, 156, 156*f*
Breast cancer
axillary staging of, 108, 158
bone metastases
lytic, 157
PET *versus* bone scan of, 114, 157
sclerotic, 157
brachial plexus involvement in, 159, 160*f*
carcinoma in situ, 156
chest wall metastases, 159, 160*f*
distant staging of, 157
estrogen receptor status, and FDG uptake, 156
and flare phenomenon, 119–120
internal mammary nodal metastases, 157, 158*f*, 158*t*, 159
invasive lobular, 156
mediastinal nodal metastases, 157, 158*f*, 158*t*
metastases, 157, 158*t*

Index

Breast cancer (*Continued*)
multifocal, 157*f*, 158
nodal staging of, 108, 158, 158*f*, 158*t*
oncological PET imaging in, 155–163
delayed, 155
dual time point, 155
false negatives, 156
false positives, 156
progesterone receptor status, and FDG uptake, 156
prognosis for, 160
recurrence, 159, 160*t*
distant, 159
elevated tumor markers and, 160
locoregional, 159, 160*f*
staging of, 156–158
sternal metastases, 159
therapy response, 160, 161*f*
tubular, 156
Breastfeeding, and FDG uptake, 36
Breast implants, FDG uptake, 52
Bronchiolitis obliterans with organizing pneumonia, and pulmonary FDG uptake, 53
Bronchoalveolar carcinoma, 144, 145*f*
Brown fat
FDG uptake, 27, 28*f*, 71–72
azygoesophageal recess, 55
combined with muscle/nodal uptake, 68*f*, 72, 74*f*
differential diagnosis of, 72–75
factors affecting, 72
infradiaphragmatic, 75
in interatrial septum, 72, 73*f*
mediastinal, 69*f*, 74*f*, 75
minimization, for oncological PET, 34
in neck, differential diagnosis of, 138*f*, 140
in neck/supraclavicular region, 69*f*, 74–75, 74*f*
paraspinal, 72, 73*f*, 75
in pediatric patients, 231*f*–232*f*, 232
and skeletal muscle uptake, differentiation of, 69*f*, 71
standardized uptake values (SUV) for, 72
supradiaphragmatic, 75
suprarenal, 75
thoracic, 75
locations of, in body, 73*f*, 74–75
Brown tumor, 221

C

Caffeine, and FDG uptake, 34
Calcified lesions, activity in, 96
Cancer antigen 15-3, blood level, and breast cancer recurrence, 160
Cancer antigen 125, blood level, and ovarian cancer recurrence, 199, 200
Cancer patient, drug toxicity in, and pulmonary FDG uptake, 53
Cancer surgery, and oncological PET imaging, 36
Carcinoembryonic antigen, blood level, in colorectal cancer, 213, 217
Carcinoid, pulmonary, 144, 148
Cardiac leads, and FDG uptake, 96
Cardiac PET, 263–274
artifacts, 96, 271*f*, 272–273
in diabetic patient, 37
hyperinsulinemic-euglycemic clamp for, 37
oral glucose loading for, 37
reduction of myocardial free fatty acid metabolism for, 37
Cardiac PET/CT, 263–274
artifacts, 96, 271*f*, 272–273
Cardiac tissue, FDG uptake, 25
caffeine and, 34
Cecum
FDG uptake, 58, 58*f*, 107, 108*f*, 212, 212*f*
peritoneal seeding to, 107, 107*f*, 108*f*
Cement, and FDG uptake, 96
Central nervous system (CNS) lesions, in HIV-infected (AIDS) patients, evaluation, FDG PET in, 250–251
Central venous line reservoir, and FDG uptake, 96
Cervical cancer
dual time imaging in, 197
early-stage, 197
nodal metastases, 196–197, 196*f*, 197*f*, 197*t*
oncological PET imaging of, 196–198, 196*f*, 197*f*
primary tumor detection, 196, 196*f*, 197*f*
prognosis for, 196, 198
radiotherapy planning for, 196
recurrence, 197
squamous carcinoma antigen in, 197
staging, 196–197, 196*f*, 197*f*
therapy response, 198
Cervical node(s), metastases to, with unknown primary, PET imaging for, 127, 128*f*
$C_f(t)$ (unmetabolized or free FDG), 19, 19*f*
Chemoradiotherapy
esophageal ulceration caused by, and therapy response imaging in esophageal cancer, 170
for head and neck cancer, therapy response imaging after, 132
Chemotherapy

and bone marrow FDG uptake, 64
and oncological PET imaging, 36
therapy response imaging after, pitfalls of, 119
therapy response imaging in, midtreatment *versus* posttreatment, 118–119
and thymic uptake, 52, 53
Child(ren). *See* Pediatric PET/CT
Cholangiocarcinoma, 90*f*, 103
distant metastases, 187
infiltrative, 187
metastatic, 187, 187*f*
nodular, 187
oncological PET imaging of, 187
perihilar, 187
primary tumor detection, 187
regional nodal metastases, 187, 187*t*
Cholangitis, and FDG uptake, 187
Cholecystitis, and FDG uptake, 60, 187
Cholestasis, and FDG uptake, 60, 60*f*, 193
Chondroblastoma, 221
Chondromyxoid fibroma, 221
Chondrosarcoma
and enchondroma, differentiation of, 221
FDG uptake, 221*f*
low-grade, FDG uptake, 220, 221
and osteochondroma, differentiation of, 221
Chronic myeloid leukemia, and bone marrow FDG uptake, 64
Chronic obstructive pulmonary disease (COPD), and FDG uptake, in intercostal muscles, 70
Cirrhosis, and FDG uptake, 187
Clinical target volume (CTV), 239–240
Clot, injected, 54*f*, 144
C_m(t) (metabolized FDG), 19, 19*f*
Coincidence(s)
definition of, 6
random (accidental), 6, 8*f*
scattered, 6–7, 8*f*
true, 6, 8*f*
Coincident photon events, 5–7, 8*f*
Cold temperature, environmental, and FDG uptake, 27, 34, 72, 75
Colon
FDG uptake, 58, 58*f*, 212, 212*f*
diffuse, 212
focal, 59, 212
nonmalignant causes of, 213
oral contrast and, 58
pattern of, 213
segmental, 58*f*, 59, 213
polyps, detection of, 212, 212*f*
primary neoplasms of, detection of, 212, 212*f*
Colon cancer
peritoneal metastasis of, 104*f*
primary, detection of, 212, 213*f*
synchronous with head and neck cancer, 128, 129*f*
Colonography, PET/CT, 213
Colony-stimulating factor therapy, and FDG uptake, 25, 26*f*
Colorectal cancer
advanced, chemotherapy response in, 217
extrahepatic metastases, 216–217
liver metastases, 216, 217
local ablative therapy for, monitoring response to, 217
prognosis for, 216–217
oncological PET imaging of, 212–219
preoperative chemoradiotherapy for, response evaluation in, 217
prognosis for, 215–216
recurrence, 213–217, 213*f*–214*f*
local, 216
peritoneal, 216
restaging, 213–214
staging, initial, 213, 213*f*
therapy response, 217
Complete metabolic response, definition of, 117
Compton scatter, 4, 6–7
Computed tomography (CT). *See also* Positron emission tomography/computed tomography (PET/CT)
of breast cancer
for nodal staging, 158, 158*t*
with recurrence, 159, 160*t*
of cervical cancer, 197
chest
breath-hold, 111
in melanoma, 182
of cholangiocarcinoma, 187, 187*t*
of colorectal cancer, 216
dynamic contrast-enhanced, of solitary pulmonary nodule, 142
in evaluation of infection and inflammation, 245
of gastric cancer metastases, 164
head, in melanoma, 182
of head and neck cancer, 128, 130*t*
for therapy response imaging, 132, 132*t*
of hepatocellular carcinoma, 187
of lymphoma, 176, 176*t*, 178
of medullary thyroid cancer, 140*t*
of osteosarcoma and soft-tissue sarcoma, 223, 225, 225*t*
of ovarian cancer, 200

Computed tomography (CT) (*Continued*)
of pancreatic cancer, 190, 190*t*
and positron emission tomography, comparison of, 3
of prostate cancer, 210
protocol for, with intravenous contrast, 96
of renal tumors, 204, 205*t*
respiratory averaged low-dose scanning, 92
of testicular cancer, 206, 207*t*
of thyroid nodules, 136–137, 137*f*
Contrast agent(s)
intravenous
and attenuation artifacts, 95, 96*f*
for PET/CT, 97
oral
and attenuation artifacts, 95, 95*f*
and colonic FDG uptake, 58
negative, 95
for PET/CT, 97
Corpus luteum cyst, 198
Corticosteroids, and brain FDG uptake, 122
Costovertebral joint, FDG uptake, 68
$C_p(t)$ (arterial plasma concentration), 19, 19*f*
C-reactive protein (CRP), 190
Crossed cerebellar diaschisis, 41, 43*f*
CT. *See* Computed tomography (CT)
CTAC. *See* Attenuation correction, CT-based
Curie (unit), 4
Cushing disease, and brain FDG uptake, 121
Cushing syndrome, adrenal hyperplasia in, and FDG uptake, 61*f*
Cyst(s)
dermoid, 198
hepatic, 105
ovarian, 198
renal, indeterminate, 204
Cystadenoma, pancreatic, serous, 192
Cystic neck masses, characterization of, 132
Cystic tumor(s), pancreatic, 191*f*, 191*t*, 192

D

DAR (differential absorption ratio, dose absorption ratio). *See* Standardized uptake value (SUV)
Degenerative disc disease, and FDG uptake, 65
Degenerative joint disease, and FDG uptake, 65
Dementia, 258–262
Dental implants, metallic, and FDG uptake, 75, 96
2-Deoxy-D-glucose, chemical structure of, 15, 15*f*
Dephosphorylation, of FDG, 25
Dermoid cyst, 199
Desmoid, FDG uptake, 222
Desmoplastic fibroma, 221
Diabetes mellitus, 148
and cardiac PET, 37
and FDG uptake, 25, 26*f*, 33
oral therapy for, and FDG uptake, 33–34
Diabetic foot, complicated, evaluation of, FDG PET in, 248, 248*f*
Diaphragmatic crus, FDG uptake, 70*f*, 71
Diaphragmatic slips, FDG uptake, 71
Diazepam
and minimization of brown fat FDG uptake, 75
and minimization of physiologic FDG uptake, for oncological PET, 34
Diet
and FDG uptake, 27, 34
for oncological PET, 34
in preparation for exam, 34
Differential absorption ratio. *See* Standardized uptake value (SUV)
Differential uptake value. *See* Standardized uptake value (SUV)
Dimercaptosuccinic acid uptake, in medullary thyroid cancer, 140*t*
Diuretics, and minimization of physiologic FDG uptake, for oncological PET, 35, 204, 205*f*
Dobutamine, in myocardial viability assessment, 271, 271*t*
Dose absorption ratio. *See* Standardized uptake value (SUV)
Dose extravasation
and axillary node uptake, 52
and standardized uptake value (SUV), 39
Dose painting, 241–242
Dose uptake ratio (DUR). *See* Standardized uptake value (SUV)
DUR (dose uptake ratio). *See* Standardized uptake value (SUV)

E

Echocardiography, in myocardial viability assessment, 271, 271*t*
EM. *See* Expectation maximization (EM)
Enchondroma, 221
Endometrial cancer, oncological PET imaging of, 201, 201*f*
Endometrioma, 199
Endometrium, FDG uptake, 64
Endoscopic ultrasound (EUS), in esophageal cancer, 166, 166*f*, 166*t*, 169

Endothelial cells, FDG uptake, 25
Ephedrine, and FDG uptake, 34
Erythropoietin (EPO), and bone marrow FDG uptake, 64
Esophageal cancer
  bone metastases, PET *versus* bone scan of, 113, 166, 166*f*, 167*t*
  distant metastases, 167–168
  FDG uptake, 165
  and FDG uptake, 56*f*
  interval metastases, 169
  locoregional metastases, 166*f*, 167–168
  neoadjuvant therapy for, therapy response imaging in, 169, 170
  nodal metastases, 166, 166*f*, 166*t*, 167*t*
    and gastrohepatic *versus* celiac nodes, 169
  oncological PET imaging in, 167–170
  primary, detection of, 165
  prognosis for, 165, 169
  recurrence, 167*f*, 169
  staging, 166*f*, 166*t*, 167–169, 167*t*
  synchronous neoplasms with, PET imaging for, 169
  therapy response, 169–170
Esophageal spasm, and FDG uptake, 55
Esophageal stricture(s), and FDG uptake, 165
Esophageal ulceration, chemoradiotherapy-induced, and therapy response imaging in esophageal cancer, 170
Esophagitis
  and FDG uptake, 165
  radiation-related, and therapy response imaging in esophageal cancer, 169–170
Esophagus, FDG uptake
  diffuse
    intense, 55
    mild, 55, 56*f*
  focal, 55, 56*f*
  patterns of, 55, 56*f*
Ewing sarcoma
  in pediatric patients, 232–233, 235*f*
  PET *versus* bone scan of, 225, 226*t*
Exercise, and FDG uptake, in skeletal muscle, 68
Expectation maximization (EM), 9
Expiration, normal, and misregistration artifact, 91–92
Extraocular muscles, FDG uptake, 71

F

^{18}F. *See* Fluorine-18
Facet disease, and FDG uptake, 65
Fasting
  and FDG uptake, 25–28, 26*f*, 33, 34
  for oncological PET, 34
FBP. *See* Filtered backprojection (FBP)
FDG. *See* [^{18}F]fluorodeoxyglucose
FDG PET. *See* Positron emission tomography (FDG PET, PET)
FDG-6-phosphate (FDG-6-P), 22, 24*f*, 25
  in malignant cells, 25
Fever of unknown origin, evaluation, FDG PET in, 250–251
[^{18}F]FDG. *See* [^{18}F]fluorodeoxyglucose
[^{18}F]fluorodeoxyglucose, 15–20
  activity
    at cellular level, 25
    in malignant cells, factors affecting, 25
    at organ level, 25, 26*f*
    at tissue level, 25
    at whole-body level, 25–28, 26*f*
  biology of, 19–20
  excretion of, 62
  intravenous administration of, 36
  metabolism of, 15, 19–20, 23–24, 24*f*
  oral administration of, 36, 36*f*
  in pediatric imaging, 232
  pharmacokinetics of, 15, 19–20
  positron (β^+) emission, 4
  synthesis of, 16–19
    electrophilic route, 16–17
    initial method of, 16, 16*f*
    later method of, 16–18, 17*f*
    nucleophilic route, 17–18, 17*f*
    quality control in, 17–18
  two-tissue compartmental model for, 19–20, 19*f*
  uptake of, 23–24, 24*f*
    aerobic glycolysis and, 28
    blood glucose level and, 25, 27*f*, 33
    body weight and, 38
    at cellular level, 25
    chemotherapy and, 36
    factors affecting, 25
    hypoxic environment and, 28
    in malignant cells, 28
      factors affecting, 25
    noninfectious/inflammatory causes of, 41
    normal sites of, 41
    at organ level, 25, 26*f*
    physiologic, minimization for oncological PET, 34–35
    at tissue level, 25
    tumor-specific factors affecting, 28–29

[18F]fluorodeoxyglucose (*Continued*)
two-tissue compartmental model for, 19–20, 19*f*
at whole-body level, 25–28, 26*f*
FH, 28
Fibroadenomas, of breast, 156
Fibroid(s), uterine. *See* Leiomyoma(s)
Fibro-osseous defects, 222
benign, in pediatric patients, 233*f*, 234
Fibrous dysplasia, 221
Field of view, 6
and standardized uptake value (SUV), 39
true, 10, 10*f*
and truncation artifact, 96
Filtered backprojection (FBP), 9–10, 11*f*–12*f*
and standardized uptake value (SUV), 39
Flare phenomenon
on bone scan, 119
with glioblastoma treatment response, 122
on PET, 119
Flip-flop phenomenon
in thyroid cancer, 139
in treated lymphoma of bone, 66*f*
Fluorine-18, 4. *See also* [^{18}F]fluorodeoxyglucose
2-Fluoro-2-deoxy-D-glucose. *See also* [^{18}F]fluorodeoxyglucose
chemical structure of, 15–16, 15*f*
Fluoromisonidazol (FMISO), 240
FMISO. *See* Fluoromisonidazol (FMISO)
Focal nodular hyperplasia, hepatic, 105
Foley catheter, 35
Follicular cyst(s), and FDG uptake, 63*f*, 64
Food and Drug Administration (FDA), good manufacturing practice guidelines, 19
FOV. *See* Field of view
Fracture(s)
benign, and FDG uptake, 64–65, 64*f*, 65*f*, 222
insufficiency, and FDG uptake, 64, 65*f*
Free breathing, and misregistration artifact, 92
Frontotemporal dementia, 259, 261*f*
Fungal infection, pulmonary, 144
FUO. *See* Fever of unknown origin

G

Gadolinium orthosilicate (GSO) scintillator, 5, 5*t*
Gallbladder. *See also* Cholangiocarcinoma
benign polyps, FDG uptake, 187
FDG uptake
focal, 59
normal pattern, 59
in wall, 59
Gallbladder cancer, and FDG uptake, 59, 187, 187*f*
Gallium scan, in lymphoma, 175
Ganglioglioma, 121
Gastric cancer
FDG uptake, 164, 165
and FDG uptake, 57*f*, 58
metastases, 164, 164*f*, 165*f*
mimics, 90*f*
mucinous, FDG uptake, 164, 165
nodal metastases, 164, 164*f*
oncological PET imaging in, 164–165
prognosis for, 164
recurrence, 164–165
signet ring cell, FDG uptake, 164, 165
therapy response, 164
Gastric remnant, FDG uptake, 165
Gastric ulcer, and FDG uptake, 57*f*, 58
Gastritis, and FDG uptake, 165
Gastroesophageal junction, FDG uptake
focal, 55, 56*f*, 165
neoplasia and, 55
Gastroesophageal reflux, and FDG uptake, 55, 58
standardized uptake value (SUV) for, 58
Gastrointestinal stromal tumors (GIST)
oncological PET imaging of, 168*f*, 170
recurrence, 170
therapy response, 168*f*, 170
Gastrointestinal tract. *See also* Bowel activity; Colon; Large bowel; Small bowel
FDG uptake, 212*f*
standardized uptake value (SUV) for, 59
PET/CT and SUV for, 92, 94*f*
G-CSF. *See* Granulocyte colony-stimulating factor (G-CSF), therapy with
Genitourinary tract, FDG excretion, 60–61
Giant cell tumor, 221, 222*f*
of tendon sheath, FDG uptake, 222
Glenohumeral joint, FDG uptake, 52*f*, 53, 68
Glioblastoma, and flare phenomenon, 110, 122
Glioma
high-grade, 122*f*
low-grade, transformation to high-grade, 121
Glipizide, and FDG uptake, 34
Glucose. *See also* Oral glucose loading
blood level of
and FDG uptake, 25, 27*f*, 121
for oncological PET imaging, 33–34, 121
and pancreatic PET, 192
and standardized uptake value (SUV), 38–39
cerebral metabolism of, factors affecting, 121

infusion, for cardiac PET, 37
metabolism of, 15–16, 19, 22, 23–24
cancer therapy targeted to, 28
in malignancy, 22–23, 28
D-Glucose, chemical structure of, 15*f*
Glucose analogues, chemical structure of, 15*f*
Glucose-6-phosphatase, 24*f*, 25
in cancer cells, 25
Glucose-6-phosphate dehydrogenase, 16
Glucose-6-phosphate (Gluc-6-P), 22, 25
Glucose transporters
GLUT1, 19, 23–24, 24*f*
in inflammatory cells, 25
in malignant cells, 25, 28
GLUT4, 19, 23–24, 26, 27*f*
GLUT. *See* Glucose transporters
Glyburide, and FDG uptake, 34
Glycolysis, 22, 26
aerobic, 28
Granulocyte colony-stimulating factor (G-CSF), therapy with
bone and splenic FDG uptake after, 58*f*, 59, 64, 175
and oncological PET imaging, 36, 175
Graves disease
and FDG uptake, in skeletal muscle, 68
thymic uptake in, 53
thyroid uptake in, 51
Gross tumor volume (GTV), 239
Ground glass opacity(ies), in lung, 144
Gynecologic tumors. *See also* Cervical cancer; Endometrial cancer; Ovarian cancer; Ovary(ies), masses
oncological PET imaging, 196–201

H

Half-life, of radionuclides, 4
HCC. *See* Hepatocellular carcinoma (HCC)
HD. *See* Hodgkin disease (HD)
Head and neck
FDG uptake, normal, on sagittal images, 47, 47*f*
PET imaging of, dedicated protocol for, 130
Head and neck cancer
characterization of, 132
distant metastases, PET imaging for, 128, 128*f*
nodal staging of, 128, 128*f*, 130, 130*f*
size-based SUV cutoffs for, 130
PET/CT of, 128*f*–130*f*, 132, 133
PET imaging for, 127–135
accuracy/comparison to other modalities, 129, 130*t*
dedicated protocol for, 130
in N0 neck, 127
prognostic significance of, 132
scan volume in, 130
postradiotherapy neck dissection in, 132
pretreatment SUV for, prognostic significance of, 128
prognosis for, 132
radiotherapy planning for, PET imaging in, 132
recurrence
magnetic resonance imaging of, 130*t*, 131
PET imaging for, 131
compared to MRI, 130*t*, 131
compared to other radionuclides, 130*t*, 131
laryngeal uptake and, 131
postoperative, 131
SUV cutoffs for, 131
tumor stunning and, 131
staging, 127–130, 128*f*, 130*f*
synchronous lesions, PET imaging for, 128, 130*f*
therapy response imaging in, 132
postchemoradiotherapy, 132
postradiotherapy, 132
tumor volume delineation in, 240
with unknown primary, PET imaging for, 127, 128*f*, 129*f*
Heart. *See also* Cardiac *entries*
FDG uptake, 42–45
perfusion imaging, nitrogen 13-labeled ammonia distribution in, 44
Hemangioma
FDG uptake, 222
hepatic, 105
sclerosing, pulmonary, 144
vertebral body, and FDG uptake, 66*f*
Hemorrhoids, FDG uptake, 212
Hepatitis, and FDG uptake, 187
Hepatobiliary tumors. *See also* Cholangiocarcinoma; Hepatocellular carcinoma (HCC)
oncological PET imaging of, 185–189
Hepatocellular carcinoma (HCC), 103
delayed imaging in, 187
extrahepatic involvement in, 185–186
FDG uptake, 25
fibrolamellar, 187
high-grade, 185, 186*f*, 187
low-grade, 105, 185, 186*f*
oncological PET imaging of, 185–189
primary tumor detection, 185–186, 186*f*

Hepatocellular carcinoma (HCC) (*Continued*)
prognosis for, 187
recurrence, 185, 187
standardized uptake value (SUV) for, 187
therapy response, 187, 187*f*
Hepatocytes, FDG uptake, 25
Hexokinase, 16, 19, 24*f*, 25
in cancer cells, 25, 28
Hiatal hernia, and FDG uptake, 58, 166
Hibernoma, FDG uptake, 222
HIF-1. *See* Hypoxia induction factor (HIF)-1
Hilar adenopathy, differential diagnosis of, 53, 71, 72*f*
Hilar node(s)
FDG uptake, 110, 148, 166
bilateral, 53, 56*f*
symmetric, 110, 110*f*
melanoma metastatic to, 183*f*
Hip prosthesis, infected, evaluation of, FDG PET in, 248–249, 248*f*, 249*f*
Histiocytes, FDG uptake, 25
Histoplasmosis, adrenal, and FDG uptake, 59
HIV-infected (AIDS) patients. *See* AIDS patients
Hodgkin disease (HD)
staging, 174
therapy response, 176–179
H-Ras, 28
Hürthle cell adenomas, 137
Hydration, for oncological PET, 34
Hyperglycemia
and FDG uptake, 25, 121
and pancreatic PET, 192
and standardized uptake value (SUV), 38–39
Hyperinsulinemic-euglycemic clamp, for cardiac PET, 37
Hypopharyngeal tumors, tumor volume delineation in, 239
Hypoxia, in tumors, and FDG uptake, 28
Hypoxia induction factor (HIF)-1, 28
stabilization, and Warburg effect, 28–29

I

Iliac node(s), 110, 110*f*
Image reconstruction, 9–10
and standardized uptake value (SUV), 39
Imatinib mesylate therapy, for gastrointestinal stromal tumors (GIST), 168*f*, 170
Immunoscintigraphy, in colorectal cancer, 216
Implantable cardioverter defibrillator, leads, artifacts caused by, 96
Implants, orthopedic, and FDG uptake, 96
IMRT. *See* Radiation therapy, intensity-modulated
Infection
evaluation of, FDG PET in, 245–256
advantages and disadvantages of, 245
in HIV-infected (AIDS) patients, detection of, FDG PET in, 250–251, 250*f*
and therapy response imaging, 119
therapy response imaging in, 253–254, 253*f*, 254*f*
Inflammation
evaluation of, FDG PET in, 245–256
advantages and disadvantages of, 245
therapy response imaging in, 253–254, 253*f*, 254*f*
Inflammatory bowel disease (IBD), evaluation, FDG PET in, 253
Inflammatory cells, FDG uptake, 25
Inflammatory pseudotumor
hepatic, 105
pulmonary, 144
Inspiration, and misregistration artifact, 91*f*, 92
Insulin/insulin therapy
and FDG uptake, 25–28, 27*f*, 33, 34*f*
in heart, 42–43
in liver, 59
in skeletal muscle, 68
infusion, for cardiac PET, 37
in myocardial viability studies, physiologic basis of, 23–24
Intercostal muscles, FDG uptake, 71
Interstitial pneumonitis, 148
Interstitial space, FDG in, 23–24, 24*f*
Intracellular space, FDG in, 23–24, 24*f*
Intraductal papillary mucinous tumor (IPMT), pancreatic, 192
Intrauterine device (IUD), and endometrial FDG uptake, 64
IPMT. *See* Intraductal papillary mucinous tumor (IPMT)
Islet cell tumors, 192, 192*f*
Isotopes, radioactive, 4

J

Joint(s), FDG uptake, nonspecific, 255

K

Kidney(s). *See also* Renal *entries*
inflammatory lesions, and FDG uptake, 205

metastases to, 204
position, on PET *versus* CT, 92
size, on PET *versus* CT, 92
Kissing spine. *See* Baastrup disease
K_{1-5} (rate constants), 19, 19*f*
Kryptofix 2.2.2, 16–19

L

Lactation, FDG uptake and excretion in, 36, 52
Langerhans cell histiocytosis, 221
in pediatric patient, 235–238, 237*f*
Lanthanum bromide (LaBr) scintillator, 5
Large bowel, FDG uptake, 58–59, 58*f*
focal, 58*f*, 59
segmental, 58*f*, 59
Laryngeal cancer
metastases of, 130
tumor volume delineation in, 239
Larynx, FDG uptake, 49*f*, 51, 131
asymmetric, 49, 49*f*
minimization, for oncological PET, 34
Lateral pharyngeal recess uptake
asymmetric, 47–48
benign and malignant, differentiation of, 49
LCH. *See* Langerhans cell histiocytosis
Lean body mass, and standardized uptake value (SUV), 38
Leiomyoma(s)
esophageal, FDG uptake, 166
pulmonary, 144
uterine, and FDG uptake, 62, 62*f*
Lewy body dementia, 261, 261*f*
Line of response (LOR), 6*f*, 7, 8, 8*f*
Lingual tonsils, FDG uptake, 47
Lipoma, FDG uptake, 222
Liposarcoma, and lipoma, differentiation of, 222, 222*f*
Liver. *See also* Hepatocellular carcinoma (HCC)
abscess, 105
adenomas, 105
artifacts in, intravenous contrast and, 96
benign lesions of, 105
dome, lesions of, mislocalization, PET/CT and, 92, 94*f*
FDG uptake, 59
focal, 103, 105–106
insulin and, 59
noise artifact and, 59
posttherapy, in lymphoma, 178
standardized uptake value (SUV) for, 59
lesions of, mislocalization, PET/CT and, 92, 94*f*
malignant lesions of, 104–105
metastases to, 103, 105, 106*f*
and flare phenomenon, 119
serosal, 107
oncological PET of, 103–107, 106*f*
position, on PET *versus* CT, 92
size, on PET *versus* CT, 92
small lesions of, 105, 106*f*
therapy response imaging for, 119
Longus colli muscle(s), FDG uptake, 49, 49*f*, 50, 71
LOR. *See* Line of response (LOR)
Lumbar spine
FDG uptake, 68–70, 69*f*
intraspinous bursa, FDG uptake, 68–70, 69*f*
Lung
bases
lesions of, mislocalization, PET/CT and, 92
nodules in, 144
PET/CT and SUV for, 92
PET/CT of, interpretation, 96
FDG uptake
diffuse, causes of, 53
false-positive results, causes of, 53
focal
causes of, 53
without CT correlate, 53, 54*f*
increased, causes of, 53
normal gradient of, 53
without CT correlate, 144
granulomatous/inflammatory processes in, 144
ground glass opacities in, 144
lesions in, coincidental detection of, 128
lymphangitic carcinomatosis, 53, 54*f*
melanoma metastatic to, 182–184, 183*f*
metastases to, 111
and benign nodule, differentiation of, 144–145
and standardized uptake value (SUV), 111
nodules in (*See also* Solitary pulmonary nodule)
benign *versus* malignant, 111
mislocalizations, PET/CT and, 93
PET/CT of, interpretation, 96
PET of, interpretation, 111
posttherapy, in lymphoma, 178
and pulmonary metastases, differentiation of, 144–145
small, with minimal or no uptake, 111
oncological PET imaging of, 111
peripheral adenocarcinoma, pleural dissemination of, 148
PET/CT of, interpretation, 96

Lung cancer. *See also* Non-small cell lung cancer; Small cell lung cancer
adrenal metastases, 115
bone metastases, PET *versus* bone scan of, 113
synchronous with head and neck cancer, 128, 129*f*
tumor volume delineation in, 239, 240
Lutetium oxyorthosilicate (LSO) scintillator, 5, 5*t*
Lutetium yttrium oxyorthosilicate (LYSO) scintillator, 5, 5*t*, 7
Lymph node(s)
axillary, FDG uptake, differential diagnosis of, 53
FDG uptake, 109*f*, 110
combined with brown fat/muscle uptake, 69*f*, 72, 74*f*
differentiation from atrial uptake, 44, 46*f*
location of, 110
pattern of, 109*f*, 110
and skeletal muscle uptake, differentiation of, 68, 69*f*, 70*f*
flat, 109*f*, 110
inflammatory and malignant, differentiation of, 109*f*, 110, 111*f*
medial neck, 137, 137*f*
metastases to, 108
oncological PET imaging of, 108–110, 109*f*, 111*f*
correlation with CT, 109*f*, 110
and standardized uptake value (SUV), 110
size of, and sensitivity of PET, 108–109
and thyroid nodules, differentiation of, 51
Lymphocyte(s), FDG uptake, 25
Lymphoma(s)
autologous stem cell transplantation for, and pretreatment PET, 179
baseline pretreatment PET in, 178
of bone, treated, flip-flop phenomenon of, 66*f*
bone marrow uptake in, 175
posttreatment, 178
cerebral involvement in, PET imaging for, 125–126
extranodal disease, detection of, 175, 176*t*
follicular, staging, 174
gastric, and FDG uptake, 166
hepatic lesions in, posttreatment, 178
low-grade, and FDG uptake, 175
lung nodules in, posttreatment, 178
marginal zone, staging, 174
minimal residual uptake in, posttherapy, 178
mucosa-associated lymphoid tissue (MALT), staging, 174
nodal disease, detection of, 175, 176*t*
oncological PET imaging in, 173–180
peripheral T-cell, staging, 174
residual posttherapy mass, 177–178
spectrum of disease, 173, 175*f*
splenic uptake in, 175
posttreatment, 178
staging, 173–176, 173*f*, 175*f*
therapy response, 176–179, 177*f*
posttreatment evaluation, 177–178, 177*f*

M

Macrophages, FDG uptake, 25
Magnetic resonance imaging (MRI)
of brain tumor recurrence, 124, 124*f*, 125*f*
of breast cancer, 157*f*, 158
of cervical cancer, 196–197, 197*t*
of colorectal cancer, 216
contrast-enhanced, for detection of breast masses, 155
coregistration, in brain tumor recurrence, 123
with dobutamine, in myocardial viability assessment, 271, 271*t*
in evaluation of infection and inflammation, 245
of head and neck cancer, 128, 130*t*
for head and neck cancer recurrence, 130*t*, 131
of hepatocellular carcinoma, 187
of medullary thyroid cancer, 140*t*
in melanoma, 182
of multiple myeloma, 225
of osteosarcoma and soft-tissue sarcoma, 223, 225
of ovarian cancer, 199*t*, 200
and positron emission tomography, comparison of, 3
Magnetic resonance spectroscopy (MRS), of brain tumor recurrence, 123
Malignancy
FDG-6-phosphate activity in, 25
FDG uptake
at cellular level, 25
at organ level, 25
at tissue level, 25
glucose metabolism in, 22–23
hypoxic environment of, and FDG uptake, 28
Mammography, in breast cancer, 158
Medial neck node(s), 137, 137*f*
Mediastinal node(s)
FDG uptake, 104*f*, 110, 148
differentiation from atrial uptake, 44, 46*f*

in granulomatous disease, 148
and standardized uptake value (SUV), 148
symmetric, 110, 111*f*
visual analysis of, 148
flat, 109*f*, 110
Mediastinoscopy, 147–148
Melanin content, and detectability of melanoma, 182
Melanoma
adrenal metastases, 182*f*
bowel metastasis, 182*f*
brain metastases, 182
distant metastases, 181, 182, 182*f*
hepatic metastases, 182
local nodal staging of, 110
lung metastases, 182, 183, 183*f*
melanin content, 182
nodal metastases, 181, 181*f*, 182*f*, 183*f*
oncological PET imaging in, 181–184
peripheral lesions in, 183
prognosis for, 182
recurrence, 182–183
sentinel node biopsy in, 182
splenic metastases, 181, 181*f*, 182*f*
staging, initial, 181–182, 181*f*–183*f*
Meningioma, 122, 122*f*
Menstrual cycle
and endometrial FDG uptake, 63
and ovarian FDG uptake, 63, 199
Mesenteric node(s), melanoma metastatic to, 183*f*
Mesothelioma, 151*f*, 152
Metallic prostheses, and FDG uptake, 75, 96
Metastatic disease
detected by PET, confirmation with anatomical imaging, 103
in liver, 104
Metformin, and FDG uptake, 33–34
MIP. *See* Maximum intensity projection (MIP)
Mislocalization of lesions
on fused PET/CT images, 91
in liver dome, 93, 94*f*
in lung bases, 93, 94*f*
Misregistration artifacts, 88–93, 104
correction for, 92
at heart–lung interface, 91*f*, 92
at liver–lung interface, 144
at lung–diaphragm interface, 91*f*, 92
peridiaphragmatic, 166
Mitochondria, dysfunction, and tumorigenesis, 28–29
Motion, and image correlation, 91, 92*f*–93*f*, 93
MRI. *See* Magnetic resonance imaging (MRI)
MRS. *See* Magnetic resonance spectroscopy (MRS)
Mucoepidermoid carcinoma, 144
Mucosa-associated lymphoid tissue (MALT) lymphoma, staging, 174
Multi-infarct dementia, 259–260
Multiple myeloma (MM), 225–226, 226*f*
Muscle, FDG uptake, minimization, for oncological PET, 34
Musculoskeletal tumors
benign and malignant, differentiation of, 220–223
biopsy, guiding, 223–226
grading, 223–226
oncological PET imaging of, 220–227
recurrence, 223–226, 224*f*
staging, 223–226, 223*f*
therapy response, 223–226, 223*f*
MYC oncogene, 28
Myelodysplastic syndromes, and bone marrow FDG uptake, 64
Myelolipoma, giant adrenal, and FDG uptake, 59
Mylohyoid muscle, FDG uptake, normal
on axial images, 47, 47*f*
on sagittal images, 47, 47*f*
Myocardial infarct/infarction, recent, and FDG uptake, 271
Myocardial ischemia, 267–268, 268*f*
Myocardial perfusion assessment, 263–264, 264*f*–267*f*, 271
Myocardial viability, assessment of, methods for, 271–272, 271*t*
Myocardial viability PET, 264–273, 268*f*, 270*f*
clinical applications of, 272–273
hyperinsulinemic-euglycemic clamp for, 37
insulin in, 37
physiologic basis of, 23–24
interpretation, 271–272
and myocardial stunning, 272
oral glucose loading for, 37
partial mismatch in, 272
in prediction of cardiac events, 268
in prediction of improvement of CHF after revascularization, 272–273
in prediction of long-term survival, 268
in prediction of perioperative complications, 268–270
in prediction of postrevascularization functional recovery, 272
in prediction of remodeling, 268
in prediction of short-term survival, 268–270
reduction of myocardial free fatty acid metabolism for, 37

Myocardial viability PET (*Continued*)
reverse mismatch in, 272
sensitivity and specificity of, 271, 271*t*
Myocardium, FDG uptake
in fasting state, 42, 43*f*
insulin and, 42–43
Myxoid tumors, 221

N

NAC images. *See* Nonattenuation-corrected (NAC) images
Nasopharyngeal carcinoma
and asymmetric uptake, 48*f*
in lateral pharyngeal recess, 49
bone metastases, PET *versus* bone scan of, 113, 128
with cervical metastases, primary tumor localization in, 127
metastases of, 130, 130*f*
Nasopharyngeal uptake, 47*f*, 48
Neutrophils, FDG uptake, 25
NHL. *See* Non-Hodgkin lymphoma (NHL)
Niacin, and myocardial glucose uptake, 37
Nicotine, and FDG uptake, 34
Nipple, FDG uptake, 52
Nitrogen-13 ammonia, in cardiac PET and PET/CT, 271–272, 271*f*
Nodular lymphoid hyperplasia, 105
Nonattenuation-corrected (NAC) images
and interpretation of PET/CT, 96–97
Non-Hodgkin lymphoma (NHL)
low-grade, therapy response, 177
staging, 173*f*, 174, 174*f*
therapy response, 176–179
Nonossifying fibroma, 221
Nonseminomatous germ cell tumors (NSGCT), 206–207
Non-small cell lung cancer
adrenal metastases, 147, 147*f*, 148
bone marrow metastases, 146, 147*f*
brain metastases, 147
FDG uptake, 25
lymphatic metastases, and pattern of uptake, 149
prognosis, 149–150
radiotherapy planning in, 150
recurrence, 150–151, 151*f*
staging, 146–149
distant, 146
mediastinal, 146
therapy response, 149–150
tumor volume delineation in, 240
NSGCT. *See* Nonseminomatous germ cell tumors (NSGCT)
Nuclear medicine, in evaluation of infection and inflammation, 245

O

Obesity
and standardized uptake value (SUV), 38, 39
and truncation artifact, 96
Oligodendroglioma, 122
Omentum, metastases to, 107
Oncocytoma, renal, and FDG uptake, 62, 206
Oncogenes, activation of, and Warburg effect, 28
Oncological PET imaging
of adrenals, 114*f*, 115
false negatives, 115
advantages and disadvantages of, 103–104, 104*f*
and anatomical localization of lesions, 103
by anatomical region, 103–116
baseline
before chemotherapy, 36
and therapy response imaging, 120, 178
of bladder cancer, 208, 208*f*
of bone marrow, 111–114, 112*f*, 113*f*
of brain, 114*f*, 115, 122–126
of breast cancer, 155–163
and breastfeeding, 36
of cervical cancer, 196–198, 196*f*, 197*f*
of cholangiocarcinoma, 187
of colorectal cancer, 212–219
correlation with anatomical imaging, 103, 104*f*
for differentiation of pulmonary metastasis and benign nodule, 144–145
and early detection, 103, 104*f*
of endometrial cancer, 201, 201*f*
of esophageal cancer, 167–170
false positives, 103
FDG administration for, 36, 36*f*
FDG in, advantages of, 22
of gastric cancer, 164–165
of gastrointestinal stromal tumors (GIST), 168*f*, 170
of gynecologic tumors, 196–201
of hepatobiliary tumors, 185–189
of hepatocellular carcinoma, 185–189
in HIV-infected (AIDS) patients, 250–251
lesion detectability on, lesion size and, 103

of liver, 103–107, 106*f*
artifacts, 105, 106*f*
correlation with CT, 106*f*, 107
false negatives, 105
false positives, 105
interpretation, 105–106
nonattenuation-corrected (NAC) images and, 105–106
of lungs, 111
of lymph nodes, 108–110, 109*f*, 111*f*
of lymphoma, 173–180
management effects of, 103
of melanoma, 181–184
of musculoskeletal tumors, 220–227
of non-small cell lung cancer, for staging, 146–149
of ovarian cancer, 198–201, 199*t*, 200*f*
of pancreatic cancer, 190–195
patient preparation for, 33–35
of peritoneum, 107–108, 107*f*, 109*f*
principles of, 103
of prostate cancer, 208–210
of renal cell carcinoma, 204–206
sensitivity of, 103
of solitary pulmonary nodule, 142–145
of spleen, 107
of testicular cancer, 206–207, 207*f*
of thoracic neoplasms, 142–154
of thyroid cancer, 136–141
timing (scheduling) of
chemotherapy and, 36
postbiopsy, 36
postradiation, 36
postradiofrequency ablation, 36
postsurgery, 36
of urologic tumors, 204–211
Oral cavity, tumors of, metastases of, 130
Oral glucose loading, for cardiac PET, 37
Oral hypoglycemic agents, and FDG uptake, 33–34
Ordered-subsets expectation maximization (OSEM), 9, 11*f*
Oropharyngeal tumors, tumor volume delineation in, 239
Orthopedic implants, and FDG uptake, 96
OSEM. *See* Ordered-subsets expectation maximization (OSEM)
Osteoarthritis
evaluation, FDG PET for, 255
joints in, FDG uptake, 68
Osteoblastoma, 221
Osteochondroma, 221
Osteomyelitis, 222
chronic, evaluation of, FDG PET in, 245–246, 247*f*
Osteosarcoma, 223–224, 223*f*, 225*t*
in pediatric patients, 232–233
Ovarian cancer
early-stage, 199
and FDG uptake, 62*f*, 63
metastases, 200*f*, 201
nodal metastases, 200*f*, 201
oncological PET imaging, 198–201, 199*t*, 200*f*
peritoneal metastases, 200*f*, 201
recurrence, 198–201
prognosis for, 200
second look laparotomy in, 199
serosal metastases, 200*f*
therapy response, 201
Ovary(ies)
FDG uptake, 62*f*, 63, 110, 111*f*
normal pattern, 62
postmenopausal, 199
in postmenopausal women, 63
premenopausal, 199
in premenopausal women, 62*f*, 63
standardized uptake value (SUV) for, 199
follicular cyst, and FDG uptake, 62*f*, 63
inflammatory processes in, 199
masses in, differential diagnosis of, 198–201, 199*t*

P

Pacemaker leads, 96
Paget disease of bone, active, 220
Palatine tonsils, FDG uptake, 47
Pancreas
cystic tumors, 191*f*, 191*t*, 192
FDG uptake
diffuse, 60
focal, 60
standardized uptake value (SUV) for, 60
intraductal papillary mucinous tumor, 192
masses
benign
and adenocarcinoma, differentiation of, 190–191
characteristics of, 190
inflammatory, characteristics of, 190
malignant, characteristics of, 190
and standardized uptake values (SUV), 190
solid pseudopapillary tumors of, 192
Pancreatic cancer
cystic, 191*f*, 191*t*, 192

Pancreatic cancer (*Continued*)
delayed imaging in, 190–191
and FDG uptake, 60, 60*f*
metastases, 193–194, 193*f*
oncological PET imaging of, 190–195
pancreatitis with, 190, 191*f*
prognosis for, 193
recurrence (postoperative), 193, 194*f*
staging, 192*f*, 193–194
standardized uptake value (SUV) for, 191
therapy response, 193
Pancreatic islet cell tumors, 192, 192*f*
Pancreatic pseudocyst, 191*f*, 192
hemorrhagic, 192
Pancreatitis, 190, 191*f*, 192
and FDG uptake, 60
with malignancy, 190, 191*f*
Papillary muscle, FDG uptake, 43–44, 44*f*–45*f*
Paracolic gutter(s), metastases to, 107
Parathyroid adenoma(s), 51–54, 137
Parathyroid hyperplasia, 51–54
Parkinson dementia, 261
Parotid lesions, characterization of, 132
Partial metabolic response, definition of, 117
Partial volume effects, and standardized uptake value (SUV), 39, 120
Patient preparation, for oncological PET, 33–35
Pediatric PET/CT, 231–238
of bone tumors, 232–233, 233*f*
brown fat and, 231*f*–232*f*, 232
patient preparation for, 225
and seizure localization, 258
of soft-tissue tumors, 234*f*–236*f*, 235–238
Pelvic lymph nodes, oncological PET imaging of, 110
Pelvis, peritoneal spread in, 107
PEM. *See* Positron emission mammography (PEM)
Peripheral nerve sheath tumor, malignant, in pediatric patient, 236*f*
Peritoneal carcinomatosis, diffuse, 108, 109*f*
Peritoneal disease, 90*f*
Peritoneal metastases, 107
and bowel activity, differentiation of, 104*f*, 108
Peritoneal spread, patterns of, 107, 107*f*, 109*f*
Peritoneum
FDG uptake, diffuse, 108, 109*f*
oncological PET imaging of, 107–108, 107*f*, 109*f*
Perivascular FDG uptake, 71, 73*f*
PET. *See* Positron emission tomography (FDG PET, PET)
PET/CT. *See* Positron emission tomography/computed tomography (PET/CT)
PET-trace FDG MicroLab, 17
Phase-transfer agent(s), 17–18
Pheochromocytoma, and FDG uptake, 60
Phosphatidylinositol 3-kinase, 28
Phosphohexose isomerase, 16
Photomultiplier tube(s), 5, 6*f*
Photons. *See also* Annihilation photons; Coincident photon events
detection of, 4–5
interactions with matter, 4
Pick disease, 259, 261*f*
Pituitary adenoma(s), 122, 122*f*
Plain radiograph(s), of multiple myeloma, 225, 226*f*
Planning target volume (PTV), 239–240
Plasmacytoma, FDG uptake, 220, 221
Pleomorphic xanthoastrocytoma, 122
Pleural disease, malignant *versus* benign, 147, 147*f*
Pleural effusion(s), malignant, 147, 147*f*
PMTs. *See* Photomultiplier tube(s)
Pneumonia, 149
lipoid, 144
therapy response, 253*f*
Polyp(s)
colonic, detection of, 212, 212*f*
in gallbladder, and FDG uptake, 59
Positron (β^+) emission, 3*f*, 4
Positron emission mammography (PEM), 155
Positron emission tomography/computed tomography (PET/CT). *See also* Pediatric PET/CT
for adaptive radiotherapy during course of treatment, 241–242
advantages of, 88
of alveolar rhabdomyosarcoma, 234*f*, 235
artifacts, 88–96
attenuation correction in (CT-based), 8, 14, 14*f*, 88
and artifactual FDG uptake around metallic prostheses, 75
and standardized uptake value (SUV), 39
of bowel, and focal FDG uptake, 58–59
of breast cancer recurrence, 159, 160*t*
cardiac (*See* Cardiac PET/CT)
of colorectal cancer, 215*f*, 216
contemporaneous correlation with, 88
in differential diagnosis of brown fat uptake, 72–74
disadvantages of, 88–96
of esophageal cancer, 166, 166*f*
four-dimensional, 1241
fused images, registration and, 96
of head and neck, 128*f*–130*f*, 132, 133
helical CT scan, 11–12

and incorrect uptake levels, 91
interpretation of, 96–97
nonattenuation-corrected (NAC) images and, 96–97
intravenous contrast for, 97
and localization of lesions, 88, 89*f*
of lungs, 111
interpretation of, 96
in lymphoma, 175, 176*t*
for staging, 173
in melanoma, 182–184
and mislocalization of lesions, 91
mislocalizations, 91, 93
in head and neck, 92*f*, 93
misregistration artifact (*See* Artifact(s), misregistration)
nonrespiratory motion and, 92*f*–93*f*, 93
of non-small cell lung cancer
for nodal staging, 146, 147*f*
for tumor staging, 146–149
oral contrast for, 97
of ovarian cancer, 201
patient positioning for, 97
patient preparation for, 97
physics of, 4–14
positive predictive value, for bone malignancy, 114
protocol for, 12
for radiosurgery planning, 241–242
respiration and, 97
respiratory gating for, 93
scout CT scan, 11–12
sensitivity of, 88
of solitary pulmonary nodule, 142
misregistration, 144
specificity of, 88
of splenic masses, 107
and standardized uptake value (SUV), 96–97
in bowel, 93
at lung bases, 93
for therapy response imaging, in head and neck cancer, 132, 132*t*
Positron emission tomography/computed tomography (PET/CT) scanner
acquisition system, 11–12
components of, 12–13, 13*f*
CT-based attenuation correction in, 14, 14*f*
data flow in, 13*f*, 14
image display, 14, 14*f*
Positron emission tomography (FDG PET, PET)
advantages and disadvantages of, 3
cardiac (*See* Cardiac PET)
data acquisition, 4–9
corrections, 8, 9*f*
equivocal findings on, confirmation of, 88, 90*f*
in evaluation of infection and inflammation, advantages and disadvantages of, 245
false positives, identification of, 88, 90*f*
findings on, without anatomical imaging correlate, 53, 54*f*
image reconstruction, 9–10, 11*f*
and standardized uptake value (SUV), 39
indications for
A level, 99
B level, 99
C level, 99
D level, 99
levels of evidence for, 99
interpretation of
certainty of, improving, 88, 90*f*
confidence in, increasing, 88, 90*f*
management effects of, 103
neurologic applications of, 257–262
noise/resolution trade-offs, 9–10, 12*f*
nononcologic applications of (*See* Infection(s); Inflammation; Pediatric PET/CT; Radiation therapy planning)
oncological (*See* Oncological PET imaging)
physical principles of, 3, 3*f*
of therapy response (*See* Therapy response imaging)
three-dimensional (3D) acquisition protocols, 8–9, 10*f*
two-dimensional (2D) acquisition protocols, 9, 10*f*
Positron emitters, 3, 3*f*
p53 protein, 28
Primary sclerosing cholangitis, 187
Progressive metabolic disease, definition of, 117
Progressive multifocal leukoencephalopathy (PML), 125–126
Propranolol, and minimization of physiologic FDG uptake, for oncological PET, 34
Prostate cancer
antiandrogen treatment for, 209, 210
bone metastases, 210
PET *versus* bone scan of, 114
FDG uptake, 25
metastatic, 209–210, 210*f*
oncological PET imaging of, 208–210
primary tumor detection, 209, 209*f*
recurrence, 209
staging, preoperative, 209
therapy response, 209

Prosthesis, infected, evaluation of, FDG PET in, 248–249, 248*f*, 249*f*
Pseudolymphoma, 105
Psoas muscle, melanoma metastatic to, 183*f*
Pulmonary embolism, FDG uptake, 53, 71, 72*f*
Pulmonary infarction, and pulmonary FDG uptake, 53
Pyelonephritis, xanthogranulomatous, and FDG uptake, 206
Pyriform sinus tumor, with cervical metastases, primary tumor localization in, 127, 128*f*

R

Radiation esophagitis, and therapy response imaging in esophageal cancer, 169–170
Radiation necrosis, cerebral, 123–126
Radiation pneumonitis, 150
  and pulmonary FDG uptake, 54, 55*f*
Radiation therapy
  of brain tumor, and PET imaging, 123–126
  for head and neck cancer, therapy response imaging after, 132
  intensity-modulated, 240, 241
  and oncological PET imaging, 36
  therapy response imaging after, pitfalls of, 120
  therapy response imaging in, midtreatment *versus* posttreatment, 118–119
Radiation therapy planning, 239–244
  advances in (future directions for), 242
  for cervical cancer, 196
  dose painting and, 241–242
  for head and neck cancer, 132
  for non-small cell lung cancer, 150
  staging PET and, 239, 240*t*
  target tumor volumes in, 239–240
  theragnostic imaging and, 241–242
  tumor volume delineation for, 239–240
Radioactive decay, 4
Radiofrequency ablation, and oncological PET imaging, 36, 217
Radioimmunotherapy, of brain tumor, and FDG uptake, 124
Radioiodine therapy, for thyroid cancer, and thymic uptake, 53
Radioiodine uptake, in thyroid cancer, 139, 139*t*
Radionuclides, for PET radiotracer synthesis, 3, 16
Radiotracers, 3
  for myocardial perfusion assessment, 263–264, 264*f*–267*f*
  quality control for, 17–18
  synthesis of, 16
Rate constant(s) (K_{1-5}), 19, 19*f*
Rectal cancer, staging, initial, 213, 213*f*
Rectosigmoid colon, FDG uptake, 58*f*, 59
Region of interest (ROI), 38
  fixed-size, centered on maximum pixel value, and standardized uptake value (SUV), 40
  maximum pixel value
    and standardized uptake value (SUV), 40
    three-dimensional isocontour at percentage of, and standardized uptake value (SUV), 40
  maximum SUV in, 40
  mean SUV in, 40
  placement method, and standardized uptake value (SUV), 40
  volumetric *versus* two-dimensional (2D), and standardized uptake value (SUV), 40
Renal cell carcinoma
  cystic, 204, 204*f*
  FDG uptake in, 204, 205*f*
  metastatic, 205*f*, 206
  oncological PET imaging, 204–206
  restaging, 206
  staging, 206
Renal collecting system activity
  false positive, 62
  reduction of, and minimization of physiologic FDG uptake, for oncological PET, 36, 204, 205*f*
Renal cyst(s), indeterminate, 204
Renal masses, 204–206
  exophytic, differential diagnosis of, 204
  solid, 204
Resperine, and minimization of physiologic FDG uptake, for oncological PET, 34
Respiration
  and PET/CT, 97
  type of, and misregistration artifact, 91–92
Respiratory averaged low-dose CT scanning, 92
Respiratory gating, 93, 242
Respiratory misregistration artifact. *See* Artifact(s), misregistration
Retrocrural node(s), FDG uptake, 70*f*, 71
Retroperitoneal nodes
  FDG uptake, differential diagnosis of, 61*f*, 62
  ovarian cancer metastases to, 201
Retropharyngeal node(s), FDG uptake, 49, 51*f*
Rhabdomyosarcoma
  alveolar, in pediatric patients, 234*f*, 235
  metastases, 235
  PET/CT for, 235

Rheumatoid arthritis (RA), 149
evaluation, FDG PET for, 255
joints in, FDG uptake, 68
Rheumatoid nodule, pulmonary, 144
Right ventricle, FDG uptake, 43
RMS. *See* Rhabdomyosarcoma
ROI. *See* Region of interest (ROI)
Rosiglitazone, and FDG uptake, 34
Round atelectasis, 143, 144*f*
RTP. *See* Radiation therapy planning

S

Sacrum, insufficiency fractures, and FDG uptake, 64, 65*f*
Salivary glands
FDG uptake, 47*f*, 48, 48*f*
malignancies of, 132
Sarcoid
FDG uptake, 222
pulmonary, 144
Sarcoidosis, 105, 107, 156, 221
evaluation, FDG PET in, 251, 252*f*
Sarcoma. *See also* Ewing sarcoma
soft-tissue, 223–224, 224*f*, 225*t*
in pediatric patients, 235
Schwannoma, FDG uptake, 222
Scintillator(s), for PET photon detection, 4–5, 5*t*
decay constant of, 4–5
energy resolution of, 5
light output of, 5, 5*t*
most commonly used, characteristics of, 5, 5*t*
stopping power of, 4
SDH, 28
Sedatives, and brain FDG uptake, 122
Seizures
and FDG uptake in brain, 122, 124
localization, 257–258, 258*f*
Seminoma, 206–207, 207*f*
Sentinel node biopsy, in melanoma, 182
Sentinel node imaging, 110
Sep-Pak silica cartridge, 17–18
Serosal implant, solid, 107, 107*f*
Sestamibi uptake. *See also* Technetium-99m sestamibi scan
in medullary thyroid cancer, 140*t*
of multiple myeloma, 225
of osteosarcoma and soft-tissue sarcoma, 225, 225*t*
in papillary/follicular thyroid cancer, 139, 139*t*
Sigmoid mesocolon, peritoneal spread and, 107
Single-photon emission computed tomography (SPECT), 6
in Alzheimer disease, 259
of brain, comparison with PET, 41
of brain tumor recurrence, 123
for myocardial perfusion imaging, 272
in seizure localization, 257
Sinogram(s), 8
Sister Mary Joseph node, 109*f*
Skeletal muscle
FDG uptake, 68–69
combined with brown fat/nodal uptake, 69*f*, 72, 74*f*
increased, causes of, 68
mimics of, 68–69, 69*f*, 70*f*
melanoma metastatic to, 183*f*
Skeletal muscle relaxants, and minimization of physiologic FDG uptake, for oncological PET, 34
Small bowel, FDG uptake, 58–59
Small cell lung cancer, 151
FDG uptake, 149
Smoking, and FDG uptake, in intercostal muscles, 71
Smoothing, 10, 11*f*
Soft palate, FDG uptake, normal
on axial images, 47, 48*f*
on sagittal images, 47, 47*f*
Soft tissue, FDG uptake, 71
Soft-tissue tumor(s)
benign and malignant, differentiation of, 222
in pediatric patients, 234*f*–236*f*, 235–238
Solitary pulmonary nodule, 142–145
dual point imaging of, 144
with FDG uptake and SUV <2.5, 145
histology of, and FDG uptake, 144
malignant, 142–143, 143*f*
scan time for, 144
small, 144
Somatostatin receptor scintigraphy, in medullary thyroid cancer, 140*t*
Spasmolytic premedication, and minimization of physiologic FDG uptake, for oncological PET, 36
SPECT. *See* Single-photon emission computed tomography (SPECT)
Spinal cord, FDG uptake, 42, 48*f*
Spine, degenerative spur in, and FDG uptake, 65, 67*f*
Spleen
artifacts in, intravenous contrast and, 96
FDG uptake

Spleen (*Continued*)
after G-CSF therapy, 176
in benign *versus* malignant lesions, 107
diffuse, posttherapy, in lymphoma, 178
diffuse increased, 59
infection and, 107
posttherapy, in lymphoma, 178
standardized uptake value (SUV) for, 59
hyalinized nodules, 107
lymphoma and, 176
metastases to, serosal, 107
oncological PET imaging of, 107
position, on PET *versus* CT, 93
size, on PET *versus* CT, 93
therapy response imaging for, 120
Squamous carcinoma antigen, in cervical cancer, 197
Src oncogene, 28
Stable metabolic disease, definition of, 117
Standardized uptake ratio (SUR). *See* Standardized uptake value (SUV)
Standardized uptake value (SUV), 23, 38–41
artifactually increased and decreased, in PET/CT, 93
attenuation artifacts due to dense material, 95
attenuation correction method and, 40
background activity ("spilling in" of) and, 40, 120
body weight and, 38
calculation of, 38–41
cutoff values, 40
definition of, 38
dose extravasation and, 40
dual time-point imaging and, 41
filtered backprojection and, 40
formula for, 38
and interpretation, 41
maximum (SUVmax), 40
and thresholding, 239
mean, 40
measurement
attenuation correction and, 40
error in, specific to therapy response, 120
for evaluation of therapy response, 118
PET/CT and, 96–97
in normal thyroid, 49
obesity and, 38, 39
partial volume effects and, 39, 120
patient size and, 38
for PET/CT, CT-based attenuation correction and, 39
plasma glucose levels and, 39
reconstruction parameter and, 39
reporting of, 41
ROI placement and, 40
significant change in, and therapy response, 117
and therapy response, 41, 117
timing of measurement and, 38–39
Sternoclavicular joint, FDG uptake, 68
Sternocleidomastoid muscle, FDG uptake, 49
Stomach. *See also* Gastric cancer
FDG uptake, 55–58
abnormal, 57*f*, 58
normal patterns, 55, 57*f*
proximal *versus* distal, 55, 57*f*, 58
standardized uptake value (SUV) for
in reflux disease, 58
without reflux, 58
Straight-line sign, in diffuse peritoneal carcinomatosis, 108, 109*f*
Subcarinal node(s), FDG uptake, differentiation from atrial uptake, 44, 46*f*
Subchondral cyst, and FDG uptake, 67*f*, 68
Sublingual glands, FDG uptake, normal
on axial images, 47, 47*f*
on sagittal images, 47, 47*f*
Submandibular glands, FDG uptake, 47, 49*f*
Submandibular node(s), FDG uptake, 47, 49*f*
Sulfonylureas, and FDG uptake, 34
Supraglottic cancer, metastases of, 130, 130*f*
SUR (standardized uptake ratio). *See* Standardized uptake value (SUV)
SUV. *See* Standardized uptake value (SUV)
Synchronous lesions
with esophageal cancer, 169
with head and neck cancer, 128, 130*f*

T

Talc granulomata, 145
Talc pleurodesis, and FDG uptake, 149
Tamoxifen, and false-positive flare phenomenon, 120
TCA cycle. *See* Tricarboxylic acid cycle
Technetium-99m depreotide scan
of solitary pulmonary nodule, 142
in thyroid cancer, 139
Technetium-99m sestamibi scan
for detection of breast masses, 155
for head and neck cancer recurrence, 130*t*, 131
Technetium-99m tetrofosmin scan, for head and neck cancer recurrence, 130*t*, 131

Technetium-99m tracers, in myocardial viability assessment, 271, 271*t*
Temperature, environmental, and FDG uptake, 28, 34, 72, 75
Temporal lobe epilepsy, 257–258, 258*f*
Teres minor muscle, FDG uptake, 71
Testes, FDG uptake, 64
standardized uptake value (SUV) for, 64
Testicular cancer
oncological PET imaging in, 206–207, 207*f*
recurrence, 207
staging, 206, 207*f*
Tetrabutylammonium bicarbonate, 17
Tetrabutylammonium hydroxide, 17
β-Thalassemia, and bone marrow FDG uptake, 64
Thallium-doped sodium iodide (NaI)(Tl) scintillator, 5*t*
Thallium-201 scan
reinjection studies, in myocardial viability assessment, 271*t*
rest-redistribution studies, in myocardial viability assessment, 271, 271*t*
Thallium SPECT, of brain tumor recurrence, 123
Thallium uptake, in thyroid cancer, 139, 139*t*
Thecoma, 199
Theragnostic imaging, 242
Therapy response
definition of, 117
measurement of, 118
midtreatment *versus* posttreatment, 118–119
mixed, 118–119, 119*f*
Therapy response imaging
of breast cancer, 160, 161*f*
of.cervical cancer, 198
of colorectal cancer, 217
definition of response and, 117
early prediction, 117
of breast cancer, 159–160
of colorectal cancer, 217
of esophageal cancer, 169
of gastric cancer, 164
of head and neck cancer, 132
of lymphoma, 176–177
of non-small cell lung cancer, 150
of esophageal cancer, 169–170
false negatives, 120
false positives, 120
of gastrointestinal stromal tumors (GIST), 168*f*, 170
of head and neck cancer, 132
hepatic lesions and, 120
of hepatocellular carcinoma, 187, 187*f*
infection and, 120
in infection and inflammation, 253–254, 253*f*, 254*f*
lack of baseline PET study and, 120
late prediction, 117
of colorectal cancer, 217
of esophageal cancer, 169
of head and neck cancer, 132
of lymphoma, 177
of non-small cell lung cancer, 150, 150*f*
low pretherapy FDG uptake and, 120
of lymphoma, 176–179, 177*f*
midtreatment *versus* posttreatment, 118–119
of non-small cell lung cancer, 149–150
and normal tissue response, 120
of ovarian cancer, 201
of pancreatic cancer, 193
posttherapy, of breast cancer, 160
principles of, 117
of prostate cancer, 209
sensitivity of, 118
specificity of, 118
splenic lesions and, 120
SUV measurement error in, 120
treatment effects of, 120
tumor heterogeneity and, 118–119, 119*f*
Thoracic neoplasms, oncological PET imaging of, 142–154
Thoracic veins, artifacts in, intravenous contrast and, 95, 96*f*
Thorax
lesions of, mislocalization, PET/CT and, 93
Three-dimensional (3D) acquisition protocols, 8–9, 10*f*
Thresholding, 239
Thrombosis, and FDG uptake, 71, 72*f*
Thymic hyperplasia, 52*f*, 53, 176
Thymoma, standardized uptake value (SUV) in, 53
Thymus
carcinoma, FDG uptake in, 53
FDG uptake, 53, 53*f*
in adults, 53, 53*f*
age and, 53
malignancy and, 53
in pediatric patients, 53
standardized uptake value (SUV) for, 53
superior mediastinal activity and, 53
Thyroglobulin level, and PET for thyroid cancer, 140
Thyroid, FDG uptake
diffuse, 51, 53*f*, 137
focal, 51

Thyroid cancer, 136–141
bone metastases, 139, 140
PET *versus* bone scan of, 114
cervical nodal metastases, differential diagnosis of, 138*f*, 140
false positives, 140
FDG uptake, 25, 136
Hürthle cell, 138
medullary, 139
PET for, comparison to other modalities, 140, 140*t*
metastases, 137–138, 138*f*
oncological PET imaging of, 136–141
papillary/follicular, 139
PET for, comparison to other radionuclides, 138–140, 139*t*
prognosis for, 139
pulmonary metastases, 140
radioiodine therapy for, and thymic uptake, 53
recurrent, 137–139, 138*f*
Thyroid hormone withdrawal, and PET for thyroid cancer, 140
Thyroiditis, FDG uptake in, 51, 53*f*, 137
Thyroid nodule(s), 136–137, 136*f*
benign, FDG uptake, 136
differential diagnosis of, 51–54
malignant, FDG uptake, 136
mimics, 137, 138*f*
PET imaging of, 136–137, 136*f*
correlation with CT, 136–137
Thyroid-stimulating hormone, recombinant, and PET for thyroid cancer, 140
Time of flight (TOF) PET scanners, 5, 7
TOF. *See* Time of flight (TOF) PET scanners
Tongue, FDG uptake, 49
Tongue base, primary tumor localization in, 127, 128*f*
Tonsillar cancer, 127
with cervical metastases, primary tumor localization in, 127, 128*f*
Tonsils, FDG uptake, normal
on coronal images, 47, 48*f*
on sagittal images, 47, 47*f*
Toxoplasmosis, cerebral involvement in, PET imaging for, 125–126
Transmission scan, 7
Tricarboxylic acid cycle, 22, 25
Truncation artifact, 91, 96
and standardized uptake value (SUV), 39
Tuberculosis, 156
in HIV-infected (AIDS) patients, 250*f*
pulmonary, 145, 149
Tumor
perivascular infiltration, and FDG uptake, 56, 73*f*
radiosensitivity of, 120
treatment resistance of, 118, 119*f*
Tumor volume, delineation for radiation therapy planning, 239–240
Two-dimensional (2D) acquisition protocols, 9, 10*f*

U

Ultrasound
in breast cancer, 158
of breasts, 155
of head and neck cancer, 128
of hepatocellular carcinoma, 187
of ovarian cancer, 199*t*
Umbilical nodule, 109*f*
United States Pharmacopeia, on PET radiotracers, 18
Ureteral activity
false positive, 61*f*, 62
focal linear, 61*f*, 62
reduction of, and minimization of physiologic FDG uptake, for oncological PET, 35, 197, 197*f*
Ureteral landmarks, in differentiation of ovarian and pelvic nodal activity, 110, 111*f*
Urinary tract, artifacts in, intravenous contrast and, 96
Urinary tract activity, reduction of, and minimization of physiologic FDG uptake, for oncological PET, 35, 110, 197, 197*f*, 206, 207*f*
Urologic tumors, oncological PET imaging of, 204–211
USP. *See United States Pharmacopeia*
Uterus
FDG uptake, normal pattern, 62
postpartum, FDG uptake, 63, 63*f*

V

Vascular dementia, 259–260
Vascular graft(s), FDG uptake, 71, 72*f*
Vascular space, FDG in, 23–24, 24*f*
Vascular wall, FDG uptake, 71
Vasculitis
evaluation, FDG PET in, 252–253
FDG uptake in, 71, 71*f*
Ventricle(s), cardiac, FDG uptake, 42–44
in fasting state, 42, 43*f*
insulin and, 42–43
metastases and, 43–44, 45*f*

Vertebrae, insufficiency fractures, and FDG uptake, 64, 65*f*
Vertebral body, hemangioma, and FDG uptake, 66*f*
VHL, 28
Vocal cord paralysis, and FDG uptake, 49, 49*f*, 137, 140

W

Warburg effect, 22, 28–29
 disruption of, cancer therapy targeted to, 28

Xanthoastrocytoma, pleomorphic, 122

Yttrium-90 radioablation, of colorectal cancer, therapy response imaging of, 217